Fundamentals of Law for Health Informatics and Information Management

Third Edition

Melanie S. Brodnik, PhD, MS, RHIA, FAHIMA
Laurie A. Rinehart-Thompson, JD, RHIA, CHP, FAHIMA
Rebecca B. Reynolds, EdD, MHA, RHIA, FAHIMA

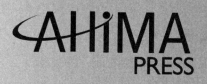
AHIMA PRESS

ISBN: 978-1-58426-530-6
AHIMA Product No.: AB241816

AHIMA Staff:
Sue Bowman, MJ, RHIA, CCS, FAHIMA, chapter contributor
Chelsea Brotherton, MA, Assistant Editor
Katherine M. Greenock, MS, Production Development Editor
Elizabeth Ranno, Vice President of Product and Planning
Pamela Woolf, Director of Publications

Cover image: ©Maxx-Studio/Shutterstock.com

American Health Information Management Association
233 North Michigan Avenue, 21st Floor
Chicago, Illinois 60601-5809
ahima.org

Brief Contents

Table of Contents

Chapter 9 Legal Health Record: Maintenance, Content, Documentation, and Disposition 169

Chapter 10 HIPAA Privacy Rule: Part I 205

Chapter 14 Patient Rights and Responsibilities 321

Chapter 15 Access, Use, and Disclosure and Release of Health Information 339

Chapter 19 Medical Staff 475

About the Volume Editors and Chapter Contributors

Melanie S. Brodnik, PhD, MS, RHIA, FAHIMA, is an associate professor emeritus of the undergraduate program in health information management and systems, and the graduate program in health informatics at The Ohio State University. She has served on the AHIMA Board of Directors, was president of AHIMA in 2004, and is currently serving on the board of directors of the Council on Accreditation of Health Informatics and Information Management Education (CAHIIM). She received the AHIMA Literary Award in 1992, the Champion Award in 2006, and the Legacy Award, in 2010; in 2006 she received the Ohio Health Information Management Distinguished Member Award, and received the AHIMA Distinguished Member Award and became a fellow of AHIMA in 2013. She has championed the issues of patient privacy, confidentiality, and security throughout her career. She has taught legal courses at Ohio State University and was editor and column writer for *Topics in Health Information Management* for 20 years. She served on the editorial review board for AHIMA's *In Confidence Privacy and Confidentiality Newsletter* from 1996 to 2002 and currently serves on the editorial review board of *Perspectives in Health Information Management*. She has authored or coauthored many publications and has presented at numerous local, state, and national professional association meetings, workshops, and conventions. She received her associate degree in medical record technology from Fullerton Junior College, a bachelor of science degree in health information management from Loma Linda University, a master's of science degree from the State University of New York at Buffalo, and her doctorate degree in educational research and evaluation from The Ohio State University.

Laurie A. Rinehart-Thompson, JD, RHIA, CHP, FAHIMA, is the director of the health information management and systems program and is an associate professor of clinical health and rehabilitation sciences at The Ohio State University. She earned her bachelor of science in medical record administration and her juris doctor from The Ohio State University. In addition to HIM education, her professional experiences span the behavioral health, home health, and acute care arenas. She has served as an expert witness in civil litigation, testifying as to the privacy and confidentiality of health information. She has chaired the AHIMA Professional Ethics Committee and served on numerous AHIMA committees, including the AHIMA Privacy and Security Practice Council and Council for Excellence in Education workgroups. She has served on the board of directors of the Ohio Health Information Management Association. A speaker on the HIPAA Privacy Rule, she is the author of AHIMA's *Introduction to Health Information Privacy and Security text.* She is also a contributing author to *Ethical Challenges in the Management of Health Information* and the following AHIMA publications: *Health Information Management Technology: An Applied Approach; Health Information Management: Concepts, Principles, and Practice; Documentation for Health Records; Documentation for Medical Practices; and the Journal of AHIMA.* She has been published in *Perspectives in Health Information Management.* She received the Ohio Health Information Management Association's Distinguished Member Award and the AHIMA Legacy Award in 2010, and became a fellow of AHIMA in 2011.

Rebecca B. Reynolds, EdD, MHA, RHIA, FAHIMA, is an associate professor and program director for the graduate program in health informatics and information management at the University of Tennessee Health Science Center (UTHSC) in Memphis. She has served on the AHIMA nominating committee and was chair of the 2010 AHIMA Education Strategy Committee. She is past president of the Tennessee Health Information Management Association and received its Outstanding New Professional Award in 1995 and Distinguished Member Award in 2004. She coordinated the HIPAA implementation program for the UTHSC system and provides HIPAA privacy and security training to all UTHSC students. She teaches the legal courses for both entry-level masters and post-professional graduate students and conducts legal workshops for attorneys, nurses, and other healthcare professionals. She served as a member of the Operations Committee of the Mid-South eHealth Alliance, which is a functioning health information exchange. She also serves on the Tennessee eHealth Network's Privacy and Security Work Group. She received her bachelor's degree in health information management from UTHSC and her master's degree in healthcare administration and doctorate in higher education administration from the University of Memphis. She received the AHIMA Legacy Award in 2010, and became a fellow of AHIMA in 2012.

Sue Bowman, MJ, RHIA, CCS, FAHIMA, is the senior director of coding policy and compliance for the American Health Information Management Association (AHIMA). Bowman's responsibilities include providing the association's strategic direction and leadership in the development, maintenance, adoption, and implementation of standards for terminologies, classifications, and associated data standards. She participates in a variety of AHIMA's activities pertaining to the advancement of healthcare data quality and the use of healthcare data standards. She has provided testimony to Congress and the National Committee on Vital and Health Statistics on ICD-10 and other issues pertaining to coding policy and the use of coded data.

Bowman participates in the development and maintenance of the ICD-10-CM, ICD-10-PCS, and CPT code sets. Bowman serves as AHIMA's representative to the Cooperating Parties, a group that sets national coding policy and guidance for the ICD code sets, impacting data reporting standards for the entire US healthcare industry. She also contributes to the development of international coding standards through her role as secretariat for a World Health Organization group directly involved in the development of ICD-11.

Bowman received a bachelor of science degree in medical record administration from Daemen College in Amherst, NY and a master of jurisprudence in health law degree from Loyola University Chicago School of Law.

Jill Callahan Klaver, JD, RHIA, recently retired from a long career of quality management and risk management consulting. She was principal of Health Risk Advantage, a Colorado-based risk management consulting firm that assists healthcare organizations in minimizing their risk of liability. Prior to this, she was senior vice president of public and industry leadership for AHIMA, where she helped plan and execute the association's policy and alliance agendas. Her leadership on health information management issues spans almost 40 years, and she is a frequent speaker on risk management, privacy, and electronic health information management topics. Her publications include numerous articles, chapters, and books, including chapter author of "Legal Issues in Health Information Management" in *Health Information: Management of a Strategic Resource* (Elsevier); author of *Privacy & Confidentiality of Health Information* (Jossey-Bass and AHA Press); and technical editor of *HIPAA by Example* (AHIMA). Jill served on AHIMA's Board of Directors from 2002 through 2007 and as the elected president in 2006. She was a member of the Confidentiality, Privacy, and Security Workgroup of the American Health Information Community (AHIC) of the US Department of Health and Human Services' Office of the National Coordinator for

Health Information Technology. She has a law degree from Loyola University of Chicago, a master's in administration (health administration concentration) from Central Michigan University, and a bachelor of science degree in medical record administration from Ferris State University.

Keith Olenik, MA, RHIA, CHP, is principal of The Olenik Consulting Group, LLC in Chicago, IL. He has over 30 years of experience working with healthcare delivery systems as a member of senior management and as a consultant. Olenik holds a bachelor of arts in health information management from the University of Kansas and an master of arts in health services management with an emphasis in computer resources management from Webster University. He is a member of AHIMA, currently serving on the Council for Excellence in Education, and previously served on the board of directors for AHIMA and the AHIMA Foundation.

In addition to these activities, he has been a speaker at various conventions and educational seminars on ICD-10, HIPAA, project management, legal health records, and electronic health record strategies.

Kim Theodos, JD, MS, RHIA, is currently an assistant professor of health studies at the University of Louisiana Monroe. She teaches classes related to health informatics, healthcare leadership, and healthcare administration in both on campus and online learning environments. She also serves as the program practicum coordinator and advisor for undergraduate health studies students. Previously, Kim taught as an associate professor of health informatics and information management at Louisiana Tech University. Kim's educational background includes a bachelor's degree in health information administration from Louisiana Tech University, a master's degree in healthcare management from University of New Orleans, and a juris doctor from Taft Law School.

Kim has volunteered in various capacities through the Louisiana Health Information Management Association, previously serving a term as president and currently serving as treasurer and secretary. She was recognized by LHIMA as distinguished member and outstanding volunteer. She also served on the AHIMA National Convention Planning Committee, serving as chair.

Acknowledgments

The editors would like to express appreciation to the many individuals who contributed to the writing, reviewing, and publication of this textbook. We are grateful for everyone's contributions and would particularly like to thank the AHIMA publications staff and book reviewers. We offer special recognition and gratitude to our chapter authors and coauthors Sue Bowman, Jill Callahan Klaver, and Keith Olenik, and first and second edition chapter authors and coauthors Elizabeth Bowman (chapter 16), Sebastian Proels (chapter 6), and Marcia Sharp (chapter 15).Without the collective contributions and expertise of these individuals, the publication of this textbook would not have been possible. We would also like to thank those who contributed to the first edition of the book, Joseph Brunetto, Denise Burke, Frances W. Lee, Julie Roth, and Dianne Wilkinson. Special thanks go to Mary McCain, professor emeritus, University of Tennessee, Memphis, who served as one of the editors and coauthor for the book's first edition. Her dedication and hard work on the book's first edition is greatly appreciated. Finally, the editors wish to thank their families for their support and patience during the revision process of the book.

AHIMA Press would also like to thank Judy A. Ferraro, RHIA, and Heather L. Merkley, RHIA, for their technical reviews of this text.

Online Resources

For Students

The AHIMA Press *Fundamentals of Law for Health Informatics and Information Management*, Third Edition student website includes a student workbook and a Check Your Understanding (CYU) answer key. Visit **http://www.ahimapress.org/Brodnik5306/** and scratch off the student sticker to reveal your unique student code to access the book website. Your password cannot be shared or transferred. Access to the website is for individuals only and will be terminated on publication of the next edition of this book.

For Instructors

AHIMA provides supplementary materials for educators who use this book in their classes. Materials include discussion questions and application exercises with taxonomy levels, test bank questions for each chapter with answers, PowerPoint slides, and a Check Your Understanding (CYU) answer key. Visit **http://www.ahimapress.org/Brodnik5306/** and click the link to download the PowerPoint files. Please do not enter the scratch-off code from the interior front cover, as this will invalidate your access to the instructor materials. If you have any questions regarding the instructor materials, contact AHIMA Customer Relations at (800) 335-5535 or submit a customer support request at https://my.ahima.org/messages.

Introduction to the Fundamentals of Law for Health Informatics and Information Management

Melanie S. Brodnik, PhD, RHIA, FAHIMA

Learning Objectives

- Differentiate between the concepts of law, and the privacy, confidentiality, and security of health information
- Discuss why protecting the privacy and confidentiality of health information is a challenge for health information management and informatics professionals
- Discuss the difference between a paper health record, a hybrid record, and an electronic health record
- Discuss the concepts of ownership and control of the health record, how these concepts relate to the concepts of health record custodianship and stewardship, and the roles and responsibilities of the custodian or steward of health records

Key Terms

- American Recovery and Reinvestment Act of 2009 (ARRA)
- American Society for Testing and Materials (ASTM)
- Business record
- Confidentiality
- Custodian
- Custodianship
- Data security
- Electronic health record

- Electronic medical record
- Enterprise information management
- Health information exchange
- Health information technology
- Health Information Technology for Economic and Clinical Health Act (HITECH)
- Health Insurance Portability and Accountability Act of 1996 (HIPAA)

- Health record
- Hybrid health record
- Information governance
- The Joint Commission
- Law
- Legal health record
- National Alliance for Health Information Technology
- Office of the National Coordinator for Health Information Technology

- Ownership
- Patient portal
- Personal health record
- Privileged communication
- Privacy
- Protected health information (PHI)
- Security
- Steward
- Stewardship
- System security

The complexities of managing data and information are expanding as the US healthcare industry faces increasing demands to share patient information and reduce healthcare costs while enhancing the quality and safety of patient care. There has been unparalleled interest in decreasing costs and improving the quality and safety of patient care by using **health information technology (HIT)**. The federal government has incentivized healthcare providers to move from paper to **electronic health records (EHRs)** and to share patient information through **health information exchanges (HIEs)**. The ability to integrate and share data and information from multiple sources could possibly save more than $300 billion per year in US healthcare costs (McKinsey & Company 2013). To achieve savings, individuals with access to health data and information have a legal responsibility to protect its access, use, and disclosure.

Over the last two decades, public and private efforts have been devoted to the legitimate sharing of information among multiple parties and across multiple boundaries in support of the industry's transition from fee-for-service to value-based healthcare delivery (Kloss 2015). Public and private collaborations have worked toward eliminating legal and economic barriers that prevent the compiling, storing, and sharing of electronic health information securely. Efforts have focused on identifying solutions and strategies that protect the privacy, confidentiality and security of electronically stored and exchanged health information. For example, the National Governors Association has published a roadmap to help states address barriers that prevent information flow between healthcare providers in a given state (Johnson et al. 2016). In addition, the federal **Office of the National Coordinator for Health Information Technology (ONC)** offers numerous guides and tools in support of nationwide sharing of health information, patient engagement, and contract negotiation between healthcare providers and EHR vendors (Henry et al. 2016; ONC 2016a; ONC 2016b).

Individuals responsible for protecting the privacy and security of health information within a healthcare organization are health information management (HIM) and health informatics professionals. They, along with healthcare administrators and providers (including physicians, nurses, dentists, and others), are challenged to understand the complexity of healthcare law and the requirements to protect the privacy, confidentiality, and security of health records and information. They must accommodate changes to laws, standards, and programmatic policies and procedures that support legal issues surrounding the delivery of healthcare and the growing use of health information and health records. It is important to have an understanding of the legal system, along with the laws, regulations, standards, and ethical considerations that arise in the delivery of safe, quality healthcare.

This chapter introduces the concept of law and the complexity of issues surrounding the growing use of HIT. It defines health information and health records and discusses the types of records commonly used in healthcare. The concepts of privacy, confidentiality, and security are discussed in terms of their significance in protecting health information. The concepts of custodial responsibility and stewardship of health records are introduced. The chapter concludes with a discussion of information and data governance as an overall means for enterprise information management.

Defining Law

Law represents a set of governing rules designed to protect citizens living in a civilized society. Law establishes order, provides parameters for conduct, and defines the rights and obligations of the government and its citizens. It controls behavior that threatens public safety and sets penalties for disobedience. There are two types of law, public and private. Public law involves federal, state, and local government and serves to define, regulate, and enforce rights and duties among individuals and businesses as related to government. For example, federal or state laws that define access, use, and disclosure of patient healthcare information represent public laws. Private law is concerned with the rules and principles that define rights and duties among individuals and among private businesses. Private law addresses issues such as contracts between two entities; for example, a contract between an EHR vendor and a hospital system.

Healthcare in the United States is a trillion-dollar industry that is highly regulated by federal and state laws, institutional accrediting bodies, professional standards of practice, and codes of ethics. These laws and standards define how healthcare is delivered, financed, and reimbursed. The laws and standards protect patients and healthcare providers by requiring accountability for services rendered, and privacy, confidentiality, and security of patient and provider health records and information. Health information may be used as evidence in legal cases when conflict arises and resolution is sought through the court system.

Health Information and Health Records

Health information refers to the data generated and collected as a result of delivering care to a patient. Its primary use is for clinical care; however, secondary uses are numerous, such as public health reporting, population health management, third-party reimbursement, quality improvement, and patient safety.

Health information is collected from multiple sources and is used for a wide variety of purposes. It is protected under the **Health Insurance Portability and Accountability Act of 1996 (HIPAA)**, which defines **protected health information (PHI)** as:

> … any information, whether oral or recorded in any form or medium, that: (1) Is created or received by a health care provider, health plan, public health authority, employer, life insurer, school or university, or health care clearinghouse; and (2) Relates to the past, present, or future physical or mental health or condition of an individual; the provision of health care to an individual; or the past, present, or future payment for the provision of health care to an individual (45 CFR 160.103).

What information is documented varies depending on several factors, including state or jurisdiction of healthcare provider, accrediting or licensing body requirements, type of healthcare provider (for example, hospital, clinic, physician practice, behavioral health center), and services rendered for the episode of care.

The information generated on a patient's episode of care comprises a patient's health record or record of care. A health record may also be known as a medical record, patient record, client record, inpatient record, outpatient record, or clinic record. The American Health Information Management Association (AHIMA) states that a **health record** "comprises individually identifiable data, in any medium, that are collected, processed, stored, displayed, and used by healthcare professionals" (AHIMA e-HIM Work Group 2010). It documents the care provided to the patient and the patient's healthcare status.

Health records are maintained in either paper or electronic formats, or a combination of both. The term **hybrid health record** refers to a record that consists of both paper and electronic records and media (for example, film, video, or imaging system) and uses both manual and electronic processes (AHIMA 2010). Electronic records may be composed of information from clinical, administrative, or financial systems, along with paper documents from internal or external sources that are scanned into the record. The data in the record may be handwritten, direct voice entry captured in a word-processing system, from provider wireless mobile devices such as phones, handheld personal computers, or any combination of these (Amatayakul 2013). Electronic and paper records may differ as summarized in figure 1.1.

If the health record is completely electronic, it is called an EHR or electronic medical record (EMR). These terms are often used interchangeably but may be defined differently depending on the organization and how the record is designed or used. To help alleviate legal barriers and facilitate adoption of EHRs and HIEs, the **National Alliance for Health Information Technology** (NAHIT), sponsored by the ONC, developed consensus-based definitions related to key HIT terms (NAHIT 2008). NAHIT's definitions for an EHR and EMR are as follows:

- **Electronic health record:** "an electronic record of health-related information on an individual that conforms to nationally recognized interoperability standards and that can be created, managed, and consulted by authorized clinicians and staff across more than one healthcare organization"
- **Electronic medical record:** "an electronic record of health-related information on an individual that can be created, gathered, managed, and consulted by authorized clinicians and staff within one healthcare organization" (NAHIT 2008, 6)

The key difference in these definitions is that the EMR is considered an electronic record housed within an organization, whereas an EHR is thought to contain data or information from more than one

Figure 1.1 Six key areas where electronic records differ from paper records

1. **Volume and Duplicability:** With advances in information technology, at least 93% of information generated today is created using digital technology. Moreover, digital information is routinely and easily duplicated. Users can easily save files and disseminate them through e-mail. Most applications used to create electronic data and files have automatic backups, which help to protect against accidental loss of data.

2. **Persistence:** It is much more difficult to dispose of electronic documents than paper documents. Paper documents can be destroyed by shredding or some other form of physical destruction. However, as noted by the court in *Zubulake v. UBS Warburg LLC*, "The term 'deleted' is sticky in the context of electronic data. Deleting a file does not actually erase the data from the computer's storage devices. Rather, it simply finds the data's entry in the disk directory and changes it to a 'not used' status—thus permitting the computer to write over the 'deleted' data. Until the computer writes over the 'deleted' data, however, it may be recovered by searching the disk itself rather than the disk's directory. Accordingly, many files are recoverable long after they have been deleted even if neither the computer user nor the computer itself is aware of their existence."

3. **Dynamic Changeable Content:** Electronic information can be more easily modified than paper information. For example, correcting a spelling error on a document created using a typewriter involves physically "whiting out" the misspelled word and replacing it with the correctly spelled word. The same process is much easier in an electronic word processing application, and often only involves the use of an automatic spell checker. Further, simply accessing or moving electronic data can alter that data by changing file creation and modification dates.

4. **Metadata:** Electronic documents contain "metadata," which is "information about the document or file that is recorded by the computer to assist the computer and often the user in storing and retrieving the document or file at a later date." File designations, create/edit dates, authorship, and edit history are all examples of metadata. Where such issues are relevant or in dispute, metadata can be useful in authenticating documents or establishing exactly when documents were created. An electronic document's metadata may not be relevant in every case, especially when there is no dispute as to who authored a document or when a document was modified. However, in *Williams v. Sprint/United Mgmt. Co.*, the court held that "When a party is ordered to maintain documents as they are maintained in the ordinary course of business, the producing party should produce the electronic documents with their metadata intact."

5. **Environment-Dependence and Obsolescence:** Unlike paper documents, electronic data may not be readable once it is moved from its "environment." For example, if a file is transferred to a different computer, that computer must have the appropriate software loaded to open that file. If it does not, then the file may not open correctly or may not be readable at all. Further, with the continual advances and upgrades of information technology, many organizations routinely migrate to new or upgraded information systems. This can make it difficult to restore electronic data or files exactly as they were maintained in previous systems.

6. **Dispersion and Searchability:** Electronic documents are easily stored in multiple locations such as on computer hard drives, servers, or portable devices such as laptops, PDAs, cell phones, or jump drives. Searching electronic documents for specific pieces of information is often less cumbersome than conducting the same search on paper. For example, a "find" or "search" function in a word processing document can quickly find all occurrences of a certain word within electronic documents regardless of their size. To find all occurrences of the same word in a large paper document could take hours of manual labor.

Source: Adapted from *The Sedona Principles, Second Edition: Best Practices Recommendations & Principles for Addressing Electronic Document Production.*

organization. For this reason, use of the term *EHR* appears to be more prevalent, although as previously mentioned, these terms are often used interchangeably.

Healthcare consumers may also maintain a **personal health record** (PHR), which is defined as "an electronic record of health-related information on an individual that conforms to nationally recognized interoperability standards and that can be drawn from multiple sources while being managed, shared, and controlled by the individual" (NAHIT 2008, 6). Healthcare providers have implemented **patient portals** that allow patients to electronically access their personal health record, and schedule appointments, communicate with their provider via e-mail messaging, and perform other functions as offered by the organization. Henry et al. (2016) reports that "there has been a significant increase in the percent of hospitals that provide patients with the ability to electronically view, download, and transmit their health information" since 2013 with an increase in patient engagement functionalities in 2015.

Whether the health record is a paper record, a hybrid record, an EMR, or an EHR, it is the legal **business record** created in the normal course of business of an organization or healthcare provider. It is used for business, legal, and compliance purposes. For example, it serves as evidence in lawsuits or other legal actions. Information detailing the contents of a health record, including what constitutes a **legal health record,** is discussed in more detail in chapter 9.

Protecting Health Records and Information

Working within healthcare requires an understanding of the American legal system, and the laws and standards that govern its delivery, financing, and reimbursement methods. Managing health data, information, and records also requires a clear understanding of laws and standards that protect the collection, access, use, exchange, and disclosure of health information and records. There is a longstanding history of state-specific and federal laws governing the privacy of health records and information. However, it was not until the passage of HIPAA (45 CFR 160, 164) in 1996 that federal rules were enacted to specifically protect patient information as a result of increasing use of information technology in healthcare. HIPAA privacy rules went into effect in 2002, followed by security rules in 2003.

Subsequently in 2009, the **Health Information Technology for Economic and Clinical Health Act (HITECH)** (42 USC 17921), part of the **American Recovery and Reinvestment Act of 2009** (ARRA), was passed to further promote the creation of a national healthcare infrastructure through adoption and meaningful use of EHR systems by healthcare providers, and the sharing of health information through HIEs.

HITECH widened the scope of privacy and security protections under HIPAA to include companies previously not affected by HIPAA. It also provided for stricter enforcement of the rule, and increased potential legal liability for noncompliance (Callahan-Dennis 2010, 6). Many of the HITECH requirements went into effect in 2010, with the remaining requirements finalized in 2013. HIPAA and HITECH are discussed in more detail in chapters 10, 11, and 12. HIPAA and HITECH are two of more than 50 federal laws and regulations addressing privacy, confidentiality, and security protections (Office of the National Coordinator for Health IT, Privacy & Security 2016).

Core to HIPAA, HITECH, and other federal and state laws related to the protection, access, use, and disclosure of health information records is an understanding of the concepts of privacy, confidentiality, and security.

Check Your Understanding 1.1

Instructions: Indicate whether the following statements are true or false (T or F).

1. An electronic personal health record contains health-related information for an individual.
2. An EHR can be managed across more than one healthcare organization.
3. HIPAA represents a private law designed to protect patient information.
4. Patient portals are used to encourage patient engagement in their care.
5. HITECH limited the scope of privacy and security protections under HIPAA.

Privacy, Confidentiality, and Security

Privacy and confidentiality have historically been key components of the patient–provider relationship. The information contained in a health record, regardless of its scope or format, can be some of the most private and sensitive information that exists about a person. In conjunction with a healthcare encounter, documentation is created to record the care that was provided, support medical decisions, and provide evidence of patient outcomes. Patients are encouraged to be truthful with their care providers regarding their mental and physical conditions, because the truth is essential to the successful delivery of appropriate healthcare. Such truths, however, can place the patient in an extremely vulnerable position when intimate clinical and behavioral secrets are revealed or discovered as patient treatment is provided, test results are reported, and future options for care are discussed. Because of this, when a patient provides information and it is documented, there is an inherent trust that it will be kept private and protected from unauthorized access (Rinehart-Thompson and Harman 2017).

The protection of individuals' health information is a central, defining obligation of healthcare providers and health information and informatics professionals. In every area of law that relates to health information, the appropriate use and disclosure of that information must be a primary consideration. Although the protection of health information is discussed extensively later in the book, its significance warrants specific discussion in this introductory chapter. An understanding of the concepts of privacy, confidentiality, and security and the differences among the three concepts is important for the management of health information from a legal perspective.

Privacy

Privacy is an important social value that, described by jurists Samuel Warren and Louis Brandeis in 1890, means the right "to be let alone" (Rinehart-Thompson and Harman 2017). It is an important aspect of an individual's freedom and legal rights to be selective about what is revealed to others (Bankert and Amdur 2006, 143). One definition, which addresses the breadth of privacy, is provided by the **American Society for Testing and Materials** (ASTM) E31 Health Informatics Subcommittee, which states:

> Privacy is a right of individuals to be let [*sic*] alone and to be protected against physical or psychological invasion or the misuse of their property. It includes freedom from intrusion or observation into one's private affairs, the right to maintain control over certain personal information, and the freedom to act without outside interference (ASTM Committee E31 on Healthcare Informatics Subcommittee E31.17 on Privacy, Confidentiality, and Access 2010, 4).

Although the US Constitution does not expressly grant the right of privacy, it does provide safeguards against government intrusion. Further, courts have interpreted the Constitution to give privacy rights with respect to religious beliefs (using the First Amendment as the basis), unreasonable searches (using the Fourth Amendment as the basis), marriage, and child-rearing. In addition, privacy rights have been further extended through such high-profile US Supreme Court cases such as *Griswold v. Connecticut* (contraception) and *Roe v. Wade* (abortion).

Although a constitutional right of privacy related to one's own health information is nonexistent, privacy protection has been established through other means such as court decisions, accrediting body standards, individual state laws, and federal laws like HIPAA and the HITECH provisions of ARRA. For example, the predominant accrediting body and standards-setting organization in healthcare is **The Joint Commission**. The Joint Commission is an independent, not-for-profit organization that evaluates and accredits more than 21,000 healthcare organizations and programs in the United States, including

- Ambulatory healthcare
- Behavioral healthcare

- Critical access hospital
- Home care and hospice
- Hospital
- Laboratory services
- Nursing care center

The accreditation standards used by The Joint Commission are designed to address an organization's level of performance in specific functional areas, such as patient treatment, patient safety, and privacy and confidentiality of information. The Joint Commission defines privacy as an individual's "right to limit the disclosure of personal information" (The Joint Commission 2016, DSCT.1). Its standards require the maintenance of information privacy, confidentiality, and security and supports efforts to ensure the integrity of data, which is the assurance that the data have not been modified without authorization or corrupted, either maliciously or accidentally (The Joint Commission 2016).

Standards of professional practice are also defined by professional healthcare organizations that offer protection of privacy rights as a main component of professional codes of ethics, as discussed in more detail in chapter 2.

Confidentiality

The terms *privacy* and *confidentiality* are often used interchangeably; however, there are important distinctions between the two terms. **Confidentiality** results from sharing private thoughts with someone else in confidence. The ASTM E31 Subcommittee on Health Informatics defines confidentiality as the "status accorded to data or information indicating that it is sensitive for some reason, and therefore it needs to be protected against theft, disclosure, or improper use, or both, and must be disseminated only to authorized individuals or organizations with a need to know" (ASTM 2010, 5).

Confidentiality, as recognized by law, stems from a relationship where information is shared between two parties such as physician and patient, attorney and client, clergy and parishioner, or husband and wife. The information or communication shared in these relationships is considered "privileged." What constitutes **privileged communication** is usually delineated by state law. Such laws in the case of healthcare providers may also further define what records of communication are privileged based on the healthcare provider's scope of practice (for example, physician, nurse, psychologist, licensed clinical social worker, or psychiatric nurse practitioner).

The concept of confidentiality of patient information resulting from a patient–provider relationship can be traced back to the fourth century BC. Hippocrates, considered the father of medicine, required Greek physicians to take the Hippocratic Oath. A modern translation of the oath includes a tenet specific to protecting the confidentiality of information shared between patient and physician:

> I will respect the privacy of my patients, for their problems are not disclosed to me that the world may know. Most especially must I tread with care in matters of life and death. If it is given me to save a life, all thanks. But it may also be within my power to take a life; this awesome responsibility must be faced with great humbleness and awareness of my own frailty. Above all, I must not play at God (MedicineNet 2011).

Confidentiality obligates healthcare providers—individuals and organizations—to protect patient information that is collected. When a patient reveals information to a physician or other provider of care, there is a presumption that this information will be considered confidential and protected as such

(Rinehart-Thompson and Harman 2017). Healthcare organizations have the dubious task of balancing individual privacy rights and the use of confidential information to perform necessary clinical or business tasks (Herzig 2010). This includes the confidentiality of all information systems and verbal communication related to financial and business records, including employee information, as well as clinical and service communication. As with privacy, The Joint Commission also offers standards in support of confidentiality. It defines confidentiality as "protection of data or information from being made available or disclosed to an unauthorized person(s) or process(es)" (The Joint Commission 2016).

Security

The concept of **security** is related to privacy and confidentiality in that it pertains to the physical and electronic protection of information that preserves these concepts. The Joint Commission definition of security reflects all administrative, physician, and technical safeguards to "prevent unauthorized access, use, disclosure, modification, or destruction of information or interference with system operations in an information system" (The Joint Commission 2016). The ASTM E31 Health Informatics Subcommittee defines security from two perspectives, security related to data and security related to systems:

- **Data security** is the result of effective data protection measures; the sum of measures that safeguard data and computer programs from undesired occurrences and exposure to accidental or intentional access or disclosure to unauthorized persons, or a combination thereof; accidental or malicious alteration; unauthorized copying; or loss by theft or destruction by hardware failures, software deficiencies, operating mistakes; physical damage by fire, water, smoke, excessive temperature, electrical failure, or sabotage, or a combination thereof. Data security exists when data are protected from accidental or intentional disclosure to unauthorized persons and from unauthorized or accidental alteration.
- **System security** is the totality of safeguards including hardware, software, personnel policies, information practice policies, disaster preparedness, and oversight of these components. Security protects both the system and the information contained within from unauthorized access from without and from misuse from within. Security enables the entity or system to protect the confidential information it stores from unauthorized access, disclosure, or misuse, thereby protecting the privacy of the individuals who are the subjects of the stored information (ASTM 2010, 3).

Systems security includes cybersecurity efforts to prevent the stealing of electronically stored information. There has been an increase in the number of cyberattacks on healthcare providers in the last year, which has required providers to enhance cybersecurity protection (Dodson and Patrick 2016). From a federal perspective, the US Code on Information Security defines information security as follows:

Protecting information and information systems from unauthorized access, use, disclosure, disruption, modification, or destruction in order to provide

- Integrity, which means guarding against improper information modifications or destruction, and includes ensuring information non-repudiation and authenticity
- Confidentiality, which means preserving authorized restrictions on access and disclosure, including means for protecting personal privacy and propriety information
- Availability, which means ensuring timely and reliable access to and use of information (National Institute of Standards and Technology 2008, A-6)

Harriet Pearson, chief privacy officer of IBM, affirmed the interdependence of privacy and security by identifying security as the way to implement an individual's expectation of privacy. "You can have outstanding security, yet violate people's perception of what their privacy ought to be. But you can't have privacy without having the right security measures in place. Privacy rests on a good security foundation always" (IBM Executive Interaction Channel 2007).

The interplay between the concepts of privacy, confidentiality and security is important since they are supported through federal and state laws accrediting body standards, and the work of numerous private and public entities concerned with the privacy, and security of EHRs and HIEs (AHIMA HIMSS HIE Privacy and Security Joint Work Group 2011).

Custodian Health Records

Ownership of the physical health record, whether paper, electronic, or hybrid, has traditionally been granted to the healthcare provider who generates the record. However, state and federal laws have long upheld the right of the patient to control the information within the record (Rinehart-Thompson 2016, 60, 63–64). Understanding who owns the health record is an important issue as healthcare providers expand their use of EHRs and HIEs. Associated with ownership of health records is the legal concept of **custodianship**. The **custodian** of health records is the individual who has been designated as having responsibility for the operational functions related to the development and maintenance of records (AHIMA e-HIM Work Group 2010). This includes the care, custody, control, and proper safekeeping and disclosure of health records, whether stored in paper or electronic format for such persons or institutions that prepare and maintain records of healthcare. An official custodian is required by both federal and state rules of evidence that permit health records to be entered as business records in legal proceedings; this is discussed further in chapter 5. The official custodian is authorized to certify (that is, verify that the record or information is what it purports to be), through affidavit or testimony, the normal business practices used to create and maintain the record (AHIMA e-HIM Work Group on the Legal Health Record 2005a, b). The custodian supervises the inspection and copying or duplication of records and can be called to testify as to the authenticity of the record.

In most healthcare organizations, those who request health information obtain it from the HIM department. The director of the HIM department (or designee) is traditionally the legal custodian of health records. In organizations that have hybrid or electronic health records, the custodian may differ depending on who is responsible for and can explain the procedures for compiling and maintaining patient information and records. This individual must also be able to validate the integrity of the information requested. See chapter 15 for a more detailed discussion of the process for releasing health information upon request or by subpoena or court order.

Regardless of the record format, patient information may be evidence in legal proceedings to allege medical negligence, assert the mental competence of an individual, or for other health or treatment issues. Individuals charged with the custodial responsibility of protecting health information act as a gatekeeper for the appropriate access, use, and disclosure of information for legitimate purposes and in conjunction with federal and state laws as well as the court system for use in legal proceedings.

Stewardship and Information Governance

With the increasing use of HIT, the role of the data or information **steward** is emerging. Similar to the role of custodianship, **stewardship** goes beyond the physical record to include "responsibilities for ensuring integrity (accuracy, completeness, timeliness) and security (protection of privacy as well as from tampering, loss or destruction) within the context of electronic information and records management"

(Davidson 2010, 42). Stewardship is a component of **information governance**. It refers to "an organization-wide framework for managing information throughout its lifecycle and supporting the organization's strategy, operations, regulatory, legal, risk, and environmental requirements" (Johns 2015, 323). When an organization engages in **enterprise information management (EIM)**, it facilitates stewardship and overall information governance by supporting the "functions used to plan, organize, and coordinate people, processes, technology, and content for managing information as a corporate asset that ensures data quality, safety, and ease of use" (Johns 2015). The role of stewardship requires leadership, responsibility, and governance to ensure the consistent application of, and compliance with policies across organization-wide distributed information systems (Dougherty and Washington 2010, 44). Whether one is identified as a custodian or steward, key to either role is understanding the legal aspects of managing enterprise-wide information while protecting the privacy, confidentiality, and security of its access, use, and disclosure.

Check Your Understanding   1.2

Instructions: Indicate whether the following statements are true or false (T or F).

1. The US Constitution expressly grants the right of privacy to individuals.
2. Confidentiality is a legal concept designed to protect the communication between two parties.
3. Security refers to the right to be left alone.
4. Ownership of a health record generated by a physician about a patient belongs to the patient.
5. A custodian of records is responsible for certifying that a record is what it purports to be.

References

AHIMA e-HIM Work Group. 2010. Practice brief: Managing the transition from paper to EHRs. Web extra. Chicago: AHIMA. http://bok.ahima.org/doc?oid=103208

AHIMA e-HIM Work Group on the Legal Health Record. 2005a. Update: Guidelines for defining the legal health record for disclosure purposes. *Journal of AHIMA.* 76(8):64A–G.

AHIMA e-HIM Work Group on the Legal Health Record. 2005b. The Legal Process and Electronic Health Records. *Journal of AHIMA* 76(9):96A–D.

AHIMA HIMSS HIE Privacy and Security Joint Work Group. 2011. The privacy and security gaps in health information exchanges. Chicago: AHIMA. http://bok.ahima.org/PdfView?oid=104470

Amatayakul, M. 2013. *Electronic Health Records: A Practical Guide for Professionals and Organizations,* 5th ed revised reprint. Chicago: AHIMA.

American Society for Testing and Materials Committee E31 on Healthcare Informatics Subcommittee E31.17 on Privacy, Confidentiality, and Access. 2010. Standard guide for confidentiality, privacy, access, and data security principles for health information including computer-based patient records. Publication no. E1869-04(2010). Philadelphia: ASTM.

Bankert, E. and R. Amdur. 2006. *Institutional Review Board: Management and Function,* 2nd ed. Sudbury, MA: Jones and Bartlett.

Callahan-Dennis, J. 2010. *Privacy: The Impact of ARRA, HITECH and Other Policy Initiatives.* Chicago: AHIMA.

Davidson, L. 2010. From custodian to steward. *Journal of AHIMA* 81(5):42–43.

Dodson, D. and R. Patrick. 2016 (December). Horizon Report. The State of Cybersecurity in Healthcare. http://www.fortifiedhealthsecurity.com/wp-content/uploads/2016/12/Fortified-Health-Security-Horizon-Report-2016.pdf.

Dougherty, M. and L. Washington. 2010. Still seeking the legal EHR. *Journal of AHIMA* 81(2):42–45.

Henry, J., Y. Pylypchuk, and V. Patel. 2016. Electronic capabilities for patient engagement among U.S. non-federal acute care hospitals: 2012-2015. *ONC Data Brief* No. 38 (September).

Herzig, T. 2010. *Information Security in Healthcare Managing Risk.* Chicago: Health Information Management and Systems Society.

IBM Executive Interaction Channel. 2007. Privacy is good for business: An interview with Chief Privacy Officer Harriet Pearson. http://www.ibm.com.

Johns, M. 2015. *Enterprise Health Information Management and Data Governance.* Chicago, IL: AHIMA.

Johnson, K., C. Kellecher, L. Block, and F. Isasi. 2016. *Getting the Right Information to the Right Healthcare Providers at the Right Time: A Road Map for States to Improve Health Information Flow between Providers.* Washington, DC: National Governors Association Center for Best Practices.

The Joint Commission. 2016. Glossary. *Comprehensive Accreditation Manual for Hospitals: The Official Handbook. CAMH* Refreshed Core, January. http://www.jointcommission.org.

Kloss, L. 2015. *Implementing Health Information Governance Lesson from the Field.* Chicago: AHIMA.

McKinsey & Company. 2013. The big data revolution in US healthcare. Center for US Health System Reform Business Technology Office. http://www.mckinsey.com/industries/healthcare-systems-and-services/our -insights/the-big-data-revolution-in-us-health-care.

MedicineNet. 2011. Definition of Hippocratic Oath. http://www.medterms.com/.

National Alliance for Health Information Technology. 2008 (April). Defining key health information technology terms. http://healthit.hhs.gov.

National Institute of Standards and Technology. 2008. An introductory resource guide for implementing the Health Insurance Portability and Accountability Act (HIPAA) Security Rule. NIST Special Publication 800-66 Revision I. http://csrc.nist.gov.

Office of the National Coordinator for Health Information Technology. 2016a (December). A shared nationwide interoperability roadmap: A year in review. https://www.healthit.gov/year-in-review.

Office of the National Coordinator for Health Information Technology. 2016b (September). EHR contracts untangled. Selecting wisely, negotiating terms, and understanding the fine print. Washington, DC. https://www .healthit.gov/sites/default/files/EHR_Contracts_Untangled.pdf.

Rinehart-Thompson, L., and L. Harman. 2017. Privacy and Confidentiality. In *Ethical Challenges in the Management of Health Information,* 3rd ed. Edited by Harman, L. and F. Cornelius. Sudbury, MA: Jones and Bartlett.

Rinehart-Thompson, L. 2016. Legal Issues in Health Information Management. Chapter 2 in *Health Information Management: Concepts, Principles, and Practice,* 5th ed. Edited by Oachs, P. and A. Watters. Chicago: AHIMA.

The Sedona Conference. 2007. *The Sedona Principles: Second Edition, Best Practices Recommendations & Principles for Addressing Electronic Document Production.* https://thesedonaconference.org/publication/The%20 Sedona%20Principles

Cases, Statutes, and Regulations Cited

Griswold v. Connecticut, 381 US 479 (1965).

Roe v. Wade, 410 US 113 (1973).

45 CFR 160.103: Definitions, Privacy rule. 2002.

45 CFR 160, 164: Standards for privacy of individually identified health information. 2002.

45 CFR 164.524–526: Amendment of protected health information. 2007.

42 USC 17921: Health Information Technology for Economic and Clinical Health Act. 2009.

Law and Ethics

Kim Theodos, JD, MS, RHIA

Learning Objectives

- Define ethics and distinguish between law and ethics
- Differentiate between ethics and morals
- Analyze ethical theories relevant to HIM practice
- Describe the role of professional codes of ethics in protecting health information
- Explain consequences of unethical behavior
- Discuss and apply the ethical decision-making process
- Examine the ethical issues surrounding bioethics

Key Terms

- Applied ethics
- Autonomy
- Beneficence
- Bioethics
- Blanchard-Peale Ethics Check
- Code of ethics
- Conflict of interest
- Deontology
- Distributive justice
- Embryonic stem cell research
- Ethical decision-making model
- Ethical principles
- Ethics
- Hospice care
- In vitro fertilization
- Justice
- Medical ethics
- Moral values
- Morals
- Nonmaleficence
- Paternalism
- Procreation
- Professional ethics
- Professionalism
- Right-based ethics
- Utilitarianism
- Virtue-based ethics

Healthcare professionals are often faced with difficult decisions that relate to various aspects of their responsibilities. Decision-making may be influenced by reasoning from a wide variety of sources, such as culture, family, religion, law, and organization. Some decisions can be made based strictly on laws or regulations, whereas other decisions require a different source of guidance or expectation. Decision makers may be presented with a situation where a law exists, but there are complicating factors that require ethical decisions to be considered. There may also be situations in which no law or regulation exists; thus, a decision must be made based on another set of criteria, or ethics. When considering professional decisions, healthcare professionals have an obligation to adhere to laws, standards of practice, and professional codes of ethics and interpretative guidelines. As new laws and regulation grow with advances in science and technology, ethical considerations in the use of such technology are also likely to evolve. It is important for healthcare professionals to understand where the law and ethics intersect when faced with decisions in support of quality patient care. This chapter will explore the relationship between law and ethics, ethical theories and principles that facilitate ethical decision making, codes of professional conduct, models of ethical decision making, and a myriad of bioethical issues that present challenges to not only patients but also healthcare professionals.

Relationship between Law and Ethics

Law and ethics are closely intertwined. As discussed in chapter 1, law refers to a set of governing rules used to protect citizens living in a civilized society. It establishes order, provides parameters for conduct, and defines the rights and obligations of the government and citizens. In contrast, **ethics** reflects a culmination of individual morality, expectations of reasonable human behavior, and obligations to act appropriately based on profession or philosophy. It can also be referred to as the "formal process of intentionally and critically analyzing, with clarity and consistency, the basis for one's moral judgement" (Glover 2017, 51). A person's ethics develop from their concepts of right and wrong. Ethics functions with a set of rules of conduct that stem from **moral values** formed through the influence of family, culture, religion, and society. Taken together, law and ethics enable the healthcare professional to offer compassionate, competent care while adhering to governing laws surrounding the delivery, financing, reimbursement, and quality of healthcare.

Applied ethics, medical ethics, professional ethics, and bioethics are all terms relating to healthcare ethics in general. **Applied ethics** is a practical application of moral standards or philosophical examination of moral situations or issues. Applied ethics can be general, relating to an individual's morals and how those apply to situations. Examples of applied ethics are decisions involving issues such as the death penalty, war, gender equality, and racial division. **Medical ethics** is a specific type of applied ethics, because it draws upon moral principles and applies those to relevant scenarios or situations in the delivery of healthcare. A common example of medical ethics can be seen during end-of-life decisions and abortion procedures. **Professional ethics** are designed to provide guidance about the ethical conduct of a profession. Healthcare has various applicable codes of ethics; several will be discussed later in this chapter. **Bioethics** addresses matters of life and death in the use of biological and medical technology.

Throughout the healthcare continuum and across all healthcare delivery models, healthcare providers are trusted with providing quality patient care that adheres to applicable state and federal laws as well as ethical principles set forth by respective professional disciplines. Health information management and informatics professionals, as protectors of patient information and gatekeepers of data, may provide legal and ethical guidance on issues related to access, availability, and integrity of healthcare data and information.

Protecting the privacy and confidentiality of patient information is a common tenet of professional codes of ethics and numerous state and federal laws. Patients have an established right to access their information and request a copy of it, request restrictions or amendments to their information, and request confidential communication regarding their care and an accounting of disclosures. Patients can exercise these rights while also controlling what happens to their information to a certain extent. Through a signed authorization for release of information, a patient can exercise their right to control their information. Honoring those rights and protecting the privacy and confidentiality of patient health information is ingrained in law, healthcare organization policy, and the code of ethics of most healthcare disciplines.

Although federal laws provide a foundation of privacy and security regulation, more detailed policy is required to truly address the legal and ethical issues that arise from advancements in technology and changing infrastructure of individual health systems or healthcare organizations. Healthcare professionals are equipped with professional codes of ethics, decision-making frameworks, and theory-based guidance, which provide groundwork to quickly and accurately assess a situation, determine viable options, and make sound decisions. Privacy and security of patient information rests solely on the shoulders of those who access it and manage it. For example, health information management and informatics professionals must understand the privacy and security rules and regulations while upholding the measures to protect patient information. Ethical considerations may emerge when determining levels and contexts of access allowed by users to patient information. Use of ethical decision-making approaches found later in this chapter may assist the health information management or informatics professional faced with such considerations. In addition, moral values play an important part in one's overall response to an ethical issue.

Ethics and Morality

As individual as humans are, so is their moral code. **Morals** concern or relate to what is right or wrong in human behavior. Much of this stems from how someone was raised or what they were taught as a young person. Some morals stem from religious affiliations, life experiences, and theology and beliefs. The totality of beliefs, experiences, and affiliations creates someone's personal morals.

Because morals stem largely from internal sources, and ethics emerge from external obligations and expectations, some experts relate an individual's morality to the extent their psychological needs have been met or are being met. Psychologist Abraham Maslow created a hierarchy of needs denoting the most basic of physiological needs of food and water in a pyramid leading up to advanced psychological decision making and awareness. His indication was that an individual cannot achieve a high level of psychological decision making if their basic needs (bottom of the pyramid) are not met (Maslow 1943). This can be linked to someone's moral and ethical decision making as well. Consider someone who was homeless or struggling to feed themselves or their family. Their need to provide basic food and shelter for themselves and their family would become a priority. Maslow's theory is based on the idea that once basic needs are met, an individual can obtain a higher level of psychological awareness and well-being.

Personally, morals guide everyday decisions and are passed on in families as children are raised with similar beliefs and moral codes. However, a professional use of morals is considered professional ethics and comes with a higher level of decision making, because professionals draw on a broader source of information. Balancing personal and professional ethics can be difficult, especially in healthcare when not all decisions are clearly right or wrong. For example, a physician may personally disagree with an individual's decision to forgo treatment or to elect to have a certain procedure; however, a person's professional ethics must guide his or her professional decisions. This personal–professional struggle can often be seen in end of life, quality of life, and procreation treatments and procedures. Several of these dilemmas and legal implications are discussed in later chapters of the book.

Consequences of Unethical Behavior

Unethical behavior comes in many forms in healthcare and has serious consequences for both employees and managers. Hourly employees may be unethical in reporting their time worked, essentially misreporting the time they worked to get paid higher wages than they earned. Falsifying a timesheet can be interpreted as stealing from the organization and should be strictly prohibited. Another unethical behavior seen in the workplace is violating company internet policies. Spending excessive company time surfing the internet instead of working is an ethical issue in many departments today. Also, employees who use the internet to visit prohibited websites, such as social media sites, would be considered unethical. The issue with these actions is related to the reduction in productivity when employees are not doing their jobs. Consequences of these behaviors could include fewer or no pay increases, poor performance reviews, and disciplinary actions such as reduction of duties or access, verbal warnings, written warnings, suspension, and termination.

Individuals in positions of authority, such as supervisors and managers, are also at risk of unethical behavior while conducting their business, because of their position and the power they possess. Nondisclosure or underreporting of incidents or breaches is an example of an unethical behavior.

A HIM or informatics professional may wish to not disclose incidents because they may fear the negative repercussions. Because they are often in the position to make decisions in the organization, healthcare vendors or companies selling items may approach them to purchase their product or service. Vendors or sales companies may offer to take the manager to lunch or offer them an item of nominal value. A manager accepting these items could appear to be taking a bribe in return for purchasing or contracting with that vendor or salesperson. HIM or informatics managers must be careful to stay in compliance with guidelines set forth by their compliance department and the AHIMA Code of Ethics, covered later in this chapter, or the state they work in if their actions are ethical. Unethical behavior may result in loss of respect; loss of credibility with peers, and loss of position in the organization.

Ethical Theories

Throughout history, philosophers and theorists have developed ethical concepts and frameworks, many of which date back hundreds of years. These ethical theories vary widely in how they are derived and applied. Some theorists take a logical approach, valuing consequences or duty over virtue. However, others hold morals and essential rights over outcome. A review of a few valid theories is important to understand how ethical standards have emerged and how they can each be applied to ethical predicaments and to the healthcare professional. The HIM and informatics professional may use one or several of these theories as they are faced with ethical dilemmas and must make difficult decisions.

Utilitarianism is an ethical theory based on the idea that the best option in an ethical decision relates to which choice provides the greatest advantage or benefits the greatest number of people. Therefore, the suitability of an ethical decision depends solely on the outcomes; fundamentally, the benefit justifies the cost or the means. This theory can apply to a healthcare organization in allocation and utilization of resources. Often, in healthcare, decisions to invest organizational funds are based on what will make the most difference financially or improve patient care. The options that result in higher reward or that effect more patients would be selected under the utilitarianism theory. However, this theory does not consider situations in which the organization is required by law to implement new initiatives that may not result in the greatest benefit. When an organization is required to comply with a law, there exists a duty to act. The outcome is not considered (Fremgen 2016).

Deontology is derived from the word duty. Another term for deontology is *duty-based ethics*. Instead of the result or outcome shaping decisions, as in utilitarianism theory, the obligation to perform your duty is the critical concept in deontology. It can be explained that the creation of duty has already weighed good versus bad, and duty exists only to do good (Allen 2013); thus individuals tend to feel it is their duty to follow the laws of their government. Duties may also arise from religious affiliations, moral obligations, or even employment relationships. One argument against the deontology theory is that duties can vary from one person to another. One person may feel an obligation to act in a certain way whereas someone else does not experience that obligation. This could lead to inconsistencies in ethical decision making (Fremgen 2016). In healthcare, a duty exists in the physician–patient relationship. Often, healthcare providers feel obligated to the patient's successful outcome, even after discharge. A physician or nurse staying after their shift ends to monitor a patient would be an example of deontology in healthcare ethics.

Right-based ethics is based on the idea that every individual has certain rights. Maintaining those rights should be the overall goal and the primary ethical consideration. Although considering every individual's rights (both legal and perceived) is an ideal approach, there may be a conflict between two individuals who both have rights. For example, an employee complains that his or her rights have been violated by a hospital policy against smoking on hospital campus. The hospital maintains a right to create policies that may restrict actions of its employees but are essential to maintain a professional and healthy environment. These two existing rights may conflict, and using rights-based ethics may not help in determining the best option (Fremgen 2016).

Virtue-based ethics can be viewed as seeking the "good life." Dating back to the philosopher Aristotle, this theory of ethics focuses on the happiness found in our intrinsic characteristics and virtues. Without considering consequences, this approach values an individual's positive moral principles that lead them to do positive things. The idea that healthcare professionals elect their profession because they possess the virtue to innately want to do good is an example of virtue-based ethics. Of course, there are times that this innate virtue is overcome by selfishness, greed, or malice found either in the individual or in others who may take advantage of a virtuous person (Fremgen 2016).

Each ethical theory has substantial benefits and strong reasoning and can influence ethical healthcare decisions. Where one theory has strong ethical undertones, another may have thorough justification. A combination of these theories is the best approach to guiding ethics in the healthcare organization.

Ethical Principles

A principle is a guiding foundation used to determine a course of action. To facilitate decision making as related to right or wrong, four **ethical principles** can be used to assist healthcare professionals in addressing healthcare-related dilemmas (Beauchamp and Childress 2012). Those principles are autonomy, beneficence, nonmaleficence, and justice. Although universally accepted as ethical principles, each uniquely provides healthcare professionals a foundation upon which decisions can be based. A thorough understanding of each principle is critical to defining ethical issues and establishing reasoning.

Autonomy

Autonomy is recognizing the right of a person to make one's own decision, or self-determination. The ability to control what happens to your own body is an integral right of a human that is protected by law but also rooted in ethics. The principle of autonomy is at the forefront of the informed consent process, which will be discussed in chapter 8. A patient must demonstrate competence to maintain autonomy and the ability to make their own decisions. Competence is derived from a patient's age, mental status, and capacity to make sensible decisions. Once a patient reaches the age of majority, they are legally able to make their own healthcare decisions unless their mental status either temporarily or permanently prevents them from making sound decisions (Beauchamp and Childress 2012).

Two challenges to a patient's autonomy include paternalism and right-to-die decisions. **Paternalism** arises when a medical professional's opinion on how the patient should act is considered above the patient's opinion or personal preferences. It often threatens to supersede a patient's autonomy. Although patients should trust their physicians and caregivers and listen to their advice and educated opinions, their ideas should not supplant the patient's ability to make independent decisions.

Beneficence

Beneficence can be defined as doing good, promoting the health and welfare of others, demonstrating kindness, showing compassion, and helping others. Compassion and kindness are at the forefront of healthcare, with beneficence guiding the activities of providers every single day (Beauchamp and Childress 2012). One major challenge a provider may face is when a patient or their family demands more care or additional services the provider knows to be futile. Consider a terminally ill patient whose family is trying to decide whether to put that patient on a ventilator and sustain their life. An ethical conflict often is realized when families request additional services or attempts at resuscitation. The caregiver's ethical principle of beneficence is challenged, weighing the idea of promoting health and welfare and showing compassion for a patient who is dying.

Nonmaleficence

All physicians take an oath upon entering practice "to do no harm." This is called the Hippocratic Oath, and it speaks directly to the next ethical principle called **nonmaleficence**. Defined as doing no harm, this principle protects patients from care that will injure or further hurt them. Although physicians and other caregivers do not typically intend to injure patients or cause harm, it does happen. Medical malpractice and negligence lawsuits often result from unintentional harm done to patients. Chapter 6 will discuss the liability assumed when such harm occurs.

Administration of certain types of medications can have both positive and negative effects. For example, powerful chemotherapy medications have very specific benefits for cancer patients that have been well-documented and researched. However, those medications can also cause severe side effects for the patients who take them. Chemotherapy patients often experience constant fatigue, nausea and vomiting, pain, and hair loss. The benefits of the medication must outweigh the side effects for nonmaleficence to stay intact.

Justice

Justice is known as the obligation to be fair in the distribution of benefits and risks. At first glance, justice may not seem related to healthcare; however, the ethical ideas of benefits and risks, the right to care, and what is owed to patients apply to the healthcare industry. The availability of high-quality healthcare to all Americans, as well as the injustice of illness and cost of treatment are all issues surrounding the principle of justice. Some identify healthcare as a "benefit" to be distributed to those who seek care, whereas others hold the idea of healthcare as a human right. If healthcare is a benefit to be distributed, someone must determine the definition of "fairness" in relation to each patient request. In addition, risk assumed by patients' actions often leads to ethical decisions. Lifelong smokers put themselves at a greater risk for certain diseases, just as skydivers take known risks when they jump out of a plane. Should risky actions be awarded the same distribution of benefits? Or should all patients expect the same distribution of benefits regardless of cost, risk, or disregard for potential danger?

Examining the concept of justice more closely, the terms *fairness* and *impartiality* emerge as indicative of the ethical challenges faced. Allocation of scarce and costly healthcare resources is a source of much debate and varying theory. **Distributive justice** focuses on fair apportionment of resources to all patients, considering several factors including ability to pay, need, equity, and potential benefit of resources. Many theorists support use of distributive justice because it includes more determinants for decision making, and it also considers the unique aspects of providing healthcare services to patients (Neuberger and Swirsky 2017, 250).

Check Your Understanding 2.1

Instructions: Indicate whether the following statements are true or false (T or F).

1. Psychologically, an individual will seek fulfillment of their basic needs before considering ethical repercussions of their actions.

2. The level of ethics increases as responsibility and position in the industry increases.

3. When a patient refuses treatment, he or she is exercising the ethical principle of beneficence.

4. The ethical principle of nonmaleficence refers to making sure rules are fairly and consistently applied to all.

Codes of Professional Conduct

Professionalism

Professionalism can be interpreted as the conduct or qualities that characterize or mark a profession or a professional person. At the center of the idea of professionalism is the profession itself. The profession is established around a core set of competencies or technical abilities. The members of a profession regulate themselves and establish their own expectations (Kirk 2007). As in any other industry, there are certain characteristics intrinsic to the HIM profession. For example, HIM professionalism reflects the expected knowledge base of the profession, the nature of the occupations within the profession, and the licenses, credentials, or certifications that often identify members of the profession. Although ethics can certainly play a role in professionalism, there is a clear distinction between the two terms. Professionalism may change based on age, education, position, or work setting, whereas ethics remain consistent across all areas and levels of practice. The ethical behavior of an HIM director is the same as that expected of a coder. Although professionalism denotes the conduct marking a profession as a whole, ethics is much more comprehensive, encompassing professional ethics, personal ethics, and morals.

Conflicts of Interest

Professional ethics may be challenged when a professional is faced with a conflict of interest. A **conflict of interest** occurs when there is a conflict between private or personal interests and the official responsibilities of a person in a leadership position. An individual may be presented with situations in which they or someone they know could benefit personally or financially from decisions made. For example, a physician practice has decided to hire an agency to clean their office after hours. The professional's spouse owns a commercial janitorial service and offers the spouse's company name as a recommendation. This would be considered a conflict of interest because the individual or someone closely aligned with the individual stands to benefit from the individual's decision or influence on the decision. The decision appears to be self-serving and unethical, and in some cases, it may even be illegal. Healthcare professionals in decision-making positions are often required to sign a conflict of interest agreement. This statement expresses the individual's understanding of conflicts of interest and gives an opportunity to disclose any known conflicts. Many states prohibit state employees or their family members from entering into contracts that would be considered conflicts of interest (Louisiana Code of Governmental Ethics 2015). The legality of an act does not correlate with the ethical nature of that same act, so because something is not prohibited legally does not mean that is ethical or that it is not a conflict of interest. Determining the ethical nature of an act takes reasoning and weighing of benefits and risks. Conflicts of interest often pit ethics against personal satisfaction or personal or financial gain. Codes of professional conduct, ethics, and interpretative guidelines can assist professionals in navigating through these types of ethical problems. In addition, in certain situations, laws have been enacted that define issues of conflict of interest.

Code of Ethics

The ideal is to uphold laws while demonstrating the moral values and ethical principles defined by one's professional code of ethics. A **code of ethics** reflects the values and principles defined by a profession as acceptable behavior within a practice setting. It represents the guiding principles by which a profession governs the conduct of its members. Health informatics and information management professionals face unique decisions related to privacy, security, and confidentiality; collection, maintenance, and storage of patient information; and integrity and accessibility of patient information (AHIMA 2011a). Since codes of ethics represent standards of ethical practice, they are often used as a benchmark for acceptable practice in malpractice, negligence, or other litigious situations. Codes of ethics are dynamic in that they change as societal and practice expectations change. A brief overview of several prominent healthcare professional associations and their codes of ethics will be discussed, including the American Health Information Management Association (AHIMA), the American Medical Association (AMA), and the American Medical Informatics Association (AMIA).

American Health Information Management Association (AHIMA)

The ethical principle of protecting patient privacy has been a cornerstone and an inherent core value and ethical obligation within the AHIMA Code of Ethics since the beginning of the profession in 1928. The discipline of HIM focuses on the process and systems for managing health information and records required to deliver quality healthcare to the public. HIM professionals work in a variety of businesses and health-related settings, and may be found in departments throughout organizations. They may have oversight responsibility for upholding federal and state laws regarding practices related to documentation, reimbursement, quality of care, employee and overall privacy, confidentiality, and security of health information. They are cognizant of the policies, procedures, rules, and regulations that allow for the legitimate fulfillment of requests for access, use, release, or disclosure of health information.

AHIMA created its code of ethics to guide conduct and decision making of HIM professionals. The code of ethics not only assists HIM professionals in their daily mission to protect patient information and improve quality of care, it also creates an expectation of patients and coworkers about what type of conduct they can anticipate from AHIMA members. With this expectation also emerges an appreciation for the HIM professional's expertise in the protecting the privacy and security of patient health information. The AHIMA Code of Ethics is firmly rooted in establishing positive relationships between HIM professionals, healthcare organizations, and the patients they serve. Figure 2.1 depicts the 11 specific ethical focuses for AHIMA and its members. Much of the code of ethics focuses on advancing the HIM profession in a positive, honorable manner through continuing education and mentoring of new professionals. Each principle is further enhanced by interpretive guidelines that can be accessed on the AHIMA website referenced at the end of the chapter. There are several examples of how the AHIMA Code of Ethics provides guidance for examining ethical issues related to complex work situations, such as pressure to upcode, underreport delinquent records, and deny professional development (Crawford 2011).

There is a need to balance the appropriate and lawful use of health information with the protection of the patient's privacy. Although all healthcare providers must be vigilant about protecting patient privacy, the HIM professional is often the individual designated by an organization to address privacy issues; protect patient information from unauthorized, inappropriate, and unnecessary intrusion; and make day-to-day operational decisions about disclosures and release of information policies and procedures. Core to the profession's *code of ethics* are Tenets I, III, and IV, which specifically address protecting the privacy and confidentiality of health information and records. The interpretive guidelines for these principles are shown in figure 2.2.

Tenet I states that the professional must "advocate, uphold, and defend the individual's right to privacy and the doctrine of confidentiality in the use and disclosure of information" (AHIMA 2011a). As shown in figure 2.2, this tenet implies that there is an obligation to maintain confidentiality of the patient's information, honor their right to privacy through ensuring proper access and use of that information, and be an active advocate for the patient's right to privacy. HIM professionals are called to actively participate in privacy and confidentiality through workforce training, consistent monitoring of safeguards, and by effectively ensuring those accessing the patient's information have such authority.

Figure 2.1 AHIMA Code of Ethics

Preamble

The ethical obligations of the health information management (HIM) professional include the safeguarding of privacy and security of health information; disclosure of health information; development, use, and maintenance of health information systems and health information; and ensuring the accessibility and integrity of health information. Healthcare consumers are increasingly concerned about security and the potential loss of privacy and the inability to control how their personal health information is used and disclosed. Core health information issues include what information should be collected; how the information should be handled, who should have access to the information, under what conditions the information should be disclosed, how the information is retained and when it is no longer needed, and how is it disposed of in a confidential manner. All of the core health information issues are performed in compliance with state and federal regulations, and employer policies and procedures. Ethical obligations are central to the professional's responsibility, regardless of the employment site or the method of collection, storage, and security of health information. In addition, sensitive information (e.g., genetic, adoption, drug, alcohol, sexual, health, and behavioral information) requires special attention to prevent misuse. In the world of business and interactions with consumers, expertise in the protection of the information is required.

Ethical Principles: The following ethical principles are based on the core values of the American Health Information Management Association and apply to all health information management professionals.

Health information management professionals:

I. Advocate, uphold, and defend the individual's right to privacy and the doctrine of confidentiality in the use and disclosure of information.

II. Put service and the health and welfare of persons before self-interest and conduct themselves in the practice of the profession so as to bring honor to themselves, their peers, and to the health information management profession.

III. Preserve, protect, and secure personal health information in any form or medium and hold in the highest regard the contents of the records and other information of a confidential nature, taking into account the applicable statutes and regulations.

IV. Refuse to participate in or conceal unethical practices or procedures.

V. Advance health information management knowledge and practice through continuing education, research, publications, and presentations.

VI. Recruit and mentor students, peers, and colleagues to develop and strengthen professional workforce.

VII. Represent the profession accurately to the public.

VIII. Perform honorably health information management association responsibilities, either appointed or elected, and preserve the confidentiality of any privileged information made known in any official capacity.

IX. State truthfully and accurately their credentials, professional education, and experiences.

X. Facilitate interdisciplinary collaboration in situations supporting health information practice.

XI. Respect the inherent dignity and worth of every person.

Source: AHIMA 2011a.

Tenet III states that the professional must "preserve, protect, and secure personal health information in any form or medium and hold in the highest regard the contents of the records and other information of a confidential nature obtained in the official capacity, taking into account the applicable statutes and regulations"(AHIMA 2011a). The HIM professional's obligation does not end with the patient's health record. Knowing all the places where patient data is stored, transmitted, and created electronically is both a challenge and an ethical obligation according to this tenet. To safeguard patient data from unauthorized access and disclosure, that data must be secured in all formats. Again, the AHIMA Code of Ethics calls

Figure 2.2 AHIMA Code of Ethics interpretive guides for protecting health information and records

I. Advocate, uphold, and defend the individual's right to privacy and the doctrine of confidentiality in the use and disclosure of information.

Health information management professionals shall:

1.1. Safeguard all confidential patient information to include, but not limited to, personal, health, financial, genetic, and outcome information.

1.2. Engage in social and political action that supports the protection of privacy and confidentiality, and be aware of the impact of the political arena on the health information issues for the healthcare industry.

1.3. Advocate for changes in policy and legislation to ensure protection of privacy and confidentiality, compliance, and other issues that surface as advocacy issues and facilitate informed participation by the public on these issues.

1.4. Protect the confidentiality of all information obtained in the course of professional service. Disclose only information that is directly relevant or necessary to achieve the purpose of disclosure. Release information only with valid authorization from a patient or a person legally authorized to consent on behalf of a patient or as authorized by federal or state regulations. The minimum necessary standard is essential when releasing health information for disclosure activities.

1.5. Promote the obligation to respect privacy by respecting confidential information shared among colleagues, while responding to requests from the legal profession, the media, or other non-healthcare related individuals, during presentations or teaching and in situations that could cause harm to persons.

1.6. Respond promptly and appropriately to patient requests to exercise their privacy rights (e.g., access, amendments, restriction, confidential communication, etc.). Answer truthfully all patients' questions concerning their rights to review and annotate their personal biomedical data and seek to facilitate patients' legitimate right to exercise those rights.

III. Preserve, protect, and secure personal health information in any form or medium and hold in the highest regard the contents of the records and other information of a confidential nature obtained in the official capacity, taking into account the applicable statutes and regulations.

Health information management professionals shall:

3.1. Safeguard the privacy and security of patients' written and electronic records and other sensitive information. Take reasonable steps to ensure that health information is stored securely and that patients' data are not available to others who are not authorized to have access. Prevent inappropriate disclosure of individually identifiable information.

3.2. Take precautions to ensure and maintain the confidentiality of information transmitted, transferred, or disposed of in the event of a termination, incapacitation, or death of a healthcare provider to other parties through the use of any media.

3.3. Inform recipients of the limitations and risks associated with providing services via electronic media (such as computer, telephone, fax, radio, and television).

IV. Refuse to participate in or conceal unethical practices or procedures and report such practices.

Health information management professionals **shall not**:

4.6. Participate in, condone, or be associated with dishonesty, fraud and abuse, or deception. For example,

- Allowing patterns of retrospective documentation to avoid suspension or increase reimbursement
- Assigning codes without physician documentation
- Failing to report licensure status for a physician through the appropriate channels
- Recording inaccurate data for accreditation purposes
- Allowing inappropriate access to genetic, adoption, or behavioral health information
- Misusing sensitive information about a competitor
- Violating the privacy of individuals
- Coding when documentation does not justify the diagnoses or procedures that have been billed
- Coding an inappropriate level of service
- Miscoding to avoid conflict with others
- Engaging in negligent coding practices

Source: AHIMA 2011a.

the professional to take an active role in managing patient information by taking steps to identify and safeguard patient information. Notably, this obligation remains throughout the patient's continuum of care, even if the healthcare provider no longer exists.

Tenet IV takes a different approach, because it addresses what an HIM professional should *not* do. Refusal to participate in, condone, or be associated with unethical behavior ensures that the professional maintains integrity, honesty, and ethics in all duties (AHIMA 2011a). Several of the unethical behaviors listed in Tenet IV have been discussed as ethical challenges in this chapter. Using the AHIMA Code of Ethics as a guide for best practice is the optimal display of professionalism and high ethical standards for a health information management professional.

Complementing the Code of Ethics Tenets I, III, and IV is AHIMA's Consumer Health Information Bill of Rights (AHIMA 2011b). AHIMA created the bill for the purpose of educating healthcare consumers about the protections and safeguards related to their personal health information. The bill validates every individual's right to lawful access of their personal health information, expectation of protection and prevention of unauthorized access, assurance of accuracy of their record; and an expectation for appropriate remedy when these privileges are violated (AHIMA 2011b). While the document is designed for healthcare consumers, it also offers those responsible for managing health information additional knowledge for ethical decision making regarding the protection and release of health information.

American Medical Association (AMA)

Ethical principles related to privacy and confidentiality have been inherent to the practice of medicine since the fourth century BC, when the Hippocratic Oath was created and "appealed to the inner and finer instincts of the physician" (American Medical Association 2007). The AMA, from its first established code of ethics in 1847 to its most recent update in 2016, has upheld the preservation of patient confidentiality through its code of medical ethics. Principle IV of the code states, "A physician shall respect the rights of patients, colleagues, and other health professionals, and shall safeguard patient confidences and privacy within the constraints of the law." The principles are then further explained in related chapters (Brotherton et al 2016). Chapter 3 of the code of ethics offers more specific guidelines on privacy, confidentiality, and medical records. Specifically, Sections 3.3.2 and 3.3.3 address electronic storage of patient records. Section 3.3.2 provides guidance for physicians when selecting an electronic system, including user access controls for authorized individuals, data integrity, and practices for releasing and sharing information electronically. Section 3.3.3 discusses the ethical obligation of a physician to both ensure confidentiality of electronic records and report breaches of confidentiality (AMA 2016). This update and revision of the AMA code of ethics addresses major changes in the healthcare industry involving the use of information technology in patient care. As the industry changes, so do the ethical codes guiding these professionals.

American Medical Informatics Association (AMIA)

Another professional group that addresses the appropriate use and protection of health information is AMIA. This not-for-profit organization supports the transformation of healthcare through science, education, research, and practice in biomedical and health informatics (AMIA 2010). Members of AMIA are asked to uphold the organization's code of professional ethical conduct, which specifically addresses the use of patient information in its first ethical guideline (see figure 2.3). The code also offers ethical guidance as related to patients, employers, colleagues, society, research, and general performance.

As with AHIMA's Code of Ethics, the AMIA guidelines focus on directing informatics professionals in serving as an expert in their organizations while meeting the needs and honoring the rights of patients.

AMIA also specifically addresses the ethical use of electronic information and research using patient information. Another goal is to ensure the accessibility and usability of patient information for colleagues and other healthcare professionals (AMIA 2013).

The first principle found in the AMIA code of ethics closely resembles the tenets of the AHIMA code. AHIMA focuses on protecting the patient's information while protecting individual patient rights, and this is paralleled in the AMIA principle found in figure 2.3. AMIA discusses the potential harm that exists when improper disclosures occur, thereby focusing on the importance of mitigating that risk. The remaining ethical code focuses on those functions integral to the informatics profession, such as research, data governance, and technological approaches to improving quality of care (AMIA 2013).

Check Your Understanding 2.2

Instructions: Indicate whether the following statements are true or false (T or F).

1. Conflicts of interest can be unethical as well as illegal.

2. A code of ethics should guide patient behavior.

3. The HIM professional's ethical duty ends when the patient's record is complete.

4. A profession's code of ethics should be created and maintained by individuals in that profession.

5. AHIMA created the Consumer Health Information Bill of Rights for the purpose of educating healthcare providers about the protections and safeguards related to health information.

Ethical Decision Making

Ethics Committee

Healthcare organizations recognize the need for a standardized approach to ethical decision making and education of their workforce. An ethics committee is commonly found in healthcare organizations.

Figure 2.3 AMIA principles of professional ethical conduct related to protecting health information

I. Key ethical guidelines regarding patients, guardians, and their authorized representatives (called here collectively "patients"):

  A. Given that patients have the right to know about the existence and use of electronic records containing their personal healthcare information, AMIA members involved in patient care should:

    1. Not mislead patients about the collection, use or communication of their healthcare information;

    2. Enable and-as appropriate, within reason and the scope of their position and in accord with independent ethical and legal standards, facilitate patients' rights to access, review, and correct their electronic healthcare information. Further, they should:

  B. Advocate and work as appropriate to ensure that health and biomedical information is acquired, stored, analyzed and communicated in a safe, reliable, secure and confidential manner, and that such information management is consistent with applicable laws, local policies, and accepted informatics processing standards.

  C. Never knowingly disclose biomedical data in violation of legal requirements or accepted local confidentiality practices, or in ways that are inconsistent with the explanation of data disclosure and use previously given to the patient. AMIA members should understand that inappropriate disclosure of biomedical information can cause harm, and so should work to prevent such disclosures. Likewise, even if an action does not involved disclosure, one should not use patient data in ways inconsistent with the state purposes, goals, or intentions of the organization responsible for these data—except as appropriate for approved research, public health or reporting as required under the law.

Source: American Medical Informatics Association 2013.

The ethics committee's function is to contemplate, analyze, and make recommendations for addressing complex ethical problems (Hurst et al. 2005) The committee must consider the mission of the organization, any religious affiliations of the organization that may impact their approach to the ethical issue or resolution of the issue, and the applicable laws or regulations. Furthermore, participants on the committee must understand all of these factors as well as the professional ethics that organizational employees may be held to (Judicial Council 1985).

In addition to an internal recognition of a need for an ethics committee, external sources have identified the value of an ethics committee as well. The Joint Commission, an accrediting body for healthcare organizations, requires accredited healthcare institutions to provide a mechanism by which the organization promotes a "culture of ethical practices and decision making." In their Governance, Leadership, and Direction standards, The Joint Commission addresses ethics from the patient rights, financial, and clinical perspectives (The Joint Commission n.d.). Even the judicial system has recognized the need for a review body within healthcare to advise providers on ethical decisions. In the first right-to-die case involving Karen Quinlan, the judges actually discussed a need for an official committee to review and assist decision making, basically denoting these issues as questions of medical ethics rather than law (*In re Quinlan*1976).

Models of Ethical Decision Making

Ethics and ethical decisions permeate every department, function, and system in healthcare today. Because all individuals have different sets of moral codes, those responsible for ethics training must standardize ethical decisions. When everyone sees right and wrong a little differently or follows different codes of ethics, it can be extremely difficult to manage the risk of someone's decisions. The privacy and security challenges found in healthcare can be approached from a legal perspective using laws such as HIPAA and HITECH as justification; however, ethical challenges should be approached using a standardized set of steps such as those described next in this section. Whereas an ethical code is a set of guidelines, a model of ethical decision making provides specific steps that can be used to approach any ethical decision. In their Ethics & Compliance Toolkit, the Ethics and Compliance Initiative (ECI) created an **Ethical Decision-Making Model** that can easily be used in healthcare ethics decision (ECI n.d.). This method of ethical decision making assumes a multistep approach.

Steps in Ethical Decision Making

1. Define the problem
2. Seek out relevant assistance, guidance, and support
3. Identify alternatives
4. Evaluate the alternatives
5. Make the decision
6. Implement the decision
7. Evaluate the decision (ECI n.d.)

The initial steps involve clarifying the ethical issue and gathering facts. Understanding the problem includes understanding whether the decision calls upon ethics, morals, laws, or other controlling regulations. Defining the ethical issue helps the decision maker clarify what specifically has to be decided. Considering the facts of the issue, as well as those individuals or stakeholders involved, is crucial to fully understanding the decision required. This process may involve making inquiries to other parties or witnesses, reviewing relevant documentation or reports, and observing behaviors or actions. Once the issue is clearly defined, applicable laws, codes of ethics, and organizational policies and procedures may help guide the decision-making process. These guidelines and best practices can assist a decision maker by providing an objective standard on which to base a decision. Applicable policies, organizational mission and vision, and affiliations must all be considered in these decisions, because they often guide decisions throughout the organization. Certain actions may be against hospital policy, and thus the best decision becomes apparent through careful review of those policies (ECI n.d.).

Once all information about the problem has been gathered, analyzed, and reviewed, all options should be considered. A decision maker must be knowledgeable of all alternatives available before determining whether they are viable options. This should be an inclusive process rather than exclusive. When evaluating options, the HIM and informatics professional must weigh expected benefits and outcomes against potential risk and challenges. This reasoning can be the most difficult aspect of the decision-making process, because many competing interests may be involved, and a complex decision may have various options or alternatives. After all alternatives are exhausted, the optimal option is determined. Once a decision is made, all focus turns to implementing that decision, educating those it will affect, and monitoring the outcome. Some decisions have subsequent effects on other individuals or situations, similar to a domino effect. Ideally, this effect would have been predicted in the evaluation step, and the individuals affected by the decision would have been prepared. However, the domino effect can be unpredictable. In this case, part of the evaluation and reflection would be centered on managing the potential negative effects or new decisions presented as a result (ECI n.d.).

Another reputable decision-making guideline is known as the **Blanchard-Peale Ethics Check** (1988). They suggest a three-prong approach to making a decision about an ethical problem. The following questions are asked:

1. Is it legal? For example, a HIM or informatics professional would examine applicable laws and regulations or company policy. In essence, if the answer to this question is "no," that resolves the ethical problem or action. That option would not be considered if it violates a law or policy.

2. Is it balanced? If the ethical action will more heavily favor one party over the other, the decision is not balanced. The HIM or informatics professional would weigh the benefits to one party versus another party to determine fairness, a term that is quite subjective. Comparing the advantage to one party against the other is one way to determine if an action or decision is fair and balanced.

3. How will it make me feel about myself? This asks the HIM or informatics professional to reference his or her own personal feelings about the decision. If a negative emotion is experienced when considering an option, perhaps that is not the optimal choice (Blanchard and Peale 1988).

These step-by-step approaches to ethical decision making assist in breaking down complex situations into manageable and understandable steps. Ethical decisions, especially in healthcare may cause emotional conflict and uncertainty. HIM and informatics decisions can range from coding to management, with multiple factors contributing to potential outcomes. Utilizing a standardized process for decision making eliminates some of the uncertainty and emotional distress when weighing alternatives and options. When uncertainty is eliminated, an HIM or informatics professional can be confident in a decision and can support that decision with sound reasoning and justification. Ethical decision making is often not a singular activity, but one that includes input for a variety of individuals, especially in cases where human health and life are concerned. With rapid advances in science and technology, the field of bioethics has emerged.

Bioethics

The term *bioethics* first emerged in the late 1960s when rapid advancements were made in biological research involving animals. Scientists identified and anticipated the rapid change in medical technology and advancement of new treatments (Khushf 2004). Bioethics in general can be defined as ethical issues that arise as a result of advancements in healthcare disease detection, medication interventions, and enhanced treatments. Bioethical concerns range from beginning-of-life decisions, including abortion and contraception, to end-of-life decisions, including euthanasia. New technologies developed to support advancements in stem cell research and reproduction have ethical considerations and are the subject of much debate. Many bioethical issues have been addressed through the courts and in some cases through laws designed to protect the privacy and security of patient information. Advancements in technologies have "extended the power to control, explain and predict human attributes and life processes ... with this power comes the ethical dilemma of 'We can do it, but should we?'" (Science Reference Services 2015). Some issues that have arisen as a result of biological and medical advances are discussed in later sections.

Ethical Dilemmas at the Beginning and End of Life

Ethical decisions relating to **procreation**, or the beginning of life, have presented themselves in determining when life begins and identifying the product of life. Many research studies have focused on the issues, risks, and expected outcomes of the science and technologies that relate to procreation. One type of procedure that is widely used is **in vitro fertilization (IVF)**, which refers to the act of fertilization outside of the woman's body. Typically, a number of the woman's eggs are fertilized with a male's sperm during IVF. The fertilized eggs are then introduced into the woman's uterus. The fertilized eggs that are not used are often frozen so that they may be used later if the procedure is not successful the first time or if the woman decides to use IVF again for a later pregnancy. Ethical issues have arisen in regard to the disposition of frozen eggs and sperm if the partners divorce or one of them dies. For example, in the case of *Davis v. Davis*, ownership and disposition of the frozen fertilized eggs after the couple decided to end their marriage arose. Mr. Davis struggled ethically with his ex-wife's wishes to donate the fertilized eggs to couples who could not conceive. The court found that the ethical concerns of Mr. Davis outweighed his ex-wife's wishes to donate the eggs, thus finding in favor of Mr. Davis's desire not to donate the eggs.

Another issue related to fertilized frozen eggs is **embryonic stem cell research**. Embryonic stem cells are harvested from unused donated fertilized embryos acquired through an IVF process. When the eggs are no longer needed, the couple may decide to donate those fertilized eggs for research purposes. Studies have shown these cells to be particularly beneficial in treating Down syndrome and Parkinson's disease as well as many degenerative diseases. The benefit of these cells versus the ethical issues surrounding their procurement has been the subject of much debate and litigation. Some argue that fertilized eggs have the potential to become human life or are even in the beginning stages of human life. Others argue that these cells have not yet become human life, and thus the benefits associated with using them for research and possibly treatment are enough to support their use.

Preventing procreation through contraception and sterilization can also involve ethics and morals. Prescription and use of contraceptives, especially by minors or in religiously affiliated institutions, is often strictly controlled or even prohibited. There are various forms of contraceptives, including pharmaceuticals, physical barriers, or other temporary implantable devices that prevent conception. A permanent form of controlling procreation is known as sterilization. Sterilization in a male patient is accomplished through a vasectomy and in a female patient through tubal ligation. Both of these procedures prevent conception by permanently altering the reproductive organs of the patient, thereby rendering them sterile. Again, some patients, providers, and institutions choose not to participate in these interventions because of their ethical, moral, or religious values.

Just as the beginning of life can create ethical situations, so can end-of-life decisions. For terminally ill patients, quality of life becomes an important consideration. Patients and families often have to decide whether to continue treatment, which may be difficult for the patient to endure, or to forgo treatment for the duration of the patient's life. Advancements in healthcare treatments have created an even more difficult paradigm of decision making as providers are able to offer more interventions that may increase life span for terminally ill patients. When no cure is possible, patients and families must decide when quality of life surpasses quantity of life; or when the quality of days is more important than the number of days remaining for their loved one. Many who choose quality of life over quantity opt for hospice care. **Hospice care** is palliative care provided to terminally ill patients, often in their home or residential living facility. Other options for end-of-life treatment and procedures may be available in particular states where voluntary euthanasia, or physician-assisted suicide, is legal.

Decisions regarding end-of-life matters are often dealt with through legal determinations, although these decisions remain incredibly difficult and many patients and families struggle with the ethical obligations involved. Family wishes and patient wishes are sometimes not synonymous. During a period of life where emotions are already high, creating an environment conducive to decision making is key. Providing useful information, access to resources and time can assist families in this process. A patient's right to self-determine care or not receive care as well as legal issues surrounding life decisions are discussed in chapter 8.

Genetics, Genetic Testing, and Gene Therapy

Contemporary medicine has advanced such that an individual's genetic code can be examined, and predictions of disease incidence can be made based on the content of that code. An individual's decision to discover those predictions is personal, but it may raise ethical issues between the individual and family members. For example, a patient with a family history of breast or ovarian cancer may undergo genetic testing to determine his or her likelihood of developing the disease. Some patients who discover they are carrying the *BRCA1* gene are at a higher risk of developing the disease, and thus, decide to have preventative procedures performed, such as removing their breasts or ovaries (Metcalfe et al. 2013). Others argue that genetic testing results in prediction of disease rather than certainty, and organ removal may not be the best course of action for an individual. Test results should not automatically result in major surgical procedures; however, more frequent screenings may be a better option (Veeravagu 2015).

Genetic testing can be done on couples to determine the likelihood of certain genetic diseases in their offspring, and the results may lead to ethical questions of whether to reproduce. Also, testing can be done on fetuses in utero. Discovering that a fetus has a particular genetic disorder may create ethical decisions to be made by the parents. Finally, gene therapy is an experimental form of gene research that is still being developed with limited use. Gene therapy involves identifying mutated genes in a patient's DNA and replacing the mutated gene with a healthy copy of the gene. Although risky, promising results have provided encouragement for continued study. However, altering an individual's genetic identity is a fiercely debated intervention and one that results in ethical, moral, religious, and in some cases, political concerns (Terry 2017, 470).

With advancements in genetic testing and treatment, more genetic information is generated. This information is considered sensitive and poses a challenge for HIM professionals to properly store, secure, and transmit such information. The Genetic Information Nondisclosure Act of 2008 (GINA) was passed to regulate the use and disclosure of genetic information specifically. GINA also created new regulations related to the use of genetic information in determination of life and health insurance. Overall, GINA prevents misuse of genetic information and provides patients with certainty of the protection of their information (Asmonga 2008).

Ethical Decision Making in HIM and Informatics

Healthcare clinicians, providers, and staff may face ethical decisions daily regarding the care provided to a patient and the patient's well-being. Ethical decisions made by HIM and informatics professionals differ from those of caregivers in that the decisions of the former are related to managing the patient's health data or information rather than their care. For example, in revenue management, coding has a direct effect on reimbursement. Concerns may arise related to assignment of correct codes and pressure to maximize reimbursement, which may result in a higher level of payment. A HIM department director with knowledge of regulatory coding rules and strong ethical judgment will manage the coding process to ensure validity of codes and correct payment, thus preventing healthcare fraud and abuse. Inquiries made to physicians for clarification can assist coders in their decisions while also enhancing the quality of the documentation in the record.

Although patients and healthcare providers or professionals may face different ethical issues, their decisions often require information or access to patient information. Maintaining patient information, anticipating patient information needs, and granting access to this information can assist patients in their decision-making process. Advancements in technology have also revolutionized the amount of data collected as well as how data is stored, shared, accessed, and disclosed. Ethical issues related to the use and protection of patient information are surfacing as a result of the increased use of electronic health records (EHRs) and biomedical data sources. Integration of medical devices and inclusion of their data creates ethical concerns related to "(1) accurate collecting and reporting of data by the devices; (2) the ability of consumers to understand the data that is presented, as well as a mechanism to ensure that consumers will not misinterpret the data; and (3) integrating the data reliably and accurately with the EHR to inform clinical decision making" (Fenton and Cornelius 2017, 378).

The challenge for health information management and informatics professionals is to work with appropriate organizational staff to ensure policies and procedures are in place when ethical issues arise.

Check Your Understanding 2.3

Instructions: Indicate whether the following statements are true or false (T or F).

1. Taking a step-by-step approach to ethical decision making can assist an HIM or informatics professional when faced with a challenging decision.
2. Stem cell research is an example of a bioethical issue.
3. GINA is an ethical code used to establish expected responses to conflicts of interest.
4. When making an ethical decision, the first step is to gather the applicable facts.
5. Ethics committees create internal recommendations for ethical decisions.

Scenario 2

Jan Geisler is the HIM director at Hillside Medical Center. The administration at Hillside has just approved the budget, which includes a new electronic health record. They assigned Jan as the project manager and give her the task of reviewing and selecting the company (vendor) with the EHR that best suits the hospital's needs. Jan immediately thinks of her college roommate, Ana. Ana also majored in HIM and now works for a large EHR vendor in California. Jan sends a quick e-mail to Ana to catch up and asks about her company's EHR system. Ana responds immediately with updated

Scenario 2 (Continued)

pictures of her family and some general information about the EHR her company sells. Ana offers for her company to fly Jan to California so she can see the system and have a live demonstration. As an added bonus, Ana writes that she cannot wait to see her friend, take her to dinner, and catch up. Jan goes to California and enjoys her time with Ana, but she is a little disappointed with the EHR system. She just doesn't think it will meet the needs of her hospital. Jan has a meeting with the chief information officer today and is expected to present her recommendations. She feels obligated to recommend Ana's company, but she also has major concerns about their product.

1. What ethical issues can be found in Ana's investigation of EHRs?

2. Was it a conflict of interest for Jan to do business with her personal friend Ana?

3. Using the ethical decision-making model described in this chapter, analyze the scenario and recommend a decision.

References

AHIMA. 2011a. Code of ethics. http://www.ahima.org.

AHIMA. 2011b. AHIMA Consumer Health Information Bill of Rights: A Model for Protecting Health Information Principles. http://www.ahima.org.

Allen, James F. 2013. *Health Law and Medical Ethics for Healthcare Professionals*. Boston: Pearson.

American Medical Association. 2007. E-history. http://www.ama-assn.org.

American Medical Association. 2016. Code of Medical Ethics. https://www.ama-assn.org/about-us/code-medical-ethics.

American Medical Informatics Association. 2010. Strategic Alignment Summary. http://www.amia.org.

American Medical Informatics Association. 2013. Code of professional ethical conduct. http://www.amia.org

Asmonga, D.D. Getting to know GINA: An overview of the Genetic Information Nondiscrimination Act. *Journal of AHIMA* 79(7):18, 20, 22.

Beauchamp, T. and J. Childress. 2012. *Principles of Biomedical Ethics*, 7th ed. New York: Oxford University Press.

Blanchard, K. and N.V. Peale. 1988. *The Power of Ethical Management*. New York: William Morrow.

Brotherton, S., A. Kao, and B.J. Crigger. 2016. Professing the values of medicine: The modernized AMA Code of Medical Ethics. *JAMA*, 316(10):1041–1042. doi:10.1001/jama.2016.9752

Crawford, M. 2011. Everyday ethics. AHIMA code of ethics guides daily work, complex situations. *Journal of AHIMA* 82(4):30–33.

Ethics & Compliance Initiative. n.d. Ethics & compliance toolkit. https://www.ethics.org/resources/free-toolkit.

Fenton, S. and F. Cornelius. 2017. *Ethical Health Informatics: Challenges and Opportunities*, 3rd ed. Edited by Harman, L. and F. Cornelius. Sudbury, MA: Jones and Bartlett Learning.

Fremgen, B. 2016. Medical Law and Ethics. 5th ed. Boston: Pearson.

Glover, J. 2017. Ethical Decision-Making Guidelines and Tools. *Ethical Health Informatics Challenges and Opportunities*, 3rd ed. Edited by Harman, L. and F. Cornelius. Sudbury, MA: Jones and Bartlett Learning.

Hurst, S., S. Hull, G. DuVal, and M. Danis. 2005. How physicians face ethical difficulties: A qualitative analysis. *Journal of Medical Ethics* 31(1):7–14. http://doi.org/10.1136/jme.2003.005835.

Judicial Council. 1985. Guidelines for ethics committees in healthcare institutions. *JAMA* 253(18):2698–2699.

Khushf, G. 2004. Handbook of bioethics: Taking stock of the field from a philosophical perspective. Boston: Kluwer Academic.

Kirk, L. 2007. Professionalism in medicine: Definitions and considerations for teaching. *Proceedings (Baylor University Medical Center)*. 20(1):13–16.

Maslow, A.H. (1943). A theory of human motivation. *Psychological Review* 50(4):370–396.

Metcalfe, K., C. Kim-Sing, P. Ghadirian, P. Sun, and S. Narod. 2013. Health care provider recommendations for reducing cancer risks among women with a *BRCA1* or *BRCA2* mutation. *Clinical Genetics,* 85(1):21–30.

Neuberger, B. J. and E.S. Swirsky. 2017. Public health and informatics. In *Ethical Health Informatics: Challenges and Opportunities,* 3rd ed. Edited by Harmen, L. and F. Cornelius. Sudbury, MA: Jones and Bartlett Learning.

Science Reference Services. 2015. Bioethics Tracer Bullet 91-4. http://www.loc.gov/rr/scitech/tracer-bullets /bioethicstb.html.

Terry, S. 2017. Genetic Information. In *Ethical Health Informatics: Challenges and Opportunities,* 3rd ed. Edited by Harmen, L. and F. Cornelius. Sudbury, MA: Jones and Bartlett Learning.

The Joint Commission International Accreditation Standards for Hospitals, 5th ed. Standards GLD.12, GLD.12.1, GLD.12.2. https://www.ethics.org/eci/research/free-toolkit/decision-making-model#filters.

Veeravagu, A. 2015. Why Angelina Jolie's Surgery Isn't for Everyone. *The Daily Beast.* http://www.thedailybeast .com/articles/2015/03/24/why-angelina-jolie-s-surgery-isn-t-for-everyone.html.

Cases, Statutes, and Regulations Cited

Davis v. Davis, 842 S.W.2d 588 (Tenn. Supr. 1992).

In re Quinlan, 70 N.J. 10, 355 A.2d 647 (1976).

Louisiana Code of Governmental Ethics, R.S. 42:1111–1121, Section III, F 1112.

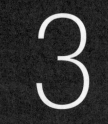
The Legal System in the United States

Laurie A. Rinehart-Thompson, JD, RHIA, CHP, FAHIMA

Learning Objectives

- Apply the relevance of law to the health information management and informatics profession and other health professions
- Differentiate between public law and private law
- Name and give examples of the four sources of law
- Identify resolutions in cases where laws conflict with one another
- Compare the branches of government and the role that each plays
- Analyze the separation of powers in a democratic society
- Compare the federal and state court systems and the appeals processes in both
- Discuss the role of nonlegal accrediting bodies, such as The Joint Commission, and differentiate their authority from that of the legal system
- Demonstrate types of alternative dispute resolution available as options to the court system

Key Terms

- Administrative agencies
- Administrative agency tribunals
- Administrative law
- Alternative dispute resolution
- Appellate court
- Arbitration
- Brief
- Case law
- Circuit courts
- Civil law
- Code of Federal Regulations (CFR)
- Common law

- Conditions of Participation
- Constitution
- Constitutional law
- Court of Claims
- Criminal law
- Department of Health and Human Services (HHS)
- District courts
- Diversity jurisdiction
- Due process of law
- Executive branch
- Felony
- General jurisdiction
- Judicial branch

- Judicial law
- Jurisdiction
- Legislative branch
- Limited jurisdiction
- Mediation
- Misdemeanor
- Opinion
- Oral argument
- Persuasive authority
- Petition for *writ of certiorari*
- Precedent
- Private law
- Procedural due process
- Public law

- *Res judicata*
- Separation of powers
- Special jurisdiction
- *Stare decisis*
- State action
- Statutory law
- Subject matter jurisdiction
- Substantive due process
- Supremacy Clause
- Trial court
- United States Code (USC)
- United States Supreme Court
- US Constitution

Law is a "body of rules of action or conduct prescribed by a controlling authority ... having binding legal force ... which must be obeyed and followed by citizens subject to sanctions or legal consequences ... (it is) a solemn expression of the will of the supreme power of the State" (Garner 2014).

To enjoy the benefits of living in a civilized society, laws must be created and followed to establish order, provide the parameters within which we lead our lives, and define the rights and obligations of both the government and its citizens. Nonetheless, laws are often broken and, because of their manmade imperfections, subject to dispute. It is therefore necessary for a legal system to not only create laws but also enforce and interpret them.

This chapter discusses the role of law in the US healthcare system, distinguish public law from private law, and introduce the student to the four sources of law and conflict of laws. It also addresses government organization with an emphasis on the judicial system; outlines the requirements of nonlegal entities such as accrediting bodies; and describes the types of alternative dispute resolution, which provide options to resolving an issue inside the courtroom.

Role of Law in the US Healthcare System

Health information management and informatics professionals and other healthcare professionals are employed in a wide range of settings, ranging from acute care hospitals to insurers and vendor corporations. Regardless of the venue, the legal system guides business decisions and practices. From wrongful disclosures of patient information to contract issues and employment matters, the law will constantly affect the decisions that health information management and informatics professionals and other health professionals make.

Public versus Private Law

In the United States, law can be divided into two types: public and private. **Public law** involves the federal, state, or local government and its relationship to individuals and business organizations. Its purpose is to define, regulate, and enforce rights where any part of a government agency is a party (Showalter 2015, 4–5). The most familiar type of public law is **criminal law**, where the government is a party prosecuting an accused who has been charged with violating a criminal statute or regulation by committing either a more serious **felony**, which is usually punishable by at least one year in prison, or a **misdemeanor**, which is a less severe crime than a felony and generally involves imprisonment of up to one year. Criminal law does not result in compensation to the injured victim. Instead, the victim is the government's chief witness. Public law also encompasses regulatory activities, which can be criminal in nature or within the realm of **civil law** (that is, noncriminal law). In healthcare, public law encompasses regulations at the state and national levels. For example, the Medicare Conditions of Participation, which involve the government and its relationship with individuals by providing health insurance for the elderly and other designated groups, is federal public law. Public law is enforced through the judicial (court) system or by government agencies.

Private law, conversely, is concerned with the rules and principles that define rights and duties among people and among private businesses. The government is not a party. Instead, private law consists of actions by one or more individuals acting in a private capacity against other individuals also acting in a private capacity. The rights and obligations of individuals in private law are generally enforced through the judicial (court) system. For example, private law applies when a contract for the purchase of a house is written between two parties. Normally, private law encompasses issues related to contracts, property, and torts (injuries). In the medical context, private law often applies when there is a breach of contract or when a tort occurs through malpractice. There are four sources of public and private law: constitutions, statutes, administrative law, and judicial decisions. Table 3.1 shows the relationship of public and private law to civil and criminal law.

Table 3.1 Relationship of public and private law to civil and criminal law

	Civil Law	Criminal Law
Public Law	X	X
Private Law	X	

Note: Public law encompasses both civil and criminal actions, but private law encompasses only civil actions.

Sources of Law

No one source or type of law governs the actions of individuals and governmental entities. Instead, the laws governing our society come from four sources:

- Constitutions (federal and state)
- Statutes (federal, state, and local)
- Administrative law, which consists of rules and regulations created by **administrative agencies**, which reside under the executive branch of a government (described later)
- Common law (court decisions)

Constitutions

Constitutional law is the body of law that deals with the amount and types of power and authority that governments are given.

The **US Constitution** defines and lays out the powers of the three branches of the federal government. The **legislative branch** (the US House of Representatives and the US Senate) creates statutory laws (statutes) such as Medicare and HIPAA. The **executive branch** (the president and staff, namely cabinet-level agencies) enforces the law. For example, the Centers for Medicare and Medicaid Services (CMS), which enforces Medicare laws, are contained within the US **Department of Health and Human Services (HHS)**, a cabinet-level agency dedicated to health policy that reports to the president. The third branch of government, the **judicial branch** (composed of courts), interprets laws that are passed by the US Congress and signed by the president. A similar system can be found at the state level, where state courts interpret laws that are passed by state legislatures and signed by their respective governors.

In addition to defining the three branches of government, the Constitution includes 27 amendments. These include the Bill of Rights (the first 10 amendments) and 17 additional amendments. The purpose of these amendments is to place restrictions on the federal government so that the most fundamental legal rights of US citizens are not infringed upon. Through the Fourteenth Amendment, these restrictions are also applied to state governments. In addition to the US Constitution, each state also has a **constitution** that lays out the powers of the branches of the state's government. The state constitution is the supreme law of each state but is subordinate to the US Constitution, the supreme law of the nation.

Due process of law, provided for by the US Constitution, places restrictions on governments and public organizations and facilities (for example, Veterans Health Administration hospitals), and it also may apply to private organizations that take on characteristics of a public organization, perform substantial public functions, or have significant government involvement (for example, a private corporation that operates a state-owned facility by contract) (Showalter 2015, 246). They are then held to government standards, such as due process. Activities by these organizations are called **state action**. There are two types of due process:

- **Substantive due process** protects individuals' legal rights and guarantees that laws are fair, reasonable, and not arbitrary; it allows for challenges to a law's content and substance.
- **Procedural due process** applies due process to the federal and state governments. It requires that government shall not take a person's life, liberty, or property without due process of law. Procedural due process intends fair legal processes and procedures.

Although due process is a hallmark of the US court system, the legal system increasingly requires that it be exercised outside the court system by companies and other entities, to ensure fairness to individuals.

In many cases, both public and private entities must apply due process through various sources of law: the Constitution, statutory law, administrative regulations, or judicial precedent.

Statutes

Statutes (**statutory law**) are enacted by a legislative body. The US Congress and state legislatures are legislative bodies, and the compendiums of statutes they create are generally referred to as codes. The **United States Code (USC)** is the compilation of all federal statutes. Commonly known healthcare laws include Medicare and HIPAA (discussed later in the text). They are statutes because they were enacted by the US Congress. Statutes can also be enacted by local bodies, such as municipalities, and are then referred to as ordinances. Table 3.2 lists all the titles within the US Code.

Table 3.2 Titles within the US Code

Title Number	Title Name
1	General Provisions
2	The Congress
3	The President
4	Flag and Seal, Seat of Government, and the States
5	Government Organization and Employees (with Appendix)
6	Domestic Security
7	Agriculture
8	Aliens and Nationality
9	Arbitration
10	Armed Forces
11	Bankruptcy (with Appendix)
12	Banks and Banking
13	Census
14	Coast Guard
15	Commerce and Trade
16	Conservation
17	Copyrights
18	Crimes and Criminal Procedure (with Appendix)
19	Customs Duties
20	Education
21	Food and Drugs
22	Foreign Relations and Intercourse
23	Highways
24	Hospitals and Asylums
25	Indians
26	Internal Revenue Code
27	Intoxicating Liquors
28	Judiciary and Judicial Procedure (with Appendix)
29	Labor

Table 3.2 Titles within the US Code (Continued)

30	Mineral Lands and Mining
31	Money and Finance
32	National Guard
33	Navigation and Navigable Waters
35	Patents
36	Patriotic and National Observances, Ceremonies, and Organizations
37	Pay and Allowances of the Uniformed Services
38	Veterans' Benefits
39	Postal Service
40	Public Buildings, Property, and Works
41	Public Contracts
42	The Public Health and Welfare
43	Public Lands
44	Public Printing and Documents
45	Railroads
46	Shipping
47	Telecommunications
48	Territories and Insular Possessions
49	Transportation
50	War and National Defense (with Appendix)
51	National and Commercial Space Programs
52	Voting and Elections
53	(Reserved)
54	National Park Service and Related Programs

Source: US House of Representatives 2016.

There are many health information management and informatics issues that can be impacted through legislation, both at the federal and state levels. An increasingly critical role of individuals responsible for the management of health information is to stay abreast of legislative activity and advocate for changes that will positively affect the future of the profession.

Administrative Law

Administrative law falls solely under the umbrella of public law. As noted, the executive branch of government is responsible for enforcing laws enacted by the legislative branch. Frequently, the legislative body (US Congress or state legislatures) gives various executive branch (administrative) agencies the power to develop rules and regulations that carry out the intent of statutes. For example, the US Congress directed the Secretary of HHS to promulgate or develop rules and regulations (administrative law) that carry out the intent of the Medicare Conditions of Participation. Additionally, the US Food and Drug Administration (FDA), another HHS agency, can develop rules that control the manufacture of drugs. Regulations developed by federal administrative agencies are published in the **Code of Federal Regulations (CFR)**. They are located online at http://www.archives.gov.

Federal and state administrative agencies can have a significant influence on health information and informatics issues. Health information management and informatics professionals should serve as advocates for changes in administrative rules and regulations that will affect the profession in a positive manner.

At times, disputes may arise from administrative law. These can often be handled within the relevant administrative agency, without resorting to litigation, through **administrative agency tribunals**, who are legal decision makers for their respective agencies. Tribunals make decisions about disputes arising from administrative law, either in lieu of the court system or in an attempt to resolve the issue before resorting to the court system. A common example would be a case dealing with workers' compensation. Such cases are settled by a state workers' compensation tribunal, such as a commissioner or hearing officer. The agency resolving the dispute through this process is also generally the same administrative agency that created the rules that are in dispute. Individuals responsible for health information would be involved in such cases to the extent that the workers' compensation board or commission subpoenas health records (Showalter 2015, 14–15).

Common Law

The fourth major source of law is **common law** (also known as **judicial law** or **case law**), which is created when a court resolves a dispute. Courts hold significant decision-making authority when resolving disputes, including interpreting constitutions; interpreting statutes and regulations and determining their constitutionality; resolving conflicting statutes and regulations; deciding cases based on binding prior judicial decisions; and creating common law where a void currently exists in the law.

The outcomes of common law decisions vary from state to state and from one part of the federal court system to another. (Court systems are discussed later in this chapter.) Two interchangeable terms relating to court decisions are *stare decisis*, a Latin term meaning "let the decision stand," and **precedent**. These principles state that lower courts within a court system are bound to follow (that is, apply) the decisions of higher courts in the same court system when determining the outcome of the case, so long as the fact pattern of the case in the higher court is similar to that of the current case. This principle applies to decisions rendered by a judge or instructions given to a jury prior to deliberations. For example, if a court heard a case and determined that a provider was liable for the wrongful disclosure of a patient's health record, lower courts within that same court system would be bound to make the same decision in future cases if the facts are similar enough to the case decided by the higher court.

Stare decisis, or precedent, is applied in only one direction. Lower courts must look to higher courts within their own court system for precedent; however, higher courts are not bound by decisions of lower courts within their court system. Likewise, courts on the same tier need not follow each other's decisions. Finally, courts within one state court system need not follow decisions made by courts in other states. District (trial) courts, the lowest level in the federal court system, must look to the decisions of their own circuit (appellate) courts and the US Supreme Court; however, circuit courts must only follow US Supreme Court decisions from similar cases. Courts that are not bound by precedent to follow each other may nonetheless look to another's decisions as **persuasive authority**, for guidance only.

Check Your Understanding | 3.1

Instructions: Indicate whether the following statements are true or false (T or F).

1. Administrative law is created by court decisions. *→ Public branch*
2. Persuasive authority occurs when a court looks to another court's decision for guidance, even if it is not required to do so.
3. The United States Code is a compilation of federal ~~court decisions~~. *Statutes*
4. Private law defines rights and duties between individuals and the government.
5. Statutes are enacted by ~~administrative agencies~~. *Legislative bodies.*

Conflict of Laws

Conflict of laws occurs when there is an inconsistency between the laws of different states arising from a legal action that involves more than one jurisdiction (a territory of legal control) (Garner 2014). For example, a medical malpractice action where the rights and obligations of the parties and the injuries incurred involved more than one state requires each state's legal system to make a determination about the extent to which the law of each state would apply. Conflict of laws may involve any of the sources of law described in the previous section. The Supremacy Clause of the US Constitution states that federal law preempts any conflicting state law.

Government Organization

The federal government and individual state governments each have a three-part system, and each of their constitutions have overriding authority. The three parts of government and the separation of powers among them are described next.

Executive Branch

The executive branch of government is charged with enforcing laws. Ultimate executive branch power rests with the chief executive (the president of the United States, federally; and each governor at the state level). Federal cabinet-level agencies (that is, those that report directly to the president) are responsible for areas that warrant high-level attention from the US government through executive agency representation. Figure 3.1 lists the agencies that make up the president's cabinet.

Administrative agencies create and issue rules and regulations that are then used to enforce the law. Each agency follows the intent of statutory law and provides administrative oversight of the industry for which it is responsible. For example, the US Department of Transportation oversees the airline industry, the US Department of Agriculture oversees the importation of crops and livestock from other countries, and HHS oversees the healthcare industry. The executive branch at both the federal and state levels of government are responsible for issuing regulations.

Federal Regulation of Healthcare

Because national healthcare policy is critical, HHS is part of the president's cabinet (figure 3.1). Some of the healthcare issues regulated at the federal administrative level are disbursement of Medicare and Medicaid funds, standards for providers receiving Medicare and Medicaid reimbursement (CMS),

Figure 3.1 President's cabinet

Executive agencies	Cabinet-rank agencies and individuals
• Department of Agriculture	• Council of Economic Advisers
• Department of Commerce	• Environmental Protection Agency
• Department of Defense	• Office of Management and Budget
• Department of Education	• United States Ambassador to the United Nations
• Department of Energy	• United States Trade Representative
• Department of Health and Human Services	• Vice President of the United States
• Department of Homeland Security	• White House Chief of Staff
• Department of Housing and Urban Development	
• Department of Justice	
• Department of Labor	
• Department of State	
• Department of the Interior	
• Department of the Treasury	
• Department of Transportation	
• Department of Veterans Affairs	

Source: White House n.d.

healthcare research (National Institutes of Health), and healthcare issues relating to specific populations, such as those represented by the Indian Health Service and the Administration on Aging. The complete list of agencies within HHS is illustrated in the organizational chart in figure 3.2.

HHS is also actively involved in combating healthcare fraud and abuse that occurs through fraudulent billing. As with other federal administrative agencies, one HHS office is the Inspector General. In conjunction with the Department of Justice, another federal cabinet-level agency, the Inspector General for HHS investigates providers that are believed to be receiving Medicare and Medicaid funds fraudulently. The tenacious efforts of the government, while costly, have proven beneficial in ferreting out criminal activity and allowing the government to recoup dollars obtained illegally by healthcare providers.

State Regulation of Healthcare

Healthcare is an important policy objective for state governments as well as for the federal government. Issues and populations that are addressed and regulated at the state administrative level are disbursement of Medicaid dollars; funding and operation of facilities for state residents with mental illnesses, developmental disabilities, and substance abuse problems; public health issues, such as naturally occurring epidemics and bioterrorism threats; regulation of facilities that receive state reimbursement, including nursing homes, mental health facilities, and facilities for the developmentally disabled and those suffering from substance abuse; and regulation of healthcare professionals, such as physicians, nurses, and allied health professionals. With a broad spectrum of responsibility and oversight, numerous statewide administrative agencies share the responsibilities of managing operational and policy issues.

Figure 3.2 Department of Health and Human Services organizational chart

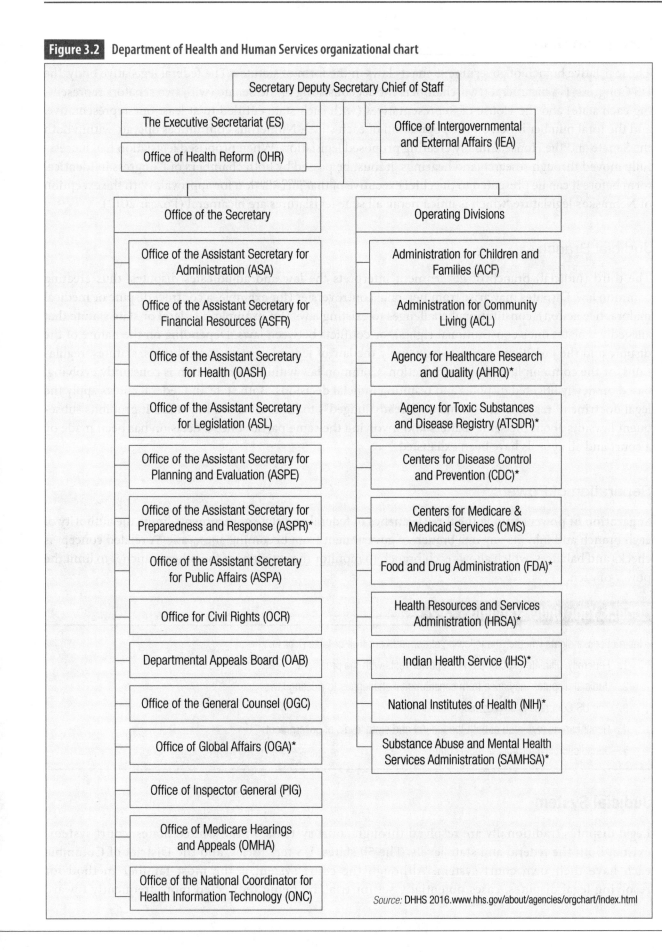

Source: DHHS 2016.www.hhs.gov/about/agencies/orgchart/index.html

Legislative Branch

The legislative branch of government enacts laws in the form of statutes. The federal legislative body, the US Congress, is a bicameral (two-chamber) model consisting of the Senate (with two senators representing each state) and the House of Representatives (with each state entitled to at least one representative, and the total number based on the population of each state). Numerous committees operate within both the Senate and the House, initially creating proposed legislation. When proposed legislation has successfully moved through research and hearings, it must be passed by both chambers of Congress in identical form before it can be presented to the chief executive of that jurisdiction for approval. With the exception of Nebraska's legislature, which is unicameral, all state legislatures are bicameral (Pozgar 2012).

Judicial Branch

The third (judicial) branch of government interprets the law and adjudicates disputes, thus creating common law. Disputes may arise from personal controversies (for example, a contract dispute or medical malpractice action), constitutional challenges to existing laws (for example, a federal or state statute that allegedly violates one's constitutional rights), or conflicts between laws. Depending on the nature of the dispute and the jurisdiction, courts may apply the law of federal or state constitutions, statutes, regulations, or the common law of that jurisdiction. Common law within a jurisdiction is constantly evolving, based on newly litigated disputes and resulting judicial decisions. Both state and federal courts apply the legal doctrine of **res judicata** ("a matter already judged") to limit excessive litigation. It prohibits subsequent lawsuits about the same matters and involving the same parties once a decision has been made by a court and all appeals have been exhausted.

Separation of Powers

Separation of powers among the three branches of federal and state governments limits the authority of each branch and inhibits any one branch of government from becoming autocratic. A related concept is checks and balances, which allows each branch to monitor the activities of the other branches to limit the power of each.

Check Your Understanding   3.2

Instructions: Indicate whether the following statements are true or false (T or F).

1. Federally, ultimate executive branch power rests with the president.
2. Judicial disputes may arise from constitutional challenges to existing laws.
3. The US Congress is a unicameral model. bicameral
4. Healthcare is regulated at both the federal and state levels of government. True
5. Jurisdiction is a territory of legal control.

Judicial System

Legal disputes traditionally are resolved through court systems. In the United States, court systems exist at both the federal and state levels. The 50 states, US territories, and the District of Columbia each have their own court system. Although the court system is the most familiar method for resolving legal disputes, cases potentially set for trial are being redirected more frequently toward

Figure 3.3	Comparison of state and federal court systems

State*	Federal
State Supreme Court	US Supreme Court
Court of Appeals	Circuit Court
Trial Court (for example, Common Pleas Court)	District Court

*This terminology may vary from state to state.

alternative dispute resolution methods, which are described later. Use of these methods decreases the burden on typically overwhelmed court systems and provides lower cost options for opposing parties to settle their differences. This section discusses both the state and federal court systems, as well as the concept of jurisdiction.

State Court System

State court systems generally use the same three-tier system that the federal courts follow, which will be described later in this chapter. However, the terminology differs slightly for each. Figure 3.3 demonstrates a side-by-side comparison of the court hierarchy in both the state and federal court systems. **Trial courts** are the lowest tier of state courts and are divided into two types. Courts of **limited jurisdiction** hear cases that pertain to a particular subject matter (for example, landlord and tenant cases or juvenile cases); or that involve crimes of lesser severity (for example, misdemeanors) or civil matters of lesser dollar amounts. Courts of **general jurisdiction** hear more serious criminal cases (for example, felonies) or civil cases that involve large amounts of money. At the trial court level, the judge or jury decides the facts of the case based on the evidence presented. For example, the party bringing a complaint or charges (the plaintiff or a prosecutor on behalf of a government entity) will present evidence that supports allegations of the defendant's wrongdoing. Likewise, the defendant, against whom a lawsuit or charges are brought, will present evidence that disproves or tends to disprove wrongdoing. Given the evidence, the judge or jury will decide what they believe the facts are in order to determine liability or guilt, or lack thereof.

The next tier is the **appellate court**. Appellate courts hear appeals on final judgments of the state trial courts. The state **supreme court** is the highest tier. It hears appeals from the appellate courts or from trial courts in states without appellate courts. Cases presented before appellate courts, including supreme courts, in both the federal and state court systems are not reenactments of the trial. A legal document (**brief**) is prepared by each party's attorney(s), who then argue the merits of the case in an **oral argument** before a panel of appellate judges. Witnesses are not called, and, generally, the facts of the case are not revisited. Appeals are designed solely to address legal errors or problems that are alleged to have occurred at the lower court. At all tiers, a court's written determination outlining the facts of the case and the legal theories followed to reach an outcome is the **opinion**.

State court judges may be elected or appointed. The rules that govern the process vary from state to state.

Federal Court System

The federal court system is arranged much the same as each state court system, with a three-level hierarchy consisting of a trial court, appellate court, and Supreme Court. Final judgments of the trial court may be appealed to the appellate level, with appellate decisions appealed to the Supreme Court of the United States.

In the federal court system, trial courts (called **district courts**) exist throughout the United States. Each state has at least one district court, with a total of 94 courts. Bankruptcy, an area of law exclusively under the jurisdiction of federal law, is a unit of the district court system with its own courts and judges. Federal appellate courts (called **circuit courts**) are distributed throughout the United States. Each court represents a specific number of the district courts. Figure 3.4 illustrates the distribution of the 11 federal circuit courts nationwide. The twelfth circuit court covers the District of Columbia, and the thirteenth circuit court (federal circuit) has the authority to hear certain appeals nationally, depending on the subject matter.

The **United States Supreme Court** is the court of final decision making. It hears appeals most commonly from the federal appellate (circuit) courts and occasionally from state supreme courts in matters involving federal statutes or the US Constitution. Because its jurisdiction is federal law and the US Constitution, most cases come from the lower tiers of the federal court system. Thousands of cases with requests for review are submitted annually to the United States Supreme Court by parties who have lost at

Figure 3.4 Geographic boundaries of US courts of appeals (circuit courts) and district courts

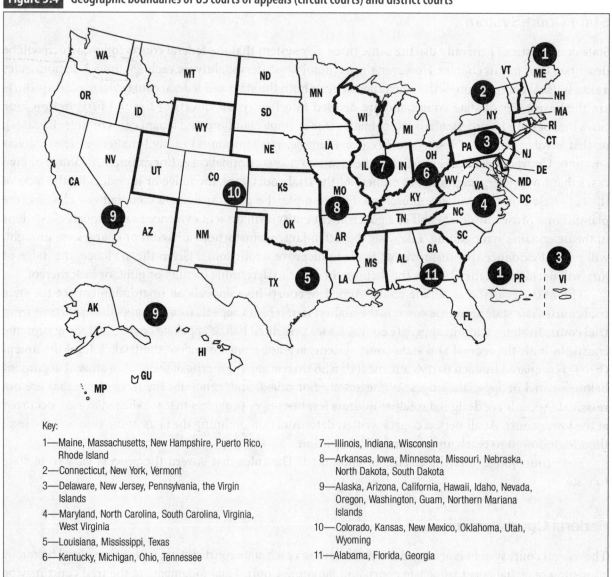

Key:

1—Maine, Massachusetts, New Hampshire, Puerto Rico, Rhode Island

2—Connecticut, New York, Vermont

3—Delaware, New Jersey, Pennsylvania, the Virgin Islands

4—Maryland, North Carolina, South Carolina, Virginia, West Virginia

5—Louisiana, Mississippi, Texas

6—Kentucky, Michigan, Ohio, Tennessee

7—Illinois, Indiana, Wisconsin

8—Arkansas, Iowa, Minnesota, Missouri, Nebraska, North Dakota, South Dakota

9—Alaska, Arizona, California, Hawaii, Idaho, Nevada, Oregon, Washington, Guam, Northern Mariana Islands

10—Colorado, Kansas, New Mexico, Oklahoma, Utah, Wyoming

11—Alabama, Florida, Georgia

Source: uscourts.gov n.d.

a lower court level and are appealing. The Supreme Court exercises considerable discretion in determining which cases it will hear. The process by which a party submits a request for the Supreme Court to hear a case is called a **petition for writ of certiorari**. The Supreme Court either denies cert (and declines to hear the case) or grants cert (and accepts the case for oral argument). As with appellate courts (including supreme courts) at the state level, the US circuit courts and the US Supreme Court do not conduct trials. Rather, they review written briefs submitted by the parties or their legal counsel and listen to oral arguments presented by each party, often interjecting questions during each side's argument.

Judges for all federal courts are nominated by the president and confirmed by the US Senate. Because federal judicial decision making shapes the political landscape of the nation into the future, the nomination and confirmation process can become highly charged.

Jurisdiction

Referred to earlier in the chapter as a territory of legal control, jurisdiction is also the legal authority that a body possesses to make decisions. A case that may be brought in the federal court system must meet two jurisdictional limitations: subject matter jurisdiction and diversity jurisdiction.

Subject matter jurisdiction is based on the content or substantive area of the case being brought. Because the jurisdiction of the federal court system is generally limited to federal laws and the US Constitution, cases brought in federal court generally must relate to either federal law or the US Constitution. For example, lawsuits may be filed to challenge laws or governmental actions that limit free speech or freedom of religion. In the state court system, most trial courts are courts of general jurisdiction, meaning that they may hear all matters of state law except for those cases that must be heard in state courts of **special jurisdiction**, where areas of the law have been carved out for resolution (for example, small claims, domestic relations, juvenile, and probate courts).

Diversity jurisdiction enables parties from different states to engage in a lawsuit in federal court, but federal statute limits the number of lawsuits brought this way by imposing two restrictions:

- No plaintiff can be from the same state as any of the defendants.
- The amount in controversy must be at least $75,000.

A landmark US Supreme Court decision, *Erie Railroad Co. v. Tompkins*, determined that, in diversity jurisdiction cases, the law of the state in which the lawsuit was filed would be applied by the court.

The federal court system and many state court systems have established a **Court of Claims,** where lawsuits against the government are brought.

Requirements of Nonlegal Entities Such As Accrediting Bodies

Nonlegal entities, especially healthcare accrediting bodies, are often viewed as having a great deal of authority. However, they are voluntary and do not have the legal authority of laws created by statute, common law, constitutions, and regulations. Nonetheless, they often wield a great deal of power and exhibit a significant presence. Accreditation is often vital to the credibility of an organization and may be a prerequisite to provider reimbursement. For example, The Joint Commission, the Healthcare Facilities Accreditation Program (HFAP), DNV GL Healthcare, and the Center for Improvement in Healthcare Quality (CIHQ) have all been granted deeming authority by HHS. This means that healthcare organizations accredited by any of these accrediting bodies will be deemed to have met the **Conditions of Participation**, rules that are required for Medicare and Medicaid certification.

In addition to the four accrediting bodies previously mentioned, other well-known accreditation organizations in the healthcare industry include the National Committee for Quality Assurance (NCQA) for managed care organizations, and the Commission on Accreditation of Rehabilitation Facilities (CARF). Because the accreditation process imposes stringent standards and involves regular on-site surveys, continuous compliance is critical to a healthcare organization's ongoing success.

Alternative Dispute Resolution

Resolution of disputes through the judicial (court) system is a complex process that exacts a toll on financial resources, time, and emotions. Although a considerable percentage of lawsuits filed eventually end in negotiation and settlement rather than proceeding to trial, many resources have already been expended by the time a case is settled. Therefore, the US legal system promotes **alternative dispute resolution**, a system that provides means other than the courts to resolve lawsuits. The two primary types of alternative dispute resolution are arbitration and mediation.

In **arbitration**, a dispute is submitted to a third party or a panel of experts outside the judicial system. This process is most effective when the parties to the dispute agree to have their differences heard and settled by an arbitrator or arbitration panel and agree that the settlement will be binding.

In **mediation**, a dispute is also submitted to a third party. However, the outcome of mediation occurs by agreement of the parties, not by a decision of the mediator. The role of the mediator is to facilitate agreement between the disputing parties.

Arbitration and mediation offer several advantages over the court system, including time and cost savings. These proceedings usually allow for more privacy than court proceedings do. Criminal misdemeanors may be handled through mediation. Smaller tort claims are often handled through arbitration. For example, a healthcare organization's wrongful disclosure of patient health information, particularly if it is not highly sensitive in nature, may be resolved by remedying the patient's injuries in an acceptable manner through arbitration or mediation rather than through a lawsuit.

Check Your Understanding	3.3

Instructions: Indicate whether the following statements are true or false (T or F).

1. In mediation, a third party makes a final decision about a dispute between parties.
2. Diversity jurisdiction enables parties from different states to engage in a lawsuit in federal court.
3. Healthcare accrediting bodies are seen as having little authority because they do not have the legal authority of laws.
4. Appellate courts hear appeals on final judgments of trial court decisions.
5. An opinion is the written argument of one of the parties in a lawsuit

Scenario 3

Public law involves government and its relationship to individuals and business organizations. One of its goals is to enforce regulations where any part of a government agency is a party. State medical boards are government entities that, among other roles, take action against physicians for behaviors that violate the law or otherwise jeopardize patient safety. One state medical board's monthly agenda included taking actions against physicians who

Scenario 3 (Continued)

- Abused alcohol and other substances that impaired their ability to practice
- Delegated medical device usage to an unlicensed individual
- Improperly prescribed medications
- Obtained health records of a former patient without authorization and by using an altered release
- Engaged in sexual misconduct with a patient
- Made misleading statements to procure a license to practice and committed felonies either related or unrelated to their practice of medicine

1. Should physician disciplinary action be within the realm of public law, or should it be a private law matter between the physician and a wronged party?

2. Should certain types of wrongdoing be subject to public law, whereas other types are subject to private law? If so, which of the previous list of offenses would you place in each category?

3. In all cases, the physicians are entitled to due process. What types of due process are they entitled to? Give examples of each.

4. Regarding felonies committed outside the individual's practice of medicine: should these be subject to state government disciplinary action in all cases? No cases? Some cases? If the latter, where do you draw the line?

References

Code of Federal Regulations. http://www.archives.gov.

Department of Health and Human Services. 2016. Department of Health and Human Services organizational chart. http://www.hhs.gov.

Garner, B.A. 2014. *Black's Law Dictionary*. Abridged 10th ed. St. Paul, MN: Thomson West.

Pozgar, G.D. 2012. *Legal Aspects of Health Care Administration*. 11th ed. Sudbury, MA: Jones and Bartlett.

Showalter, J.S. 2015. *The Law of Healthcare Administration*. 7th ed. Chicago: Health Administration Press.

US Courts. n.d. Geographic boundaries of US courts of appeals (circuit courts) and US district courts. http://www.uscourts.gov.

US House of Representatives. 2016. United States Code. uscode.house.gov.

White House. n.d. The Cabinet. http://www.whitehouse.gov.

Cases, Statutes, and Regulations Cited

Erie Railroad Co. v. Tompkins, 304 US 64 (1938).

Legal Proceedings

Laurie A. Rinehart-Thompson, JD, RHIA, CHP, FAHIMA

Learning Objectives

- Identify the role of procedural laws in the legal system
- Identify the parties to a lawsuit
- Demonstrate the methods of discovery
- Identify requirements of e-Discovery amendments in the Federal Rules of Civil Procedure
- Analyze the differences between a court order and a subpoena
- Examine the purposes and limitations of a subpoena
- Compare the individuals involved in a trial
- Organize the steps in a trial
- Examine the legal appeals process
- Explain the processes for the collection of judgment

Key Terms

- Admissibility
- Answer
- Appeal
- Appellant
- Appellee
- Authentication
- Bailiff
- Bench trial
- Beyond a reasonable doubt
- Burden of proof
- Cause of action
- Civil procedure
- Class action
- Clerk of court
- Closing argument
- Complaint
- Counterclaim
- Court order
- Court reporter
- Criminal procedure

- Cross appeal
- Cross-claim
- Default judgment
- Defendant
- Deliberations
- Deponent
- Deposition
- Directed verdict
- Discoverability
- Discovery
- Dismissal
- e-discovery
- Equity
- Expert witness
- Federal Rules of Civil Procedure (FRCP)
- Federal Rules of Criminal Procedure (FRCrP)
- Garnishment
- Hung jury

- In camera inspection
- Interrogatories
- Joinder
- Judgment lien
- Judicial search warrant
- Jury instructions
- Lay witness
- Litigation
- Mental examination
- Motion to quash
- Opening statement
- Parties
- Peremptory challenges
- Petitioner
- Physical examination
- Plaintiff
- Pleadings
- Preponderance of evidence
- Pretrial conferences
- Pro se

- Procedural law
- Request for admissions
- Request for production of documents or things
- Respondent
- Service
- Settlement
- Shadow record
- Subpoena
- *Subpoena ad testificandum*
- *Subpoena duces tecum*
- Substantive law
- Summons
- Trial
- Verdict
- *Voir dire*
- Writ of execution

A working knowledge of the procedural aspects of the law is essential for any healthcare professional. For example, individuals who are responsible for the integrity of the health record or electronically stored information (ESI), both inside and outside a healthcare organization, may be involved with procedures such as responding to and/or attending civil or criminal legal proceedings relating to accidents, workers' compensation, malpractice, physical abuse, or other criminal activity.

This chapter takes the reader through legal proceedings from the discussion of parties to a lawsuit and pre-trial procedures to the trial, and post-trial processes. The emphasis is on civil proceedings, although criminal proceedings are also addressed.

Procedural Law

Substantive law, defines the rights and obligations that arise between two or more parties, and includes torts (chapter 6) and contracts (chapter 7). Of equal importance is **procedural law**; that is, the court's rules that guide a lawsuit from the time it begins through completion, whether it ends in a **trial**, where facts are presented before a jury or judge; ends with a **settlement**, an agreement that avoids trial; or results in **dismissal**, which denies relief to the party initiating a lawsuit. Of further importance is the uniformity with which cases are handled. Procedural rules are the mechanisms used to guide substantive law in dispute resolution. Because most legal healthcare cases are civil rather than criminal, they will follow the rules of **civil procedure** (procedural law) to guide the lawsuit. Criminal cases follow the rules of **criminal procedure**, which is procedural law that guides criminal cases.

In federal court, judges who preside over civil and criminal cases at the trial level (U.S. district courts) follow federal rules that have been approved and periodically amended over the years by the US Supreme Court and the US Congress. Civil cases adhere to the **Federal Rules of Civil Procedure (FRCP)**, which are outlined in table 4.1, whereas criminal cases adhere to the **Federal Rules of Criminal Procedure (FRCrP)**. The FRCP encompass 11 categories and 86 rules, whereas the FRCrP encompass 11 categories and 61 rules. Both sets of rules address procedural processes from the time a lawsuit is filed until its conclusion. Individual states follow their own rules of civil and/or criminal procedure, which often are adaptations of the federal rules. Furthermore, regions within a state court system may follow their own sets of specific local rules. Just as rules govern cases at the trial court level, appellate and bankruptcy rules govern procedures in appellate and bankruptcy courts.

Plaintiff(s) may take legal action against the same defendant(s) both civilly and criminally. For example, a defendant who is charged criminally for assaulting a victim ("the government" versus the defendant) can also be sued civilly by the victim in pursuit of monetary damages. The case caption then becomes the "victim/plaintiff" versus the defendant. In healthcare the majority of cases are civil in nature; thus, the remainder of the chapter will focus on civil legal proceedings.

Parties to a Lawsuit

Parties are the individuals or organizations involved in a lawsuit. The party that initiates a lawsuit to enforce his or her rights and/or another's obligations is the **plaintiff**. The individual or organization that is the object of the lawsuit, and against whom a lawsuit is brought, is the **defendant**. There may be multiple plaintiffs and defendants, although a large number of people who have been similarly wronged may be categorized for certification (that is, approval and identification) as a class (Rule 23 of FRCP) and represented legally thereafter as a class. **Class action** lawsuits often proceed for groups of consumers to file lawsuits against a large and generally powerful entity for alleged wrongdoing.

Table 4.1 Outline of the federal rules of civil procedure

Category	Category description	Rules in category	General content in category
I	Scope	1 and 2	Category I describes the purpose of the rules and their role in governing civil action in federal district courts.
II	Commencement of civil suits	3 to 6	Category II contains the rules that provide for the commencement of a civil suit, including the filing, summons, and service of process (legal notice).
III	Pleadings and motions	7 to 16	Category III provides for civil suit pleadings, motions, and defenses and counterclaims. The complaint is the plaintiff's pleading. The answer is the defendant's pleading.
IV	Parties	17 to 25	Category IV describes the capacities in which a party or parties can be sued. It maintains the provisions describing the mechanisms for the filing of countersuits, joinder claims, class action lawsuits, and other actions.
V	Discovery	26 to 37	Category V contains the rules governing discovery (e-Discovery included). In general, the discovery rules help ensure that neither party is subjected to surprises at trial. In many states, discovery can occur only through formal request. In contrast, the FRCP requires parties to divulge certain information without a formal discovery request.
VI	Trial	38 to 53	Category VI provides for the plaintiff's right to a trial by jury or by the court. Additionally, this category contains the rules that describe how cases are assigned for trial, how actions are dismissed, and how subpoenas are handled. On December 1, 2006, FRCP 45 (subpoenas) was amended to conform with the e-discovery rules.
VII	Judgment	54 to 63	Category VII maintains the provisions governing legal judgment and costs. "Judgment" is the decree and any other order from which an appeal lies. Category VII judgment rules maintain provisions for establishing new trials, amending judgments, and the enforcement of judgments.
VIII	Provisional and final remedies and special proceedings	64 to 71	Category VIII contains the series of rules that provide for the final provision or remedy of a case. The rules covered in this category include seizure of property, injunctions, offers of judgment, and execution of judgments.
IX	Special proceedings	72 to 76	Category IX contains the rules governing special civil action proceedings, such as condemnation of real and personal property, magistrate judges, and pretrial orders.
X	District courts and clerks	77 to 80	Category X provides direction concerning the business and operations of the district courts. The rules covered in this category include hours of operation, filing of pleadings and orders, trials and hearings, orders in chambers, procedures for books and records maintained by the clerk, the role of stenographers, and transcripts as evidence.
XI	General provisions	81 to 86	Category XI explains to which proceedings the rules apply (United States district courts vs. state courts) and provides direction on their general applicability, jurisdiction and venue, local rules applications, and judges directives.

Source: Baldwin-Stried Reich et al. 2012.

Pretrial

From the time a lawsuit is filed until the date a trial is scheduled, a number of procedures will take place. This period of time is the pretrial phase of a lawsuit. The following sections address pretrial elements.

Commencement of a Lawsuit

Litigation refers to the legal proceedings that accompany a lawsuit. The first step in litigation is the commencement, or filing, of a lawsuit (that is, a legal action) by one or more plaintiffs against one or more defendants. The filing is documented via a **complaint**. Courts vary in their jurisdictions (a concept discussed in chapter 3); therefore, the plaintiff's attorney (or the plaintiff himself, if he or she is acting **pro se** through self-representation) must file the complaint in the appropriate court. Failure to do so will result in dismissal of the case and often refiling of the case in the proper court.

Once a complaint is filed, a copy is served on the defendant along with a **summons**, which gives the defendant notice of the lawsuit and explains the defendant's procedural obligations. Through the summons and complaint, the defendant is informed of the nature of the case, a list of each **cause of action** (facts that give the plaintiff[s] the right to some type of legal remedy [Garner 2014]) and the amount of damages being sought. The defendant must respond to the complaint by filing an **answer** within the time frame specified by the court. Failure to answer may result in an automatic or **default judgment** by the court against the defendant. Usually, however, the defendant answers the complaint in one of several ways: by denying, admitting, or pleading ignorance to the allegations, or by bringing additional legal actions. The defendant can also ask the court to dismiss the plaintiff's complaint, but not without substantial reason.

The parties to a lawsuit are not finalized when the complaint is filed. Rather, a number of subsequent actions may occur. A **counterclaim** is a claim by a defendant against a plaintiff. A **cross-claim** is a claim by one party against another party who is on the same side of the main litigation (Garner 2014). For example, two physicians may be named as codefendants by a plaintiff. One physician may then sue the other physician in a cross-claim, thus bringing a legal action against the other physician. **Joinder** is an action by a defendant to bring in (join) an outsider as a codefendant. For example, an orthopedic surgeon who is sued for negligence by a plaintiff patient who received a hip replacement may "join" the manufacturer of the hip replacement device, claiming that the manufacturer was negligent in its production of the device.

Under rules of civil procedure, **pleadings** are documents generated by parties involved in a lawsuit, including complaints and answers (Garner 2014). They are central to the litigation process. It is the responsibility of a government official, often a **clerk of court**, to officially maintain documents associated with legal actions filed in that court system.

An entire body of case law addresses what constitutes adequate **service** of a summons and complaint upon a defendant. Although service may be personal, by mail, or by publication, court requirements vary by jurisdiction, and proof of service may be required. Further, adequate time is required to allow the defendant(s) to sufficiently respond to a summons and complaint. Although this seems like a mundane area of law, it has been the subject of numerous historic and lively lawsuits and court decisions. For example, service was disputed but found by the court to have occurred where a summons was placed on a defendant's car bumper after he was touched with the summons but refused to take it (*Nielsen v. Braland*, 1963). Likewise, a court found that service had been accomplished when a summons and complaint were placed under the windshield wiper of a defendant's car after the defendant refused to acknowledge it by remaining seated in the car with the windows rolled up while the summons was read to him. The documents were dislodged and lost when the defendant drove away (*Trujillo v. Trujillo*, 1945).

Check Your Understanding 4.1

Instructions: Indicate whether the following statements are true or false (T or F).

1. A cross-claim is a claim by a defendant against a plaintiff.
2. Joinder involves bringing an outsider into a lawsuit as a codefendant.
3. Procedural law encompasses a court's rules that guide a lawsuit.
4. Notification of a lawsuit occurs through service of a summons.
5. Class action lawsuits proceed for groups of consumers.

Discovery

Following the commencement of a lawsuit, the next pretrial stage is **discovery**. Discovery is both a process and a time period. It occurs during the period leading to trial and allows all parties (generally via their legal counsel) to use various strategies to discover or obtain information held by other parties and, subsequently, to assess the strengths and weaknesses in each party's case. The idea behind the civil discovery process is that the parties should go to trial with as much knowledge about the facts of the case as possible. Although discovery is time-consuming, information obtained as a result of the process can be invaluable in determining the course a case should take and whether negotiation and settlement is preferable to trying the case before a judge or jury. In fact, careful legal work during the discovery process may be significant toward winning a case through either trial or settlement, and it may prevent the need for an expensive trial. Health information evidence presented at trial is usually obtained through the pretrial discovery process.

Discovery is distinguishable from **discoverability**, which refers to limits on parties to discover pretrial information held by another. For information to be discoverable, it must relate to the subject matter of the pending case. For example, if a plaintiff is claiming damages for a back injury as a result of a car accident, then information such as the plaintiff's medical bills and health records related to the accident clearly relate to the case. However, if the plaintiff had other injuries to his back before or after the car accident, records about those injuries would relate to the case as well, because they could identify other sources of the plaintiff's claimed injuries. Whether a piece of information is discoverable depends on specific federal and state rules of evidence, statutes, and case law. For example, state law may protect physician–patient, spousal, or attorney–client communications from discoverability (that is, access by other parties) during the discovery period of a lawsuit.

Discoverability is also distinguishable from **admissibility**, which refers to evidence that is allowed to be admitted in a court of law and considered by the judge or jury in making a final determination about a case (Garner 2014). Admissible evidence is often more restricted than discoverable evidence. Stated another way, more information is generally discoverable than is admissible. Information that has been obtained during the discovery period may or may not be admissible for consideration by a judge and jury during trial. Admissibility of evidence is an issue that is limited to the trial and will be discussed further in chapter 5.

The majority of the discovery rules apply only to parties involved in a case—in other words, the plaintiff(s) and defendant(s). However, since the business records of nonparties are subject to discovery under Rule 45 of the FRCP, it is important for organizations to be prepared to identify, protect, and produce the information requested. This section discusses e-discovery as well as types of discovery: depositions, interrogatories, requests for production of documents or things, physical or mental examination of a party, and requests for admissions.

E-Discovery

In general, the discovery process includes obtaining information, whether paper or ESI. The discovery process differs depending on whether the format is paper or electronic. To address the increasing use of ESI in the discovery process, the FRCP were amended in 2006 to provide uniform rules for the preservation, collection, and production of ESI in federal civil cases. These and subsequent amendments to the rules are referred to as electronic discovery or **e-discovery**. The rules provide for early involvement of the court in managing when and how the courts make arrangements for the discovery of ESI with regard to scheduling, scope of discovery, preservation obligations, waiver of privilege, form of production for ESI, and the burdens that may be applied via subpoenas, and for deriving answers to interrogatories (described later) from electronically produced materials. About half of all states have adopted the federal e-discovery rules or have e-discovery rules of their own. Key e-discovery amendments are summarized in figure 4.1.

HIM Role in E-Discovery

Individuals responsible for the management of health records, ESI, and/or information systems should be involved in the pretrial conference to discuss the scope of information being requested (AHIMA 2013).

Figure 4.1 Summary of key e-discovery amendments

Scheduling orders (Rule 16(b)), which outline key deadlines that apply to the case, may address the disclosure and discoverability of electronically stored information. They may also address agreements regarding how parties will handle privileged information that is inadvertently produced.

Initial disclosures (Rule 26(a)) are mandatory disclosures of certain basic information that must be provided before a formal discovery request and should include a copy or description and location of any electronically stored information that may be used to support parties' respective claims or defenses. For example, if an electronic health record (EHR) will be used as evidence in a case, the initial disclosure should describe that record and provide its location.

Reasonable access (Rule 26(b)(2)) allows for discovery of ESI to be limited if that information is not reasonably accessible because of undue burden or cost. What constitutes reasonably accessible can vary from case to case and court to court.

Discussion between two parties (Rule 26(f)) supports the requirement that very early on in the case, parties must confer with one another about a variety of issues, such as the nature of any claims and defenses, settlement possibilities, arrangements for initial disclosures, preservation of discoverable information, and the development of an overall discovery plan. Amendments to the rules now specifically require the parties to address "any issues relating to disclosure or discovery of electronically stored information, including the form or forms in which it should be produced." An understanding of an organization's document retention policies and the intricacies and capabilities of its information technology system is important to facilitating this process.

Interrogatories and Production of documents (Rules 33 and 34) now both contemplate the production of ESI. With respect to ESI, if a request does not specify the form for producing such information, the responding party must produce it in the form in which it is ordinarily maintained or in a form that is reasonably usable. Further, a party need not produce the same ESI in more than one form.

Failure to make disclosures (Rule 37(f)) says a court may not impose sanctions on a party for failing to provide ESI lost as a result of the "routine, good-faith operation of an electronic information system." What constitutes good faith will vary from case to case and court to court. However, once there is reasonable notice of potential or actual litigation, an organization or party may need to suspend the routine destruction of electronic data that are potentially relevant to the litigation in order to satisfy the good faith standard.

Testing or sampling of documents (Rule 45) allows, in cases where large volumes of documents may contain relevant evidence, the testing or sampling of those documents to determine whether relevant evidence exists. The rules for subpoenas have been amended to allow for the testing and sampling of ESI.

Source: National Court Rules Committee 2016a.

The parties need to decide what information needs to be preserved and the format in which it will be presented. In the past, paper records were simply retrieved and copied for discovery purposes. Now, all information created in a health record—both electronic and paper—is potentially open to discovery unless otherwise directed by the court. Depending on how an organization has defined its business or legal health record (LHR) (discussed in chapter 9), a request for the "complete patient record" may encompass a wider range of information (including copies printed from an electronic health record [EHR] system) than that which was typically considered to be part of the paper health record.

With ESI, e-discovery involves information and data from source systems outside of those which are usually printed or viewed electronically, such as native file formats, computer files, erased files, and e-mails. It is important to be informed early in the discovery process if electronic information will be needed and to know the locations of all components of ESI in order to produce the information as requested. To assist organizations and vendors who provide technology services and products designed to help organizations find and manage information required by the court, a group of interested parties (attorneys, vendors, and other stakeholders) developed the **Electronic Discovery Reference Model (EDRM)** to address the complexity of e-discovery (EDRM 2016). The EDRM defines the process of e-discovery by using terminology that is meaningful to both healthcare providers and vendors. The model assists vendors in mapping their products and services to steps in the e-discovery process so that they can efficiently locate and prepare relevant ESI (figure 4.2). Whether discovery entails paper or ESI, several discovery methods and tools may be used by parties in the discovery phase of a lawsuit, which are discussed next.

Deposition

A **deposition** is a formal proceeding by which oral testimonies of individuals are obtained. Prior to a deposition, a **deponent** is directed to appear at an appointed time and place to testify under oath. Attorneys for both the plaintiff(s) and defendant(s) are present and the deponent's testimony is transcribed by a **court reporter**. Deposed individuals may be parties to the lawsuit or independent witnesses. An attorney will be present to act on behalf of the deponent and will interject objections when legally impermissible questions are asked by an opposing attorney who is conducting a cross-examination. The accuracy of one's testimony at a deposition is important because the deposition is not only a discovery method; the court reporter's transcript may be read into evidence at trial if the individual is unable to testify at trial or if opposing counsel wishes to use it to impeach or discredit a witness. Thus, consistency between the deposition and trial testimony is crucial to the credibility of a witness.

Testimony is generally required to establish the authenticity or genuineness of paper records (including health records), electronic records (including EHRs), or other ESI that is introduced as evidence. (See appendix 4A for a sample subpoena.) **Authentication** is verification of the record or ESI's validity (that is, it is the record of the individual in question and it is what it purports to be) and, therefore, it is reliable and truthful as evidence. Because individuals who document in a health record do not typically falsify their entries, the truthfulness of a health record is generally not questioned. As will be further discussed in chapter 5, rules of evidence generally permit health records to be used as evidence if it can be established that the records were created in the regular course of business (that is, they qualify as business records). Parties to litigation may agree about (stipulate to) a record's authenticity and allow it to be entered into evidence without requiring an individual to personally appear in court and testify. The parties may further agree to allow a photocopy of the record to be introduced into evidence instead of the original. This generally requires written certification that the photocopy being provided is an exact copy of the original. EHRs and other ESI create challenges to authentication. At a deposition, as well as at trial (discussed later), the deposed health information management and informatics professional may be asked to respond in more detail regarding how the EHR is organized. Additionally, because all changes

Figure 4.2 Electronic discovery reference model

The EDRM diagram represents a conceptual view of the e-discovery process, not a literal, linear, or waterfall model. One may engage in some but not all of the steps outlined in the diagram, or one may elect to carry out the steps in a different order than shown here.

The diagram also portrays an iterative process. One might repeat the same step numerous times, honing in on a more precise set of results. One might also cycle back to earlier steps, refining one's approach as a better understanding of the data emerges or as the nature of the matter changes.

The diagram is intended as a basis for discussion and analysis, not as a prescription for the one and only right way to approach e-discovery.

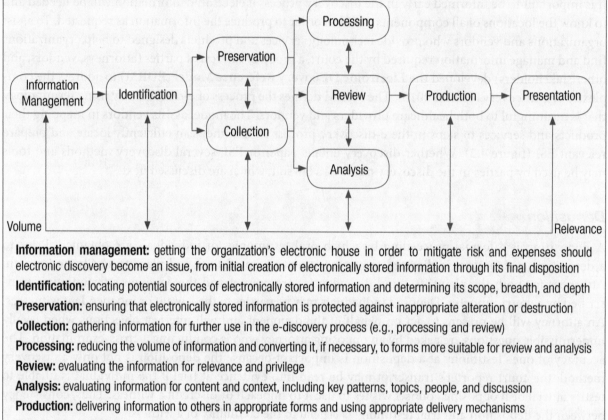

Information management: getting the organization's electronic house in order to mitigate risk and expenses should electronic discovery become an issue, from initial creation of electronically stored information through its final disposition

Identification: locating potential sources of electronically stored information and determining its scope, breadth, and depth

Preservation: ensuring that electronically stored information is protected against inappropriate alteration or destruction

Collection: gathering information for further use in the e-discovery process (e.g., processing and review)

Processing: reducing the volume of information and converting it, if necessary, to forms more suitable for review and analysis

Review: evaluating the information for relevance and privilege

Analysis: evaluating information for content and context, including key patterns, topics, people, and discussion

Production: delivering information to others in appropriate forms and using appropriate delivery mechanisms

Presentation: displaying the information before audiences (e.g., at depositions, hearings, and trials), especially in native and near-native forms, to attempt to persuade or elicit further information

Source: edrm.net 2009.

to an EHR are recorded, he or she may be asked to explain logs that reflect electronic document creation, revision, and access (Dimick 2011).

HIM Role in Depositions

An individual who is called as a witness to testify as to the authenticity of a health record or ESI may expect the types of queries outlined in figure 4.3. Further, health information management and informatics professionals are frequently deposed to answer questions about logs that contain metadata regarding information in the EHR that was created, edited, authenticated, and accessed (Dimick 2011). At times attorneys may ask additional questions during authentication determination that are not appropriate.

Figure 4.3	Types of witness queries

- What is your position/title?
- Who is the custodian of health records?
- How long has the "custodian" of health records been employed? (if applicable)
- Do you currently have possession of the record(s) in question?
- How and when was the record prepared?
- Is there health information from another organization contained in the patient's record?
  - Was this information received in the normal course of business?
  - Can you attest to the recordkeeping practices of another organization?
- How was this set of documents arrived at?
- For electronic records, what were the search parameters?
- From what systems, and from what areas of each system, were electronic documents produced?
- Can you describe the logs that record when and by whom data were created, edited, authenticated, and accessed?
- What does a system's definition of an "edit" encompass?
- How are logs organized, and what types of information do they contain?

Sources: Reynolds 2010; Dimick 2011.

It is inappropriate for an attorney to ask questions of a medical nature of an individual who is testifying to establish the authenticity of a health record or ESI. Examples of such inquiries include those that solicit personal opinion; seek the purpose of a medication or treatment regimen; or require interpretation of the health record. Other situations—such as asking the testifying individual to read entries that may be deemed illegible by others—are questionable and must be addressed on a case-by-case basis. If the individual is familiar with the practitioner's handwriting and is able to read the entries, guidance should be sought from the attorney acting on his or her behalf as to whether the attorney will object to the request and whether or not to proceed. If the individual is not comfortable with his or her ability to read the entries, however, this should be clearly stated and the request declined. It is acceptable to respond "I don't know" if the answer to a question is not known.

Interrogatories

Written **interrogatories** provide a mechanism for questions to be presented to parties in the lawsuit and answered in writing during a more extensive time frame than that provided by a deposition. Because responses to written interrogatories may be prepared by a party's attorney or the attorney's legal staff instead of the party directly, these responses may provide less illuminating information than that provided directly by a party via a deposition. Nonetheless, the party must attest to the truthfulness and accuracy of responses to written interrogatories.

Request for Production of Documents or Things

A **request for production of documents or things** is a discovery method to gather tangible items and information, including electronic or paper health records, or other ESI, related to a case.

As the healthcare industry moves toward EHRs and key evidence is contained in other electronic documents such as e-mails, the legal concept of e-discovery has evolved. The US Supreme Court amended the FRCP to address the discovery of electronic records and to increase involvement by courts in the discovery process, creating a new paradigm with respect to the production of documents as a discovery method.

Physical or Mental Examination of a Party

When the physical or mental condition of a party is in question, the opposing party may request an independent **physical examination** or an independent **mental examination**. If the court determines that there is good cause for this request, such an examination will be ordered (Showalter 2014). For example, a defendant may request that a physical examination be performed on the plaintiff in a personal injury lawsuit if the nature and extent of the injuries claimed are in question.

Request for Admissions

A **request for admissions** asks the opposing party to make certain admissions that will diminish the amount of time and money that would otherwise be spent proving those facts (Showalter 2014). Although it is unlikely that an opposing party will admit to facts that would dramatically damage his or her case, this discovery device is nonetheless useful for eliciting facts that are not in dispute. For example, if asked to do so, a plaintiff may admit to the fact that he is no longer receiving medical treatment related to the injuries he allegedly suffered in an accident that gave rise to the lawsuit. Admission of such a fact is more efficient than obtaining this information through a deposition or a subpoena for the production of health records.

Check Your Understanding 4.2

Instructions: Indicate whether the following statements are true or false (T or F).

1. Admissibility refers to evidence that parties can obtain during the pretrial period.
2. An independent mental examination may be requested as a type of discovery.
3. Interrogatories are prepared for both independent witnesses and parties to a lawsuit.
4. A deposition does not occur under oath.
5. Discovery allows parties in a lawsuit to use strategies to obtain information held by other parties.

Tools to Compel Discovery

The legal system uses two important tools to facilitate discovery and evidence at trials. Court orders and subpoenas are described later, as are warrants and searches, which are important in criminal cases.

Court Orders

A **court order** is a document or verbal mandate issued by a judge that compels certain action, such as testimony or the production of documents such as health records or ESI. For example, a court order may command a hospital to disclose health records or ESI when the hospital, for whatever reason, refuses to disclose them pursuant to an authorization. Possessing greater legal force than a subpoena, valid court orders must be complied with, and failure to do so may result in a citation for contempt of court citation with possible accompanying jail time. If there is any question as to whether an organization has received a court order or a subpoena, legal counsel should be consulted. If a document requesting the production of health records or ESI is determined to be a court order, it must be complied with regardless of the presence or absence of patient authorization.

Subpoenas

A **subpoena** is a legal tool used to compel one's appearance at a certain time and place to testify or produce documents or other tangible items either during discovery or at trial. A subpoena can be civil, criminal, or administrative. It is generally issued by the clerk of court or by an attorney for one of the parties in the name of the court having jurisdiction over the case (a court order, conversely, is issued by a judge).

The subpoena is often confused with a court order because both are official in nature and may be issued to compel testimony or the production of documents. A subpoena is designated with a seal of the court and in the name of the presiding judge, which also appears on a court order, thus causing confusion between the two documents. A subpoena compels a timely response and requires proper service; failure to respond may result in a court order compelling attendance or a contempt of court citation. It is often served by law enforcement or sent via US Postal Service and is not to be disregarded. Nonetheless, because it is issued by the court or an attorney and generally not by the judge presiding over the case, it does not have the same force and effect as a court order. In most cases where health records or ESI are requested, a subpoena must be accompanied by patient authorization to be valid. Patient authorization, however, is not always required.

Because of the federal government's emphasis on reducing fraud and abuse in healthcare, the Office of the Inspector General (OIG) for the US Department of Health and Human Services has been given certain powers to compel both testimony and the production of documents without patient authorization as part of its investigations (5 USC 552a (App. 3 sec. (6)(a)(4))). The False Claims Act, discussed in chapter 18, and the Health Insurance Portability and Accountability Act (HIPAA) Privacy Rule, discussed in chapters 10 and 11, both allow administrative subpoenas that can be enforced by the federal court system. Grand jury subpoenas, which are issued to obtain evidence for consideration by grand juries in criminal cases, also may not require an individual's authorization. Requirements vary based on jurisdiction.

There are two forms of subpoenas. A **subpoena ad testificandum** primarily seeks an individual's testimony. In a medical malpractice case, this type of subpoena is more likely to be directed toward physicians and other healthcare providers involved in the plaintiffs' care than toward health information management and informatics professionals. A custodian of health records would rarely expect to receive a subpoena that is primarily interested in his or her testimony. Rather, records custodians (who are often referred to legally as such) will likely find themselves served with a **subpoena duces tecum** (see appendix 4.A for a sample), which instructs the recipient to personally appear at a deposition or in court, with documents in hand. Such subpoenas may direct the recipient to produce and bring originals or copies of health records, laboratory reports, x-rays, or other records. Copies of records requested by this type of subpoena may often be substituted, so long as appropriate steps have been taken to authenticate them. If copies may not be substituted and the original is ordered to remain with the court, the healthcare organization representative should confirm that the original record is in the custody of the court and obtain a receipt verifying this. Additionally, a copy of the health record should be retained at the healthcare organization in case the information is needed for patient care. For either form of subpoena, the individual who receives a subpoena should verify its validity.

States have different rules governing responses to subpoenas and the production of health records or ESI in litigation. State law and local court rules should be consulted to determine whether a specified amount of time is required between service of a subpoena and the requested appearance; to determine the acceptability of mailing health records in response to a subpoena; and to become familiar with other legal procedural requirements. Component state associations of the American Health Information Management Association (AHIMA) may have legal handbooks that outline state requirements and the appropriate response to a *subpoena duces tecum*. Discussed next are the elements of a valid subpoena, objections to subpoenas, and duties in responding to subpoenas.

Elements of a Valid Subpoena

A subpoena must be examined for validity before the recipient complies with it. For state cases, the required elements vary from state to state and are often present on a state prescribed form. Compliance with federal requirements is necessary for subpoenas issued in federal cases. Elements of a valid subpoena commonly include

- The name of the court from which the subpoena was issued
- The caption of the action (that is, names of plaintiff[s] and defendant[s])
- Assigned case docket number (to validate the case)
- Date, time, and place of requested appearance
- The information required, such as testimony or the specific documents sought in a *subpoena duces tecum*
- The form in which that information (including electronic information) is to be produced
- The name of the issuing attorney
- The name of the recipient being directed to disclose the records
- The signature or stamp of the court/official or judge authorized to issue the subpoena (Reynolds 2010)

The authorization of the person whose records are to be disclosed is nearly always required, although there are exceptions, as described previously. If, in the case of a *subpoena duces tecum,* an authorization is required but does not accompany the subpoena, the subpoena should be declined and an authorization requested and received before the records are produced. If records requested per subpoena contain information that is specifically protected by state or federal law (for example, mental health or substance abuse information), the patient must specifically authorize the disclosure of those records. If requested records have been appropriately destroyed according to the organization's policies and in compliance with applicable laws, a certificate of destruction should be produced in lieu of the records.

Objections to Subpoenas

Certain protections are provided to persons who are subpoenaed. Like the specific requirements for subpoena content, these protections can vary based on the jurisdiction and type of subpoena. Subpoenas issued in federal civil cases include the following protections:

- The party issuing the subpoena must take reasonable steps to avoid imposing an undue burden or expense on the person subject to the subpoena.
- A person commanded to produce and permit inspection and copying of designated books, papers, documents, or tangible things, or inspection of premises need not appear in person at the place of production or inspection unless commanded to appear for a deposition, hearing, or trial (FRCP 45(d)).

Although the recipient of a subpoena must respond in a timely manner to avoid a contempt of court action, the subpoena may warrant an objection. A person who is commanded to produce records for inspection or copying may, within 14 days of being served with the subpoena, provide a written objection to the party or attorney designated in the subpoena. Once written objections have been made, a court determines whether the subpoenaed information must be produced and issues an order accordingly.

Formal written objections to subpoenas are often made in a **motion to quash**. A motion to quash is a document filed with the court that asks the judge to nullify the subpoena for any number of reasons. Under FRCP 45(c) and (d), a court must quash or modify the subpoena if it

- Fails to provide adequate time for compliance (FRCP 45 (d))
- Requires (per FRCP 45(c))
    - A non-party to travel to a trial, deposition or hearing beyond the rule's geographical limit, which is over 100 miles of where the subject resides, is employed, or regularly transacts business in person
    - A party or party's officer to travel to a trial beyond the rule's geographical limit, which is outside the state where the subject resides, is employed, or regularly transacts business, or if the travel requires substantial expense
    - The production of documents, ESI, or tangible things beyond the rule's geographical limit of 100 miles of where the subject resides, is employed, or regularly transacts business in person
- Discloses privileged information that is not subject to any exception or waiver (FRCP 45(d)) (privileges are discussed in detail in chapter 5)
- Imposes an undue burden on the subject (FRCP 45(d))

An example of an unduly burdensome subpoena that might be objected to is one that constitutes a "fishing expedition" for a broad range of documents that might not exist, but if they do, may benefit the requesting party's case (McLendon 2011). Two cases involving motions to quash related to privilege and undue burden are outlined in figure 4.4.

The risk of subpoenas that may be deemed unduly burdensome increases with EHR systems that are capable of producing many types of data and metadata (data about data). As previously discussed, subpoenas may also be objected to based on the absence of patient authorization. The HIPAA Privacy Rule, discussed in chapters 10 and 11, protects records that have been subpoenaed from covered entities, such as health plans, healthcare clearinghouses, and healthcare providers, when patient authorization is not required. Specifically, records may be produced according to a subpoena only if

- The covered entity has received satisfactory assurance from the party seeking the information that reasonable efforts have been made to ensure that the individual whose records have been subpoenaed has been given notice of the request.

Figure 4.4 **Motions to quash subpoenas**

Motion to Quash Based on Privilege:

In *Fabich v. Montana Rail Link, Inc.*, the state court denied the plaintiff's motion to quash on grounds of privilege because the plaintiff waived privilege by putting his own condition at issue by filing a claim for damages. However, the court provided that any specific records the plaintiff objected to producing to the defendant could instead be produced directly to the court. This is an **in camera inspection** and the judge personally reviews disputed records in his or her chambers and decides whether they are discoverable or admissible.

Motion to Quash Based on Undue Burden:

In *Smith v. Rossi*, a party moved to quash a subpoena for medical records on the grounds that complying with the subpoena would be unduly burdensome. The plaintiff claimed that the defendants' subpoenas were oppressive and unreasonable because the defendants had already received all of his medical records. However, because there was doubt as to whether this was true, the court denied the plaintiff's motion to quash and noted that the records were relevant to the defendant's defense.

- The covered entity has received satisfactory assurance from the party seeking the information that reasonable efforts have been made to secure a qualified protective order, limiting the use and disclosure of the protected information in the record (45 CFR 164.512(e)).

Court decisions may impose additional duties on providers to protect health information beyond statutory and regulatory protections. Individuals responsible for managing healthcare data and information must be aware of fiduciary duties to protect health information that may be imposed by such case law.

If a subpoena is invalid or otherwise unreasonable, an organization's legal counsel should be consulted regarding the legal mechanics of objecting to the subpoena according to court rules and in a manner that communicates with the party issuing the subpoena.

HIM Role in Responding to Subpoenas

While the law provides protections for persons who are subject to subpoenas, it also imposes certain duties in responding to subpoenas. The duties are specified by the applicable rules of civil procedure for the court in which the case is being heard. A person responding to a subpoena for documents must "produce them as they are kept in the usual course of business" or "organize and label them to correspond with the categories in the demand" (FRCP 45(e)). The organization must clearly define what constitutes a health record that is kept in the usual course of business. For example, is e-mail or text message communication from a patient included in the record? What about x-ray films or audio/video recordings made for patient care? If so, through what process are these items integrated into the record? Once an organization has defined the content of records kept in the usual course of business, it must have a system to ensure all records commanded by the subpoena have been produced. This can be challenging in settings where shadow records, hybrid records, or electronic records are used. A **shadow record** is a duplicate record sometimes kept for the convenience of the provider or organization (Burrington-Brown 2003). The shadow record should be an exact duplicate of the original health record and contain no documentation that is not in the original record, but in practice it is sometimes easy for staff to inadvertently file paperwork in a shadow record instead of the original record. When this happens, the original record becomes incomplete. As a result, the custodian of records risks representing that a true and complete copy of a patient's record has been produced in response to a subpoena when this is not the case.

Release of information staff, also covered in chapter 15, must know how and be able to access and reproduce both paper and ESI components. It is important to remember that all information stored, created, or accessed within the organization, including e-mail, voice mail, text messages, metadata, back-up tapes, and legacy information systems may be requested (Baldwin-Stried Reich et al. 2012).

Under FRCP, a subpoena may specify the form or forms in which the health record or ESI is to be produced (FRCP 45(a)). If no specification is made, the records must be produced in the form(s) in which they are ordinarily maintained or in a form that is reasonably usable. However, the same rules provide some protection against producing ESI that is not reasonably accessible because of undue burden or cost. Further, the rules provide that ESI need not be produced in more than one form (FRCP 45(e)).

Not all states have implemented e-discovery frameworks similar to that of the FRCP. If a subpoena is issued for a case being tried under state law, state rules establish the records custodian's duties in responding to that subpoena. Therefore, individuals responsible for the management of health information must be familiar with the subpoena requirements and discovery rules for their particular state. Courts also interpret and apply state and federal rules, so awareness of judicial decisions is equally important.

Individuals who respond to subpoenas may also have a duty to claim a privilege on behalf of the individual whose records have been subpoenaed. As will be discussed in chapter 5, privileges protect certain information from being disclosed in court. Under the FRCP, if a records custodian withholds information based on a privilege, the custodian still must provide a description of the withheld information that is sufficient enough that the demanding party has enough information to contest the claim of privilege.

Warrants and Searches

Health records and ESI frequently are necessary as evidence in civil cases, such as medical malpractice actions; however, they can also play a significant role in criminal cases, such as healthcare fraud and abuse investigations (to be discussed in chapter 18). In criminal cases, obtaining evidence (including health records) often involves law enforcement actions such as warrants and searches. A **judicial search warrant** is a judge's written order authorizing a law enforcement officer to conduct a search of a specified place and to seize evidence (FRCP 41).

Protections against unreasonable searches and seizures are provided by the Fourth Amendment of the Constitution (US Const. amend. IV), which deals largely with criminal cases but also applies to administrative and regulatory searches and seizures. It provides that

The right of the people to be secure in their persons, houses, papers and effects, against unreasonable searches and seizures, shall not be violated, and no warrants shall issue, but upon probable cause, supported by oath or affirmation, and particularly describing the place to be searched, and the persons or things to be seized.

Although the HIPAA Privacy Rule (42 USC Sec. 1320), discussed in chapters 10 and 11, requires that governmental interests in preventing and stopping healthcare fraud and abuse be balanced against an individual's privacy interests, it generally does not prevent the disclosure of one's health information when it is provided to a government agency or law enforcement agency for the investigation of criminal or quasi-criminal activities. This is illustrated by the cases in figure 4.5.

State constitutions and statutes must be consistent with federal law. A search that is conducted without obtaining a proper warrant is permissible under urgent circumstances or incident to an arrest. Warrantless searches are unique because they proceed without the special statutory or legal protections built into most other types of searches. To be constitutional, a warrantless search may be executed only in circumstances where an urgent need for a health record or ESI exists. These are rare and limited.

Figure 4.5 **Privacy interests versus criminal investigations**

Privacy Interests:

In a well-publicized case involving the health records of Rush Limbaugh, *Limbaugh v. Florida*, a Florida court of appeals considered "whether the authority of the State to seize medical records in a criminal investigation by search warrant is limited by a patient's right of privacy." The court ruled that state statutory patient health record privacy protections relating to subpoenas are superseded by the State's authority to seize such otherwise protected records under a validly issued and executed search warrant.

Criminal Investigation:

A Pennsylvania court held that the confidentiality provisions of the state's Drug and Alcohol Abuse Act did not prevent a search warrant from being issued and executed for patient health records maintained by an outpatient drug and alcohol clinic for a criminal investigation of the billing practices of that clinic (*In re Search Warrant App. No. 1254, 2004*).

Pretrial Conferences

From the time a lawsuit is filed and throughout the discovery period, when determined necessary by the parties and judge involved in a case, the parties and their attorneys will meet with the court to discuss the status of the case, the upcoming trial, and potential settlement negotiations. These meetings are **pretrial conferences.** Many times, a case is settled before it reaches trial. This saves time, money, and emotional hardship on the parties. A settlement may be reached between or among the parties to a lawsuit with or without intervention from a third party.

Check Your Understanding   4.3

Instructions: Indicate whether the following statements are true or false (T or F).

1. A subpoena is another name for a court order.
2. A court order is issued by a judge.
3. In most cases, a subpoena for health records must be accompanied by patient authorization.
4. Written objections to subpoenas may be made in a motion to quash.
5. A *subpoena duces tecum* primarily seeks an individual's testimony.

Trial

If the parties fail to negotiate a settlement during the pretrial phase of a lawsuit, or if the case is not dismissed, it will proceed to trial. The following sections describe the players in a trial and trial procedures.

Players in a Trial

The environment of a courtroom during trial is often very different from the overflowing courtrooms depicted by producers in action-packed TV legal dramas. There are, nonetheless, essential players involved in the trial itself.

The judge presides over the trial and the courtroom, making critical decisions regarding the admissibility of evidence, which will guide the outcome of a case. The judge makes decisions of law (for example, evidentiary decisions) and instructs the jury regarding the law of that jurisdiction. In a trial without a jury (**bench trial**), the judge also serves as the fact finder.

The **jury** is the fact-finding body that hears evidence given by the parties (if they testify) and other witnesses, observes evidence presented by both sides, and hears the opening statements and closing arguments of each side. Importantly, the jury decides facts based on the perceived credibility of the evidence, but it does not decide law (for example, it does not determine which evidence shall be admitted and which shall not). Because opposing parties present conflicting evidence, it is the role of the jury to determine which evidence—in the form of testimony or physical evidence—is more believable and will be given greater weight in the jury's final decisions. The evidence that they choose to believe, therefore, becomes "fact" in the jurors' minds as they render their decision regarding the outcome of the case, such as liability or guilt. The number of jurors and alternates who are seated is determined by the FRCP for federal cases and by individual state rules of civil procedure for cases tried in state courts.

Parties in a trial include the plaintiff and defendant, accompanied by their respective attorneys, unless a party is acting pro se. Both the plaintiff and defendant have the right to be present during the course of the trial.

Witnesses are individuals called by each of the parties to provide evidence supporting that party's case. A hostile or adverse witness is one who demonstrates such animosity or prejudice toward the party that called the witness to the stand that the witness can be declared hostile during the trial and subsequently cross-examined and treated as though he or she had been called by the opposing party (Garner 2014). Plaintiff(s) and defendant(s) may also become witnesses, taking the witness stand to testify. The Fifth Amendment of the US Constitution protects a criminal defendant against self-incrimination, including the right not to testify. A prosecutor who brings to the jury's attention the fact that a criminal defendant declined to testify during a trial has compromised the defendant's constitutional rights, and the statement may be grounds for a mistrial.

Generally, individuals called to the witness stand are **lay witnesses**, testifying based on their own observations. A second type of witness, an **expert witness**, is called to testify based on subject matter expertise rather than personal observations (an expert witness generally was not present when the situation that prompted the lawsuit occurred). Individuals with considerable health information management and informatics experience may be called as expert witnesses in cases involving the alleged wrongful disclosure of information, for example, and asked to proffer their opinions based on their experience and knowledge in the area.

The **bailiff**, assigned to a particular court, is responsible for maintaining order and decorum in the court as well as managing the schedule of the judge. Depending on state law, the bailiff may or may not be required to be a peace officer.

Although not a player in the trial and not present in the courtroom, the clerk of court is responsible for maintaining all court records, including pleadings that are generated as the case proceeds to trial. Often this is an elected position.

A court reporter is present during the entire trial and is responsible for providing a verbatim transcript of the trial. The transcript provides key information when statements made during trial become a point of contention and, possibly, the basis for a successful appeal.

Trial Procedures

Following the pretrial period, if the parties have been unable to negotiate a settlement, the case goes to trial. (See figures 4.6 and 4.7 for the sequence of civil and criminal trials, respectively.)

A jury is selected through a process called **voir dire** or, if a jury is waived, a judge hears the case (bench trial). The number of jurors assigned to a case will vary based on whether the case is civil or criminal and in what jurisdiction the case is being tried. Attorneys are given discretion to excuse potential jurors "for cause" (for example, a prosecutor may excuse an individual in a death penalty case if the individual states that he or she will not vote for the death penalty on moral or religious grounds). Further, attorneys are given a limited number of **peremptory challenges**, which allow jurors to be excused for unstated reasons. Attorneys may not use their peremptory challenges on prejudicial grounds that excuse jurors based on such protected classes as race, gender, religion, and ethnicity, although it is difficult to prove whether an attorney has done so. In the landmark US Supreme Court case of *Batson v. Kentucky*, the court held that using peremptory challenges to dismiss jurors solely on the basis of race was unconstitutional.

When the trial begins, the attorney for each side gives an **opening statement** that outlines the evidence that will be heard. Evidence is then presented. The plaintiff's attorney is the first to call witnesses and present evidence. After the plaintiff's witnesses have been questioned by the plaintiff's attorney, the defense attorney has the opportunity to cross-examine them. After the plaintiff has rested his or her case, the defendant's attorney calls witnesses and presents evidence. After the defense witnesses have been questioned by the defendant's attorney, the plaintiff's attorney has the opportunity to cross-examine them. During the questioning of witnesses, objections are made by each side to prevent the admission of certain statements into evidence. At trial, the types of queries that may be expected and the appropriateness

Figure 4.6   Sequence of a civil trial

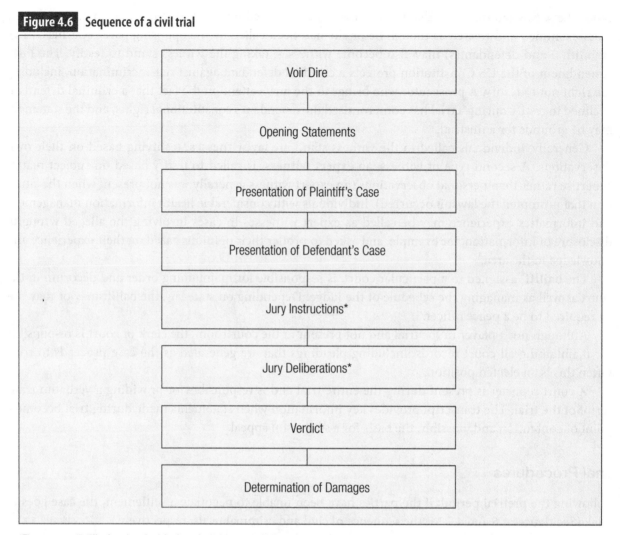

Voir Dire

Opening Statements

Presentation of Plaintiff's Case

Presentation of Defendant's Case

Jury Instructions*

Jury Deliberations*

Verdict

Determination of Damages

*The process will differ for a bench trial, where the judge acts as both judge and jury.

of questions do not differ from queries at depositions. When the appropriateness of a question is doubtful, a legal objection may be made and the judge will make a ruling as to whether or not it is to be answered. As with depositions, the custodian of health records and/or ESI or another designated individual may be called as a trial witness by one or more parties to testify as to the authenticity of a health record or ESI being sought as evidence.

Physical evidence, such as paper records (including health records) or electronic records (including EHRs) or other ESI, exhibits, or objects, is submitted to the court as evidence to be considered by the fact finders. As each side rests its case, the attorneys for the opposing party may make a motion for a **directed verdict**, requesting the judge to determine that, at that point in time, the case is over and favorable to the requesting party. Although not generally granted by the judge, a directed verdict signifies that the plaintiff failed to present the minimal evidence necessary to prove his case (even without the opposition presenting its case) and could not win the case as a matter of law. After both sides have presented and rested their cases, each presents a **closing argument** urging the jury to find in its favor.

The **burden of proof** (that is, sufficiently proving or establishing the requisite degree of belief for each element of a case) usually belongs to the plaintiff (Garner 2014). In civil cases, the burden of proof

Figure 4.7	Sequence of a criminal trial

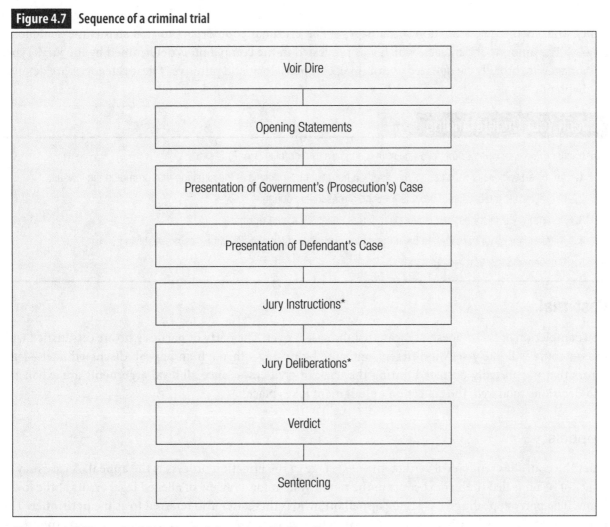

Voir Dire

Opening Statements

Presentation of Government's (Prosecution's) Case

Presentation of Defendant's Case

Jury Instructions*

Jury Deliberations*

Verdict

Sentencing

*The process will differ for a bench trial, where the judge acts as both judge and jury.

is the **preponderance of evidence** standard, which requires the plaintiff to provide evidence proving it is "more likely than not" that each element of the case was met and that the defendant committed the alleged wrongdoing. This civil standard is lower than the burden of proof for criminal cases, whereby the prosecution must prove **beyond a reasonable doubt** that the defendant committed the act(s) alleged. A higher burden of proof is required for criminal cases because the stakes (jail or prison) are higher than the stakes in civil cases, which generally involve monetary damages.

The jury is given legal **jury instructions,** which are the rules that are to be used to decide the case, by the judge. It then conducts private **deliberations,** which are discussions and careful thought about the case. Finally, it renders a **verdict** (decision). In criminal cases, a unanimous vote is required to either convict or acquit a defendant. Any split in votes results in a **hung jury,** where neither a conviction nor an acquittal is achieved. By contrast, civil cases often require only a certain majority in order to render a verdict of liability or no liability. This varies from state to state and is established by the FRCP in federal cases. A defendant is never declared innocent by the court, because a determination would indicate certainty that the defendant did not commit the act or acts alleged. Rather, "not guilty" or "not liable" verdicts indicate that the government or plaintiff did not present sufficient evidence to meet its burden of proof.

The final step in a trial where the defendant(s) have been judged liable by the jury, or a judge in a bench trial, is the determination of damages. (The criminal counterpart to this step is the sentencing phase.) The amount of damages, which was requested in the complaint, is determined by the jury. Types of damages are broadly categorized as nominal, compensatory, and punitive. These categories are detailed in chapter 6.

Check Your Understanding   4.4

Instructions: Indicate whether the following statements are true or false (T or F).

1. An expert witness is called to testify based on her own observations of the situation that prompted the lawsuit.

2. In civil cases, the burden of proof is "beyond a reasonable doubt."

3. Peremptory challenges are dismissals of jurors based on stated reasons.

4. A defendant is not permitted to be in the courtroom when the plaintiff's witnesses are testifying.

5. A bench trial is a trial without a jury.

Post-trial

The completion of a trial does not mean that the case is over. The party or parties who are dissatisfied with the outcome will likely seek a different outcome by raising—through an appeal, discussed later—legal errors that purportedly occurred during the trial. In civil cases, once all legal arguments are exhausted and decisions rendered, the collection of judgment takes place.

Appeals

After the court has rendered a verdict, the next stage in the litigation process is the **appeal**. A case may or may not be appealed to the next court in the tiered system for a review of alleged legal errors at the lower court. The party appealing a case is the **appellant**, who is thereafter also referred to as the **petitioner**. The party against whom a case is appealed is the **appellee**, who is thereafter also referred to as the **respondent**. There is not always a clear winner and loser at the conclusion of a trial. For example, a verdict may be rendered against the defendant, but the plaintiff may not believe that the amount of damages awarded was sufficient. In such cases, a **cross appeal** may occur, whereby the respondent, in addition to the petitioner who initially filed, files an appeal. In any event, appeals must be based on alleged errors or disputes of law, such as a judge admitting evidence contrary to the rules of evidence. Errors of fact, such as a jury believing an untruthful witness, cannot form the basis of a permissible appeal.

Collection of Judgment

The final stage of litigation, if there is a verdict of liability, is the collection of the judgment. Judgments may be in **equity**, and the defendant is required to do or to refrain from doing something. However, more commonly, judgments are money awards that require collection. Because awarded damages may number in the millions of dollars, it may not be feasible for the defendant(s) to write a single check to satisfy the judgment. One method of collecting the award methodically and gradually is via **garnishment** of wages. Through this court-ordered method, a percentage of the defendant's wages are routinely set aside and paid to the plaintiff toward full satisfaction of the judgment. Another method, a court-ordered **writ of execution**, directs the appropriate law enforcement official to seize the defendant's real or personal property to satisfy the debt owed to the plaintiff. This may be accomplished by accessing the defendant's bank account or by holding a sale subsequent to seizure of the property. Likewise, a **judgment lien** may be placed on the defendant's property, encumbering it and preventing the debtor/defendant from taking any money from its sale until the judgment owed to the plaintiff has first been paid. Although the judgment lien method depends on the defendant selling the property and may not occur in time to benefit the plaintiff, it can nonetheless pose a surprise to a debtor/defendant who wishes to sell his or her property years after a judgment was rendered and, perhaps, all but forgotten.

Physicians and other healthcare professionals, as well as healthcare organizations, carry malpractice insurance as protection against lawsuits where they are named as defendants and either a settlement is reached or a court finds them liable. Depending on the terms of the malpractice insurance policy and the type of wrongdoing alleged, the defendant may or may not be covered. Some malpractice insurance policies may exclude wrongdoing that is found by the courts to be intentional. If a defendant is found liable or reaches a settlement on a legal matter that the policy covers, it will be the insurance company that pays the award to the plaintiff rather than the defendant. As a result, however, the defendant can expect that his or her malpractice insurance premiums will increase. If an individual is a defendant in multiple lawsuits, the malpractice insurer may discontinue coverage at some point, deeming the individual no longer insurable.

Check Your Understanding | 4.5

Instructions: Indicate whether the following statements are true or false (T or F).

1. The party that appeals a lower court's decision is the appellee.
2. Garnishment is a court-ordered collection of money damages that is awarded to the plaintiff through a set-aside of the defendant's wages.
3. A civil judgment is always expressed in dollar amounts.
4. Appeals must be based on alleged errors or disputes of fact.
5. A judgment lien is an encumbrance placed on a defendant's property.

Scenario 4

During a school field trip to a local orchard, 13-year-old Johnny Chapman fell out of a tree while picking apples. That evening, his parents took him to the emergency room at Woodville Hospital, where he was diagnosed with a fractured ulna. He was admitted and surgery was necessary. Johnny was discharged after a two-day stay. Johnny's parents subsequently sued the school system and two of the three parent chaperones who had volunteered for failing to safeguard Johnny during the field trip and failing to seek emergency medical care.

Three months later, the health information department director at Woodville Hospital, Jay Forshall, was subpoenaed with directions to bring Johnny's record to a deposition the following day. The deposition was being held in Columbia City, which was 125 miles away. Jay complied with the subpoena by preparing Johnny's medical record. Woodville Hospital's health record was hybrid, so Jay printed out the electronic components from the hospital's electronic health record system and collected the remaining components that existed on paper.

Jay drove to Columbia City the following morning. During the deposition, legal counsel for the Chapmans proceeded to ask Jay about Johnny's medical record. Jay was asked to verify that the record was Johnny's and that it was prepared in the usual course of business. He was then asked about the contents of the record. One question posed to him was whether Tylenol, which had been

Scenario 4 (Continued)

administered to Johnny at the hospital, was given to lessen Johnny's pain. Jay stated that he presumed legal counsel's statement was true, as that is a common reason for Tylenol to be given. Jay was also asked to read an otherwise illegible note that the physician, Dr. Fogle, had written on the discharge instruction sheet. Dr. Fogle was a visiting physician, and Jay was not familiar with her handwriting. Nonetheless, he tried his best to assist legal counsel in deciphering the note.

Jay was not involved in the case any further following the deposition. Several months later, he read in the newspaper that the case had gone to trial. One of the parent chaperones who was initially sued never responded to the complaint and did not participate in any of the proceedings, including the trial. A jury rendered a verdict against the school system and the three parent chaperones, with all being required to pay money damages.

1. A verdict was rendered against three parent chaperones. How was the third parent included in the case?

2. Based on the facts, was Jay Forshall required to provide Johnny's records in response to the subpoena? Why or why not? What factors did you take into consideration?

3. Were all of the questions asked of Jay Forshall during the deposition appropriate? If your answer is no, what questions were inappropriate? Why?

4. Identify other legal procedural issues associated with this case.

References

AHIMA. 2013. E-Discovery litigation and regulatory investigation response planning: Crucial components of your organization's information and data governance processes. *Journal of AHIMA.* 84(11): expanded web version.

Baldwin-Stried Reich, K., K. Ball, M. Dougherty, and R. Hedges. 2012. *e-Discovery and Electronic Records.* Chicago: AHIMA Press.

Burrington-Brown, Jill. 2003. On the line: professional practice solutions. *Journal of AHIMA* 74(1): 62.

Dimick, C. 2011. Preparing for a deposition on an EHR: New types of information lead to new types of questions. *Journal of AHIMA* 82(3):44–45.

EDRM. 2016. EDRM at Duke Law School. www.edrm.net.

Garner, B.A. 2014. *Black's Law Dictionary.* Abridged 10th ed. St. Paul, MN: Thomson West. McLendon, Kelly and Lowe, M. 2011. *The Legal Health Record: Regulations, Policies, and Guidance.* Chicago: AHIMA Press.

Reynolds, R. 2010. *Tennessee Health Information Management Association Legal Handbook,* 11th ed. Winchester, TN: THIMA.

Showalter, J.S. 2014. *The Law of Healthcare Administration.* 7th ed. Chicago: Health Administration Press.

Cases, Statutes, and Regulations Cited

Batson v. Kentucky, 476 US 79 (1986).

Fabich v. Montana Rail Link, Inc., MT Dist., 2005 ML 135.

In re Search Warrant App. No. 1254, 852 A.2d 408 (PA Super. 2004).

Limbaugh v. Florida, 887 So.2d 387 (2004).

Nielsen v. Braland, 264 MN 481, 119 N.W.2d 737 (1963).

Smith v. Rossi, 115 A.D. 2nd 899; NY App. Div. (1985).

Trujillo v. Trujillo, 71 CA App. 2nd 257, 162 P.2d 64 (1945).

45 CFR 164.512(e): HIPAA. 2006.

5 USC 552a (App. 3 sec.(6)(a)(4)): The Privacy Act of 1974.

42 USC 1320: HIPAA. 1996.

FRCP 23: Class Action. 2009.

FRCP 41: Dismissal of Action, 2001.

Federal Rules of Civil Procedure (FRCP): FRCP 45(a)

Federal Rules of Civil Procedure (FRCP): FRCP 45(c)

Federal Rules of Civil Procedure (FRCP): FRCP 45(d)

Federal Rules of Civil Procedure (FRCP): FRCP 45(e)

Resources

National Court Rules Committee. 2016. Federal Rules of Criminal Procedure. 2016 ed. As amended through Dec 1, 2015. https://www.federalrulesofcriminalprocedure.org/table-of-contents/.

National Court Rules Committee. 2017. Federal Rules of Civil Procedure. 2017 ed. As amended through Dec. 1, 2016. https://www.federalrulesofcivilprocedure.org/frcp/.

National Court Rules Committee. 2017 Federal Rules of Evidence 2017 ed. https://www.rulesofevidence.org/.

US Const. Fourth Amendment: Search and Seizure.

Appendix 4

Sample Subpoena Duces Tecum (Civil)

SUBPOENA DUCES TECUM (CIVIL) –
ATTORNEY ISSUED VA CODE §§ 8.01–413, 16.1–89, 16.1–265;
Commonwealth of Virginia Supreme Court Rules 1:4, 4:9

Case No:..

....

HEARING DATE AND TIME

.... Court

....
COURT ADDRESS

.... V./In re: ....

TO THE PERSON AUTHORIZED BY LAW TO SERVE THIS PROCESS:
You are commanded to summon

....
NAME

....
STREET ADDRESS

....
CITY   STATE   ZIP

To the person summoned: You are commanded to make available the documents and tangible things designated and described below:

A certified copy of any and all records reflecting treatment, including office visits, ER records,
....
diagnoses, histories and physicals, discharge summaries, consultations, operative reports, pathological reports,
....
x-ray reports and films, lab reports, echocardiogram reports and tapes, EKG reports and tracings, doctors, orders,
....
progress notes, nurses notes and any outpatient records concerning X, Date Of Birth, Social Security Number
at .... at ....
LOCATION   DATE AND TIME

to permit such party or someone acting in his or her behalf to inspect and copy, test or sample such tangible things in your possession, custody or control

This Subpoena Duces Tecum is issued by the attorney for and on behalf of

....
PARTY NAME

....
NAME OF ATTORNEY   VIRGINIA STATE BAR NUMBER

....
OFFICE ADDRESS   TELEPHONE NUMBER OF ATTORNEY

....
OFFICE ADDRESS   FACSIMILE NUMBER OF ATTORNEY

....
DATE ISSUED   SIGNATURE OF ATTORNEY

Notice to Recipient: See page two for further information.

Return of service (see page two of this form)

FORM DC-498 7/00
(MASTER, PAGE ONE OF TWO)

To the person summoned:

If you are served with this subpoena less than 14 days prior to the date that compliance with this subpoena is required, you may object by notifying the party who issued the subpoena of your objection in writing and describing the basis of your objection in that writing.

To the person authorized to serve this process: Upon execution, the return of this process shall be made to the clerk of court.

NAME:	
ADDRESS:	
....	
☐ PERSONAL SERVICE	Tel. No. ....

Being unable to make personal service, a copy was delivered in the following manner:

☐ Delivered to family member (not temporary sojourner or guest) age 16 or older at usual place of abode of party named above after giving information of its purport. List name, age of recipient, and relation of recipient to party named above:

....

....

☐ Posted on front door or such other door as appear to be the main entrance of usual place of abode, address listed above. (Other authorized recipient not found.)

☐ not found

...., Sheriff

.... by ...., Deputy Sheriff

DATE

CERTIFICATE OF COUNSEL

I, ... , counsel for ...., hereby certify

that a copy of the foregoing subpoena duces tecum was ....

DELIVERY METHOD

to .... , counsel of record for ....,

on the .... day of .... , ...

_____

SIGNATURE OF ATTORNEY

FORM DC-498 7/00
(MASTER, PAGE TWO OF TWO)

Evidence

Jill Callahan Klaver, JD, RHIA

Learning Objectives

- Explain the significance of health information as evidence
- Distinguish between the types of evidence
- Describe the concept of admissibility and authentication of evidence
- Explain the evidentiary rule of hearsay and exceptions to the rule
- Identify the components of the best evidence rule
- Describe the principle of privilege, the types of communication it applies to, and when it may be waived
- Discuss how evidence may be protected through the concept of legal hold and other administrative controls
- Explain spoliation and the concern it raises in legal cases
- Discuss legal protections applied to incident reports and peer review records

Key Terms

- Admissibility
- Apology statutes
- Authenticated evidence
- Best evidence rule
- Business records exception
- Direct evidence

- Documentary evidence
- Evidence
- Federal Rules of Evidence
- Fiduciary duty
- Hearsay
- I'm Sorry Laws

- Incident reports
- Legal hold
- Metadata
- Peer review
- Physician–patient privilege
- Privilege

- Privileged communication
- Relevant evidence
- Spoliation
- Triggers
- Waiver of privilege
- Weight of the evidence

Health information is routinely relevant in legal proceedings, whether that information is being used to allege a physician's negligence, assert an individual incompetence, show physical damages from an accident, or address any number of other legal issues. Individuals charged with the responsibility of protecting health information in paper and/or electronic form must understand how patient information is used as evidence in litigation. Healthcare professionals must understand federal and state health privacy, procedural, and evidentiary laws along with organizational policies and practices that foster compliance with those laws. This chapter introduces key evidentiary rules that impact how health records and other types of electronically stored information (ESI) are used as evidence, in addition to evidentiary rules, apology statutes, protection of evidence and related medical documentation, incident reports, and peer review records.

Health Information as Evidence

Just as a variety of rules govern the trial process discussed in chapter 4, many additional federal and state rules specifically govern when and how evidence may be used during the trial process. **Evidence** is used to prove or disprove the facts of a case (Garner 2014). It may be presented in the form of oral testimony, contained in written or electronic documents, or presented through pictures, devices, and objects. To manage how evidence is used during cases, both federal and state laws provide frameworks that govern the admission of evidence during litigation. Generally, if a case is presented in federal court because it involves a federal law (for example, the False Claims Act), or if the parties are from different states, the **Federal Rules of Evidence** (FRE) apply. These rules were initially passed by Congress in 1975 and consist of 11 articles and 42 rules (National Court Rules Committee 2016). If a case is tried in state court, then the rules of evidence for that state apply. State rules are often similar to the federal rules, although the degree of similarity varies from state to state.

Health information, whether in paper or electronic record format, is an important kind of evidence that is relied upon in a variety of legal cases. If a plaintiff wishes to prove injury by the defendant in a personal injury case, health information will be used to establish the extent of the plaintiff's injuries. In a medical malpractice case, health information will be used to establish the standard of care that applied to the defendant's conduct and to establish whether the defendant's conduct caused the plaintiff's injuries. Similarly, if an injured worker wishes to claim benefits for a work-related injury, health information evidence will be used to prove the extent of the worker's injury. Individuals applying for federal disability benefits will use health information to establish that they qualify as disabled.

Courts will review health information evidence in cases involving custody, especially when the health of a child or custodial parent is at issue. Health information evidence will also be used in cases where an individual's competence is at issue, such as in guardianship or commitment proceedings, which are discussed in more detail in chapter 8. Health information is central in criminal proceedings as well. Prosecutors use health information to prove injuries to victims in murder, manslaughter, criminal assault and battery, and abuse cases. It may also be used to establish a defendant's claim of self-defense in such cases. Health information may also be used in white-collar crime cases, such as criminal fraud and abuse. Figure 5.1 illustrates the use of health information as evidence in several types of legal proceedings.

To use health information as evidence in a trial, it is usually obtained during the pretrial discovery process as discussed in chapter 4. Whether the information is discoverable or admissible will depend on procedural and evidentiary rules discussed later in this chapter in the section on admissibility.

Types of Evidence

There are several major types of evidence:

- **Direct evidence** is "real, tangible or clear evidence of a fact, happening or thing that requires no thinking or consideration to prove its existence," offered through direct testimony by a witness (such as a visible injury in a criminal trial for battery)
- **Demonstrative (real or physical) evidence** is actual objects, charts, diagrams, maps, video, pictures, photographs, models, illustrations and other devices that are supposedly intended to clarify or prove the facts for the judge and jury—how an accident occurred, actual damages, medical problems, or methods used in committing an alleged crime; considered the most trustworthy and preferred type of evidence (such as a broken IV pump in a case involving harm through a medication error)
- **Documentary evidence** is evidence in written form, not oral, (original records, letters, e-mails, photographs) used to prove a fact included in the information imparted (such as medical record documentation that describes a patient fall)

| Figure 5.1 | Cases illustrating use of health records as evidence |

Medical Malpractice:

In *Kohl v. Tirado,* the plaintiff alleged that his podiatrist had committed malpractice by failing to diagnose a fractured ankle and provide appropriate treatment. The health records kept by the podiatrist were instrumental in determining whether the podiatrist had failed to diagnose the fracture and whether the podiatrist's overall treatment was reasonable.

Child Custody:

In the Matter of J.B., the respondent appealed the trial court's order terminating her parental rights to her son. Specifically, the respondent argued that her mental health records should not have been admitted into evidence because they were protected from disclosure under a state statute. The appellate court disagreed, finding that the records were admissible under a statutory exception. (Admissibility will be discussed later in this chapter.) The court also noted that the contents of the records indicated that the respondent's mental health issues seriously impeded her ability to provide minimally acceptable parenting for her son.

Criminal Manslaughter:

In *Connecticut v. Abney,* the defendant was convicted of manslaughter after she stabbed her ex-boyfriend. She claimed that the stabbing occurred in self-defense and sought to admit her own health records showing past treatment for injuries that she alleged were previously caused by her ex-boyfriend. Admission of health records would bolster the defendant's claim of self-defense by suggesting the defendant's state of mind at the time of the stabbing. The trial court excluded these records, but the appellate court disagreed, ruling that the records were relevant to her claim of self-defense.

White-Collar Crime:

In *United States v. Syme,* health records were instrumental in the appellate court's finding that there was insufficient evidence to convict the defendant of intentionally billing Medicare for medically unnecessary ambulance services of a nursing home resident. The specific ambulance service at issue occurred on August 3, 1994. In determining that transporting the resident via ambulance was not medically necessary, the prosecutor's expert witness testified that he had reviewed the resident's nursing home records for January 20 and March 17, 1994. Those records showed that the resident was able to walk and sit up on her own, suggesting that absent an emergency, ambulance transportation would not be appropriate. However, the court found this evidence to be insufficient because other health records dated between March 17 and August 3, 1994, were not reviewed. The court determined that during those four months, the resident's condition could have deteriorated, thus making transportation via ambulance medically necessary.

- **Circumstantial (indirect) evidence** is "evidence in a trial which is not directly from an eyewitness or participant and requires some reasoning to prove a fact," used most often in criminal trials (such as testimony from someone who saw the defendant exit the patient's room and flee just before a Code Blue was called, in a case involving an attack on a patient) (Garner 2014).

Evidence is often in written form or "writing," such as medical reports and records. With the onset of electronic health records (EHRs), and other forms of electronically stored information (ESI), courts take a broad view of what constitutes writing. The general definition of writing includes "writings and recordings consisting of letters, words, or numbers, or their equivalent, which are set down by handwriting, typewriting, printing, photostatting, photographing, magnetic impulse, mechanical or electronic recording, or other forms of data compilation" (FRE 1001(1)). Generally, photographs include still photographs, x-ray films, videotapes, and motion pictures (FRE 1001(2)). As with writings, photographic evidence must be authenticated and trustworthy. Authentication of material presented through the discovery process related to depositions and during a trial is discussed in chapter 4.

Evidence may also take the form of direct or oral testimony. (See chapter 4 for information about expert witnesses.) Oral testimony is provided when a witness is deposed or questioned at a hearing or trial. Often, testimonial evidence and documentary evidence are combined. For example, a witness on the stand may refer to a document to refresh his or her recollection of an event, or the witness may be asked to read or explain the contents of writing to the court. Sometimes, documents may not be presented at all unless they are accompanied by witness testimony. *Fred's Stores of Tennessee v. Brown* involved a negligence claim brought by the parents of a 10-year-old girl who was injured after a bicycle assembled by Fred's broke as it was being ridden by the girl. At trial, authenticated health records were entered into evidence, but the physicians who created those records were never deposed and were never called to testify about the contents of those records. Although the court noted that presenting unexplained health records could cause the judge and jury to be confused, it noted, "The health records were introduced without objection at the beginning of trial. If Fred's believed that the testimony in the documents might require expert explanation, the time to make the objection was then. Therefore we find that the records could be used by the trial judge, subject to a reasonable layperson's limits on what may be gleaned from such records."

Evidentiary Rules

Rules of evidence, such as those relating to relevance and admissibility, are governed by state and federal rules of evidence. These rules establish a comprehensive framework for the admissibility and use of evidence during trials. Key evidentiary rules are discussed next.

Admissibility

Admissibility, part of the discovery process as discussed in chapter 4, refers to evidence that may be admitted in a court of law. It is important to distinguish between discoverability and admissibility. Evidence that is discoverable during the pretrial process may not necessarily be admissible at trial. Generally, only **relevant evidence** is admissible at trial (FRE 402). Evidence is relevant if it tends to make the existence of any fact more probable or less probable than it would be without that evidence (FRE 401).

Even if evidence is relevant, it may still be excluded from a trial on a number of grounds. For example, if a piece of relevant evidence also happens to be unfairly prejudicial, confusing, or misleading, or if it is needlessly redundant, then the court must conduct a balancing test before allowing the piece of evidence to be admitted. The probative value of this evidence must substantially outweigh the dangers of unfair prejudice and/or undue delay associated with presenting that evidence (FRE 403). Figure 5.2 provides two examples where the issue of admissibility and authentication of evidence are discussed.

If evidence appears to be relevant, it still must be authenticated. As introduced in chapter 4, the evidence itself must be shown to have a baseline authenticity or trustworthiness. As a general rule, **authenticated evidence** is present if there is "evidence sufficient to support a finding that the matter in question is what its proponent claims" (FRE 901(a)). Generally, this is established by a record custodian's affidavit that the record was

- Documented in the normal course of business (following normal routines)
- Kept in the regular course of business
- Made at or near the time of the matter recorded
- Made by a person within the business with knowledge of the acts, events, conditions, opinions, or diagnoses appearing in it (AHIMA e-HIM Work Group on Maintaining the Legal EHR 2005)

Whereas the authentication requirements established by the FRE are agreeable with paper health records, establishing the authenticity of electronic records, especially EHRs, or ESI presents additional challenges for individuals responsible for the management and integrity of health information.

| Figure 5.2 | Cases concerning admissibility and authentication of evidence |

In *Broek v. Park Nicollet Health Services,* a wrongful death action was brought by the plaintiff regarding the death of her husband. The plaintiff appealed the trial court's decision to admit certain health records of her husband, who had been diagnosed with a ventricular septal defect as a teenager. Specifically, the records noted that her husband experienced an episode of dizziness while playing basketball several months before his sudden cardiac arrest, but he had not sought any treatment at that time. In upholding the trial court's decision, the appellate court noted that evidence is not unfairly prejudicial merely because it is damaging to one party's case.

In *American Color Graphics v. Rayfield Foster,* the appellate court determined that health records were improperly admitted into evidence because they had not been properly authenticated. In this case, the plaintiff wished to demonstrate the extent of his claimed injuries by offering a variety of health records and reports into evidence. However, the doctors and psychologists who compiled the reports were not deposed and did not testify at trial. Under Alabama discovery rules, if copies of health records and bills are certified and sealed, they may be admitted "without further need for authenticating testimony".

Some of the reports offered into evidence contained the following certification by the treating physician: "I hereby certify that the attached is a true and correct copy of the health records kept on file in my office." With respect to these records, the court stated, "Because none of the language on any of these documents reference that these reports were compiled in the regular course of business and at a time consistent with the regular course of business, we conclude that their certifications fail and they were improperly admitted into evidence". Other reports offered contained this certification:

> I hereby certify and affirm in writing that the attached is a true and complete copy of the records regarding treatment of [the plaintiff], which are kept in the office of [the physician], in my custody and control. I further certify that I am the legal custodian and keeper of the records. The attached records were made in the regular course of business and it was in the regular course of business for such records to be made at the time of the events, transactions, or occurrences to which they refer, or within a reasonable time thereafter.

The appellate court found that the certification language followed the requirements of Alabama law. However, because a notary public did not seal those records, the court still found that they had been improperly admitted.

Electronic documents can sometimes be easily modified and, depending on the system used, those modifications are not always apparent. It is not possible to visually detect alterations in an EHR the way one could do in a paper health record. Tracing alterations may be possible with the use of the EHR's **metadata** (data about the data) or audit trails that can "tell who accessed the record, which information was reviewed, and how and when the document was modified" (McLean et al. 2008). Drury et al. (2014) have suggested that "digital record systems especially EHRs, may as a matter of routine, merit testing for reliability and trustworthiness as a precondition" of validity (FRE 901(b)(9)) and admissibility (FRE 803(6)).

It is important that individuals designated as record or information systems custodians be aware of the both FRE along with state rules for authenticating evidence. These individuals should also be able to describe how an electronic system monitors or manages modifications or different versions of electronic information to satisfy the court that the electronic documents should be admitted into evidence. Indicators of the potential reliability of electronic records or ESI as evidence are summarized in figure 5.3.

Even if evidence has been properly authenticated under the rules for a particular jurisdiction, the evidence itself may not necessarily be error-free. For example, incorrect information may inadvertently be documented in a patient record, a provider may fail to document enough information in the record, or conflicting information may be present in the record. In such cases, courts generally find that those errors or inconsistencies relate to the **weight** (or importance, or credibility) **of the evidence**, not its admissibility. In other words, the court may still admit the record into evidence, but the jury will then determine how much weight to give that record as they decide the factual issues of the case. If the jury determines that the record contains errors, they may find the record to be untrustworthy and, therefore, discount the information in the record.

Figure 5.3	Indicators of the reliability of electronic records or ESI

Reliability

- Validation of computer systems to ensure accuracy, reliability, consistent performance, and the ability to conclusively discern invalid or altered records
- The ability to generate accurate copies of records in both human readable and electronic form
- Protection of records to enable their accurate and ready retrieval throughout the records retention period
- Use of hardware, software, records management procedures (including trusted third party storage of electronic records) and/or third party notarization and time certification, to ensure reliability as to the identity of the creator and the time of creation of an electronic record, and to ensure that the electronic record has not been altered since the time of creation
- Limiting system access to authorized individuals, and use of authority checks to ensure only those individuals who have been so authorized can use the system, electronically sign a record, access the operation or device, alter a record, or perform the operation at hand
- Use of appropriate controls over systems documentation, including adequate controls over the distribution, access to, and use of documentation for system operation and maintenance; and established written policies that hold individuals accountable and liable for actions involving creation of electronic records, and where appropriate, the use of system audit trails that track creation, use, modification, and disposition of electronic records

Sources: Adapted from Cavanaugh et al. 2000; AHIMA e-HIM Work Group on Maintaining the Legal EHR 2005.

Hearsay

Hearsay is a written or oral statement made outside of court that is offered in court as evidence to prove "the truth of the matter asserted" (FRE 801(a)). For example, if a nurse in a malpractice case against Dr. Jones testifies, "Doctor Smith said that Doctor Jones committed malpractice," the nurse's statement would constitute hearsay. It is testimony about a statement that was made outside of court, and it was offered to prove the truth of Dr. Jones's negligence. This evidentiary concept is applicable to health information because much documentation in the health record is hearsay. As a general rule, hearsay is not admissible as evidence unless one of several hearsay exceptions applies (FRE 803). Some exceptions are described in the following sections.

Business Records Exception

Because health records consist of out-of-court statements that are often used in court to prove the truth of the claim, they technically constitute hearsay. However, a major exception to the prohibition against using hearsay as evidence is the **business records exception** (FRE 803(6)). Under this rule, a record of an act, event, condition, opinion, or diagnosis (in any form: memorandum, report, or data compilation) is not hearsay if it meets the following requirements:

- A record was made at or near the time by, or from information transmitted by, a person with knowledge.
- A record was kept in the course of a regularly conducted activity of a business, organization, occupation, or calling, whether or not for profit.
- Making the record was the regular practice of that business activity.
- All these conditions are shown by the testimony of the custodian or another qualified witness, or by a certification that complies with Rule 902(11) or (12) or with statute permitting certification.
- The opponent does not show that the source of information or the method or circumstances of preparation indicate a lack of trustworthiness.

Other Exceptions

There are 23 other hearsay exceptions, in addition to the business records exception that involve health information (National Court Rules Committee 2016). Examples of two of these exceptions include

- Statements made for purposes of medical diagnosis or treatment that describe medical history; past or present symptoms, pain, or sensations; or the inception of or general character of the cause are exceptions to the rule (FRE 803(4)).
- Records or data compilations, in any form, of births, fetal deaths, deaths, or marriages, if the report was made to a public office pursuant to requirements of law, are also exceptions from the hearsay rule (FRE 803(9)).

A case that involved both the business records exception to hearsay rule and the exception pertaining to statements made for purposes of medical diagnosis or treatment is summarized in figure 5.4.

Figure 5.4   Case summary illustrating exceptions to hearsay

In *American Color Graphics v. Rayfield Foster,* the plaintiff in that case filed a workers' compensation claim against the defendant-employer. To demonstrate the extent of his injuries, the plaintiff sought to admit a detailed medical report by a physician who had examined him after he had filed his claim. However, the plaintiff did not call the physician to testify as a witness. The defendant argued that the report was inadmissible because it constituted hearsay—it was an out-of-court statement offered to prove the truth of the plaintiff's work-related injuries. At issue was whether the report met either the business records exception or the statements for purposes of medical diagnosis or treatment exception to the hearsay rule. The defendant argued that the report did not meet the business records exception because it was not kept in the regular course of business, but was prepared specifically in anticipation of litigation (that is, it was prepared specifically for use at trial). In finding that the report constituted hearsay and met neither of the two exceptions at issue, the court stated:

- We first note that according to the case action summary, Foster filed his case on April 8, 1999. Plaintiff's exhibit 2(A), the medical examination report of Dr. Allen, is dated June 28, 1999—almost three months after he first filed his complaint. See plaintiff's exhibit 2(A). Furthermore, in support of its motion *in limine*, ACG submitted to the trial court a copy of Foster's deposition, in which he admitted that, although he visited Dr. Allen on a number of occasions after he had back surgery in 1997 and although he paid for his consultations through his wife's insurance, he was referred to Dr. Allen by his own attorney.

- Although Dr. Allen's report constitutes a statement "made for purposes of medical diagnosis or treatment and describing medical history, or past or present symptoms, pain, or sensations, or the inception or general character of the cause or external source thereof" and, according to its certification, constitutes a report of conditions, opinions, or diagnoses, made the day of the examination by Dr. Allen, certified by the custodian of records within one day thereafter, allegedly kept in the course of regularly conducted medical business, in the regular practice of medical evaluators to make such report, all as shown by the certification of the custodian of records and the sealing thereof by a notary public, we are not as convinced that the source of the information does not indicate a lack of trustworthiness in the sense that it has been prepared solely in anticipation of, and preparation for, litigation…

- Given the fact that the date of Dr. Allen's evaluation and Foster's own testimony that it was his attorney who sent him to Dr. Allen for consultation, we cannot conclusively say that plaintiff's exhibit 2(A) was not prepared in anticipation and preparation for the lawsuit Foster filed against ACG.

- Thus, we conclude that Dr. Allen's medical report constitutes inadmissible hearsay; the trial court erred in admitting plaintiff's exhibit 2(A) into evidence.

Check Your Understanding 5.1

Instructions: Indicate whether the following statements are true or false (T or F).

1. Circumstantial evidence requires reasoning to prove a fact.
2. To determine whether a piece of health information is admissible, one can only rely on the FRE.
3. To use health information as evidence, it must be discoverable and admissible based on procedural and evidentiary rules.
4. Relevant evidence will always be admitted into evidence.
5. Courts make the automatic assumption that written evidence is trustworthy.

Best Evidence Rule

Under the **best evidence rule**, to prove the contents of a writing, recording, or photograph, the original writing, recording, or photograph is required (FRE 1002). The rule serves mainly to protect against intentional perjury or simple faulty memory regarding the contents of writings, recordings, and photographs. Original means the writing or recording itself or a negative or any print of a photograph. With the healthcare industry's trend toward keeping EHRs instead of paper, the issue of what constitutes an original of an EHR is important. With respect to data stored in a computer or similar device, the best evidence rule states that a printout or other output readable by sight and shown to reflect the data accurately constitutes an original (FRE 1001(3)).

The best evidence rule also permits the use of duplicates in lieu of the original unless

- A genuine question is raised as to the authenticity of the original.
- Under the circumstances, it would be unfair to admit the duplicate in lieu of the original (FRE 1003).

Therefore, authenticated copies of health records are often used at trial rather than the original patient health record. However, original health records or their duplicates are not always available—records may be lost, destroyed by accident or in accordance with records retention laws, stolen, and so on. In such cases, the best evidence rule provides that other evidence of the record's contents may be admissible if

- All originals have been lost or have been destroyed (unless done so in bad faith).
- No original can be obtained by any available judicial process or procedure.
- At a time when an original was in possession of the opposing party, that party was put on notice, by the pleadings or otherwise, that the contents would be a subject of proof at the hearing, and that party does not produce the original at the hearing.
- The writing, recording, or photograph is not closely related to a controlling issue (FRE 1004).

Lipschitz v. Stein involved a malpractice claim brought by the plaintiff against his eye doctor. One basis of the claim was that the doctor negligently delayed diagnosis of postoperative eye problems because he did not see the plaintiff until 11:45 a.m., when the appointment was supposed to be at 9:00 a.m. According to the plaintiff, the delay in diagnosis and treatment caused permanent injury to the plaintiff's eye. Although the plaintiff testified that he arrived at the defendant's office at 9:00 a.m., a receptionist working for the defendant testified that the plaintiff did not arrive until 10:00 a.m. The receptionist based her testimony on a patient log, but the actual patient log was never entered into evidence. The appellate court ruled that the receptionist's testimony violated the best evidence rule because the best evidence of what was contained in the patient log was the patient log itself, not the receptionist's memory of what was contained in the log. Notably, the pretrial records of the case suggested that the log was not produced by the defendant because the receptionist had altered the times listed on the log. As a result, the appellate court awarded the plaintiff a new trial.

Privilege

To foster the free exchange of information in circumstances where open communication is essential, the law has created the concept of privilege. In essence, **privilege** means that certain specified communications are secret and cannot be forcibly revealed except under special circumstances. **Privileged communication** is shared communication between two parties. Examples of privileged communications that are recognized by law include physician–patient, clergy–parishioner, psychologist–client, attorney–client, and husband–wife. In protecting the concept of privileged communication, the concept of **fiduciary duty** may come into play. A fiduciary (a person or business) who has the power and obligation to act for another individual under circumstances of trust and confidence has the responsibility to protect this individual (USLegal 2016). Actions that do not protect the individual, such as wrongfully releasing a health record, may constitute a breach of fiduciary duty. The next section addresses aspects of the application of privileges, including physician–patient privilege, waiver of privilege, and privilege between patients and other providers.

Physician–Patient Privilege

Courts have long recognized that health records are private and "deserve the utmost constitutional protection" (*Mapes v. District Court*, 1991). The **physician–patient privilege** is a common tool for protecting that privacy in the context of litigation. Although it varies from state to state and is not provided for by every state, the physician–patient privilege generally legally protects confidential communications between physicians and patients related to diagnosis and treatment from being disclosed during civil and some misdemeanor litigation. The rationale behind the privilege is that it encourages patients to fully disclose all relevant information to their physicians without fear of the information being made public during a trial. Originating with the Hippocratic Oath, the American Medical Association's Principles of Ethics continue the professional tradition of confidence between a physician and patient unless provided otherwise by law.

Generally speaking, the patient (or his/her legally authorized representative) is the holder of the privilege, and must assert that privilege in order to prevent his/her health information from being disclosed in court. However, case law may impose a duty on a physician or hospital to claim the privilege on behalf of the patient. For example, in *Wesley Medical Center v. Clark*, the hospital sought to protect certain records from disclosure in court based on the physician–patient privilege. The Kansas Supreme Court recognized that the hospital did not meet the statutory definition of holder of the privilege; however, the court stated:

> While it is true that the physician, or in this case the hospital, is not the holder of the privilege that does not mean that a physician, absent statutory authority, may reveal, ex parte, information subject to the privilege without the knowledge and consent of the patient or holder of the privilege. Similar restraints apply to confidential records of hospitals and other treatment facilities unless otherwise provided by statute. Records in the possession of Wesley, which are subject to the physician-patient privilege under Kan. Stat. Ann. 60-427(b), would not ordinarily be discoverable without notice to and the consent of the holder of the privilege (*Wesley Medical Center v. Clark*, 1983).

| Figure 5.5 | Privileged communication and fiduciary duty |

In *Fierstein v. DePaul Health Center,* the plaintiff sued the defendant for breach of fiduciary duty for wrongful release of her health records. In that case, the plaintiff's ex-husband (through his attorney) issued a subpoena to DePaul Health Center. The subpoena ordered DePaul's custodian of records to appear at a deposition and to bring any and all records pertaining to a hospitalization of the plaintiff. The subpoena was accompanied by a letter stating that the records custodian would not need to appear at the deposition if the requested records were mailed to the ex-husband's attorney's office prior to the deposition. The records custodian testified that she telephoned the ex-husband's attorney's office and was told that the plaintiff's attorney had authorized the release of the records. The records custodian executed an affidavit and mailed the records to the ex-husband's attorney. The plaintiff subsequently sued DePaul for breach of fiduciary duty for wrongful release of her health records. She testified that she never authorized the release of her records or waived any privilege protecting the records. Further, the attorney's office testified that no one had ever represented that the plaintiff had authorized the release of her records.

After hearing the evidence, a jury awarded the plaintiff $10,000 in actual damages and $375,000 in punitive damages. The trial court reduced the punitive damage award to $25,000. The Missouri Court of Appeals (Eastern District) upheld the decision of the trial court, stating, "If a physician discloses any information, without first obtaining the patient's waiver, then the patient may maintain an action for damages in tort against the physician." (Waiver is discussed later; torts are discussed in chapter 6). A key factor in the court's decision was that the plaintiff was never given the opportunity to object to the release of her records. The Court of Appeals also upheld the trial court's decision to reduce the punitive damage award, finding that $25,000 in punitive damages was appropriate to deter the defendant from similar future conduct.

An example of breach of fiduciary duty for wrongful release of health records is summarized in figure 5.5.

As noted earlier, the existence of privilege statutes varies from state to state. The scope of privilege also varies, although certain common principles apply. Information is not generally considered privileged when it is obtained by a physician in a social situation that is outside the treatment setting. Likewise, information that is subject to public observation (for example, the fact that an individual is bleeding) is not privileged. Information obtained during an employment or pre-employment physical exam is generally not privileged because it lacks a contractual physician–patient relationship. More discussion of this contractual relationship can be found in chapter 7. Other parameters that may be defined by state law include

- Whether privilege survives the presence of a third party during a physician–patient communication
- The survival of privilege even when a third party is paying the patient's medical bill
- The survival of privilege even when a patient is unwilling to be treated (for example, emergency mental health treatment) or unable to give express consent (explained in chapter 8)
- What constitutes a physician–patient relationship

Waiver of Privilege

Like the hearsay rule discussed previously, physician–patient privilege is riddled with exceptions. One of the most common exceptions involves **waiver of privilege**. Specifically, "when a party claims damages for physical or mental injury, he or she places the extent of that physical or mental injury at issue and waives his or her statutory right to confidentiality to the extent that it is necessary for a defendant to discover whether plaintiff's current medical or physical condition is the result of some other cause" (*Fabich v. Montana Rail Link, Inc.,* 2005). However, "This waiver is not unlimited, and the defendant may only discover records related to prior physical or mental conditions if they relate to currently claimed damages. The plaintiff's right to confidentiality is balanced against the defendant's right to defend itself in an informed manner. A defendant 'is not entitled to unnecessarily invade plaintiff's privacy by exploring totally unrelated or irrelevant matters'" (*Fabich v. Montana Rail Link, Inc.,* 2005). The waiver of privilege may apply to both health records and to testimony about a patient's condition or treatment.

Another exception to the physician–patient privilege involves using the results of blood alcohol tests at trials for driving while under the influence. An individual on trial for driving while under the influence of drugs or alcohol cannot claim the physician–patient privilege to prevent the results of drug and alcohol tests from being admitted as evidence. Likewise, in a proceeding to determine whether an individual's mental capacity is such that he or she needs to be committed, that individual cannot use the physician–patient privilege to prevent testimony and health records regarding mental capacity from being admitted into evidence.

Privilege between Patients and Other Providers

The concept of privilege extends beyond the physician–patient relationship to relationships between patients and other types of providers. Privileges exist between patients and their psychologists, therapists, counselors, social workers, optometrists, dentists, and so on. The scope of these privileges is defined by state statutes and regulations, but generally prohibits providers from disclosing treatment information without patient authorization unless specific circumstances exist. For example, state laws generally allow psychologists to reveal client information to appropriate authorities when there is reasonable belief that the client presents a clear and present danger to the health and safety of himself or herself, another individual, or the public at large. See Kansas Administrative Regulation 102-1-10a(g) for an example of how psychologists can be permitted to release otherwise privileged information in the setting of danger to others. As with physician–patient privileges, patients or clients of nonphysician providers can waive their privilege rights. For example, under Kansas law, an individual waives the privilege between himself or herself and a licensed social worker by bringing charges against the licensed social worker. However, the waiver is valid only to the extent that the otherwise privileged information is relevant to the case (Kan. Stat. Ann. 65-6315(a)(3)).

Apology Statutes

Related to privilege (which belongs to the patient) are **apology statutes** that protect communications made by providers to patients (and perhaps patients' relatives) from being admitted as evidence in court. When healthcare providers apologize for unanticipated outcomes following medical procedures or treatments, the apologies may be perceived as admissions of fault rather than merely as compassionate or sympathetic expressions. Informally referred to as "I'm Sorry Laws," over 30 states have enacted these protective statutes that vary in scope. For example, Ohio and Georgia deem all statements or conduct that express apology or sympathy inadmissible as an admission of liability, and Colorado law specifically excludes statements of fault from admission. Vermont law excludes only oral apologies or statements of regret. California and Texas protect sympathetic statements made relative to an accident, but allow statements of fault to be admitted into evidence (American Medical Association Advocacy Resource Center 2015). Although the intent of apology laws is to protect healthcare providers, defense counsel may prefer that apologies be admitted because juries often view compassionate defendants more favorably.

Check Your Understanding 5.2

Instructions: Indicate whether the following statements are true or false (T or F).

1. The physician–patient privilege may be waived when a party claims damages by the physician and puts his physical or mental condition at issue.

2. Apologies from providers to patients for medical mistakes are often protected by state law from use as evidence of wrongdoing by the provider.

3. It is the physician who holds the physician–patient privilege.

4. The physician–patient privilege is used to encourage full disclosure of relevant information by patients to their physicians.

5. The best evidence rule prohibits the use of a duplicate record in lieu of the original.

Protection of Evidence

With data and information governance policies and practices in place, the organization should have knowledge of what information they have, where data is located, how long data should be retained, and what information is needed to respond to a legal, investigatory, or other event (Kearney 2014). In the evidentiary discovery and e-discovery process (see chapter 4) the healthcare organization has a legal duty to preserve all potential information whether in paper or electronic format that may be relevant in threatened or impending litigation (AHIMA 2013). This includes preserving information in anticipation of litigation based on certain "**litigation triggers,**" such as

- Adverse events: for example, improper administration of medication or unanticipated death of a patient, visitor, employee
- Sentinel events: for example, process variations that carry significant risk of death or serious physical or psychological injury
- Birth Injuries: for example, infants suffering injury, disfigurement, or death as a result of complications from delivery
- Medical device injury or harm: for example, errors that can occur in regard to malfunctioning or wrong use of medical device (Baldwin-Stried Reich et al 2012)
- To preserve information, organizations rely on the legal concepts of legal hold and spoliation as well as policies and practices related to record retention and destruction, disaster recovery and business continuity, and management of the discovery process.

Legal Hold

A **legal hold** (also known as a preservation order, preservation notice, or litigation hold) basically suspends the processing or destruction of paper or electronic records. It may be initiated by a court if there is concern that information may be destroyed in cases of current or anticipated litigation, audit, or government investigation. Or, it may be initiated by the organization as part of their pre-litigation planning and duty to preserve information in anticipation of litigation. Individual circumstances of the litigation, investigation, or audit may determine the requirements for the legal hold.

If a legal hold is issued or put into place for a paper health record or documents, it is standard practice to physically lock up the record or other related documents that may be involved in litigation to protect the integrity of the documentation and evidence. In a digital or electronic environment, an equivalent practice must also be implemented. Organizational policies and procedures should encompass the process for communicating a hold to those responsible for all systems that contain relevant information, so that data or no one system is purged in violation of the hold.

Policies and procedures should also identify the individual or individuals who are responsible for implementing a legal hold, suspending destruction, and determining when the legal hold can be lifted (AHIMA e-HIM Work Group on e-Discovery 2006). This responsibility typically falls to the custodian of records or information systems, who are usually a health information management and health information technology professionals. It is essential that the custodians have a process to ensure that others with access to the information that is the subject of the legal hold are aware of the need to suspend any destruction of relevant information.

Spoliation

Spoliation is "the intentional destruction, mutilation, alteration or concealment of evidence" relevant to a legal proceeding (AHIMA e-HIM Work Group on e-Discovery 2006). It is a legal concept applicable to both paper and electronic information. When evidence is destroyed that relates to a current or pending civil or criminal proceeding, it is reasonable to infer that the party had consciousness of guilt or another motive to avoid the evidence. In *Coleman Parent Holding Inc. v. Morgan Stanley & Co., Inc.*, the jury was instructed to find an adverse inference for the spoliation of evidence.

Spoliation of evidence has long been a concern of courts. The modern legal doctrine addressing spoliation of evidence began in 1959 (Eng 1999). It is this doctrine that drives the duty to preserve documents in the context of litigation. Various state and federal laws, such as the Sarbanes-Oxley Act of 2002, which enforces corporate accountability, broaden the reach of the spoliation doctrine from mere litigation matters to pending federal or state agency investigations.

Some jurisdictions have recognized a spoliation tort action, which allows the victim of destruction of evidence to file a separate tort action against the spoliator (Matthiesen 2016). This action, though, has been inconsistent in its application due to lack of clarity on whether the tort can be filed simultaneously with the civil action. In addition, some courts have required evidence of bad faith (that is, intentional destruction of evidence) for a plaintiff to successfully proceed (see figure 5.6). Other courts, further, have disallowed spoliation claims in conjunction with primary lawsuits alleging negligence rather than intentional wrongdoing. Courts will allow the spoliator to rebut the inference of guilt through explanations that demonstrate a lack of bad faith. A good legal hold process, as outlined in the previous section, and sound policies on retention and destruction can prevent spoliation.

In 2003 and 2004, a series of legal cases (the *Zubulake* cases) related to e-discovery and spoliation, provided for the application of the Sedona Guidelines in the courtroom setting by Judge Shira Scheindlin of the federal district court for the Southern District of New York (The Sedona Conference 2007). Among the principles established were:

- "Electronic documents are no less subject to discovery than paper records, and this is true not only of electronic documents that are currently in use, but also of documents that may have been deleted and now reside only on backup disks" (*Zubulake v. UBS Warburg*, 217 FRD 309)
- There exists a "duty to preserve backup tapes" (*Zubulake v. UBS Warburg*, 220 FRD 212)
- "When evidence is destroyed in bad faith, i.e., intentionally or willfully, that fact alone is sufficient to demonstrate relevance for purpose of sanction for spoliation of evidence; by contrast, when the destruction is negligent, relevance must be proven by the party seeking sanctions" (*Zubulake v. UBS Warburg*, 229 FRD 422)

Figure 5.6 Spoliation as a tort action

Phillips v. Covenant Clinic involved a wrongful death action brought by the plaintiff after her father suffered cardiac arrest and died on his way from a physician clinic to a hospital for medical testing. The plaintiff sought discovery of her father's record from the physician clinic, and was informed that the record was missing. Witnesses for the clinic testified that the clinic record was delivered to the hospital and disappeared at some point thereafter.

In a motion to the court, the defendants argued that the plaintiff failed to establish a causal relationship between the physicians' purported breach of the standard of care and her father's death. The plaintiff countered that the defendants' failure to produce the record entitled her to an inference that the missing medical record contained evidence unfavorable to the defendants.

The court agreed that intentional destruction of or failure to produce relevant records supports an inference that the records would have been unfavorable to the party responsible for their destruction or nonproduction. However, the court went on to note that the inference can only be based on the intentional destruction of evidence, stating, "It is not warranted if the disappearance of the evidence is due to mere negligence, or if the evidence was destroyed during a routine procedure."

Further, the court stated that the missing evidence must have been in control of the party who would ordinarily be responsible for its production. In granting summary judgment in favor of the defendants, the court found that no facts suggested that the clinic had intentionally destroyed the record. Without the inference provided by spoliation of evidence, the plaintiff was unable to establish the case.

These principles were strengthened in a 2010 opinion by Judge Scheindlin, where failures among the defendants to produce documents were found to be negligent in some instances and grossly negligent in others, thus warranting the application of sanctions (*The Pension Committee of the University of Montreal Pension Plan, et al., v. Banc of America Securities, LLC, et al.*, 05 Civ. 9016 (SAS), opinion and order filed January 11, 2010).

With respect to the preservation of records as evidence, one court observed that the duty to preserve evidence applies both to the period of time preceding litigation, when such litigation is anticipated, as well as the time period of the litigation process itself (*Silvestri v. General Motors*).

Spoliation of electronic records should be prevented through the same standards as those used for paper records; however, there are some differences. Data that have been deleted appropriately or inappropriately from an electronic record can often be recovered using software tools. It is important that policies outline the proper steps for making changes to electronic documentation. Most importantly, procedures for making corrections must be followed to eliminate the inference that information was intentionally altered. EHR systems must have functionality that meets the organization's requirements for making corrections. Inaccurate entries are far more likely to result in a malpractice claim than spoliation is.

Retention and Destruction of Health Information

Data and information governance policies and procedures related to the retention and destruction of health information and records should offer guidance and direction to a healthcare provider when protecting information as part of the discovery and e-discovery processes mentioned previously in this chapter. A healthcare provider must have knowledge of where its information is stored, how long it is kept, when it may be destroyed, and whether the information is in paper or electronic form. How long data or information is kept is a matter of legal and regulatory requirements, and business needs reflective of the type of healthcare entity (e.g., clinic, critical access hospital, minors, hospital) (Baldwin-Stried Reich et al. 2012).

Guidelines should identify where information may be found, such as backup tapes, instant messages, voicemail, word processing drafts, and shadow records, as well as when parts or all of the legal health record, audit trails, metadata, e-mails, and other business records should be destroyed. A healthcare provider must also ensure that any vendor or contractor possessing provider records is aware of the discovery rules and has the ability to comply with the rules, including the ability to preserve information and protect it from spoliation (AHIMA e-HIM Work Group on e-Discovery 2006). Guidelines should also address long-term digital preservation where data and information from old media are transferred to new media or from one information system to a new system (Kloss 2015). Further discussion of record retention and destruction issues is found in chapter 9, "Legal Health Record: Maintenance, Content, Documentation, and Disposition."

Disaster Recovery and Business Continuity

As with retention and destruction guidelines, a healthcare provider must have plans that address how health information in either paper or electronic format will be preserved in the event of a natural or man-made disaster. The plan should provide for how the provider will return to normal operation as quickly as possible, with attention to prevention of loss and restoration of access to records including legal discovery within a reasonable time frame (AHIMA 2006).

Managing the Discovery Process

Managing the discovery process along with the e-discovery and evidentiary rules is challenging. Provider methods and formats used to retain, manage, store, and destroy paper and electronic records must be understood as well the processes for producing and protecting information for litigation purposes (Baldwin-Stried Reich 2012). Organizational policies and procedures should be written to clearly define the organizations responsibility in protecting the information from modification or destruction and to ensure that privileged information is not being furnished inappropriately.

Check Your Understanding 5.3

Instructions: Indicate whether the following statements are true or false (T or F).

1. Spoliation is the accidental destruction of evidence.
2. The purpose of a "legal hold" is to prevent spoliation of potential evidence.
3. Organizations with electronic information should develop guidelines to identify where information may be hidden or not readily apparent.
4. A legal hold requires the preservation of both paper and electronic records.
5. A record retention schedule that outlines when records may be destroyed enable an organization to destroy records regardless of a legal hold.

Protection of Related Medical Documentation

Not all documentation related to patient care is made solely in the health record. In some circumstances, usually when there has been a medical error or some other unexpected adverse event, additional documentation is made in incident reports and peer review records. As discussed later, incident reports and peer review records are part of facility processes designed to document, investigate, and learn from errors and other unexpected events. The law, to varying degrees among different states, generally protects these records from disclosure in court.

Incident Reports

Incident reports are the means through which occurrences that are inconsistent with a healthcare facility's routine patient care practices or operations are documented (Dunn 2003, 46, 49). For example, an incident report should be generated if a nurse administers an incorrect dosage of medication to a patient or if a visitor slips and falls on a freshly mopped hospital hallway. The purpose of an incident report is to document the facts of the incident so that an internal investigation of that incident may be conducted. The main goals of incident reporting are to

- Describe the unexpected occurrence or incident
- Provide the foundation for an investigation of the occurrence or incident
- Provide information necessary for taking remedial or corrective action
- Provide data useful for identifying risks of future similar occurrences (Dunn 2003, 49)

Incident reports involving patient care provide a basis for investigating the incident. Specific requirements for incident reporting are addressed through state laws most often found in risk management statutes. Chapter 17 provides a discussion of the legal requirements related to risk management programs.

From an evidentiary standpoint, incident reports should not be placed in a patient's health record, nor should documentation in the record refer to an incident report having been completed. Most state laws consider incidents reports as "privileged" provider communication and thus protect incident reports from being admitted into evidence during legal proceedings. The rationale for protecting incident reports is based on the belief that providers or organizations will be more frank in their investigations of incidents, which will help reduce the likelihood of similar incidents in the future. The state law protection or "privilege" of incident report documentation can be waived, however, if the health record contains or refers to the incident report. In those situations, the incident report could be considered admissible as evidence, because the privilege has been waived via including that information in the health record.

After an incident has occurred, documentation in the health record should occur in the same manner as it is routinely completed for patient care. In other words, all the information relevant for a patient's treatment, such as a description of what occurred, the results of evaluation, and the treatment provided, should be documented by those providing care (Dunn 2003, 57). The health record generally should not refer to names (unless necessary for patient care), nor should it make excuses or cast blame for any incident (Dunn 2003, 57).

It is important to note that not all state law privileges or protections for incident report documentation prevent the records from being admitted into evidence. From a plaintiff's standpoint, incident reports or related documentation may be critical to proving a negligence claim. The plaintiff may therefore seek a court order or ruling that allows documentation to not only be discovered but also be admitted into evidence. In such situations, the court will often weigh the rights of the plaintiff against the policy behind the incident reporting protection or privilege law. If the court determines that the information contained in the incident report is necessary to the plaintiff's case, it may admit the incident report into evidence despite the existence of the privilege. Alternatively, the court may conclude that the documents at issue fall outside the scope of the privilege or that the defendant waived the privilege in some way (for instance, by referring to the incident report in the health record). Individuals who manage health information should be aware of incident reporting laws and court decisions that are applicable in their own states. Figure 5.7 illustrates such a situation.

| Figure 5.7 | Admission of incident report as evidence |

In *Riverside Hosp., Inc. v. Johnson,* the plaintiff's wife was hospitalized for lymphoma but suffered a hip fracture during her hospital stay after leaving her bed without assistance. She died several months later as a result of lymphoma. The plaintiff sued on behalf of his wife's estate, alleging that Riverside failed to accurately assess his wife's risk of falling and then failed to implement appropriate measures to prevent her from falling. The jury returned a verdict against Riverside and one of its nurses in the amount of $1 million.

The defendants believed that certain evidence was improperly admitted during trial and appealed the judgment. Specifically, the defendants argued that the trial court erred in allowing a quality care control report (QCCR) and a quality management services (QMS) database report, which were used to document factual information about the plaintiff's wife's fall (date, place, time, circumstances, severity, and so forth, of the fall). The defendants argued that the documents constituted incident reports and were therefore protected from being admitted into evidence under Virginia law. The court ruled that the documents fell outside the scope of the Virginia privilege law. According to the court, the documents were not "generated by a peer review or other quality care committee referred to in the statute". Nor were the documents created during a deliberative process involving the overall evaluation of patient safety conditions and the design of initiatives to improve the healthcare system. The court went on to state:

> Factual patient care incident information that does not contain or reflect any committee discussion or action by the committee reviewing the information is not the type of information that must 'necessarily be confidential' in order to allow participation in the peer or quality assurance review process.

The court concluded that the reports were health records of the hospital, made and kept in the normal course of operation of the hospital, and were therefore not protected by the Virginia privilege law from disclosure in court.

Peer Review Records

Another type of documentation that is generated outside of the health record involves documentation of peer review activities. **Peer review** involves a broad range of activities undertaken by a peer review committee to ensure that a facility provides quality care and may include such activities as the review of quality and safety issues and determinations of medical staff credentials, by using physicians to review the care of other physicians. Individual state law generally defines the specific scope of peer review activities. It may also provide statutory protection to peer review documentation from being disclosed in court or in preliminary proceedings. For example, in Kansas, hospital peer review activities include

- Evaluating and improving the quality of healthcare services rendered by healthcare providers
- Determining that health services rendered were professionally indicated or were performed in compliance with the applicable standard of care
- Determining that the providers of professional health services in this area considered the cost of healthcare rendered reasonable
- Evaluating the providers' qualifications, competence, and performance or taking action in disciplinary matters
- Reducing morbidity or mortality
- Establishing and enforcing guidelines designed to keep healthcare costs within reasonable bounds
- Conducting research
- Determining whether a hospital's facilities are being properly utilized
- Supervising, disciplining, admitting, determining privileges for, or managing members of a hospital's medical staff
- Reviewing the professional qualifications or activities of healthcare providers

Figure 5.8 Use of peer review reports as evidence

In *Adams v. St. Francis Regional Medical Center,* the plaintiffs brought a wrongful death suit against the defendants after their daughter died from a ruptured ectopic pregnancy at the defendant hospital. One issue in the case was the admissibility of several reports, including disciplinary reports of a nurse who treated the plaintiffs' daughter. The defendant objected to the admission of the reports based on peer review privilege.

The court recognized that, based on a literal reading of the Kansas peer review statute (detailed earlier), the disciplinary reports were protected from discovery. This, however, did not end the court's inquiry. According to the court, the privilege had to be weighed against the plaintiffs' right to "due process and the judicial need for the fair administration of justice." The court concluded that, based on the facts of the case, the peer review privilege was outweighed by the plaintiffs' right to have access to all relevant facts to their case. The court specifically noted, "Forms and documents containing factual accounts and witnesses' names are not protected simply because they also contained the officers' or committee's conclusions or decision-making process." Instead, the court can simply order the redaction (removal) of the parts of the documents containing analysis but still grant plaintiffs access to portions of documents containing relevant facts.

- Evaluating the quantity, quality, and timeliness of healthcare services rendered to patients in the facility
- Evaluating, reviewing, or improving methods, procedures, and treatments being utilized by inpatient and outpatient staff (Kan. Stat. Ann. 65-4915(d)).

As with incident reporting, it is common for plaintiffs to attempt to discover and admit peer review records into evidence during cases alleging negligence. As mentioned previously, state law may provide a peer review privilege generally protecting these records from being used in litigation. The rationale behind the privilege is that providers will be more candid in admitting fault or identifying problems if they know that this information will not later be used against them in court. By encouraging complete candor, hospitals are better able to identify, respond to, and prevent acts falling below the acceptable standard of care. However, whether the privilege will apply to keep records from being introduced as evidence depends on the facts of the particular case. In some states, hospital peer review committees carefully label all committee documents as peer review materials to try to ensure that the materials are protected; however, merely labeling the information as such does not mean that courts will always consider all materials protected. See figure 5.8 for a case involving the use of peer review records as evidence. It is again important for individuals responsible for managing health information to understand the scope of the peer review privilege law that applies in their states.

Check Your Understanding 5.4

Instructions: Indicate whether the following statements are true or false (T or F).

1. Incident reports are created for patient treatment purposes and should be a part of the health record.
2. State law may protect incident reports from being admitted into evidence.
3. The purpose of an incident report is to hide the fact that the incident occurred by documenting on the report rather than documenting anything in the health record.
4. Peer review involves activities undertaken to ensure the provision of quality care.
5. Plaintiffs commonly attempt to discover and admit peer review records into evidence during negligence cases against health care providers.

Scenario 5

A member of the hospital's medical staff has been accused of improperly billing Medicare for treatments done in his office that were not medically necessary. A subpoena for copies of patient records was received, but the subpoena does not include a patient authorization for release of records. In addition, the subpoena requests all "peer review committee" records pertaining to this physician. Consider the following questions:

1. What must you check before releasing the patient records?

2. What legal concept described in this chapter will determine admissibility of the hospital records into evidence?

3. The defendant's lawyer objects to the subpoena, arguing that the patient records are "hearsay". To resolve this issue, identify at least one element will likely be required in your testimony.

4. Your hospital attorney objects to the subpoena of the peer review committee materials, citing state law that protects peer review records from discovery. What legal concept describes this protection?

5. While acting on the subpoena, you discover that one of the patient records (which are electronic) has had major sections deleted. Your review of the audit trails determines that a hospital staff member was responsible for the deletions. Under what legal concept could the hospital be subject to liability for the deletions? What should have been done to protect the records?

References

AHIMA. 2013. E-Discovery litigation and regulatory investigation response planning: Crucial components of your organization's information and data governance processes. *Journal of AHIMA* 84(11): expanded web version.

AHIMA e-HIM Work Group on e-Discovery. 2006. Practice brief: The new electronic discovery civil rule. *Journal of AHIMA* 77(8):68A–H.

AHIMA e-HIM Work Group on Maintaining the Legal EHR. 2005. Practice brief: Maintaining a legally sound health record—Paper and electronic. *Journal of AHIMA* 76(10):64A–L.

American Medical Association Advocacy Resource Center. 2015. Apology inadmissibility laws: Summary of state legislation. http://www.ama-assn.org/ama/pub/advocacy/state-advocacy-arc.page?.

Baldwin-Stried Reich, K., K. Ball, M. Dougherty, and R. Hedges. 2012. *e-Discovery and Electronic Discovery*. Chicago: AHIMA Press.

Cavanaugh, F., W. Rishel, P. Spitzer, and J.P. Tomes, eds. 2000. *Comprehensive Guide to Electronic Health Records*. New York: Faulkner and Gray.

Drury, B., P. Trites, R. Gelzer, and P. George. 2014. Electronic health records systems: Testing the limits of digital records' reliability and trust. *Ave Maria Law Review* 12(2):257–289.

Dunn, D. 2003. Incident reports: Their purpose and scope. *AORN Journal* 78(1):46, 49.

Eng, K. 1999. Legal update: Spoliation of electronic evidence. *Boston University Journal of Science and Technology Law*. 5:L13.

Garner, B.A. 2014. *Black's Law Dictionary*, 10th ed., abridged. St. Paul, MN: Thomson Reuters.

Kearney, D. 2014. How to prepare the record for an e-discovery request. *Journal of AHIMA* 85(2):52–53.

Kloss, L. 2015. *Implementing Health Information Governance*. Chicago: AHIMA Press.

Matthiesen, Wickert & Lehrer, S.C. 2016. Spoliation of evidence in all 50 states. https://www.mwl-law.com/wp-content/uploads/2013/03/spoliation-of-laws-in-all-50-states.pdf.

McLean, T., L. Burton, C. Haller, and P. McLean. 2008. Electronic medical record metadata: Uses and liability. *Journal of the American College of Surgeons* 206(3):405–411.

National Court Rules Committee. 2016. *Federal Rules of Evidence.* Michigan Legal Publishing Ltd, https://www.rulesofevidence.org/.

The Sedona Conference. 2007. The Sedona Principles: Best practices recommendations and principles for addressing electronic document production. 2nd ed. http://www.thesedonaconference.com/.

USLegal. 2016. Breach of fiduciary duty law & legal definitions. http://definitions.uslegal.com/b/breach-of-fiduciary-duty/.

Cases, Statutes, and Regulations Cited

Adams v. St. Francis Regional Medical Center, 264 KS 144, 955 P.2d 1169 (1998).

American Color Graphics v. Rayfield Foster, AL Civ. App., 838 So.2d 374 (2001).

Broek v. Park Nicollet Health Services, MN App. Unpub. (2003).

Coleman Parent Holding Inc. v. Morgan Stanley & Co., FL Dist. Ct. App. 892, So. 2d 496 (2004).

Connecticut v. Abney, 88 CT App. 495; 869 A.2d 1263 (2005).

Fabich v. Montana Rail Link, Inc., MT Dist., 2005 ML 135.

Fierstein v. DePaul Health Center, MO Ct. App. E.D., 24 S.W.3d 220 (2000).

Fred's Stores of Tennessee v. Brown, MS App., 829 So. 2d 1261 (2002).

In the Matter of J.B., 172 N.C. App. 1; 616 S.E.2d 264 (2005).

Kohl v. Tirado, 256 GA App. 681, 569 S.E.2d 576 (2002).

Lipschitz v. Stein, NY App. Div., 10 A.D.3d 634, 781 NYS.2d 773 (2004).

Mapes v. District Court, 250 MT 524; 822 P.2d 91 (1991).

The Pension Committee of the University of Montreal Pension Plan, et al., v. Banc of America Securities, LLC, et al., SDNY, 05 Civ. 9016 (2010).

Phillips v. Covenant Clinic, 625 N.W.2d 714, Iowa (2001).

Riverside Hosp., Inc. v. Johnson, 272 VA 518, 636 S.E.2d 416 (2006).

Silvestri v. General Motors, 4th Cir., 271 F.3d 583, 591 (2001).

United States v. Syme, 3rd Cir., 276 F.3d 131 (2002).

Wesley Medical Center v. Clark, 234 KS 13, 669 P.2d 209, 220–221 (1983).

Williams v. Sprint/United Management Company. 230 F.R.D. 640 (D. Kan. 2005).

Zubulake v. UBS Warburg, SDNY, 217 FRD 309 (2003).

Zubulake v. UBS Warburg, 220 FRD 212 (2003).

Zubulake v. UBS Warburg, 229 FRD 422 (2004).

FRE 401: Definition "Relevant Evidence." 1975.

FRE 402: Relevant Evidence Generally Admissible; Irrelevant Evidence Inadmissible. 1975.

FRE 403: Exclusion of Relevant Evidence. 1975.

FRE 801: Definitions. 1975.

FRE 803: Hearsay Exceptions; Availability of Declarant Immaterial. 1975.

FRE 901: Requirement of Authentication or Identification. 1975.

FRE 1001(1): Definitions. 1975.

FRE 1002: Requirement of Original. 1975.

FRE 1003: Admissibility of Duplicates. 1975.

FRE 1004: Admissibility of Other Evidence of Contents. 1975.

Kansas Administrative Regulation 102-1-10a(g): Unprofessional conduct. Misrepresenting the services offered or provided. 2002.

Kan. Stat. Ann. 60-427(b): Privileged communications. Physician/patient. 2000.

Kan. Stat. Ann. 65-4915(d): Peer review officer or committee. 2000.

Kan. Stat. Ann. 65-6315(a)(3): Confidential information and communication exception. 2000.

Sarbanes-Oxley Act of 2002. Public Law 107-204, 116 Stat. 745.

Resources

K&L Gates. 2016. Current Listing of states that have enacted e-discovery rules. http://www.ediscoverylaw.com/state-district-court-rules/.

Tort Law

Laurie A. Rinehart-Thompson, JD, RHIA, CHP, FAHIMA

Learning Objectives

- Differentiate between the various types of torts
- Compare the legal theories of health institution liability
- Select the appropriate causes of action and defenses associated with the improper disclosure of health information
- Discuss liability of the health information professional
- Contrast factors used to determine statutes of limitation
- Appraise situations when criminal liability applies to healthcare situations
- Compare and contrast the effectiveness of various tort reform measures

Key Terms

- Act of God
- Actual causation
- Affidavit of merit
- Affirmative defense
- Agency
- Assault
- Assumption of risk
- Battery
- Breach of confidentiality
- Breach of duty
- Causation
- Charitable immunity
- Collateral source payment
- Comparative negligence
- Compensatory damages
- Contingency fee
- Contract law
- Contributory negligence
- Corporate negligence
- Criminal negligence
- Damages
- Defamation

- Discovery rule
- Economic damages
- Emotional distress
- False imprisonment
- Fiduciary duty
- Foreseeability
- General damages
- Good Samaritan statutes
- Gross negligence
- Health Insurance Portability and Accountability Act of 1996 (HIPAA)
- Immunity
- Intentional infliction of emotional distress
- Injury
- Intentional torts
- Invasion of privacy
- Joint and several liability
- Liability
- Libel
- Malfeasance

- Malpractice
- Medical malpractice
- Medical malpractice insurance
- Misfeasance
- Negligence
- Negligent infliction of emotional distress
- No-fault insurance
- Nominal damages
- Noneconomic damages
- Nonfeasance
- Ordinary negligence
- Partial/modified comparative negligence
- Proximate causation
- Punitive damages
- Pure comparative negligence
- Reasonably prudent person
- *Res ipsa loquitur*
- Rescue doctrine
- *Respondeat superior*

- Secondary liability
- Slander
- Special damages
- Standard of care
- Statute of limitations
- Statute of repose
- Strict liability
- Structured settlement
- Sudden emergency doctrine
- Tolled
- Tort
- Tort law
- Tort reform
- Tortfeasor
- Trier of fact
- Unavoidable accident
- Vicarious liability
- Writ
- Wrongful death

A **tort**, which is derived from the Latin *tortes,* or "twisted," is a civil wrong for which a court will determine liability. **Liability** is a legal obligation or responsibility that one party in a civil lawsuit has to another party, as determined by a court of law. Under tort law, the **tortfeasor** (the party who committed the tort) will be ordered by the court to provide a remedy in the form of **damages,** generally monetary compensation, to the party who was harmed. **Tort law** can be divided into three broad groups: a wrong involving the person or individual rights, a wrong involving the rights to personal property, and a wrong involving the rights to real property. Certain actions are both criminal and tortious. For example, theft of an individual's property is a crime against the state that may subject the defendant to criminal prosecution and imprisonment. The same wrongful act may give rise to a civil action for a conversion, entitling an individual to recover money damages against the individual who committed the criminal act. In a criminal proceeding, the state is responsible for prosecution of the case, and the objective of the suit is to punish the wrongdoer. In a civil action, the plaintiff is responsible for pursuing legal action, and the objective is to recover money damages to compensate for the loss.

We, as a society and a culture, decide the types of conduct that are considered acceptable or unacceptable. The development and evolution of tort law over the years has followed the path of social reform and the development of public policy. More than any other area, the law of torts reflects our social and cultural views as to what is acceptable and unacceptable conduct with respect to morality, fairness and reasonableness.

An understanding of tort law is important to health law in general, because it is the area of the law on which most healthcare lawsuits are based. This chapter will introduce types of tort legal actions, or causes of action, with a focus on negligence because it is the predominant type of wrong alleged in tort legal actions. The reader will also be introduced to causes of action for improper disclosure of health information, types of immunity from liability, statutes of limitation, and the distinction between tort and contract actions. The chapter will conclude with a discussion of criminal liability in healthcare and issues associated with medical malpractice.

Types of Torts

The US concept of torts originated in the common law of England, where the right to recover damages for a wrongful act depended on whether the king was willing to issue a **writ**, a formal written order issued by one with administrative or judicial jurisdiction over a case. Unless the plaintiff could identify a writ that applied to his or her situation, no remedy was available. In general, two writs were available for tortious conduct: trespass and trespass on the case. An action for trespass generally involved a direct and intentional interference with one's personal protected interest (such as bodily harm) or a property interest (such as harm to a person's possessions). A defendant who committed a trespass was imprisoned or fined. Trespass on the case evolved from trespass and was directed toward remedying conduct that was not necessarily intentional or directed toward the plaintiff's interest. For example, if a tortfeasor intentionally threw an object at victim A, a trespass action could result; however, if victim B was unintentionally struck by the object, he could bring a trespass on the case action.

The US legal system of today generally distinguishes between intentional torts (derived from trespass), which involve a deliberate or intentional act, and unintentional acts or negligence (derived from trespass on the case), in which the defendant does not necessarily intend to cause harm, but harm is a foreseeable consequence of the defendant's conduct. A third type of tort, strict liability, will also be discussed in this chapter.

Intentional Torts

Battery, assault, false imprisonment, and intentional infliction of emotional distress are all examples of **intentional torts**. There are defenses to each of these torts. Other torts, which may also be intentional, are relevant to health information. They include defamation, invasion of privacy, breach of confidentiality, and infliction of emotional distress, and they will be discussed as causes of action for improper disclosure of health information in the next section of this chapter.

Battery

Battery is intentional and nonconsensual contact. A certain amount of personal contact is inevitable in society and must be accepted as implied consent; in these situations, there is no tort. Examples include unavoidable contact in crowded venues and touching someone's arm to get their attention. Unless the recipient of the contact is known to be particularly sensitive, the appropriateness of a touching is based on how a reasonable and ordinary person would respond. The relationship between the person making the contact and the person being touched must also be considered. In general, lesser contact is expected or tolerated between strangers.

A defendant may be liable not only for contact that physically harms the plaintiff but also for relatively minor contacts that are offensive or insulting. Thus, spitting in the plaintiff's face or forcibly removing his or her hat may constitute battery. The law does not require that the defendant intended a certain result, but merely that the defendant intended a "touching." A defendant may be liable for battery where he or she intended only a joke or even a compliment, such as when a woman is kissed without her consent or the defendant makes a misguided effort to offer assistance. In the medical context, performing a procedure on a patient without the patient's consent (and presuming no exception allows it, such as a medical emergency) could give rise to a cause of action for battery. Patient consent is detailed in chapter 8. In some circumstances, the intent to commit a battery on one person may be transferred to a third person. If the defendant intended to commit a battery on one person but caused an unintended harmful contact to a different person, intent is transferred and the actual victim may be entitled to recover damages as if the defendant intended to affect him or her.

Assault

Assault is conduct causing apprehension that a harmful or offensive contact will occur, but it does not require actual contact. The harm is the plaintiff's mental apprehension that he or she may be the victim of a battery or other impermissible contact. Shaking a fist under another's nose, pointing a weapon, or even holding a weapon in a threatening position may constitute an assault. Mere words may also allow a plaintiff to recover for an assault. Hostile words that arouse apprehension in the plaintiff, such as threatening words or behaviors, may lead to the plaintiff's apprehension and a right to recover for assault.

False Imprisonment

False imprisonment is the intentional confinement of a person against that person's will. To be a viable legal action, it must include confinement of a person against his or her will, with absence of a reasonable means of escape, and no legal authority on the part of the person who is confining the other person.

A cause of action for false imprisonment may occur when an individual is hospitalized against his or her will, although legal exceptions exist regarding individuals in need of mental health treatment who pose harm to themselves or others, and individuals with certain contagious diseases. A familiarity with relevant state laws is necessary to appropriately address this type of situation.

Intentional Infliction of Emotional Distress

Intentional infliction of emotional distress is a common law tort for intentional conduct that results in extreme emotional distress. The elements are

- An intentional or reckless act (the defendant does not have to intend that emotional distress will occur; acting with reckless disregard is sufficient to meet this element)
- Extreme and outrageous conduct that is beyond the standards of civilized decency or is utterly intolerable in a civilized society
- The act of the defendant must have actually caused the emotional distress
- The emotional distress suffered by the plaintiff must be "severe"

Emotional distress may include manifestations such as sleeplessness, anxiety, irritability, or the emotional inability to perform activities or go places that the plaintiff was capable of prior to the conduct. To prove emotional distress, the plaintiff must demonstrate that he or she has suffered from one or more manifestations that have negatively impacted his or her life.

Defenses to Intentional Tort Claims

Potential defenses to intentional torts, depending on the specific tort alleged, include consent by the plaintiff (for example, a patient agreed to remain hospitalized); privilege by virtue of a relationship (for example, a parent spanks a child, but it is not considered battery because of the parent–child relationship); and necessity including self-defense or defense of others (for example, a person is not liable for assault or infliction of emotional distress if he was responding to protect himself or someone else).

Check Your Understanding | 6.1

Instructions: Indicate whether the following statements are true or false (T or F).

1. The law provides exceptions to false imprisonment liability where involuntarily hospitalized patients pose harm to themselves or others.
2. A tort is a civil wrong.
3. Liability refers to a legal obligation or responsibility.
4. Intentional infliction of emotional distress is a tort that results in extreme emotional distress to the plaintiff.
5. Assault is an intentional tort that involves nonconsensual contact with the plaintiff.

Negligence

Negligence is unintentional conduct that involves acting or failing to act in a way that a reasonably prudent person would act under the same circumstances, resulting in harm or injury to another (57A Am. Jur. 2d Negligence 2004). In other words, negligence is careless conduct. The law recognizes that when one person commits negligence and injures another, the injured person is entitled to compensation for his or her injuries.

Standard of care is what an individual is expected to do or not do in a particular situation (57A Am. Jur. 2d Negligence 2004). Standards of care may be established by statute or ordinance, judicial decision, professional associations, or practice (57A Am. Jur. 2d Negligence 2004). However, when none exists to define what is reasonable in a particular situation, the **trier of fact** (judge or jury) must determine what a reasonably prudent person would have done in the defendant's situation, and compare it to the defendant's behavior. Generally, a **reasonably prudent person** is a hypothetical person that a community believes exhibits ideal behavior in a particular situation and can differ from one situation to another (*Restatement of Torts* 1965). Negligence has not occurred if the defendant's behavior meets or exceeds the reasonably prudent person standard. However, if the defendant's conduct does not meet the reasonably prudent person standard, negligence has occurred. Negligence may occur even where an individual has evaluated alternatives and their consequences and has exercised his or her best possible judgment. Therefore, a person can be found negligent when he or she fails to protect against a risk that he or she knew could happen. Furthermore, negligence can occur where it is known, or should have been known, that a particular behavior would place others in unreasonable danger.

The standard of care in healthcare is similar to the standard of care generally, but the defendant is being compared to a reasonable provider in the same line of practice (Showalter 2015). As technology has enabled healthcare providers in remote locations to access more sophisticated medical resources for their patients, the community standard of care has given way to prevailing national standards.

Malpractice is the misconduct of professional persons including healthcare providers, attorneys, accountants, and others. **Medical malpractice** is misconduct by a healthcare provider against a patient. Medical malpractice can encompass both negligence and intentional torts, as well as breach of contract (which is discussed in chapter 7). Medical malpractice and negligence are often used interchangeably because negligence is the basis for most (but not all) medical malpractice lawsuits. However, they are not synonymous, because medical malpractice is a broader concept than negligence.

This section will discuss the types and degrees of negligence, elements required to prove negligence, damages awarded when negligence is proven, negligent infliction of emotional distress and *res ipsa loquitur*, defenses to negligence claims, and negligence theories under which healthcare organizations may be held liable.

Types of Negligence

Negligence can be categorized as

- **Nonfeasance:** failure to perform an act that a person is under a duty to do and that a person of ordinary prudence would have done under the same or similar circumstances (example: a patient presents with signs of a fracture, but the physician does not order an x-ray)
- **Misfeasance:** improper performance of an act that a person might lawfully do, or active misconduct that causes injury to another (example: a surgeon inadvertently nicks a patient's bladder while performing abdominal surgery)
- **Malfeasance:** performance of a wrongful act that may be unlawful (Pozgar 2016) (example: use of a joint replacement that an orthopedic surgeon knows will be problematic for the patient) (see 57A Am. Jur. 2d Negligence 2004)

Degrees of Negligence

Negligence can be categorized by the degree of wrongdoing. **Ordinary negligence** is the failure to exercise ordinary care. **Gross negligence** is very great or excessive negligence that implies an extreme departure from the ordinary standard of care and shows a reckless disregard for the rights of others. If defined as such by criminal statute, acts of gross negligence that demonstrate reckless or willful indifference to another's safety are acts of **criminal negligence**.

Elements of Negligence

To recover damages caused by negligence, the plaintiff must demonstrate that all four of the following elements of negligence are present:

- **Duty of care:** Did the defendant owe the plaintiff a duty of care? For example, did a physician–patient, nurse–patient, therapist–patient, or other relationship exist at the time of the alleged wrongful act?
- **Breach of duty:** Did the defendant deviate from his or her duty? The plaintiff must demonstrate that the defendant failed to exercise reasonable care under the given circumstances, either by acting or failing to act.
- **Injury:** Did the plaintiff suffer an injury as a consequence of the defendant's breach? Injury includes both physical and mental suffering.
- **Causation:** Is there a causal connection between the defendant's breach and the plaintiff's injury? There are two types of causation: cause in fact (actual causation) and proximate causation. **Actual causation** is determined by the "but–for" test: but for the defendant's action, the result would not have happened. For example, but for running the red light, the collision would not have occurred. **Proximate causation** is an event sufficiently related to a legally recognizable injury so as to be held as the cause of that injury. In other words, it is an act that results in injury through a natural, direct, uninterrupted consequence and without which the injury would not have occurred. In other words, there was **foreseeability** (that is, it was foreseeable that the defendant's actions would result in the plaintiff's injury) (57A Am. Jur. 2d Negligence 2004).

The four elements of negligence are outlined in figure 6.1.

Damages

A tort plaintiff may be entitled to several types of damages, which are intended to compensate a plaintiff for physical and monetary injuries. Damages can be divided into three broad categories: nominal

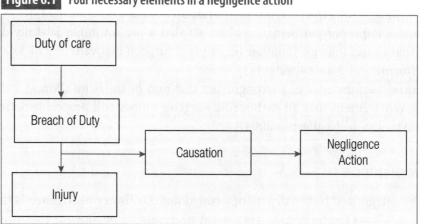

Figure 6.1 Four necessary elements in a negligence action

damages, compensatory damages, and punitive damages. **Nominal damages** are awarded simply to recognize wrongdoing by the defendant. They may be awarded when there is no substantial injury suffered by the plaintiff requiring compensation, or if the plaintiff has failed to demonstrate a dollar amount (Garner 2014).

Compensatory damages are the most common type of damages, and they compensate the plaintiff for losses incurred. They are divided into economic damages (special damages) and noneconomic damages (general damages). **Economic damages (special damages)** arrive out of the special circumstances of the event or person injured. Medical treatment costs and lost wages are the main types of special damages at issue in a personal injury tort claim. In contrast, **noneconomic damages (general damages)** directly result from the tort. For example, pain and suffering and emotional distress are part of general damages. Although economic damages can be readily verified through medical bills and lost wages, it is much more difficult—virtually impossible, in fact—to quantify intangible noneconomic damages.

Punitive damages exceed compensatory damages and are intended to punish and deter certain types of conduct, including tortious conduct. Such damages are most likely to be requested and awarded where the actions of the defendant(s) were reckless, wanton, careless, fraudulent, or so egregious as to warrant excess action by the court. In a 2014 case, a Louisiana court ordered two pharmaceutical companies, Japanese Takeda Pharmaceutical and its American counterpart Eli Lilly, to pay $9 billion in punitive damages because a diabetes drug, Actos, was linked to cancer. The punitive damages (although later reduced to $36.8 million by the court) were awarded by the jury after it learned that the cancer risks of the drug had been hidden (Fackler and Pollack 2014). Punitive damages may not be awarded without compensatory damages.

Negligent Infliction of Emotional Distress

Associated with negligence is **negligent infliction of emotional distress**. Negligent infliction of emotional distress should not stand alone as a cause of action, and even when it accompanies a negligence claim, it is often disfavored because it is vague and the value attached to it is undefined. As a result, it can easily be inflated.

Check Your Understanding 6.2

Instructions: Indicate whether the following statements are true or false (T or F).

1. The standard of care is what an individual is expected to do or not do in a particular situation.
2. Misfeasance is the failure to act per one's duty or according to the way a reasonably prudent person would act.
3. The two types of causation are actual and proximate.
4. Punitive damages punish the wrongdoer for tortious conduct that was committed.
5. Negligence is the second most common basis for medical malpractice lawsuits, following intentional torts.

Res ipsa loquitur

Generally, negligence is not inferred or presumed from an injury, and the plaintiff has the burden of proof and must prove all elements of his or her case. The exception to this rule is the doctrine of *res ipsa loquitur* (the thing speaks for itself), where the facts or circumstances accompanying an injury may permit an inference, of negligence by the defendant (57B Am. Jur. 2d Negligence 2004). This doctrine places the burden of proof on the defendant to show that he or she was not negligent. The classic example of *res ipsa loquitur* is a surgery where a surgical team leaves surgical instruments in a patient's body, resulting in injury. Such events do not "ordinarily occur in the absence of negligence."

The three elements of the *res ipsa loquitur* doctrine are

- Injury of a kind that ordinarily does not occur in the absence of someone's negligence
- Injury caused by an agency or instrumentality within the exclusive control of the defendant
- Injury not due to any voluntary action or contribution on the part of the plaintiff (57B Am. Jur. 2d Negligence 2004)

For example, in *Hake v. George Wiedemann Brewing Co.* (1970), the doctrine of *res ipsa loquitur* was applicable where a beer keg exclusively handled and controlled by the defendant rolled off an exterior second story stair platform, striking and injuring the plaintiff, who was walking underneath.

The doctrine may be applied in suits against hospitals to recover for injuries sustained by patients while they received treatment or care in the hospital. However, courts have held that it is inapplicable when the patient's condition might be due to some other cause than the alleged injury or accident on hospital premises, or when the evidence is insufficient to show that the injury was caused by the instrumentality alleged.

For example, in *Reese v. Bd. of Directors of Memorial Hosp. of Laramie Co.* (1998), a patient who alleged that she suffered a herniated disk because hospital employees failed to properly support her head and neck during oral surgery could not recover from the hospital on a *res ipsa loquitur* theory. Although the plaintiff identified several acts by hospital employees that allegedly constituted negligence, the evidence permitted a reasonable inference that her injury could have stemmed from other causes, including turning wrong or sneezing.

Several courts have warned that the *res ipsa loquitur* doctrine should be applied with caution and only under limited circumstances. In *Williams v. American Medical Systems* (2001), the plaintiff sued the manufacturer of a medical device implanted by the plaintiff's doctor. The court held that the *res ipsa loquitur* doctrine was not applicable where there was an intermediary cause that produced or could have produced the injury. Since the device was implanted by the plaintiff's doctor, it failed the *res ipsa loquitur* doctrine test because the device left the exclusive control of the manufacturer (defendant). The value of a *res ipsa loquitur* jury instruction to a plaintiff is that it permits the jury to infer negligence on an issue where the plaintiff may not have actual, discrete evidence or proof of negligence. Thus, mere control of an instrumentality permits an inference of negligence even though actual proof of negligence is lacking. Without the instruction, in certain circumstances it might be exceedingly difficult or impossible for a plaintiff to prove negligence.

Defenses to Negligence Claims

Defendants may raise a number of affirmative defenses in response to plaintiffs' negligence claims. An **affirmative defense** is one for which the defendant bears the burden of proving he or she is entitled to rely on them. Affirmative defenses to negligence claims are discussed next.

Contributory Negligence

The doctrine of **contributory negligence** bars a plaintiff from recovering any damages from the defendant if the defendant is able to prove that the plaintiff's conduct contributed in part to the injury that the plaintiff suffered. Contributory negligence has long been criticized because even if the defendant is

90 percent to blame for the plaintiff's injury and the plaintiff is only 10 percent to blame for his or her injury, the defendant is still relieved from having to pay damages to the plaintiff. Because it places such a high burden on the plaintiff, most states do not recognize this doctrine as an affirmative defense. For example, if a physician's mismanagement of a patient's diabetes was determined to be 90 percent the cause of the patient's negative outcome, but the patient was found to have contributed 10 percent to his own injury by failing to take his medication one time, the physician would not be liable and the patient would receive no monetary damages.

Comparative Negligence

Under the **comparative negligence** doctrine, a defendant demonstrates that the plaintiff's conduct contributed in part to the injury the plaintiff suffered. Unlike the doctrine of contributory negligence, in which the negligent plaintiff is completely barred from recovering damages, comparative negligence merely reduces the plaintiff's recovery by some amount based on his or her percentage of negligence. Using the previous example, if the defendant is liable for 99 percent of the injury and the plaintiff is liable for 1 percent, the defendant must pay 99 percent of the damage award.

Comparative negligence can be further divided into pure and partial or modified types. **Pure comparative negligence** permits a plaintiff to recover for the percentage of the defendant's negligence. Thus, referring to the plaintiff who was introduced in the previous section and was 10 percent to blame, the plaintiff would recover 90 percent of his or her losses (the amount caused by the physician), versus zero recovery per the theory of contributory negligence. **Partial or modified comparative negligence** allows a plaintiff to recover only if the plaintiff's negligence is "not greater than" or "not as great as" the defendant's negligence. For example, the plaintiff must be 50 percent or less at fault to recover. If the defendant is less than 50 percent negligent, then the defendant pays nothing. In the example given, the plaintiff would recover because he was less than 50 percent at fault, whereas the defendant was greater than 50 percent at fault.

Assumption of Risk

Assumption of risk is an affirmative defense that bars a plaintiff from recovering on his or her negligence claim if the defendant proves that the plaintiff had actual knowledge of a danger; understood and appreciated the risks associated with the danger; and voluntarily exposed himself or herself to those risks (57B Am. Jur. 2d Negligence 2004)

In the medical context (for example, in defending a medical malpractice claim), a defendant would be more likely to rely on contributory or comparative negligence principles (such as a plaintiff's failure to follow up as ordered or failure to follow other important medical advice) than on assumption of risk. The reason for this is that the assumption of risk defense usually contemplates a voluntary exposure by way of an affirmative act. True voluntariness is generally lacking in a patient who seeks medical care, as opposed to an individual who chooses an activity such as skiing or snowboarding. In the latter examples, a defendant who is sued following a skiing or snowboarding accident may be able to demonstrate the plaintiff's voluntary exposure.

Other Affirmative Defenses

According to the **sudden emergency doctrine, a person is relieved** of liability if, without prior negligence on his part, that person is confronted with a sudden emergency and acts as an ordinarily prudent person would act under the circumstances. (*Herr v. Wheeler,* 2006). An **unavoidable accident** is an occurrence that could not have been foreseen or anticipated in the exercise of ordinary care and that results without the fault or negligence of either the defendant or the plaintiff. **Act of God** refers to disasters that are not human related and not reasonably foreseeable. Damage from a natural cause, without any negligence by the defendant, does not result in liability. Contributory negligence and assumption of risk affirmative defenses may be barred by the **rescue doctrine**, which states that if a tortfeasor creates a circumstance that places a victim in danger, the tortfeasor is liable for the harm caused not only to the victim but also to any person injured in an effort to rescue the victim. This principle was demonstrated in *Wagner v. Int'l Railway* (1921), in which a railway company was held liable for injuries sustained by a rescuer who had fallen from a beam while searching for the body of his cousin, who had fallen from the train they were riding.

Theories of Healthcare Organization Negligence Liability

Healthcare organizations, including hospitals, have seen a growing exposure to negligence liability as they have assumed greater responsibility for monitoring the quality of care provided to patients and the medical staff who provide that care. Although hospitals were historically shielded from liability under the doctrine of **charitable immunity** due to their role as charitable organizations, this protection was gradually eliminated through state legislation and case law. *Darling v. Charleston Community Memorial Hospital* (1965), described in more detail in chapter 17, is a landmark case credited with significantly eroding charitable immunity protection. The courts have used two doctrines to establish liability: corporate negligence and *respondeat superior.*

Corporate Negligence (Primary Liability)

A healthcare organization may be held primarily liable (that is, liable in its own right) under the **corporate negligence** doctrine. Under this doctrine, the organization holds itself out as a provider of healthcare services and, therefore, also holds itself out as an entity subject to a lawsuit in an event of negligence. Under the corporate negligence doctrine, a healthcare organization owes its patients the duty to use reasonable care to maintain safe and adequate facilities and equipment; select and retain competent medical professionals; oversee all persons who practice medicine within the hospital; and formulate, adopt, and enforce rules and policies that ensure quality care for all patients (40A Am. Jur. 2d Hospitals and Asylums 2008). A plaintiff seeking to establish liability under the corporate negligence doctrine must prove that the healthcare organization deviated from the standard of care, it had actual or constructive notice of the defects or procedures that created the harm, and its act or omission was a substantial factor in bringing about the harm (40A Am. Jur. 2d Hospitals and Asylums 2008).

Respondeat superior/Vicarious Liability (Secondary Liability)

Generally, a healthcare organization is liable to patients for the torts of its employees (including nurses and employed physicians) under the doctrine of *respondeat superior* (Latin for "let the master answer"), also referred to as **vicarious liability** or **secondary liability**. Under this doctrine the organization holds itself out as responsible for the actions of its employees, provided that these individuals were acting within the scope of their employment or within the organization's direction at the time they conducted the tortious activity in question (40A Am. Jur. 2d Hospitals and Asylums 2008).

With respect to hospitals, the legal status between physicians and the hospitals in which they practice must be considered. Most commonly, physicians are granted privileges to practice in a hospital as independent contractors of the hospital rather than employees. A hospital is not held liable for the negligence of a physician with the status of independent contractor when the hospital (1) does not control the method or manner of the services the physician provides, and (2) provides meaningful notice of an independent contractor status to the patient, acknowledged at the time of admission. A hospital is, however, liable for the torts of independent contractors in the following situations:

- When the hospital contracts to provide medical services to a patient and has those services provided by an independent contractor
- When the hospital had reason to know that negligence would occur
- When the hospital holds out to the patient or the general public that the physicians associated with it are its employees, even if they are not. In this situation, liability would be premised on legal doctrines of **agency**, where individuals appear to others to be agents or representatives of the hospital or entity in which the individuals are providing services (40A Am. Jur. 2d Hospitals and Asylums 2008).

Some jurisdictions have enacted statutes that specifically provide that hospitals will not be held liable for negligent acts of healthcare professionals who are not agents or employees of the hospital. In *Fletcher v. South Peninsula Hosp.* (2003), the Alaska Supreme Court affirmed that a hospital was not liable for the negligent acts of an independent contractor surgeon, because the plaintiffs went to see a specific doctor for care, and the hospital repeatedly provided the plaintiffs with a disclaimer stating that the surgeon was an independent contractor and not an employee or agent of the hospital.

Strict Liability

Under the legal theory of **strict liability** (liability without fault), a person is responsible for the damage and loss caused by his or her acts and omissions regardless of fault. Although this theory prevailed historically, in more recent times, liability without fault has become limited to cases where abnormally dangerous activities are carried on. Examples include nuclear power plants and zoos that house wild animals. For example, under this theory, if a person was injured by an incident at a nuclear power plant, regardless of whether the defendant was at fault, the law would hold the facility strictly liable for injuries because operating a nuclear power plant is inherently an extremely hazardous activity.

The doctrine of strict liability in tort law can also be applied to product liability cases. To prevail on a product's liability claim, the plaintiff need only prove that he or she was injured by a defective product, regardless of the care taken to prevent the defect. Negligence is not required (Showalter 2015).

Check Your Understanding 6.3

Instructions: Indicate whether the following statements are true or false (T or F).

1. Per the theory of *respondeat superior*, a hospital is liable in its own right to the patients it serves.
2. Per the doctrine of *res ipsa loquitur*, an inference or presumption of the defendant's negligence is permitted.
3. Contributory negligence completely bars recovery by a plaintiff whose conduct contributed to the plaintiff's injury.
4. Assumption of risk is a viable defense by physicians in most medical malpractice cases.
5. Per the theory of corporate negligence, a hospital is liable in its own right.

Causes of Action for Improper Disclosure of Health Information

Civil causes of action encountered in healthcare settings are generally based on negligence or intentional torts (including previously discussed causes of action, such as battery, assault, false imprisonment, and intentional infliction of emotional distress). Improper disclosure of health information may lead to liability. The most serious consequence for improper disclosure of health information is criminal liability, which is generally defined statutorily. This section focuses on the more common causes of action that may be brought in connection with an improper disclosure of health information, including defamation (libel and slander), invasion of privacy, breach of confidentiality, infliction of emotional distress, negligence, and liability associated with the Health Insurance Portability and Accountability Act (HIPAA).

Defamation

Defamation of character is a false communication about a person to someone else that harms the first person's reputation. The false communication may be either oral or written. If oral, the defamation is called **slander**; if written, it is called **libel**. To prove a cause of action for defamation, the plaintiff must show the following:

- The defendant made a false and defamatory statement about the plaintiff.
- The statement was not a privileged publication (that is, made appropriately and in good faith to persons with a legitimate reason to know) and was made (published) to a third person.
- The conduct was an act of negligence or contained a higher degree of intent.
- Actual or presumed damages resulted.

Proof of special damages (such as economic losses) are not required when the plaintiff's reputation is at stake, including when the defendant allegedly accuses the plaintiff of a crime, accuses the plaintiff of carrying a loathsome disease, uses words that affect the plaintiff's professional or business activities, or calls a woman unchaste (Pozgar 2016). These types of attacks are inherently presumed to be damaging to a person's reputation, although an exception is granted to protect healthcare professionals against libel claims if they communicated information regarding loathsome diseases to comply with required reporting laws regarding communicable diseases.

There are several defenses available to defendants accused of defamation. First, there is no liability if the statement is true. In other words, truth is a defense. Second, a defendant may use the defense of privilege if the communication was made in good faith at an appropriate time and in an appropriate manner to persons who have a legitimate reason for receiving the communication (such as judicial proceedings or public safety). The defense of privilege is grounded in the law's recognition that certain privileged communications take priority over statements that may allegedly be defamatory. Authorization for the disclosure of information is also a defense. Finally, lack of publication to a third party is a viable defense. This means that the information has not been disseminated orally or in print (paper or electronic).

Invasion of Privacy

A person's right to privacy is "the right to be let alone—the right to be free from unwarranted publicity and exposure to public view, as well as the right to live one's life without having one's name, picture, or private affairs made public against one's will" (Pozgar 2016). The right to privacy also includes the right to control personal information (Pozgar 2016). To establish a claim for **invasion of privacy**, a plaintiff must establish a duty to not invade the privacy of or disclose confidential medical information of a patient, breach of that duty, and damages from the breach.

Courts recognize that absolute privacy cannot be practical in the healthcare setting, but they hold healthcare providers and personnel liable for negligent invasion of a patient's right of privacy. Courts are particularly sensitized to this right in instances because patients often cannot adequately protect their rights, because of illness, altered states of mind, unconsciousness, or immobility. In the healthcare setting, invasion of privacy can include disclosure of health information; the taking of photographs for medical, research, proprietary, or other purposes; and the presence of witnesses (for example, students) to a medical treatment or procedure.

Defenses to invasion of privacy claims include the patient's authorization or consent to the disclosure or other action that was taken; privilege, where legitimate interests are served by the disclosure or other action; and waiver, where the patient made public or otherwise placed his or her medical condition at issue.

Breach of Confidentiality (Fiduciary Duty)

A **fiduciary duty** is an obligation to act in the best interests of another party and is based on a special relationship of trust, confidence, and responsibility in certain obligations. This includes a duty by healthcare providers to maintain the confidentiality of patient information (in addition to the requirements imposed by HIPAA and detailed in chapters 10 and 11). To establish a claim for **breach of confidentiality** because of the unauthorized disclosure of a person's private information, a plaintiff must establish the following elements:

- Existence of a duty to not disclose health information
- A breach of the duty
- Damages

Breach of confidentiality and invasion of privacy have obvious similarities but are grounded in different principles. Invasion of privacy is grounded in principles of protecting privacy, whereas breach of confidentiality focuses on the special relationship—fiduciary in nature—between patients and healthcare providers.

Several cases have explored tortious conduct under the breach of confidentiality theory. For instance, in *Biddle v. Warren General Hospital* (1999), the Ohio Supreme Court held that "an independent tort exists for the unauthorized, unprivileged disclosure to a third party of nonpublic medical information that a physician or hospital has learned within a physician-patient relationship." In *Biddle*, several patients sued Warren General Hospital on learning that the hospital had entered an agreement with a law firm to screen patient intake forms to determine and pursue eligibility for Social Security reimbursements of medical expenses. Similarly, the Virginia Supreme Court in *Fairfax Hospital v. Curtis* (1997) concluded that a healthcare provider owes a duty of reasonable care to the patient to protect and preserve the confidentiality of patient information communicated to the provider in the course of treatment. A breach of that duty was held to be a tort. In *Anderson v. Strong Memorial Hospital* (1988), a New York court recognized breach of fiduciary duty as a valid claim in a case where an identifiable picture of the silhouette of the plaintiff was published in connection with an article about an AIDS diagnosis.

Defenses to breach of confidentiality claims include the patient's authorization or consent to the disclosure; privilege, where legitimate interests are served by the disclosure (for example, the safety of an individual or group of people); and waiver, where the patient made public or otherwise placed his or her medical condition at issue.

Infliction of Emotional Distress

Causes of action for the negligent or intentional infliction of emotional distress may be brought when a person whose health information has been improperly disclosed can establish that the improper disclosure caused emotional harm or injury. To recover under these causes of action, the injured person must establish that in making a nonprivileged disclosure, the defendant negligently, recklessly, or intentionally engaged in "extreme and outrageous conduct" that caused severe emotional distress (*Restatement of Torts* 1965).

A person who unintentionally causes emotional distress to another person is liable for causing injury to the other person if he should have realized that his conduct involved an unreasonable risk of causing the distress and, from the facts known, should have realized that the distress might result in illness or bodily harm (*Restatement of Torts* 1965).

A person whose health information has been improperly disclosed may also be able to allege that the disclosure amounted to an intentional infliction of emotional distress. To recover, a plaintiff must show that, in making the disclosure, the defendant intentionally or recklessly engaged in "extreme and outrageous conduct" that caused severe emotional distress (*Restatement of Torts* 1965, 46; *Johnson PPA v. Atlantic Health Services, P.C.*, 2000).

An authorization from a patient that permits the disclosure of that individual's health information may protect a defendant from liability in a claim for infliction of emotional distress.

Negligence for Improper Disclosure

Some states provide for improper disclosure of an individual's health records to be analyzed through a simple negligence inquiry, described earlier. Other states, however, have malpractice statutes to support lawsuits that relate to improper disclosure of personal health information (*Berger v. Sonneland*, 2000). In *Berger*, the court recognized the validity of a malpractice claim that alleged unauthorized disclosure of confidential health information.

Liability of Individuals Responsible for Protecting Health Information

The **Health Insurance Portability and Accountability Act of 1996 (HIPAA)** and state and federal privacy laws also impose liability for the improper use or disclosure of health information. Although violation of HIPAA is not a cause of action, civil and criminal liability may result from the improper use or disclosure of health information and for violation of other HIPAA provisions. As revised under the Health Information Technology for Economic and Clinical Health Act (HITECH), the minimum civil monetary penalty for a HIPAA violation is $100 per violation, with a $1.5 million fine per calendar year for identical violations (AHIMA 2013). On the other hand, damages for tort claims discussed previously are generally not controlled by statute. Instead, they are litigated under common law principles before a jury. Individuals responsible for protecting health information should explore professional liability insurance because they, in addition to their organization, may be named individually as defendants for the wrongful disclosure of patient information based on one or more of the theories discussed in this chapter.

Immunity from Liability

In addition to the various tort defenses previously described, **immunity** is a defense to tort liability that is extended to a particular group of persons or entities. There are two important aspects of an immunity defense. First, the defense of immunity does not deny the existence of the alleged tort; it merely denies any resulting liability. Second, immunity extends to only a limited group of people or entities. Immunity occurs because of the status or position of the defendant, not because of the facts of the case. The decision to extend immunity to a particular group of persons or entities is based on public policy. Therefore, others outside the group who engage in substantially similar conduct may be held liable for a tort.

Historically, immunity barred tort actions against governments, public officers, and charities, and it also barred litigation between spouses as well as parents and children. Today, the most important of these immunities is the immunity granted to governmental entities. Many of the other grounds for immunity have been eliminated. For example, immunity of charitable organizations as well as immunity between spouses no longer exists in most, if not all, states.

Governmental immunity, which is also referred to as sovereign immunity, originated from the common law idea that "the King can do no wrong." Certainly, under modern standards, this is flawed. Nevertheless, this defense continued as both the federal government and individual state governments were held to have immunity, absent consent, from tort liability. Additionally, the Eleventh Amendment to the United States Constitution prohibits a person or entity from suing a state in federal court.

Over time, courts and legislatures have adopted certain exceptions to governmental immunity. For example, in 1946 Congress adopted the Federal Tort Claims Act (28 USC 1346(b)), which generally permits tort claims against the federal government for its negligence. However, the act does not extend governmental liability to intentional torts. Additionally, immunity exists where the government acts with due care in carrying out a statute or regulation and for acts or omissions within the discretionary function of a federal agency or employee.

All states now consent to lawsuits under certain circumstances, and most states have statutes that govern the tort liability of state and local governmental entities and employees. These statutes typically establish a general governmental immunity but provide certain exceptions for particular types of activities. Some examples of exceptions include acts or omissions where the governmental agency is acting in a proprietary or private capacity, and acts or omissions outside the scope of a governmental employee's job duties.

Another type of immunity from liability is related to states' **Good Samaritan statutes** that provide legal immunity for ordinary negligence committed by persons who assist others in medical emergencies. The purpose of these statutes is to encourage individuals to provide good-faith emergency assistance, without fear of liability, in settings where lifesaving technology is not available. Such statutes vary from state to state, with some granting immunity only to specified healthcare professionals, and others granting immunity to "any person." Because Good Samaritan laws eliminate otherwise applicable common law rights of victims to be compensated for their injuries, these statutes raise a number of constitutional questions.

Check Your Understanding 6.4

Instructions: Indicate whether the following statements are true or false (T or F).

1. Fiduciary duty is the obligation to act in the best interests of another party.
2. To successfully claim breach of confidentiality, a plaintiff must establish that the defendant had a duty not to disclose the information.
3. Libel is spoken defamation.
4. Privilege is a defense to an invasion of privacy claim.
5. Good Samaritan statutes encourage good-faith emergency assistance by providing immunity if ordinary negligence is committed by those who assist in medical emergencies.

Statute of Limitations

A **statute of limitations** is a statutory enactment that places time limits on certain claims. For example, if a person is injured by the negligence of another, a statute of limitations will require an action to be brought against that person within a certain time period. The purpose of a statute of limitations is, first, to allow an injured person a reasonable amount of time in which to bring an action for recovery, and second, to allow claims to be resolved while evidence is reasonably available and fresh. It is important that lawsuits be brought before "evidence has been lost, memories have faded, and witnesses have disappeared" (*Order of Railroad Telegraphers v. Railway Express Agency,* 1944).

Generally, there are three steps involved in an application of a statute of limitations. First, one must identify the appropriate statutory period of limitations. Next, one must determine when that particular statutory period commenced or began to run. Finally, one must determine whether some condition or event suspended or postponed the operation of the statute of limitations.

Unlike the defense of immunity, a statute of limitations defense often varies depending on the type of tort claim asserted. For instance, intentional tort claims are usually subject to a different statutory limitations period than negligence claims. Additionally, although medical malpractice may be viewed as a form of negligence, many states have adopted special limitations periods for medical malpractice claims. Also, when a statute creates a cause of action, such as with claims for wrongful death, that particular statute will often contain its own limitations period.

The statutory period varies with the type of tort claim and the state in which the claim is filed. Each state has a comprehensive set of legislatively imposed periods of limitation related to torts. Thus, a malpractice claim arising in Ohio may have a different period of limitations than a similar malpractice claim arising in Florida.

Although a particular statute of limitations provides a time frame in which to bring an action, in some situations the parties involved may have contractually agreed on a different period of limitations. Unless such a contractual period is specifically disallowed by statute or public policy or is otherwise unreasonable, courts will usually enforce the agreement. For example, in *Thompson v. Ulysses Cruises, Inc.* (1993), a passenger on a cruise ship was injured when she slipped and fell. The court enforced a one-year limitations period contained on the five-page ticket that the passenger received.

Once the appropriate statute of limitations has been identified, one must next determine when the statutory period commenced or began to run. If a statute of limitations does not specifically identify when the period begins to run and the claim involves a single act or omission causing injury, the general rule is that the period begins to run when the act or omission causing injury is complete. Thus, if one commits an assault on another, the statutory period of limitations for an intentional tort begins to run at the time of the assault. On the other hand, if the injury is one that accrues over time, such as by exposure to a toxic chemical, the statute generally will not begin to run until the last exposure. As with most rules, there are certain exceptions to the general rules regarding the running of a statute of limitations. The tolling of a statute of limitations, as well as the statute of repose, are discussed next.

Tolling the Statute of Limitations

A statute of limitations may be impacted by several types of situations. A statute of limitations period may be **tolled** (postponed, suspended, or extended) primarily because of

- Inability to discover the injury (the discovery rule)
- Death of the injured individual

- Disability of the injured individual
- Wrongdoing by the individual or entity causing the injury

The discovery rule provides that, if the nature of an injury is inherently undiscoverable, a person exercising reasonable diligence will not be barred by the statute of limitations from bringing a lawsuit. An injury is inherently undiscoverable if it is unlikely to be discovered within the specified period of limitations. For example, during surgery a surgical team may inadvertently leave a surgical sponge inside a patient. Although the patient may experience some symptoms, he or she may have no reason to suspect that those symptoms are the result of negligent conduct. By the time the patient discovers the connection between the symptoms and the surgery, the statute of limitations may have expired. Thus, the discovery rule will toll the statute of limitations until the patient knows, or in the exercise of reasonable diligence should have known, of the injury.

When a person is injured by a tort and later dies, the statute of limitations will be affected. For example, a cause of action may occur before the death of the injured person and the time for commencement of an action has not expired, but the person did not sue prior to death. In most cases, the statute of limitations will be tolled for a period of time to allow an executor or administrator to be appointed and to bring an action. This, however, is different from a claim for **wrongful death**, a distinct claim with a separate statute of limitations that may be filed in addition to a tort claim to compensate the deceased individual's survivors.

If the injured individual is legally under a disability (such as minors and mentally impaired individuals), the statute of limitations is usually tolled until the disability has been removed. For example, if one commits a tort against a minor child, the statute of limitations will not begin to run until the child becomes an adult under the law of the state.

Finally, a statute of limitations may be tolled because of the wrongful actions of the tortfeasor-defendant. For example, if the tortfeasor attempts to conceal wrongdoing, the statute of limitations will be tolled. Additionally, a tortfeasor may be prevented from asserting a statute of limitations defense. For example, presume that two people are involved in a car accident. The person responsible for the accident promises to settle any and all claims. In the meantime, however, the statute of limitations expires. A court may prevent the wrongdoer-defendant from asserting a statute of limitations defense due to the promises made to the other person. Finally, a defendant can also waive a statute of limitations defense if it is not specifically asserted against the opposing party. For example, an injured person initiates a lawsuit by filing a complaint and sets forth a number of claims. If the defendant fails to assert the statute of limitations defense in answering the complaint, the defense is deemed to have been waived.

Statute of Repose

Many states, in the course of enacting tort reform measures, retain existing statutes of limitations for malpractice cases (for example, one year in Ohio) and personal injury cases (for example, two years in Ohio) but then add a maximum time period within which to discover and file a claim, subject to certain exceptions. Such a maximum limitation, beyond which legal action cannot be tolled, is called a **statute of repose.** For example, Ohio Revised Code 2305.113 contains a statute of repose provision that limits the discovery and filing of claims to four years under most circumstances. Important exceptions to a statute of repose include foreign objects (for example, a surgical instrument). Furthermore, certain classes of individuals, such as minors and persons of unsound mind, are subject to existing provisions of Ohio law that toll, or extend time limitations for bringing claims. Thus, the statute of repose does not apply to and does not run against individuals who are minors until they reach the age of majority.

Torts and Contracts

The focus of this chapter is torts, the causes of actions (that is, claims) that may be brought under tort principles, and defenses to tort claims. Another body of law often found in the healthcare context is contract law. **Contract law** is the body of civil law relating to agreements between parties, most often in the context of business or commercial relationships. Whereas the law of tort focuses on negligence or intentional wrongs committed by one party against another, the law of contract focuses on agreements between parties and the enforcement of such agreements. One critical difference between tort and contract law is that, by definition, negligence does not factor into the analysis and resolution of contract disputes. Contract law will be discussed in detail in chapter 7.

Criminal Liability in Healthcare

Wrongful acts committed in the healthcare environment generally lead to civil liability. However, wrongdoing in this arena can also constitute a criminal violation. One context in which criminal penalties may result is violation of the HIPAA Privacy Rule. Criminal violations of HIPAA privacy provisions are subject to penalties set forth in the United States Code at 42 USC 1320d-6(a). The key inquiry in a criminal violation is whether it was committed knowingly, which means either purposefully committing the act or acting in willful disregard of the existence of a statutory provision or scheme. Maximum penalties for criminal violations are set forth in 42 USC. 1320d-6(b). The imposition of penalties relating to federal crimes is subject to the Federal Sentencing Guidelines, which require the judge to consider the offense level and the defendant's criminal history in sentencing the defendant. Criminal penalties for knowingly committing privacy violations include the following:

- A fine of not more than $50,000, imprisonment for not more than one year, or both
- If the violation is committed under false pretense, the fine is not more than $100,000, imprisonment is for not more than five years, or both
- If the violation is committed with the intent to sell, transfer, or use personal health information for commercial advantage, personal gain, or malicious harm, the fine is not more than $250,000, imprisonment is for not more than 10 years, or both

The Office for Civil Rights of the US Department of Health and Human Services refers cases to the Department of Justice when criminal investigation is warranted. As of 2016, nearly 600 referrals had been made (OCR 2016), with fewer than 50 criminal prosecutions. In what is generally considered to be the first HIPAA privacy criminal prosecution, *U.S. v. Gibson* (2004), a covered entity employee was charged with illegal disclosure of a patient's personal health information to fraudulently obtain and use credit cards in the patient's name. Pursuant to the foregoing penalties, because the improper disclosure was for personal gain, the defendant was potentially subject to a fine of up to $250,000 and incarceration for up to 10 years. Pursuant to a plea agreement, the defendant was sentenced to 16 months in prison with three years of supervised release and more than $9,000 in restitution.

Criminal liability for wrongdoing in the healthcare context may result in other circumstances, just as criminal liability may result in business and other societal settings. For example, criminal liability issues may arise in antitrust, conspiracy, personal injury, health and safety, and fraud. Fraud, specifically fraudulent healthcare billing, has been aggressively pursued by the federal government. Led by the Office of Inspector General (OIG) for the US Department of Health and Human Services, healthcare providers have been and continue to be aggressively investigated and prosecuted for receiving payments through fraudulent activity. This will be discussed further in chapter 18.

Medical Malpractice Issues

This section addresses two interconnected issues: the overall rising cost of medical malpractice insurance and the ensuing cycle of medical malpractice insurance "crises" in certain states; and various state tort reform measures enacted to address medical malpractice, litigation, and malpractice insurance concerns.

Rising Cost of Medical Malpractice Insurance and Crisis Cycles

Physicians, as a rule, are covered by **medical malpractice insurance** to protect themselves from medical malpractice lawsuits, primarily medical negligence. The geographic region in which a physician practices, as well as the physician's specialty, affects malpractice insurance premiums. Specialty areas that are of particular risk for lawsuits, and hence higher medical malpractice premiums, include obstetrics and gynecology, and neurosurgery.

During the first decade of the 21st century, the medical malpractice insurance industry was identified as being in crisis. At its height in 2003, dramatic percentage increases every year resulted in soaring medical malpractice premiums. As a result, many states were labeled as "crisis states" (figure 6.2). The unaffordability of medical malpractice insurance in crisis states caused physicians to relocate, restrict their practices by discontinuing high-risk procedures or treatments, retire, or otherwise leave the practice of medicine. This left affected regions bereft of physicians in certain high-risk specialty areas. However, critics have pointed out that this crisis was not unique and that, in fact, medical malpractice crises cycle. The fact that medical malpractice insurance crises also occurred in the 1970s and the 1980s has been highlighted (Medical Liability Monitor 2010).

What is to blame for these cycling crises that are characterized by dramatic insurance premium increases? A number of factors have been suggested. At the forefront are excessive awards rendered by sympathetic juries who respond to the demands of aggressive personal injury attorneys. Others point to excess profit by insurance companies. In addition, inflation, lack of choice in insurance market

Figure 6.2	Medical liability crisis states in 2003
1. Arkansas	12. New York
2. Connecticut	13. North Carolina
3. Florida	14. Ohio
4. Georgian	15. Oregon
5. Illinois	16. Pennsylvania
6. Kentucky	17. Rhode Island
7. Massachusetts	18. Tennessee
8. Mississippi	19. Washington
9. Missouri	20. West Virginia
10. Nevada	21. Wyoming
11. New Jersey	

Source: Japsen 2003.

competition, changes in stock market returns that force insurance companies to make up for the losses elsewhere, and interest rates have each been blamed for forcing insurance premiums in a dramatically upward direction (LeBlang 2006).

Types of Tort Reform Measures

To lessen the strain on the healthcare industry, state and local legislatures have initiated measures in response to costly malpractice premiums, costly litigation, and mounting judgment awards. Various states, including crisis states, have instituted tort reform measures to control claims, causes of action, and judicial remedies to control malpractice costs.

Tort reform encompasses the variety of measures intended by legislatures to control the costs and perceived injustices associated with tort claims. With regard to medical malpractice, such reforms are intended to diminish the number of lawsuits and large jury verdicts, stabilize the market, and ultimately reduce premiums for physicians. Nationally, federal tort reform measures have been proposed. However, because torts are generally a matter of state law and federal tort reform faces potential constitutional challenges, efforts to control tort damage award payments have generally been left to the individual states. California is often identified as a model for its progressive tort reform measures under the 1975 Medical Injury Compensation Reform Act (MICRA), the legislative response to California's insurance crisis in the 1970s.

Tort reform measures include caps on noneconomic and punitive damages, affidavits of merit, limits on attorney contingency fees, consideration of collateral source payments, structured settlements, limits on statutes of limitations periods, joint and several liability, and no-fault systems.

Noneconomic and Punitive Damages

Noneconomic compensatory damages reimburse injured plaintiffs for losses that do not have a cash value, such as pain and suffering or emotional distress. Punitive damages punish defendants who are deemed to have acted maliciously or outrageously. Awarding noneconomic and punitive damages tends to be an emotionally charged and troubling process for juries and a significant challenge for the legal system. How does one attach a dollar value to a plaintiff's pain or disfigurement, or the diminished value of the quality of the relationship between the plaintiff and a family member due to the defendant's acts? Quite clearly, these sums cannot be computed. Plaintiffs and their attorneys, understandably, place high dollar values on noneconomic damages in an effort to recoup as much as possible. In turn, sympathetic juries award requested amounts to plaintiffs that often far exceed the actual harm. The effect is that professional malpractice insurance premiums are driven upward, creating incentives for would-be plaintiffs to file lawsuits. As a result, noneconomic compensatory and punitive damages have been targeted by many state legislatures, with monetary caps and/or stricter standards of proof put into place to stem the rising tide of jury awards.

Affidavit of Merit

To deter excessive or frivolous litigation, some jurisdictions require that an **affidavit of merit** accompanies a complaint to establish the sufficiency and validity of that complaint. In effect, it is a pretrial screening device. In Ohio, any complaint that contains a medical claim, dental claim, optometric claim, or chiropractic claim must include an affidavit of merit by an expert witness relative to each defendant in the complaint for whom expert testimony is necessary to establish liability. The affidavit of merit must include all of the following, pursuant to Ohio Civ. R. 10(D)(2)(a):

- A statement that the affiant has reviewed all medical records reasonably available to the plaintiff concerning the allegations in the complaint
- A statement that the expert is familiar with the applicable standard of care
- The opinion of the expert that the standard of care was breached by one or more of the defendants and the breach caused injury to the plaintiff

Limits on Attorney Contingency Fees

A **contingency fee** is the amount of money a plaintiff's lawyer receives based on the percentage of the money awarded to the plaintiff. It is commonly one-third of the total recovery. As opposed to charging the client an hourly fee, a contingency fee structure allows plaintiffs who otherwise could not afford a lawyer to seek redress in court without any financial investment. The contingent fee system is unique to the US legal system and has been heavily criticized because it allows lawyers to take riskier cases and encourages them to make excessive demands and seek cases that may be settled quickly with minimal time invested. Many states have implemented reform measures to curb the abuse of contingency fee arrangements by enacting statutes to limit the contingent fees in medical liability cases to certain percentages or provide that a court must review or approve the amount of the fees.

Collateral Source Payment

A **collateral source payment** is income a plaintiff in a tort case receives from a source other than the defendant(s). Under the general collateral source rule, defendants were prohibited from presenting evidence that a plaintiff received compensation for his or her injuries from any other source. Tort reform measures in many states allow courts to consider collateral source payments. One example of a collateral source payment issue in the medical malpractice context is where an injured plaintiff might recover twice if he or she received $100,000 in medical care for his or her injury under Medicare benefits and then attempted to recover the costs of medical care against the person who caused the injury. The intended effect of collateral source laws is to diminish the damages awarded by juries who are now aware of other financial resources that the plaintiff has.

Structured Settlements

In personal injury or tort settlements, parties may agree to a **structured settlement** arrangement in which the claim is paid in installments rather than in one lump sum, which can create an attractive windfall for eager plaintiffs and their attorneys. Often the defendant will purchase one or more annuities to guarantee the future payments. There is no set form for a structured settlement arrangement. In the United States, a structured settlement can significantly reduce taxes from the settlement and may even be tax-free.

Limits on Statute of Limitations Periods

As described earlier in the chapter, a statute of limitations is a statutory enactment that places time limits on certain claims. Some states have shortened the statute of limitations time periods for personal injury cases, including medical malpractice, in an effort to decrease the number of lawsuits filed.

Joint and Several Liability

Per **joint and several liability,** any one of the several codefendants in a lawsuit may be held liable for the entire amount of a judgment if the other defendants do not pay their portion. The rule of joint and several liability has sometimes been referred to as the "deep pocket" rule because of the perception that plaintiffs are inclined to sue multiple defendants to find the most financially lucrative target. For example, under this theory, financially lucrative Defendant A may be required to pay 100 percent of the damages, even though it is only 60 percent responsible, because the non–financially lucrative Defendant B is unable to pay its 40 percent share. Tort reform measures replace the rule of joint and several liability with one of proportionate liability, which means that a tortfeasor is liable only for its share or proportion of the injury it caused. Several states have enacted some form of joint and several liability reform legislation.

No-Fault Systems

No-fault insurance is an insurance contract under which insureds are indemnified (compensated) for losses by their own insurance company, regardless of fault in the incident generating losses. The term *no-fault* is most commonly used in the context of state automobile insurance laws in which a policy-holder (and his or her passengers) are not only reimbursed by the policyholder's own insurance company without proof of fault but also restricted in the right to seek recovery through the civil justice system for losses caused by other parties. Thus, in states that have adopted no-fault systems, minor accident and injury claims are generally resolved without litigation. However, in instances of catastrophic injuries or damages, no-fault states still permit an individual to bring claims where basic no-fault principles would not adequately protect or compensate the injured party.

Check Your Understanding   6.5

Instructions: Indicate whether the following statements are true or false (T or F).

1. The affidavit of merit allows a greater number of personal injury lawsuits to be filed.
2. A statute of limitations places time limits on certain claims.
3. A tolled statute of limitations is one that has been delayed or suspended.
4. Wrongful acts committed in the healthcare environment can lead only to civil liability.
5. Collateral source payments are payments received by the plaintiff from sources other than the defendant.

Scenario 6

Mrs. Stevenson was treated at the emergency room at Matthews Health, suffering from severe abdominal pain, nausea, and vomiting. The emergency room physician palpated her abdomen but did not order laboratory tests. She was discharged home with a diagnosis of indigestion and given medicine to lessen her symptoms. A day later, she returned to the emergency room with excruciating abdominal pain and worsening nausea and vomiting. At that time, she was diagnosed with a ruptured appendix, peritonitis, and septicemia. In this life-threatening condition, she was taken to surgery for an appendectomy and was given strong antibiotics for the next several weeks. Mrs. Stevenson filed a lawsuit against Matthews Health and the emergency room physician who discharged her home. Her attorney wants to seek economic and non-economic compensatory damages, and punitive damages. Consider the following:

Scenario 6 (Continued)

1. What cause of action will the lawsuit be based on? What elements must be proved?

2. If you were Mrs. Stevenson's attorney, what type(s) of damages would you seek?

3. Mrs. Stevenson receives monthly disability payments. If she wins her lawsuit, what tort reform measure applies to the fact that she receives these payments?

4. What other tort reform measures might be applicable to this case?

References

40A Am. Jur. 2d Hospitals and Asylums (2008).

57A Am. Jur. 2d Negligence (2004).

57B Am. Jur. 2d Negligence (2004).

American Health Information Management Association. 2013. Analysis of Modifications to the HIPAA Privacy, Security, Enforcement, and Breach Notification Rules Under the Health Information Technology for Economic and Clinical Health Act and the Genetic Information Nondiscrimination Act; Other Modifications to the HIPAA Rules. http://www.ahima.org.

Fackler, M. and A. Pollack. Jury Awards $9 Billion in Damages in Drug Case. *New York Times*. April 8, 2014. Available at http://www.nytimes.com/2014/04/09/business/international/japanese-drug-maker-ordered-to-pay-6-billion-over-cancer-claims.html?_r=0.

Garner, B.A. 2014. *Black's Law Dictionary*, abridged 10th ed. St. Paul, MN: Thomson West.

Japsen, B. AMA says Illinois, 5 other states join malpractice crisis. *Chicago Tribune*. March 4, 2003. Available at http://articles.chicagotribune.com/2003-03-04/business/0303040162_1_malpractice-coverage-malpractice-insurance-high-risk-specialties.

LeBlang, T.R. 2006. The medical malpractice crisis—Is there a solution? *Journal of Legal Medicine* 27(1):1–16.

Medical Liability Monitor. 2010 (October). Vol. 35, No 10. http://medicalliabilitymonitor.com.

Office for Civil Rights. 2016 (May 31). Enforcement highlights. https://www.hhs.gov/hipaa/.

Pozgar, G.D. 2016. *Legal Aspects of Health Care Administration*. 12th ed. Sudbury, MA: Jones and Bartlett.

Restatement of Torts (Second). 1965. Philadelphia, PA: American Law Institute.

Showalter, J.S. 2015. *The Law of Healthcare Administration*, 7th ed. Chicago: Health Administration Press.

Cases, Statutes, and Regulations Cited

Anderson v. Strong Memorial Hospital, 140 Misc.2d 770, 531 N.Y.S. 2d, 735 (1988).

Berger v. Sonneland, 101 WN. App. 141, 1 P.3d 1187 (2000).

Biddle v. Warren General Hospital, 86 Ohio St. 3d 395 (1999).

Darling v. Charleston Community Memorial Hospital, 33 Ill.2d 326, 211 N.E. 2d, 253, 14 A.L.R. 3d 860 (IL Sept. 29, 1965).

Fairfax Hospital v. Curtis, 249 VA 531; 457 S.E.2d 66 (1997).

Fletcher v. South Peninsula Hosp., 71 P.3d 833 (Alaska 2003).

Hake v. George Wiedemann Brewing Co., 23 Ohio St. 2d 65 (1970).

Herr v. Wheeler, 634 S.E.2d 317, 320 (Va. 2006).

Johnson PPA v. Atlantic Health Services, P.C., 2000 WL 1228275 (Conn. Super. Aug. 21, 2000).

Order of Railroad Telegraphers v. Railway Express Agency, 321 U.S. 342 (1944).

Reese v. Bd. of Directors of Memorial Hosp. of Laramie Co., 955 P.2d 425 (Wyo. 1998).

Thompson v. Ulysses Cruises, Inc., 812 F. Supp. 900 (S.D. Ind. 1993).

U.S. v. Gibson, No. CR04-0374RSM, 2004 WL 2237585 (W.D. Wash. August 19, 2004).

Wagner v. Int'l Railway, 232 N.Y. 176 (1921).

Williams v. American Medical Systems, 248 Ga. App. 682, 684 (2001).

28 USC 1346(b): Federal Tort Claims Act. 1946.

42 USC 1320d-6(a): Wrongful disclosure of individually identifiable health information: Offense. 1996.

42 USC 1320d-6(b): Wrongful disclosure of individually identifiable health information: Defense. 1996.

Ohio Civ. R. 10(D)(2)(a).

OH Rev. Code 2305.113: Medical malpractice actions. 2006.

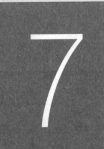

Corporations, Contracts, and Antitrust Legal Issues

Jill Callahan Klaver, JD, RHIA

Learning Objectives

- Describe the most important benefits of forming as a corporation
- Analyze the key differences between a for-profit and not-for-profit corporation
- Articulate the key responsibilities of the governing board of a typical healthcare organization
- Describe the basic elements of a valid contract
- Discuss potential defenses against allegations of nonperformance (breach) of a contract
- Describe the purposes of a hold harmless/indemnification clause
- Articulate key areas of risk associated with health information technology contracts
- Describe the physician–patient relationship as a contract
- Distinguish the parameters of three major federal antitrust statutes
- Explain contract and antitrust issues associated with medical staff

Key Terms

- Acceptance
- Adhesion contract
- Antitrust
- Arbitration
- Boilerplate
- Breach of contract
- Bylaws
- Clayton Act
- Compensatory damages
- Consideration
- Contract

- Corporation
- Due diligence
- Duty of loyalty
- Duty of responsibility
- Economic credentialing
- Exculpatory contract
- Federal Trade Commission (FTC) Act
- Fiduciary duty
- For-profit corporation

- Hold harmless/ indemnification clause
- Horizontal restraint of trade
- Injunction
- Joint ventures
- Learned intermediary
- Noncompete agreement
- Not-for-profit corporation
- Offer
- Owners
- Partnership

- Per se antitrust violation
- Piercing the corporate veil
- Rule of reason analysis
- Shareholders
- Sherman Antitrust Act
- Sole proprietorship
- Specific performance
- *Ultra vires* act
- Vertical restraint of trade
- Warranties

On an ongoing basis, healthcare organizations must make business decisions that have legal implications. One decision is the legal form that an organization will take. Although small organizations assume legal forms such as partnerships and sole proprietorships, healthcare organizations commonly take the form of corporations. This chapter will discuss the structure and legal status of a corporation, as well as the myriad legal obligations associated with it.

Regardless of the form that a healthcare organization takes, individuals within the organization have some level of contracting authority. From a provider standpoint, the physician–patient relationship itself is a contract. From a business standpoint, the authority to enter into contracts is most often held by healthcare administrators, managers, and department directors. Although contracts are diverse and created to carry out an organization's business purposes, prevalent today are health information technology (HIT) contracts, which have proliferated in response to the federal government's incentive program to adopt the electronic health record (EHR).

In addition to contracting authority, decisions made by individuals in healthcare organizations may have potential antitrust or compliance implications. The goal of this chapter is to describe some basic, yet significant, legal concepts that affect the healthcare organization as a business and that may have implications for health information management (HIM) and informatics-related functions.

Healthcare Corporations

Most healthcare organizations are formed as **corporations**. A corporation is an artificial "being" created under the authority of a state statute (a business corporation act). These state laws permit groups of persons (or even individuals in some states) to incorporate an enterprise for any lawful purpose. The purposes of the corporation and the limits of its authority are stated in the articles of incorporation, filed with the state. Articles of incorporation function like a constitution for the corporation. The Internal Revenue Service (IRS) has certain requirements for the articles, as do various states. Typically, however, the IRS requirements include:

- Name and address of the corporation
- Name and address of the registered agent for the corporation (person or entity authorized to accept legal documents on behalf of the corporation)
- Overall purpose of the corporation (which is often written very broadly to permit flexibility in the future, for example, "to engage in any lawful purpose")
- Whether the corporation is organized as for-profit or not-for-profit (which are discussed later in this chapter)
- Whether the corporation will engage in political or legislative activity (since these activities are barred in not-for-profit corporations organized under IRS code section 501(c)(3))
- How the corporation will distribute its assets upon dissolution (IRS 2016)

Healthcare organizations may take various legal forms, such as a **partnership** (for example, two or more physicians who agree to practice together) or even a **sole proprietorship** (a simpler legal form with a single owner who elects not to insulate his or her personal assets through the use of a corporation or other legal form). In a partnership, two or more parties, such as two physicians, agree to share the risks and the rewards of the enterprise. In a general partnership, the general partners usually share the profits or losses equally, and they are personally responsible for any liabilities or debts of the partnership. Decisions are made through consensus and agreement of the partners. But partnerships may also be classified as limited partnerships, in order to limit the potential liabilities attributable to some of the investors or limited partners. Limited partners have greater liability protection but also limited powers. They generally do not participate in the day-to-day management of the business.

Healthcare organizations can also be sole proprietorships, such as where a single physician owns and operates a physician practice. In this structure, the physician is fully responsible for the debts and liabilities of the organization but is entitled to all the profits.

Joint ventures are another form of partnership. They are created for a very specific purpose and are designed to have a limited lifespan. Joint ventures are sometimes seen when two separate healthcare corporations come together to provide a shared service, such as a dialysis center or a radiation therapy center.

Advantages of a Corporation

So why do most healthcare organizations or practices form as a corporation? The main advantage of a corporation is that it is a legal entity or "person" under the law. As such, it is separate from the owners or incorporators. This generally shields the owners from personal liability for the debts of the corporation, although the corporation itself can both sue and be sued. Unlike a sole proprietorship or a limited partnership, a corporation can continue to exist despite the death of an owner. **Owners** in a corporation are **shareholders** or stockholders, meaning they own shares in the corporation. In for-profit corporations, owners can generally transfer their interests (shares) to others, without having to obtain permission to do so. Corporations can be either publicly or privately-held. A publicly-held corporation sells ownership shares to the public, while a privately-held corporation is privately owned and does not sell or offer stock shares to the general public. Private companies generally have relatively few shareholders, as compared to the thousands of shareholders that publicly-traded companies have. The fact that publicly-held corporations are beholden to many shareholders (owners) can affect control of the corporation and its decision-making options, since there are potentially far more owners to whom the key executives are accountable.

A corporation is taxed as an individual entity separate from the owners, meaning that the owners are taxed only on the income they actually receive from the corporation, and not all of the corporation's profits. Corporate income tax rates are generally lower than personal income tax rates. The limited liability for owners and investors also makes it easier for the corporation to attract investors. However, the liability protections offered by a corporation to its owners are not absolute. If a corporation is used for certain nefarious purposes, such as fraud or crime, those protections can be pierced and the owners may be liable for those bad acts. This concept is described as "**piercing the corporate veil**," and for a court to do this, three elements must be present:

- Complete domination of the corporation by its owners
- Such control was used to commit fraud or perpetrate a wrong, violate a statutory or other duty, or commit a dishonest or unjust act
- Corporate control was the proximate cause of the injury that is the subject of the suit (Fletcher 1983)

If the court finds these three elements, the protections of the corporation will be pierced and the owners can be found directly liable for actions that are the subject of the suit.

For-Profit and Not-for-Profit Corporations

Healthcare organizations can be formed as for-profit or not-for-profit corporations. A **for-profit corporation** is allowed to distribute its income to the shareholders, directors, officers, and other individuals for their private gain. A **not-for-profit corporation** may not distribute its income for the private gain of individuals. A not-for-profit can certainly make money, but it must use that income for the purposes of the corporation. It is allowed to pay reasonable salaries to its members, directors, and employees. Making a profit is not the primary purpose of not-for-profit corporations. They usually have very specific social or beneficial purposes set forth in their charter. As a result of both their not-for-profit status and their beneficial purpose, they typically receive preferred treatment under tax laws as long as their actions adhere to their approved charter.

A charitable corporation is one form of a not-for-profit corporation—and perhaps the most common form that US hospitals adopt as their purpose—but it is not the only form. If formed for a charitable or benevolent purpose, charitable corporations are completely exempt from a variety of federal and state

Figure 7.1 Factors used to determine whether a hospital meets the community benefit standard

- Whether the hospital maintains a governing body that includes community leaders (and not just hospital staff and physicians and other insiders)
- Whether the hospital has an open medical staff that permits all qualified physicians to practice there
- Whether the hospital has a full-time emergency department that is open to all, regardless of their ability to pay
- Whether the hospital provides nonemergency care to all persons able to pay (including through Medicare and Medicaid programs)
- Whether the hospital uses its surplus money to improve the quality of care, expand its facilities, and improve its medical education and training programs
- Whether, in the absence of some or all of the five factors above, there are other favorable factors that demonstrate benefit to the community
- Whether the hospital serves a broad cross-section of its community through charitable care or research

Source: Adapted from Peregrine 2009.

taxes. Because tax exemption is such a significant benefit, certain requirements must be met to qualify for it. Not only must the charitable corporation be organized and operated for a charitable purpose, but its net earnings must not benefit a private individual or corporation, which would, in effect, amount to an impermissible "profit." Instead, the charitable corporation must benefit the public or the community (this is referred to as the "community benefit standard," adopted in 1969 by the IRS (26 USC 501(c)(3)). For the healthcare organization to be tax exempt it must meet at least five specific criteria set forth by the IRS as noted by Peregrine (2009) in figure 7.1.

In recent years, the charitable-purpose element of not-for-profit hospitals, which allows for tax-exempt status, has been challenged in part based on aggressive and inflated billing practices, particularly against the uninsured, who have no insurers to bargain on their behalf. Challenges can also be based on the amount of charity care provided. The Illinois Supreme Court, for example, in *Provena Covenant Medical Center v. Department of Revenue* (2010), decided that the tax-exempt status of a not-for-profit hospital should be revoked because the amount of charity care provided by the hospital was too low to justify tax exemption.

To address further controversy whether nonprofit hospitals provide sufficient community benefits to warrant favored tax status, the Patient Protection and Affordable Care Act of 2010 (Public Law 111-148) added Section 501(r)(3) through (r)(6) to the Internal Revenue Code. This section requires not-for-profit hospitals to meet four additional requirements to qualify for tax-exempt status of 501(c)(3):

- Conduct community needs assessment every three years and implement a strategy to meet needs
- Establish a written financial assistance and emergency medical care policies
- Limit amounts charged for emergency or other medically necessary care to individuals eligible for assistance under the hospital's financial assistance policy
- Make effort to determine if an individual is eligible for assistance under hospital policy before engaging in collection action (James 2016; 26 U.S.C 501)

State corporation acts determine the qualifications a corporation must meet in order to maintain its not-for-profit status, including state community benefits requirements (Hilltop Institute 2015). These vary somewhat from state to state. State corporation laws also vary in the duties and responsibilities assigned to the members of the corporation or governing body, but the detailed responsibilities of the corporation's governing body (often called board of trustees or board of directors) can be found in the corporate bylaws.

Responsibilities of the Governing Board

Bylaws refer to the internal rules of an organization or company. They describe the powers granted to the governing body, as well as their duties. Initial corporate members or owners of the organization or company set up the initial bylaws. Bylaws generally cannot be modified by the governing body unless the members or shareholders grant them that authority. In healthcare organizations, governing bodies are generally responsible for developing a strategic plan for the organization, setting broad policy, appointing medical staff members and delineating their clinical privileges, hiring and guiding the chief executive officer, and overseeing the overall performance of the organization (its clinical performance as well as overall administrative and financial performance). Governing body members may also have fundraising responsibilities in some organizations. The role is one of fiduciary oversight, not as an agent or employee of the corporation. They are generally not personally liable for the actions of corporation employees; however, they can be held responsible for failing to carry out their fiduciary duties properly. Fiduciary duty is further described later.

The bylaws often describe the actual makeup of the governing body, such as numbers, types of members (number of community members versus hospital administrators or medical staff members, which, as noted earlier, is a key factor in meeting the community benefit standard), terms of service, qualifications, duties of governing body officers, number of meetings and methods of calling for meetings and making decisions, whether governing body members are compensated, and so on. It is in a healthcare organization's best interests to select governing body members who can lend their expertise (for example, successful leaders in other industries and consumer members who represent the patient population being served).

The bylaws may provide for certain committees within the governing body. Often, committees made up of subsets of the full governing body are used to facilitate the completion of work between full meetings. Generally, these committees cannot operate and make decisions autonomously; rather, they make recommendations to the full governing body. The full body can then either accept or reject the recommendations. Some of the most commonly seen governing body committees in healthcare organizations include finance, building and grounds, human resources, corporate compliance, professional staff relations, and the executive committee. The executive committee is a key committee because it is often empowered to act on behalf of the full board in between official meetings, except where the bylaws have reserved specific decision-making authority to the full board. A governing body has specific responsibilities related to fiduciary duty and restructuring of the organization if necessary.

Fiduciary Duty

As noted previously, final decision-making authority generally rests with the full governing body. Individual trustees or board members cannot absolve themselves of their responsibility for decisions by arguing that they were not part of that committee and therefore are not responsible for that decision. They are responsible for all governing body decisions. They have a **fiduciary duty** to the corporation and its members and shareholders, and in the case of a not-for-profit corporation, they may have a duty to the community at large. Commentators often describe these duties as a duty of loyalty and a duty of responsibility (Showalter 2015).

The **duty of loyalty** means that board members must put the interests of the corporation ahead of their own personal interests. This does not bar a board member from ever benefiting from the corporation, such as by supplying certain services to the corporation, but the governing body must use great care to ensure that such arrangements are fair, fully disclosed, and the result of competitive bidding where possible. This is the reason behind conflict-of-interest policies in most corporations—such policies guard against practices that would call into question a board member's loyalty.

The **duty of responsibility** means that board members must act with due care in exercising their duties. They must attend meetings regularly, ensure that they understand the decisions under consideration, and perform **due diligence** (meaning they must exercise a legally acceptable level of care) in hiring key staff or appointing medical staff and in overseeing the performance of the corporation. This does not mean that board members must not rely on the reports and assessments provided by the senior administrative staff, but they need to be active in asking appropriate questions and be willing to seek professional, independent advice when they suspect a problem.

An example may help clarify the difference. ABC Hospital's governing body selected a new chief executive officer who ultimately proved to be engaging in billing fraud. Was its selection a breach of its fiduciary duties? The answer depends on whether the decision was made with due care, in a responsible manner. If the governing body conducted an appropriate search for the position, checked relevant references and the candidate's background, and did not have undisclosed conflicts of interest in hiring the new CEO, it probably would not be liable for a breach of its fiduciary responsibilities. On the other hand, if ABC Hospital's governing body failed to conduct an appropriate candidate search and instead hired the friend of one of the board members on his recommendation alone, failing to check references and therefore never discovering evidence of past criminal activity by this candidate, the board members could be open to potential liability.

As long as board members fulfill their duties of loyalty and responsibility, they are generally protected from personal liability for their decisions. Corporate bylaws often indemnify the board members from personal liability for board decisions as well as some statutes. For example, the State of Tennessee has several statutes that provide protection to the board. The Tennessee Code for Nonprofit Corporations (T.C.A. 48-58-502) provides the authority to indemnify a board member of a corporation when the individual acts in the best interest and in good faith on behalf of the corporation. This means that if a board member faces a personal suit arising out of his or her board decisions, the corporation will pay for the associated expenses. However, the code also limits the immunity of members of the board for breach of their fiduciary duty (T.C.A. 48-58-601). Many corporations purchase insurance (directors' and officers' insurance) to protect their governing body and key officers from personal liability. But insurance will not protect board members from liability for gross negligence, intentional acts, or crimes.

Any decision by the governing body (or by corporation executives) that goes beyond the express or implied powers of the corporation is considered to be an ***ultra vires* act**, meaning "beyond the power of the corporation." *Ultra vires* acts are usually void and can be challenged. Governing body members (and corporation executives) can be held personally liable for any financial losses suffered by the corporation as an outcome of an *ultra vires* act that was taken with knowledge that the action was beyond their power or that was made in bad faith. The content of the minutes of the governing body can be extremely important in determining whether board members have satisfied their duties of loyalty and responsibility.

Restructuring an Organization

Governing body members may be called on to make decisions about the restructuring of an organization that occurs in the form of a merger, an acquisition, or a consolidation. Although these types of restructuring are not uncommon in the healthcare arena, because of organizations' needs to maintain financial stability or enhance marketability through a broader range of services, they are major undertakings that cannot be pursued without considering all the legal restrictions and ramifications, such as state corporation law and antitrust laws (discussed more fully later in this chapter). Mergers involve the absorption of one corporation by another, where theoretically, both corporations are similar in size and are in agreement.

As an example, Riverview Hospital and Hilltop Hospital decide to merge. Riverview Hospital no longer exists as a separate entity but is now part of Hilltop Hospital. Acquisitions result in a similar consequence (that is, one company is subsumed by another), but they are often a takeover of a smaller organization by a larger organization. Consolidations involve the creation of a new corporation made up of two or more organizations that previously existed but then were dissolved (Showalter 2015). For example, Riverview Hospital consolidates with Hilltop Hospital. Both hospitals cease to exist, with a newly formed corporation—Rivertop Hospital—coming into existence.

Although individual department directors and managers may not be directly involved in the formation of the corporation or in governing bodies, they are sometimes called on to work on teams considering new joint ventures, or they may present information to the governing body. By understanding the overall corporate structure of the organization, and by appreciating the responsibilities of governing body members, they can help anticipate potential problems, questions, and the need for providing complete and accurate information for use in decision making.

Check Your Understanding 7.1

Instructions: Indicate whether the following statements are true or false (T or F).

1. Governing body members are protected from personal liability associated with the decisions they make on behalf of the corporation.
2. "Piercing the corporate veil" enables the owners of a corporation to be shielded from liability for wrongdoing committed through the corporation.
3. Fiduciary duty includes the duty of loyalty and the duty of responsibility.
4. A not-for-profit corporation is prohibited from making money.
5. A healthcare organization may not form as a partnership.

General Principles of Contracts

Healthcare administrators, directors, and managers often have the authority to enter into **contracts.** A contract is a legally enforceable oral or written agreement. Corporations may also enter into contracts, and the articles of incorporation may specify who has the authority to approve contracts on behalf of the corporation, such as the chief executive officer. Contracts to purchase items or services are among the most common examples of contracts for which health information management and informatics professionals may be responsible (Rhodes and Hughes 2003). Sometimes an individual's contracting authority is limited by a dollar amount, with contracts involving greater sums requiring a higher level of approval. But because executing contracts is often part of one's job description, it is important to understand at least the basic principles of contracts, which are discussed next. Many healthcare organizations use in-house counsel or outside legal counsel to advise on contractual matters, and it is also common to see corporate compliance officers and risk managers involved in reviewing potential contracts as well. The next section will cover elements of a contract, breach of contract, health information technology contracts, and physician–patient relationship as a contract.

Elements of a Contract

To be legally enforceable under civil law, a contract must comply with any applicable state and federal statutes and regulations, and it must meet the following conditions:

- It must describe an agreement between two or more persons or entities

- The agreement must include
  - A valid **offer** (a communicated promise by one of the parties to do [or not do] something if the other party agrees to do [or not do] something)
  - **Acceptance** of the offer (reflecting a meeting of the minds on terms that are sufficiently definite and complete)
  - **Consideration** (what each party will receive from the other party in return for performing the obligations described in the contract)

Oral contracts, while valid if they meet these criteria, can be difficult to prove. Each party may claim a different recollection of the agreement. That is why requiring written contracts for important or high-value contracts is a wise practice.

In addition, the parties to the contract must be competent; that is, they must have the legal and mental capacity to contract (Pozgar 2016). Contracts can be either express (actually written or spoken) or implied. For example, if a patient makes an appointment to seek care at her physician's office, that act implies her offer—that if the office grants her that appointment, she will pay for the services she seeks. The physician's office confirming the appointment implies its acceptance of her offer.

Breach of Contract

Once a contract is effective, violations of one or more of its terms can result in a lawsuit alleging **breach of contract**. To prevail, the plaintiff seeking to prove the breach of contract must show that a valid contract was executed, the plaintiff met the requirements of the contract, the defendant failed to meet the requirements, and as a result, the plaintiff suffered an economic loss. Nonperformance issues and the remedies available in those situations are discussed below. The problems associated with breach of contract demonstrate why clear and complete contract terms are so important. If there was no true meeting of the minds, the contract would be considered invalid. Clear contract terms can help prevent nonperformance of both parties, by leaving no room for misinterpretations of the contract's terms.

Defenses for Nonperformance of a Contract

Not every instance of nonperformance will result in a finding of breach of contract. Defenses that can be raised for nonperformance include

- Fraud: If the nonperforming party has been misled on a material fact or term of the contract and has been harmed by the misrepresentation, a breach of contract lawsuit will fail
- Mistake of fact: If both parties to the contract have relied on the mistake
- Duress: If unlawful threat or pressure was used to force a party to execute the contract
- Illegality: If the contract was for illegal purposes or against public policy (see later for additional information)
- Impossibility: If the contract required acts that were impossible to perform

Additional contracts that may fall under illegality nonperformance include exculpatory contracts and adhesion contracts. **Exculpatory contracts** contain clauses that seek to excuse a party in advance from any potential liability. For example, if a hospital admission consent form required the patient to waive in advance his or her right to sue the hospital in the event of a poor outcome, courts would generally void this clause or severely restrict its application, because such agreements do not serve the public good. Another type of contract or clause that may be found against public policy are **adhesion contracts**, which, because the bargaining power between the parties is so unequal, essentially force the weaker party to agree to unfavorable terms because it cannot do without the stronger party's services. As an example, if a hospital were the only available medical facility within hundreds of miles, and it forced patients to sign an agreement to pay in full for all services before leaving the premises, such a provision would likely be struck down because of the unequal bargaining power of the parties.

It is important to keep in mind, however, that for a breach of contract lawsuit to go forward, it must be initiated within the statute of limitations (time period) for enforcing contract rights.

Remedies

If a breach of contract is found, the court's goal is to make the injured party whole. There are several potential remedies for breach of contract:

- **Compensatory damages (money damages):** These damages attempt to return to the injured party the money it would have had, in the absence of the breach. But note that the injured party has a duty to mitigate, or reduce, the damages caused by the breach; it cannot simply do nothing so that the damages continue to increase.
- **Specific performance:** In some situations, an order requiring the breaching party to honor its contractual obligations is more desirable to the injured party than money damages. As a result, the court may order the breaching party to fulfill its obligations under the contract. This is often done via **injunction**, where the court orders a party to stop doing something (or in the case of a mandatory injunction, to do something) in order to prevent irreparable harm to the other party.
- **Arbitration:** It is increasingly common for contracts to call for arbitration of disputes as an alternative to lawsuits. In arbitration, a neutral party is agreed upon by the parties, hears the facts, and resolves the dispute. Arbitration may be binding or nonbinding on the parties. In other words, the contract may specify that the arbitrator's decision must be honored by the parties, or it may simply make the arbitrator's decision advisory in nature, with the option to proceed to lawsuit if an agreement cannot be reached.

Contract Provisions

Certain clauses are often found in contracts to help insulate and protect the parties from economic harm. Two of the most common provisions are hold harmless/indemnification clauses and warranties.

Hold Harmless/Indemnification Clauses

The purpose of **hold harmless/indemnification clauses** is to either transfer or assume liability. For example, the indemnitor (party assuming liability) may agree to hold the other party harmless against claims arising from the indemnitor's own actions or failures to act. This means that if actions (or inactions) result in harm to the other party, the indemnitor will seek to make that party whole, often through some sort of compensation. Or, the parties may agree to hold each other harmless for each other's actions/inactions. These clauses can be useful in clarifying each party's obligations under the contract, but if not understood and carefully executed, they can greatly expand one's potential liability under the contract (for example, by making one party potentially liable to indemnify the other party).

One often sees these clauses in contracts between healthcare organizations and vendors that provide products such as EHR systems or equipment for diagnostic purposes. For example, the contract might read, "Hospital agrees to indemnify, defend, and hold harmless the Vendor and its officers, directors, agents, and employees from and against any and all demands, claims, and damages to persons or property, losses and liabilities, including reasonable attorney's fees, arising out of or caused by Hospital's negligence or willful misconduct."

Hold harmless and indemnification clauses can have a substantial impact on potential liability; thus, they should be reviewed closely by legal counsel.

Warranties

All contracts include representations or **warranties** of some sort, which are statements of facts existing at the time the contract is made. These statements are made by one party to induce the other party to enter into the contract. Typically, these statements relate to the quality of goods or services purchased or leased. For example, a software company may warrant that its product will perform as described in its technical manuals for a period of x years. If within that period the software fails to perform as described in the manual, the software company agrees to fix the problem or replace the software.

Warranties can be express, as in the example just described, where a statement is made from the seller to the buyer to promise performance or describe goods or services. Warranties may also be implied by law. For example, the Uniform Commercial Code section 2-314 states in part: "(1) Unless excluded or modified ... a warranty that the goods shall be merchantable is implied in a contract for their sale if the seller is a merchant with respect to goods of that kind" (15 UCC 2-314-15). And for the goods to be considered merchantable, they must be "fit for the ordinary purposes for which such goods are used." Section 2-315 describes an implied warranty of "fitness for a particular purpose," meaning that when the seller has reason to know any particular purpose for which the goods are required, and the buyer is relying on the seller's skill or judgment to furnish suitable goods, there is an implied warranty that the goods being sold will be fit for such purpose, as long as the buyer's reliance on that skill or judgment is reasonable.

Warranties may also be disclaimed by the seller by doing so in the contract. This is just one of many reasons why persons involved in negotiating contracts should seek assistance from counsel to understand the potential impact of the terms they are considering.

Health Information Technology Contracts

HIT contracts have been the subject of substantial concern as healthcare organizations and independent healthcare providers such as physicians adopt EHRs and other information technologies. What places the purchaser and subsequent user of an HIT product in an even more difficult position is that information sharing about vendor HIT defects is often curtailed through vendor contracts. Some commentators have noted that the terms within HIT contracts are inadequate to protect purchasers or lessors from liability—even from problems directly attributable to the software or hardware. Healthcare organizations sometimes sign purchase/lease contracts without adequate review or negotiation of terms, accepting the **boilerplate**, or standard, vendor-written terms, which highly favor the HIT vendor.

Koppel and Kreda (2009) reported serious liability concerns resulting from contractual terms that shift liability to the system users—even when the users are following vendor instructions for use. To address liability, vendors may rely on the doctrine of "learned intermediaries" and on warranties prohibiting claims against their own products' fitness. **Learned intermediary** is a defense doctrine that "companies have a duty to warn physicians directly about potential adverse effects caused by their products, while physicians must serve as 'learned intermediaries' who interpret this information and advise patients appropriately" (Gemperli 2000). This doctrine is commonly used as a defense for pharmaceutical companies and medical device manufacturers (Arnold and Duncan 2014).

With increased awareness of EHR and HIT-related problems, healthcare providers must understand how to protect themselves when entering into contracts for major EHR and HIT applications (American Medical Association 2013, Texas Medical Association 2011). The American Medical Informatics Association (AMIA) Board of Directors appointed a task force to provide recommendations ranging from stakeholder responsibilities and defect reporting to meaningful use standards and unintended consequences of HIT, in an effort to help resolve issues related to vendor–user contracts and subsequent interactions (Goodman et al. 2010). In addition, the Office of the National Coordinator for Health Information Technology (2013) published a guide, "EHR Contracts: Key Contract Terms for Users to Understand," to assist providers in better understanding vendor contracts.

Concern regarding HIT contracts points to the need for careful review of contracts by someone familiar with contract law and, ideally, HIT issues. There are many issues that could affect HIT purchasers and HIT vendors that both parties need to address.

Physician–Patient Relationship as a Contract

Courts have found that the physician–patient relationship itself is a form of contract. The physician agrees to provide services in exchange for payment. This contract can either be express (for example, a patient signs a consent to have the physician treat him and agrees to pay the bill) or implied (an unconscious patient is brought into the urgent care center, and the physician treats him). This contract imposes certain duties on the physician to treat the patient. However, physicians are not obligated to treat those with whom they have not established this contract. In other words, they do not have to treat those with whom they have not established a physician–patient relationship. A physician attending a party has no obligation to respond to or treat someone because that person has talked about his or her symptoms with the physician. Also, a physician offering informal consultation to a colleague about a patient the colleague is treating has no contractual obligation to the patient who is the subject of that informal consultation. However, if the consultation was more formal (for example, the consultant examined the patient, a specimen, or a tissue sample), and the physician was billing for those services, courts would find that a contractual relationship exists.

Physician warranties to a patient about the certainty of a particular outcome can also give rise to claims of breach of warranty contract. If, for example, the physician says to the patient, "You should have this surgery. And don't worry, I promise you will be pain-free a week after the knee replacement," and the patient relies on that promise and therefore has the surgery, the existence of pain beyond a week after the surgery would be grounds for a breach of contract lawsuit.

The existence of a physician–patient relationship as a form of contract is not everlasting. The relationship can be terminated by action of either party, such as when the patient ceases treatment or dies, when the parties mutually agree to end the relationship, when the patient dismisses the physician, or when the physician dismisses the patient from his or her care. The physician must exercise care in terminating a physician–patient relationship to prevent claims based on abandonment of care. If, for example, a physician terminates the patient from his or her practice abruptly, without giving the patient time to secure another source of care, this can be considered abandonment. But if the physician notifies the patient in writing, gives him or her adequate time to secure other care and agrees to see the patient in the meantime, and cooperates in sharing relevant information with the new care provider once selected by the patient, the physician can likely prevent claims of abandonment.

Reasons vary for termination of physician–patient relationships. Some patients simply do not like the physician they have selected and therefore elect to leave the practice. Some physicians choose to terminate relationships with patients who repeatedly refuse to follow their medical advice or who are verbally abusive to the practice staff. Abandonment cases do make it clear, however, that once a physician–patient relationship has been established, a clear, careful stepwise approach to terminating the relationship will make abandonment claims more defensible.

Check Your Understanding 7.2

Instructions: Indicate whether the following statements are true or false (T or F).

1. A hold harmless clause may provide for compensation by one individual to another.
2. A breach of contract judgment always requires monetary compensation.
3. An acceptance of an offer reflects a meeting of the minds regarding the contract terms.
4. To be valid, a contract must be in writing.
5. Mistake of fact is a potential defense for nonperformance of a contract.

General Principles of Antitrust Law

To understand how **antitrust** (which can be considered "anti-monopoly") laws affect healthcare organizations, it is important to have a basic understanding of three federal antitrust statutes: the Sherman Antitrust Act, the Clayton Act, and the Federal Trade Commission Act. All of these are discussed in this section, along with examples of how they operate in healthcare organizations. These statutes seek to protect the public against trusts and monopolies that are so large they have the power to control a market and thereby restrict free trade and freedom of choice. If, for example, a single healthcare organization controlled all healthcare services in a single market, the consumer would be at the mercy of the pricing and practices of the monopoly, simply because the monopoly controlled the market. This can result in inflated prices, and even in poor quality, because there essentially is no competition.

The Sherman Antitrust Act

The general purpose of the **Sherman Antitrust Act** (15 USC 1-7), passed in 1890, is to prevent restraints of trade among the states (or with foreign countries). It does so in Section 1 of the act by declaring that "every contract ... or conspiracy, in restraint of trade or commerce among the several states, or with foreign nations, is ... illegal." Section 2 of the act seeks to prevent monopolies in a market. Restraints of trade can be classified as either horizontal or vertical. In a **vertical restraint of trade**, two or more entities at different levels in a distribution chain act together to restrain trade (for example, a manufacturer of hospital supplies collaborates with a wholesaler to keep prices artificially high). In a **horizontal restraint of trade**, competitors agree to fix prices, divide the market (for example, "I will serve residents on the west side of town only; you serve them on the east side"), or try to exclude others from competing in the same market. Section 1 of the act applies to joint actions (two or more parties), whereas Section 2 can apply to a single organization. For example, if a healthcare organization attempts to create a monopoly, even if the actions it takes are solely its own and not in concert with any other organization, it can be found in violation of the Sherman Act. This act as well as the Clayton Act are also discussed in chapter 18 in regard to issues related to corporate compliance, fraud, and abuse.

The Clayton Act

Because the language of the Sherman Act was very broad, and therefore was being used in unintended ways (notably union busting), Congress passed the **Clayton Act** (15 USC 12 et seq) 24 years later, in 1914. The Clayton Act exempted union activities from antitrust laws and prohibited acquisitions or mergers that lessen competition. It also prohibited, among other things, discriminatory pricing practices (where different purchasers are given different prices for commodities of like grade and quality, where the effect of that pricing practice is to lessen competition; but note that there are many important exceptions to this prohibition), tying arrangements (exclusive dealing contracts where the selling party requires the buyer to not use or deal in the goods or commodities of a competitor, where the effect lessens competition), and mergers and acquisitions that reduce competition.

The Federal Trade Commission Act

The **Federal Trade Commission (FTC) Act** (15 USC 41-58), also passed in 1914, gave the FTC broad powers to act against organizations engaging in unfair methods of competition, or unfair or deceptive acts that affect commerce (including advertising). Practices that could apply to healthcare organizations include

- Failing to reveal material facts about a product
- Making false claims and misrepresentations
- Offering misleading prices
- Disparaging a competitor's product by making misleading or untrue assertions
- Presenting advertising that is intended to attract a customer who will then be switched to a higher-priced product (Showalter 2015)

Rule of Reason and Per Se Violations

Not all restraints of trade are actual antitrust violations. For example, by virtue of having a superior product or services, an organization may lawfully dominate a local market. If antitrust challenges are raised for activities that are *not* automatically considered to be antitrust violations (automatic violations are called **per se antitrust violations** and include price fixing, division of markets, group boycotts, and tying arrangements), courts apply a **rule of reason analysis** to determine whether an antitrust violation exists. This analysis considers the geographic markets affected and the product/service market involved, the nature of the industry, the motivation for the allegedly illegal activity, and the impact of the activity on the industry.

Enforcement and Applicability to Healthcare Organizations

The Sherman Act offers both civil and criminal penalty options, whereas the Clayton Act offers only civil remedies. The FTC Act, on the other hand, is enforced only by the FTC and offers no private right of action. In any event, certain types of common activities within healthcare organizations can give rise to possible antitrust concerns:

- Health planning, which can raise restraint of trade issues
- Shared services, which can raise possible issues of price fixing or group boycott

Figure 7.2 Healthcare antitrust safety zones

- Mergers involving small hospitals (where one has fewer than 100 beds and average census of fewer than 40 patients)
- Joint ventures for expensive or high-tech equipment
- Joint ventures to offer specialized services
- Efforts to provide medical data
- Provision of healthcare fee/price information to purchasers of health services
- Surveys about prices, wages, and benefits
- Joint purchasing arrangements between healthcare organizations
- Exclusive and nonexclusive joint ventures with physician networks
- Multiprovider networks (although these are evaluated under the rule of reason)

Source: Showalter 2015, 470.

- Utilization review, which can involve possible group boycott
- Medical staff privileging/credentialing, which can involve possible group boycott (and is discussed later in this chapter)
- Third-party payer contracts or managed care organizations, which can involve possible price fixing, group boycott, and monopolization
- Mergers and consolidations, which can involve possible monopolization of a market (Showalter 2015, 462)

In 1996, the Department of Justice and the FTC provided additional guidance for healthcare organizations by publishing "Statements of Antitrust Enforcement Policy in Health Care." The paper recognized the benefits of economy of scale in hospital mergers and set in force nine "safety zones" of activity that will ordinarily not be challenged by these federal agencies. These safety zones are outlined in figure 7.2. It is important for healthcare executives to understand the kinds of activities that can raise the specter of antitrust, so that assistance can be sought in structuring these activities in ways that do not violate the law.

Check Your Understanding 7.3

Instructions: Indicate whether the following statements are true or false (T or F).

1. Antitrust violations are generally governed by individual state laws.
2. The Federal Trade Commission allows hospitals to offer misleading prices on their services in order to be competitive with others in their geographic area.
3. There are nine safety zones in healthcare that the federal government will generally not challenge as antitrust violations.
4. Joint ventures to offer specialized services will often be challenged as antitrust violations.
5. The Sherman Act is the oldest of the three major federal antitrust statutes.

Contract and Antitrust Issues Associated with the Medical Staff

The **medical staff** of a healthcare organization is comprised of individuals who have been credentialed and granted clinical privileges to provide care to patients in the organization. The process of credentialing and delineating medical staff privileges is discussed in chapter 19. Antitrust-related claims sometimes arise out of a denial of staff privileges or a restriction of credentials, such as denying privileges to "all chiropractors." In this kind of litigation, the plaintiff seeks to prove anticompetitive effects from the action denying membership or privileges. The potential monetary damages associated with successful claims can be substantial; thus, care must be exercised not only in drafting medical staff bylaws and associated rules and regulations, but also in adhering to them at all times when considering medical staff applications and requests for privileges.

Broad medical staff bylaws language that seeks to exclude an entire class of practitioners can be seen as a group boycott, which, if proven, is a per se violation of antitrust laws, as noted previously. Even individual denials can raise antitrust issues when existing medical staff members seek to limit the number of certain types of potential competitors on staff (for example, the credentials committee chair is a neurosurgeon, and he takes action to ensure that all other neurosurgeon applications for staff membership and privileges are denied to ensure his own market share).

Some organizations consider the volume of certain types of cases treated by that physician or surgeon in deciding whether to grant specific privileges, sometimes because they want to secure the loyalty of that practitioner in using the hospital's facilities. This is sometimes referred to as **economic credentialing** (if that information is unrelated to clinical performance issues), and the appropriateness of using volume data is a matter of dispute. However, the issues of quality and volume are not completely unrelated. In some situations, the number of certain types of procedures performed is arguably linked to clinical performance and quality issues. Certain medical specialty societies have stated that the number of procedures performed is a relevant consideration in granting initial and renewal privileges (American Society for Gastrointestinal Endoscopy 2002).

The tension between physician loyalty and economic credentialing—and ultimately a hospital's bottom line—has been apparent in the proliferation of physician-owned hospitals, where community hospitals have resisted the referral of more profitable patients by physicians to facilities where those physicians have an ownership stake. In certain instances, physician privileges have been revoked via economic credentialing based on perceived loss of loyalty and financial conflict of interest. However, the Patient Protection and Affordable Care Act of 2010 has significantly limited the ability of physicians to invest in hospitals, which may reverse the tendency for physicians to have a stake in owning a hospital.

Medical staff bylaws must clearly state the process for granting medical and professional staff membership, and clinical privileges, and the process required for thorough investigation of all applicable qualifications and clinical performance. The bylaws should include a mechanism to request and hold a fair hearing in the event a physician wishes to challenge an adverse decision. Having some sort of internal mechanism for impartial review of the decision (by elevating those disputes to the full medical executive committee and ultimately to the organization's board of directors) can aid in preventing antitrust-related litigation, by helping to ensure that the decision is not based on anticompetitive motivations.

Antitrust issues arise not only with independent medical staff members but also with employed physicians and other professionals. Employment agreements can be found to be anticompetitive if they are too restrictive in their terms. **Noncompete agreements**, in which an individual agrees not to compete directly or work for a competitor for a certain period of time after leaving his or her employment, can be subject to antitrust litigation if they are too restrictive. This does not mean that all noncompete agreements are invalid, but they must be narrowly drawn to avoid an effect that restrains trade. See figure 7.3, which discusses a case related to noncompete agreement that was found to be too restrictive by the court.

Figure 7.3 Case of restrictive noncompete agreement

In *Emergicare Systems Corporation v. Bourdon*, Emergicare contracted to provide emergency physicians, including Dr. Bourdon, to Longview Regional Hospital for a period of years. In October 1991, Emergicare wrote to Bourdon to confirm that it would terminate the agreement with Longview on November 8, 1991, and accordingly, Dr. Bourdon's agreement with Emergicare would also terminate. Bourdon then contacted Longview and arranged to stay on as an emergency physician, through a new arrangement with Metroplex Emergency Physicians. Emergicare then sued Bourdon and Metroplex, alleging that Bourdon breached a covenant not to compete with Emergicare. The trial court ruled in favor of Bourdon and Metroplex, noting that the covenant sought to restrict Bourdon from working within five miles of any clinic operated by Emergicare, whether the physician ever worked in that clinic or not. The covenant also sought to restrict Bourdon from working in any emergency department where Emergicare provided services for one year following termination of Emergicare's contract. On appeal, the appellate court affirmed the trial court's decision, finding the noncompete agreement "too restrictive" and thus an unreasonable restraint of trade.

Check Your Understanding   7.4

Instructions: Indicate whether the following statements are true or false (T or F).

1. Economic credentialing is the granting of medical staff privileges based on quality of care indicators.

2. Antitrust claims are valid only if they relate to an entire group of individuals who have been denied privileges at a healthcare organization.

3. Bylaws should include a mechanism to request and hold a fair hearing in the event a physician wishes to challenge an adverse decision.

4. Courts uphold all noncompete agreements in order to protect the livelihood of organizations that have had an employee or a contractor leave for other opportunities.

5. The number of procedures performed by a provider may be linked to clinical performance and quality issues when determining medical staff privileges.

Scenario 7

After several years serving as a respected department director in the local hospital, you have been invited to join the board of directors of a local clinic that serves the homeless in your community. It is organized as a not-for-profit corporation. You begin attending board meetings. Over the course of the first year of your appointment, you notice that the clinic's executive director is heavily involved in local political activities, and she places political literature in the clinic waiting areas and exam rooms as reading material. You also hear rumors that she is funneling donated funds intended for the clinic into the campaign funds of some of her political friends, one of whom serves as alongside you as a member of the board of directors. When you approach her to ask about this, she reminds you that she is a 51 percent owner of the corporation and therefore she has the control to decide how best to direct all funds. You are disgusted by this response and lose the enthusiasm for your appointment, and you begin to skip board meetings.

1. What risks are posed by this scenario
   a. To the corporation?
   b. To the board of directors collectively?
   c. To you personally?

Scenario 7 (Continued)

2. What duty is the "political friend" director violating?

3. What duty are you violating?

4. What recommendations should you make to the board of directors to manage the risks and violations you have identified?

5. Which of your behaviors should you change to protect yourself against potential liability?

References

American Medical Association. 2013 (February 25). Ways EHRs can lead to unintended safety problems. http://www.amednews.com/article/20130225/profession/130229981/4/.

American Society for Gastrointestinal Endoscopy. 2002. Methods of granting hospital privileges to perform gastrointestinal endoscopy. *Gastrointestinal Endoscopy* 55(7):780–783.

Arnold, K. and S. Duncan. 2014 (October 14). The Learned Intermediary Doctrine: A Historical Review. Law360. http://www.law360.com/articles/587180/the-learned-intermediary-doctrine-a-historical-review.

Fletcher, W. 1983. *Cyclopedia of the Law of Private Corporations*, section 43.10.

Gemperli, M. 2000. Rethinking the role of the learned intermediary: The effect of direct-to-consumer advertising on litigation. *JAMA* 284(17):2241.

Goodman, K., E. Berner, M. Dente, B. Kaplan, R. Koppel, D. Rucker, D. Sands, and P. Wunkelstein. 2011. Challenges in ethics, safety, best practices, and oversight regarding HIT vendors, their customers, and patients: A report of an AMIA special task force. *Journal of the American Medical Informatics Association* 18:77–81. http://jamia.oxfordjournals.org/content/jaminfo/18/1/77.full.pdf.

Hilltop Institute. 2015. Hospital community benefit program state law profiles comparison. http://www.hilltopinstitute.org/hcbp.cfm.

Internal Revenue Service. 2016 (November). Publication 557, Tax-Exempt Status for Your Organization. https://www.irs.gov/uac/about-publication-557.

James, J. 2016 (February). Health Policy Brief: Nonprofit Hospitals' Community Benefits Requirements. *Health Affairs*. http://healthaffairs.org/healthpolicybriefs/brief_pdfs/healthpolicybrief_153.pdf.

Koppel, R., and D. Kreda. 2009. Health care information technology vendors' hold harmless clause. *JAMA* 301(12):1276–1278.

Office of the National Coordinator for Health Information Technology. 2013. EHR Contracts: Key Contract Terms for Users to Understand. https://www.healthit.gov/sites/default/files/ehr_contracting_terms_final_508_compliant.pdf.

Peregrine, M. 2009. Overview of the "community benefit" standard of federal tax exempt status. Washington, DC: American Healthcare Lawyers Association. http://publish.healthlawyers.org. https://www.healthlawyers.org/Events/Programs/Materials/Documents/ArchivedProgramMaterialFolders2009-2011/AM11/AHLAResources/publicinterest/OverviewCommunityBenefit_Peregrine.pdf.

Pozgar, G. 2016. *Legal Aspects of Health Care Administration*, 12th ed. Sudbury, MA: Jones and Bartlett.

Rhodes, H. and G. Hughes. 2003. Practice brief: Letters of agreements and contracts. Chicago: AHIMA. Online extra.

Showalter, J.S. 2015. *The Law of Healthcare Administration*, 7th ed. Chicago: Health Administration Press.

Texas Medical Association. 2011. EHR Buyer Beware: Issues to Consider When Contracting with EHR Vendors. https://www.texmed.org/Template.aspx?id=22484&terms=EHR%20buyer%20beware%20Issues%20to%20Consider.

Cases, Statutes, and Regulations Cited

Emergicare Systems Corporation v. Bourdon, 942 S.W.2d 201 (Tex. App. 1997).

Provena Covenant Medical Center v. Department of Revenue, 2010 WL 966858, 10 (2010).

15 UCC 2-314-15: Uniform Commercial Code.

15 USC 1-7: Sherman Act of 1890.

15 USC 12-27: Clayton Act of 1914.

15 USC 41-58: Federal Trade Commission Act of 1914.

26 USC 501(c)(3): Exemption from tax on corporations, certain trusts, etc. 2014.

Patient Protection and Affordable Care Act (2010). Public Law 111–148.

T.C.A. 48-58-502: Authority to indemnify. 1987.

T.C.A. 48-58-601: Limitation of and immunity from actions for breach of fiduciary duty. 1986.

Consent to Treatment

Jill Callahan Klaver, JD, RHIA

- Distinguish between express and implied consent
- Identify the components of informed consent
- Differentiate between the various types of advance directives
- Discuss the consent rights and limitations of competent adults, incompetent adults, and minors
- Describe the legal basis for challenging consent
- Discuss how consent should be documented
- Identify different types of consent forms

Key Terms

- Advance directive
- Age of majority
- Agent
- Capacity
- Competent adult
- Consent
- Do not resuscitate (DNR) order
- Durable power of attorney (DPOA)
- Durable power of attorney for healthcare decisions (DPOA-HCD)
- Emancipated minors
- Express consent
- Federal Policy for the Protection of Human Subjects (Common Rule)
- General consent
- Good Samaritan statute
- Implied consent
- Informed consent
- Incompetent adult
- Institutional review board (IRB)
- Living will
- Long form
- Minor
- National Research Act of 1974
- Non compos mentis
- Patient Self-Determination Act (PSDA)
- Power of attorney (POA)
- Principal
- Short form
- Therapeutic privilege
- Uniform Anatomical Gift Act (UAGA)
- Uniform Health-Care Decisions Act (UHCDA)

One of the most valued rights in American society is the right to control one's own body, especially when it comes to medical decision making. Individuals have the right to consent or refuse consent to medical treatment, whether that treatment is minor or lifesaving. However, rights surrounding consent are not absolute and can be affected by factors such as age, competence, and emergency circumstances. The law governing consent is found in both state and federal statutes as well as case law. Before giving consent, individuals have the right to be fully informed of a treatment's risks, benefits, and alternatives. A provider who fails to fully discuss these issues with a patient may be held liable for negligence based on lack of informed consent. If an intervention is performed on a patient with no consent at all, the provider may be held liable for battery. Healthcare providers and individuals responsible for the management of health information must be knowledgeable about the ethical and applicable legal principles of consent and with consent law applicable in their states. This chapter introduces the concept of consents, parties to consents, how advance directives relate to consents, legal challenges to consents, and issues related to who should document that a consent has been provided and forms of consent.

Types of Consent

When thinking about consent in healthcare, most people think of the patient signing a form that gives a healthcare provider permission to perform a test or procedure. However, **consent** is a broad process that can be in written or unwritten form and can vary in terms of how much information is provided. In most cases, consent involves a patient's acknowledgement that he or she understands a proposed intervention, including that intervention's risks, benefits, and alternatives. In other cases, such as emergency circumstances or legal matters, consent may be provided through the operation of law rather than individual choice. The types of consent are express consent, implied consent, and informed consent, but there are exceptions to informed consent.

Express Consent

Express consent refers to consent that is communicated through words, whether written or spoken. An individual may show express consent through written documentation or by orally agreeing to an intervention. Although both forms of express consent are valid, written consent is more desirable than oral consent from an evidentiary standpoint. The passage of time, a medical condition, or sheer forgetfulness can affect an individual's ability to recall the details of an orally expressed consent. In disputes where consent is an issue, this can lead to conflicting accounts as to the information discussed by a provider or questions raised by a patient during the oral consent process. When written consents are used, the evidence regarding the information provided is stronger. However, just because a consent is in written format does not mean that the patient's consent was informed. Express consents, whether oral or written, must provide the patient with enough information to make an informed decision regarding medical treatment. A detailed discussion of informed consent is found later in this chapter.

Implied Consent

Implied consent refers to consent for medical treatment that is communicated through a person's conduct or some other means besides words. For example, most physicians do not directly ask the patient for express written or oral consent prior to conducting a basic physical examination or minor office procedure. However, the patient still communicates consent through his or her conduct: scheduling and arriving for the appointment and submitting to the exam or procedure without objection. Implied consent is most appropriate for interventions that are noninvasive and very low risk. As interventions become more invasive or risky, providers should obtain a patient's express written informed consent. For implied consent to be valid from an evidentiary standpoint, the patient's conduct and surrounding circumstances must create a reasonable belief that consent was given.

Another form of implied consent occurs in emergency situations where an individual may be unconscious or otherwise lacks capacity to communicate consent. In these cases, consent is implied by the law rather than the patient's words or conduct, and lifesaving treatment can proceed, unless there are advance directives in place that clearly express wishes to the contrary. The law creates a presumption that incapacitated individuals would consent to medical treatment and protects providers who treat these individuals from lawsuits based on lack of consent. Implied consent is limited in nature, and consent in this kind of situation is discussed in greater detail later in this chapter. Many states also have implied consent laws related to operating motor vehicles. These laws are aimed at protecting the public and typically state that by obtaining a license to operate a vehicle, drivers imply consent to a breath, blood, or urine test at the request of a law enforcement officer (Oregon Department of Motor Vehicles n.d.).

Informed Consent

Whether given orally or in writing, a patient's consent should be an **informed consent, which** means the patient should have a basic understanding of what medical procedures or tests may be performed and the risks, benefits, and alternatives for those tests or procedures. It also implies that the individual who is being asked to give his or her informed consent is competent to give such a consent and that the consent must be voluntary. However, the amount of information provided during the consent process can vary. Sometimes information provided to the patient is tailored to a specific test or procedure and is quite detailed. In other cases, such as when it is not known what interventions may be necessary, the information provided to the patient is more generalized. For example, when patients are admitted to the hospital, they often sign a **general consent** form authorizing hospital staff to perform the underlying tests and interventions necessary for overall medical care. This general consent must be supplemented with informed consents for the more invasive tests, operations, and other interventions that care may entail.

Requirements

The type and amount of information that should be disclosed to a patient during the consent process is determined by the applicable standard of care, including the Centers for Medicare and Medicaid Services (CMS) Hospital Guidelines requirements. In other words, a provider should give the patient the same information that a reasonable provider would disclose under the same or similar circumstances. Communication between the patient and provider is paramount to obtaining informed consent. The American Medical Association (AMA) suggests that physicians should disclose and discuss

- The patient's diagnosis, if known
- The nature and purpose of a proposed treatment or procedure
- The risks and benefits of a proposed treatment or procedure
- Alternatives (regardless of their cost or the extent to which the treatment options are covered by health insurance)
- The risks and benefits of the alternative treatment or procedure
- The risks and benefits of not receiving or undergoing a treatment or procedure (AMA n.d.).

The communication process also involves answering any questions a patient may have about a proposed intervention or lack of intervention. Patients may wish to consider the questions presented in figure 8.1.

Documentation of informed consent is important to ensure a complete and accurate health record that is legally sound and evidences quality patient care. Although the informed consent process itself may span several days by being initiated before a treatment or procedure is actually scheduled, the signed consent form becomes part of the patient's health record. For quality and legal purposes, the presence of signed informed consent forms for procedures should be verified by operating room or special procedures room staff before the physician is permitted to begin the procedure. The presence of a signed consent form in a patient's health record is also important for CMS and Joint Commission surveys. The Joint Commission requires that an executed informed consent be placed in the patient's health record prior to surgery, unless it is not possible to do so because of an emergency.

| Figure 8.1 | Questions for patients to ask as part of achieving informed consent |

- What is the condition, disease, or problem called?
- How do you recommend treating it?
- What are the risks of this type of treatment?
- What are the benefits?
- What is the complication (morbidity) rate for this treatment?
- What is the mortality (death) rate for patients in my condition using this treatment?
- What other treatments are available? Why are those not recommended?
- What will happen if I don't do anything?
- How many patients have you cared for with this problem? How many patients have you performed this surgery or this test on?
- What is your success rate in treating this problem?
- If I undergo this treatment, will it prevent me from using an alternative treatment if needed?
- Are you board certified in the specialty that treats this disease or condition?
- What can I expect if I undergo this treatment?
- Will I be able to work and/or care for myself?
- Will my activities be restricted?
- How much pain or discomfort will I be in?
- Will this treatment cause other problems?
- What kind of side effects should I expect?
- What should I do if I experience side effects?
- Will you personally perform the surgery, test, or procedure?
- Is anesthesia necessary?
- Who will be the anesthesiologist?
- What can I expect if I don't undergo this treatment?
- What are the alternatives to this treatment?
- What are the potential risks, complications, or side effects associated with the alternative treatment?

Source: The Foundation for Taxpayer and Consumer Rights n.d.

Informed Consent for Human Subjects Research

The potential to misuse human subjects in research activities and, hence, the need to protect those subjects are historical issues. The Nuremberg Code was a response to the harmful use of concentration camp prisoners by Nazi physicians for experimentation without the consent of those individuals. Although the code did not become law in the United States, it remains a powerful statement on the ethical use of human subjects. In the United States, the US Public Health Service used male African American sharecroppers (again without their consent) for a harmful study in which treatment was often denied, in what is known as the Tuskegee Syphilis Study (1932–1972). This ultimately led to the **National Research Act of 1974** (Pub. L. 93-348), which required the Department of Health, Education, and Welfare (now the Department of Health and Human Services [HHS]) to codify its policy for the protection of human subjects into federal regulations. This act also created a commission that generated the Belmont Report, a "statement of basic ethical principles that should assist in resolving the ethical problems that surround the conduct of research with human subjects"

(NIH 1979). These studies and others demonstrate the international historical misuse of human subjects, and the importance of protections against this.

Today, research on human subjects is governed by the **Federal Policy for the Protection of Human Subjects (Common Rule)**, which emanated from the joint promulgation of regulations from several federal agencies and, specifically, from HHS Regulation 45 CFR Part 46, based on the Belmont Report. In 1991, the portion of the HHS regulations that focused on the protection of human subjects (45 CFR 46(a)) was adopted by a number of federal departments and agencies involved in human subject research either as research bodies themselves or as agencies that fund research conducted by others. The US Food and Drug Administration imposes additional requirements at 21 CFR Parts 50 and 56. Requirements of the Common Rule include

- Compliance assurances by organizations conducting research
- Requirements for informed consent
- Special protections for vulnerable populations, such as prisoners, pregnant women, children, mentally disabled persons, and economically or educationally disadvantaged persons (45 CFR 46.101–46.112)

If a proposed medical intervention is related to a research study, then the Common Rule imposes specific requirements designed to protect participants in that research. Under this rule, any research on human subjects must be approved by an **institutional review board (IRB)**. An IRB is a committee of at least five members with varying backgrounds that determines the acceptability of proposed research in accordance with institutional policies, applicable law, and standards of professional practice and conduct (45 CFR 46.107). Among other standards, the Common Rule requires researchers to obtain informed consent from study participants. The informed consent document required by the IRB and signed by the patient is typically a separate document from the consent form for the procedure being performed. The latter consent form is to be included in the individual's health record. The basic elements of an informed consent for human subjects research include

- A statement that the study involves research, an explanation of the purposes of the research and the expected duration of the subject's participation, a description of the procedures to be followed, and identification of any procedures which are experimental
- A description of any reasonably foreseeable risks or discomforts to the subject
- A description of any benefits to the subject or to others which may reasonably be expected from the research
- A disclosure of appropriate alternative procedures or courses of treatment, if any, that might be advantageous to the subject
- A statement describing the extent, if any, to which confidentiality of records identifying the subject will be maintained
- For research involving more than minimal risk, an explanation as to whether any compensation and an explanation as to whether any medical treatments are available if injury occurs and, if so, what they consist of, or where further information may be obtained
- An explanation of whom to contact for answers to pertinent questions about the research and research subjects' rights, and whom to contact in the event of a research-related injury to the subject
- A statement that participation is voluntary, refusal to participate will involve no penalty or loss of benefits to which the subject is otherwise entitled, and the subject may discontinue participation at any time without penalty or loss of benefits to which the subject is otherwise entitled (45 CFR 46.116)

When appropriate and required by an IRB, additional informed consent elements may be required, such as study withdrawal procedures, costs to participants, and potential conflicts of interest (45 CFR 46.116(b)).

It is important to note that consent to participate in research also involves consent to disclose medical information related to that research. Medical information includes written documentation about an identifiable individual and it also includes an individual's bodily materials, such as blood and tissue samples. Unless a waiver is granted by an IRB, researchers must obtain consent prior to using human tissue specimens for research (NCI n.d.a.). IRB-approved informed consent may include restrictions on the rights of participants to access their health information during the study process, which should be noted in patients' health records. Thus, study participants must consent not only to the medical intervention itself, but also to the use and disclosure of their medical information for purposes of the research study, including possible restrictions on their rights of access.

The Privacy Rule of the **Health Insurance Portability and Accountability Act** (HIPAA), which went into effect in 2003, also addresses informed consent for research through its authorization requirements. Although a separate informed consent document for research is often preferable, HIPAA allows an organization's IRB or privacy board to permit compound authorizations that combine informed consent with an authorization for the use and disclosure of a research subject's health information. Types of authorizations permitted for research under HIPAA, including revisions per the Health Information Technology for Economic and Clinical Health Act (HITECH), are discussed more fully in chapter 11.

Exceptions to Informed Consent

In most situations, healthcare providers who fail to properly obtain informed consent prior to performing a medical intervention run the risk of liability for battery or negligence. Lawsuits for battery are most often based on performing an intervention with no permission at all (such as performing a tubal ligation without consent during a Caesarean section). Negligence lawsuits are often based on failure to fully inform the patient of a risk, benefit, or alternative, resulting in harm to the patient (such as failing to inform a patient that nonsurgical options exist for managing a medical condition, causing the patient to undergo unnecessary surgery). Both types of lawsuits will be discussed later in the chapter. In some situations, it is not feasible for a healthcare provider to obtain informed consent prior to performing an intervention. To accommodate such situations, the law has established exceptions to the general requirement that informed consent is necessary.

Emergency Situations

As discussed earlier, the law permits a presumption of consent during emergency situations, whether the patient is an adult or a minor. However, that presumption of consent is not unlimited. Healthcare providers should rely on that presumption only to address true emergencies, such as conditions posing a threat to the patient's life or the risk of permanent loss of function. Aspects of the patient's care that can await the patient's express consent should do so. For example, an emergency room physician would not proceed with an elective procedure unrelated to the emergency, simply because the person accompanying the unconscious patient to the emergency room indicates that the patient would like that procedure done. Most states have some form of a **Good Samaritan statute** that protects various types of healthcare providers from liability for failing to obtain informed consent before rendering care to adults or minors at the scene of an emergency or accident. The rationale for Good Samaritan laws is that they are necessary to ensure that providers are not deterred from rendering aid at accident scenes for fear of being sued for battery or negligence. An example of a Good Samaritan law is provided next:

Any physician or surgeon, registered professional nurse or licensed practical nurse licensed to practice in this state or licensed to practice under the equivalent laws of any other state and any person licensed as a mobile emergency medical technician may:

1. In good faith render emergency care or assistance, without compensation, at the scene of an emergency or accident, and shall not be liable for any civil damages for acts or omissions other than damages occasioned by gross negligence or by willful or wanton acts or omissions by such person in rendering such emergency care;
2. In good faith render emergency care or assistance, without compensation, to any minor involved in an accident, or in competitive sports, or other emergency at the scene of an accident, without first obtaining the consent of the parent or guardian of the minor, and shall not be liable for any civil damages other than damages occasioned by gross negligence or by willful or wanton acts or omissions by such person in rendering the emergency care. (Mo. Rev. Stat. 537.037; subsections 3 and 4 omitted)

Governmental Action

Sometimes an individual's consent to a medical exam or intervention is not freely given, but is instead ordered by a court or through some other governmental action. This situation most often arises when the welfare of the public outweighs the individual's right to withhold consent.

Criminal Cases

In many states, drivers who have been pulled over must consent to blood alcohol tests when asked to do so by police officers. For example, in Oregon, if an individual refuses to consent, the government may suspend his or her driver's license for a certain period (for example, one to three years) and may use the refusal to consent as evidence against the individual in court in a driving under the influence case (Oregon Department of Motor Vehicles n.d.). The justification is that the government's interest in protecting the public from drivers under the influence outweighs an individual driver's right to refuse consent. This exception may also be interpreted as an implied consent, as described earlier in the chapter.

The government may also order individuals to undergo specific medical tests or interventions when certain infectious diseases may be involved (such as HIV or hepatitis B). For example, under Kansas law, if an individual has been convicted of a crime that may have involved the transmission of bodily fluids from one person to another, a court may order that individual to submit to infectious disease tests (KS Stat. Ann. 65-6009). Again, the government's interest in protecting the public from certain infectious diseases outweighs certain individuals' right to refuse consent to tests for infectious disease.

Civil Cases

In cases where the mental or physical condition of a party is at issue, courts may order a party to submit to physical or mental examinations. Courts must have "good cause" for ordering these exams and generally must specify the time, place, manner, conditions, and scope of such examinations, as well as identify the physician who will conduct the examination (for example, see MO Rev. Stat. 510.040).

Cases Involving Mental Competence

States generally have detailed laws regarding procedures for making competency determinations and committing or providing other means of treatment for mentally ill individuals. Generally, these laws provide for involuntary examinations, treatment, and detainment of individuals with mental illness who are in danger of causing harm to themselves or others (for example, see KS Stat. Ann. 59-2953, 2954). The laws also provide the framework for conducting court-ordered mental evaluations where there is a reasonable basis for the belief that an individual is **non compos mentis** (not of sound mind) and may no longer have legal competence to make their own decisions. If an individual is found to be mentally ill, then the courts may order appropriate treatment (for example, see KS Stat. Ann. 59-2966). Here, the government's interest in protecting the mentally ill individual as well as others who may be placed in danger by that mentally ill individual outweighs that individual's right to refuse medical examinations and treatment.

Courts may order psychiatric or psychological examinations of defendants in criminal cases when determining whether the defendant is competent to stand trial (for example, see KS Stat. Ann. 22-3302). Likewise, if a defendant pleads an insanity defense, he or she will be required to submit to psychiatric or psychological examinations to substantiate the claim of insanity (for example, see MO Rev. Stat. 522.030).

Waiver

Although legal cases have recognized the ability of a patient to waive the right to informed consent, this practice subjects a provider to legal risks that are simply better avoided altogether by securing an informed consent. Waiver of informed consent must be initiated by the patient, associated only with low-risk treatments, completed only if the patient affirms that he or she would subject himself or herself to the treatment regardless of information that informed consent would provide, and carefully documented in the health record. Providers are advised to encourage patients to complete the informed consent process rather than avoiding it.

A more common type of waiver relates to individuals serving as subjects in research studies. Under the Common Rule, the informed consent requirement for human subjects research may be waived or altered if approved by an IRB. For approval to be granted, the IRB must find and document that

- The research involves no more than minimal risk to the subjects
- The waiver or alteration will not adversely affect the rights and welfare of the subjects
- The research could not practicably be carried out without the waiver or alteration
- Whenever appropriate, the subjects will be provided with additional pertinent information after participation (45 CFR 46.116(d))

Regarding access to information without patient consent, an IRB may waive the informed consent requirement when a research study involves a retrospective review of charts. For example, researchers are studying whether a certain intervention has been successful for patients presenting to the emergency room, and they want to review five years of emergency department visits. Such a study may qualify for waiver of informed consent, because retrospective data collection poses minimal risk to the health of subjects, and locating and obtaining signatures from subjects who have visited the emergency department over the past five years may not be practicable. Again, the final decision regarding whether consent would be waived rests with the IRB.

Therapeutic Privilege

The **therapeutic privilege** is a doctrine that has historically allowed physicians to withhold information from patients in limited circumstances, stemming from the historical paternalistic nature of medicine, whereby physicians had a duty to avoid things that would "discourage a patient and depress his spirits" (AMA Council on Ethical and Judicial Affairs 2006). It has been applied in extreme situations in which a provider believes that the risk of physical or psychological injury to the patient resulting from full disclosure outweighs the patient's right to be fully informed.

However, with today's emphasis on patient autonomy and individuals' right of access to their health information, the use of therapeutic privilege is discouraged in all but very extreme cases. In 2006, the AMA Council on Ethical and Judicial Affairs revised its Code of Medical Ethics to better support the patient's right of self-decision regarding healthcare, thus deemphasizing the use of the therapeutic privilege. The updated code states:

> The patient's right of self-decision can be effectively exercised only if the patient possesses enough information to enable an informed choice. The patient should make his or her own determination about treatment. The physician's obligation is to present the medical facts accurately to the patient or to the individual responsible for the patient's care and to make recommendations for management in accordance with good medical practice. The physician has an ethical obligation to help the patient make choices from among the therapeutic alternatives consistent with good medical practice. Informed consent is a basic policy in both ethics and law that physicians must honor, unless the patient is unconscious or otherwise incapable of consenting and harm from failure to treat is imminent. In special circumstances, it may be appropriate to postpone disclosure of information.

> Physicians should sensitively and respectfully disclose all relevant medical information to patients. The quantity and specificity of this information should be tailored to meet the preferences and needs of individual patients. Physicians need not communicate all information at one time, but they should assess the amount of information that patients are capable of receiving at a given time and present the remainder when appropriate. (AMA Council on Ethical and Judicial Affairs 2006)

Check Your Understanding 8.1

Instructions: Indicate whether the following statements are true or false (T or F).

1. A person must give permission to receive medical treatment through express consent.
2. Healthcare providers should encourage patients to waive consent.
3. Informed consent should include alternatives to the proposed treatment or procedure.
4. The law permits a presumption of consent during emergency situations.
5. IRBs may waive the informed consent requirement for research that only involves retrospective record of patient records.

Advance Directives

As discussed previously, communication between the physician and the patient is a key element of informed consent. However, sometimes the patient's health status may make communication impossible, such as when a patient is incapacitated by a head injury or a stroke. Through advance directives, the law provides a means for individuals to communicate their healthcare wishes in advance, should they become incapacitated. Specifically, an **advance directive** is a legal document that specifies an individual's healthcare wishes in the event that he or she has a temporary or permanent loss of competence. Some advance directives appoint a specific friend, family member, or other person to make healthcare decisions on behalf of an individual should that individual lose competence. Other advance directives leave specific instructions restricting the use of ventilators, artificial nutrition and hydration, and other types of life support. Specific types of advance directives are discussed next.

Powers of Attorney

A **power of attorney** (POA) is a legal instrument used by a principal (person) to grant legal authority to one or more agents to make certain legal and financial decisions on behalf of the principal. The **principal** is the individual who signs the POA, and the **agent** is the person designated by the principal to make certain decisions or perform certain acts on the principal's behalf. The specific authority granted to the agent is listed in the POA instrument. For example, a principal may designate an agent to sign real estate contracts or transfer money on the principal's behalf, or make healthcare decisions, as discussed later in the chapter. The agent's authority to act on behalf of the principal may be broad or may be limited to a specific task or transaction. Specific rules for how the POA must be drafted are defined by each state. Generally, they must be written, signed, witnessed, and executed by an adult.

Durable Power of Attorney (DPOA)

Unless a POA is durable, it is only effective when the principal has capacity. **Capacity** indicates that an individual is mentally competent and is in control of himself or herself. If the principal becomes incapacitated, then the agent's authority is also incapacitated. So, in the previous example, the agent's authority to sign real estate contracts or transfer money on the principal's behalf would be terminated upon the principal's incapacitation. This situation can be prevented by executing a **durable power of attorney** (DPOA). A DPOA is a POA that remains in effect even after the principal is incapacitated. Some DPOAs are drafted so that they only take effect when the principal becomes incapacitated. These are sometimes called springing POAs, because they only "spring" into effect upon the principal's incapacitation. State law defines the specific language required to create a DPOA versus a POA, but it generally includes an express statement that the agent's authority is not terminated by the principal's incapacity.

Durable Power of Attorney–Healthcare Decisions (DPOA-HCD)

Powers of attorney and DPOA most often deal with financial, real estate, and other legal transactions, but they generally do not cover healthcare decisions. State law creates a separate, but similar, framework for appointing agents to make healthcare decisions on behalf of principals. A **durable power of attorney for healthcare decisions** (DPOA-HCD) is a legal instrument through which a principal appoints an agent to make healthcare decisions on the principal's behalf in the event the principal become incapacitated. It is important to note that not every state calls this type of instrument a DPOA-HCD. It is sometimes referred to as a medical power of attorney or a healthcare proxy. Depending on the wording of the instrument, the agent may have power to make healthcare decisions on behalf of a principal while the principal is still competent, but often the agent's power is not effective until the principal becomes incompetent.

The determination of whether a patient is incompetent is typically made by a physician or judge. Again, to be durable, the instrument must contain specific language defined by state law. For example, Kansas law requires DPOA-HCDs to contain the words, "'this power of attorney for healthcare decisions shall not be affected by subsequent disability or incapacity of the principal' or 'this power of attorney for healthcare decisions shall become effective upon the disability or incapacity of the principal,' or similar words showing the intent of the principal that the authority conferred shall be exercisable notwithstanding the principal's subsequent disability or incapacity" (KS Stat. Ann. 58-625).

In addition to the language required for durability, state law also defines other aspects of DPOA-HCDs. For example, both the principal and the agent(s) must be adults for DPOA-HCDs to be valid. A DPOA-HCD can grant the agent authority to make all healthcare decisions on behalf of the principal, or it may be limited to only certain decisions. With respect to exercising the authority granted, the agent steps into the shoes of the principal. Any decisions made by the agent are treated as though they were made by the principal. The agent not only has the power to make the healthcare decisions specified in the DPOA-HCD, but also has the power to exercise the principal's corresponding HIPAA privacy rights related to those treatment decisions (see chapter 10 for discussion of personal representatives).

Once executed, the principal should inform friends and family about the DPOA-HCD document and provide copies to the appointed agents as well as to any healthcare providers the principal plans on visiting. Different states tend to recognize each other's properly executed DPOA-HCDs. Therefore, providers may rely on DPOA-HCDs that were properly executed in other states. Healthcare providers should store copies of DPOA-HCDs prominently in the patient's record, and are required to do so by the laws of many states. If the provider uses an electronic health record (EHR), then the EHR must be set up to refer or link to the existence of the DPOA-HCD. Some states, such as Arizona, have created a secure advance directive registry, a website that permits individuals to store their DPOA-HCD and other advance directives online (Arizona Secretary of State 2015). Individuals then provide healthcare providers and others with passwords to access the online advance directive.

Revoking a DPOA-HCD

The process for revoking a DPOA-HCD varies by state law, but generally involves some form of express communication showing the principal's intent to revoke the instrument. This communication must be made to the agent as well as to healthcare providers who have been previously notified about the document's existence. In cases where spouses are appointed as agents, some DPOA-HCDs contain specific language that automatically revokes the instrument if the principal and the agent become separated or divorced. If a principal executes a second DPOA-HCD naming new agents or granting different powers, then the previous DPOA-HCD is automatically revoked. The law generally protects agents and providers who are unaware that a DPOA-HCD has been revoked and in good faith rely on the instrument to make decisions. Sample DPOA-HCDs for each state are widely available on the Internet through state government and consumer advocacy websites.

Living Wills

A living will is a document executed by a competent adult that expresses that individual's wishes to limit treatment measures when specific health-related diagnoses or conditions exist and the individual cannot communicate on his or her own behalf. In some states, a living will may only take effect when two or more physicians certify in writing that a patient has a terminal condition. A terminal condition generally connotes a condition where an individual is likely to die in the near future, with or without treatment. Since permanent unconsciousness or confusion caused by accidents or diseases such as Alzheimer's may not qualify as terminal, it is important to note that these conditions may be outside the scope of a living will. However, court cases have held that individuals can execute other advance directives that exceed limitations set by state terminal condition living will statutes (Missouri Bar 2014).

In other states, conditions governed by living wills are broader and encompass "seriously incapacitating" illnesses or conditions, persistent unconsciousness with no reasonable expectation of recovery, or "permanent confusion." The types of treatment limited by living wills typically involve life-prolonging procedures, such as artificially supplied nutrition and hydration, cardiopulmonary resuscitation (CPR), and use of respirators.

The technical process for executing living wills varies from state to state. Common requirements are that living wills must be written, signed, and dated by the individual executing the will; executed by adults; and witnessed or acknowledged before a notary public or other witnesses not related to the individual executing the will. Not every state uses the term *living will* to define this type of advance directive. Sometimes the terms *healthcare directive* or *advance care plan* are used in lieu of living will. Once an individual has executed a living will, it is important that he or she communicate its existence to close friends, family, and healthcare providers. An individual should keep a copy of his or her living will in an easily accessible place, and healthcare providers must store copies of living wills in the front of a patient's paper record or make them immediately accessible in an EHR system. The process of revoking a living will varies from state to state, but generally involves some express act or statement indicating an intent to revoke. This may involve oral or written statements or physically gathering and destroying copies of the living will. In some states, healthcare providers are required to document the revocation of a living will in the patient's health records (Missouri Bar 2014).

It is common for individuals to have both a DPOA-HCD and a living will. If such an individual is incapacitated and is also diagnosed with a condition specified in the principal's living will, it can be difficult to determine whether treatment decisions should be made according to the living will or according to the agent's judgment. Some DPOA-HCDs directly address this issue by specifically stating that the agent either does or does not have the power to act in contradiction to the wishes outlined in a living will. State law may also limit an agent's ability to contradict or revoke a properly executed living will. In situations where irresolvable conflict exists, a judge may enter an order regarding treatment after being presented with evidence at a hearing.

Sample living wills and other related advance directive plans are widely available on the Internet through state government and consumer advocacy websites. Some examples include the Ohio Hospice & Palliative Care Organization, "Choices: Living Well at the End of Life" (2004), Tennessee Department of Health's Advance Directives Resources (n.d.a) and Advance Directives for Health Care Decision Making (n.d.b), and the Kansas Legal Services (2016).

Do Not Resuscitate Orders

Generally, healthcare facility staff and paramedics will perform cardiopulmonary resuscitation (CPR) on any individual whose heart or breathing has stopped. However, individuals may wish to forego CPR for a variety of reasons, such as the belief that it will only prolong the dying process and cause unnecessary discomfort and emotional distress (State of California Emergency Medical Services Authority 2013). A **do not resuscitate (DNR) order** is a specific type of advance directive in which an individual states that healthcare providers should not perform CPR if the individual experiences cardiac arrest or cessation of breathing (NCI n.d.b).

The framework for DNR orders is addressed by state law and can vary from state to state. The individual may sign a state-approved consent form specifically tailored to requesting a DNR order. State law typically requires additional signatures from physicians and witnesses. The language required on a DNR consent form varies from state to state but generally describes CPR and indicates the individual's desire not to have CPR performed. The Joint Commission requires that all accredited acute care facilities have institutional policies regarding advance directives and DNR orders, and that they be included in the health record.

Since DNR orders are only utilized in emergency circumstances, it is important that the existence of a DNR order can be immediately communicated to healthcare providers. This is usually accomplished by issuing DNR patients an approved bracelet or some other form of identification that makes it immediately clear to healthcare providers that a valid DNR order is on file for that individual. DNR orders must be kept in the individual's health record, whether that record is paper or electronic.

Individuals have the right to revoke a DNR order at any time. The individual's revocation of the DNR order can be expressed in a variety of ways, such as writing void across the order or by removing or damaging the DNR identifier. Sometimes a DNR order can be affected by a patient's transfer from one facility to another. Some states may allow the order to transfer with the patient, whereas others may require a new order to be issued at the new facility. State law also addresses whether a DNR order is valid during the patient's actual transport from one facility to another. The law may also permit facilities to suspend a DNR order during surgery or when a patient's heart or breathing has stopped because of an unforeseen external event, such as choking or a car accident (Illinois Department of Public Health 2010). As part of the informed consent process, providers and patients should have detailed discussions of circumstances where DNR orders are and are not effective. Some facilities have mandated policies that require patients and physicians to reconsider the desire for a DNR order prior to certain surgeries or other medical interventions (American College of Surgeons 2014).

Patient Self-Determination Act

Advance directives clearly play an important role in the informed consent process. They are the means through which individuals can ensure that their healthcare wishes are carried out even after they are incapacitated or incompetent. To raise public awareness about the use of advance directives, Congress passed the **Patient Self-Determination Act** (PSDA) as part of the Omnibus Budget Reconciliation Act of 1990. The law, which became effective in December 1991, requires healthcare institutions (that is, hospitals, nursing facilities, hospice programs, and home health agencies) that bill Medicare or Medicaid for services to provide adult patients with information about the various types of advance directives. Specifically, providers are required to

- Provide to all adult patients, residents, and enrollees written information on their rights, under state law, to make decisions concerning medical care, including the right to execute an advance directive, as well as maintain the policies of the provider regarding implementation of advance directives
- Document in the health record whether the individual has an advance directive

- Educate the staff and the community about advance directives
- Not condition the provision of care, or otherwise discriminate, on the basis of whether an individual has an advance directive
- Ensure compliance with state law respecting advance directives (General Accountability Office 1995)

Further, the PSDA requires that the Department of Health and Human Services provide public education about advance directives and oversee provider compliance with the law's requirements. In recent years, public education websites have been created to expand the public's knowledge of advance directives and end-of-life care. See, for example, the website, *The Conversation Project* (2016). In 2015, the US General Accountability Office (GAO) reported that many individuals now have advance directives but the prevalence of directives varies by provider type and individual demographic characteristics (GAO 2015).

Uniform Anatomical Gift Act

During the past several decades, medical technology has made significant improvements in the ability to harvest and successfully transplant human organs. The need for organ transplantation is great—as of February 2015, more than 122,071 individuals were on organ transplant waiting lists, according to the US government's official organ donor website (HHS 2015). However, there is a shortage of organs available for transplantation, with an average of 22 people dying each day waiting for a transplant. One of the key barriers to organ donation involves obtaining consent of individuals to donate their organs and enforcing such consent when individuals closely associated with the decedent object.

The legal processes for organ donation are defined by state law. However, consistency among state laws has been promoted through the adoption of the **Uniform Anatomical Gift Act** (UAGA), promulgated by the National Conference of Commissioners on Uniform State Laws (NCCUSL). The UAGA provides suggested standards for all aspects of organ donation, including who may make anatomical gifts and how intent to make anatomical gifts should be expressed. The first UAGA was created in 1968 and was adopted by all 50 states. It created an opt-in system for organ donation where individuals are not considered to be organ donors unless they have specifically indicated a desire to donate. Since then, the act has been revised several times to account for changes in medical technology and laws but has always retained the opt-in element. States have been inconsistent in the degree to which they have adopted subsequent revisions to the UAGA, resulting in confusion and barriers in the transplant process. The most recent revision to the UAGA was distributed in 2009 (Uniform Law Commission 2009). The revised act is shown in figure 8.2.

The UAGA permits an anatomical gift by any person designated to make decisions about the decedent's remains, and where there is more than one person in this class of persons, so long as no objections by other class members are known. If an objection is known, the UAGA permits a majority of the members of the class of persons who are reasonably available to make the gift. The objections of any class members who are not reasonably available do not have to be considered. (Uniform Law Commission 2009).

Again, states are not required to adopt the revised provisions of the UAGA, and the process for obtaining informed consent for organ donation for each state must be followed. The desire to donate organs can be expressed in a number of ways, such as through registering at the Department of Motor Vehicles or leaving specific instructions in an advance directive. Where an individual has left no

---

Figure 8.2 Uniform Anatomical Gift Act (UAGA)

1. Honors the choice of an individual to be or not to be a donor and strengthens the language barring others from overriding a donor's decision to make an anatomical gift (Section 8)

2. Facilitates donations by expanding the list of those who may make an anatomical gift for another individual during that individual's lifetime to include health-care agents and, under certain circumstances, parents or guardians (Section 4)

3. Empowers a minor eligible under other law to apply for a driver's license to be a donor (Section 4)

4. Facilitates donations from a deceased individual who made no lifetime choice by adding to the list of persons who can make a gift of the deceased individual's body or parts the following persons: the person who was acting as the decedent's agent under a power of attorney for healthcare at the time of the decedent's death, the decedent's adult grandchildren, and an adult who exhibited special care and concern for the decedent (Section 9) and defines the meaning of "reasonably available" which is relevant to who can make an anatomical gift of a decedent's body or parts (Section 2(23))

5. Permits an anatomical gift by any member of a class where there is more than one person in the class so long as no objections by other class members are known and, if an objection is known, permits a majority of the members of the class who are reasonably available to make the gift without having to take account of a known objection by any class member who is not reasonably available (Section 9)

6. Creates numerous default rules for the interpretation of a document of gift that lacks specificity regarding either the persons to receive the gift or the purposes of the gift or both (Section 11)

7. Encourages and establishes standards for donor registries (Section 20)

8. Enables procurement organizations to gain access to documents of gifts in donor registries, health records, and the records of a state motor vehicle department (Sections 14 and 20)

9. Resolves the tension between a healthcare directive requesting the withholding or withdrawal of life support systems and anatomical gifts by permitting measures necessary to ensure the medical suitability of organs for intended transplantation or therapy to be administered (Sections 14 and 21)

10. Clarifies and expands the rules relating to cooperation and coordination between procurement organizations and coroners or medical examiners (Sections 22 and 23)

11. Recognizes anatomical gifts made under the laws of other jurisdictions (Section 19)

12. Updates the [act] to allow for electronic records and signatures (Section 25)

Source: Uniform Law Commission 2009.

instructions regarding donations, state law may provide a hierarchy of persons who can consent to organ donation on behalf of the deceased. For example, Kansas law (KS Stat. Ann. 65-1734) states that when there is no notice of contrary wishes by the decedent, the following individuals (in the order of priority stated) may give all or any part of the decedent's body for donation:

- The agent for healthcare decisions established by a durable power of attorney for healthcare decisions, if such power of attorney conveys to the agent the authority to make decisions concerning organ donation
- The spouse
- The decedent's surviving adult children
- The decedent's surviving parents
- The persons in the next degree of kinship under probate law
- A guardian of the person of the decedent at the time of such person's death
- The personal representative of the decedent

Check Your Understanding 8.2

Instructions: Indicate whether the following statements are true or false (T or F).

1. Unless it is designated as durable, a power of attorney is only effective when the principal has capacity.

2. If it is considered a springing DPOA for healthcare decisions, the agent will have decision-making power in all circumstances.

3. A durable power of attorney for healthcare decisions expresses an individual's wishes to limit treatment measures when specific health-related diagnoses or conditions exist and the individual cannot communicate on his own behalf.

4. The technical process for executing a living will is standardized nationally.

5. The Patient Self-Determination Act requires hospitals that are Medicare providers to document in the health record whether an individual has an advance directive.

6. The Uniform Anatomical Gift Act permits an anatomical gift by any person designated to make decisions about a decedent's remains, as long as no objections are known.

7. A decision to be an organ donor can only be made by an adult (person of legal age).

Parties to Consent

The rights and processes surrounding informed consent operate differently depending on whether the individual is a competent adult, an incompetent adult, or a minor child. A **competent adult** is an individual who is mentally capable and is at or above the age of majority. An **incompetent adult** refers to an individual who is at or above the age of majority but is incapacitated due to illness or injury, either permanently or temporarily. The **age of majority** is the legal recognition that an individual is considered responsible for, and has control over, his or her actions. These actions include consenting to or refusing medical treatment, voting, entering into binding contracts, enlisting in the armed forces, marrying, buying alcohol, and other actions defined by state law. In most states, the age of majority is 18 years. Exceptions include states such as Alabama and Nebraska (19 years) and Mississippi (21 years). Some states, such as Nevada, base the age of majority upon graduation from high school or a designated age, whichever occurs earlier. An incompetent adult is an individual who is no longer capable of controlling his or her actions because of illness, injury, or disability. Control over this individual is through an agent or guardian. A **minor** is generally defined as an individual who is under the age of majority and whose rights are usually exercised through a parent or other legal guardian. There are, however, certain circumstances that allow minors to exercise their own decision-making rights. The rights and processes surrounding informed consent are discussed in more detail below.

Competent Adults

Absent the exceptions discussed above, competent adults have a general right to consent to or refuse medical treatment. As "right to die" court decisions have ruled, a competent adult's right to refuse consent to medical treatment applies even when the treatment is lifesaving. Treatment may be refused for any reason, whether it is religious, financial, or personal. The right to refuse treatment stems from more than a century of court decisions recognizing the profound importance of bodily integrity. In 1891, the United States Supreme Court observed, "[n]o right is held more sacred, or is more carefully guarded by the common law, than the right of every individual to the possession and control of his own person, free from all restraint or interference of others, unless by clear and unquestionable authority of law" (*Union Pacific R. Co. v. Botsford*, 1891).

For decades, courts have specifically applied the notion of bodily integrity in the context of medical care. In 1910, Benjamin Cardozo, who would later become a Supreme Court Justice, stated, "Every human being of adult years and sound mind has a right to determine what shall be done with his own body, and a surgeon who performs an operation without his patient's consent commits an assault, for which he is liable in damages" (*Schloendorff v. Society of New York Hospital*, 1914). When the refusal to consent is based on a religious belief, the First Amendment's freedom of religion clause provides additional authority for refusing treatment. Perhaps the most recognized example of refusing medical care based on religious beliefs occurs when Jehovah's Witnesses refuse consent to certain types of blood transfusions.

In general, the right to refuse consent to medical care has two important prerequisites: adulthood and competence. To be an adult, one must have reached the age of majority. Although the standards vary from state to state, competence can generally be described as an individual's overall ability to understand, process, and communicate information adequately enough to meet essential life needs, such as food, clothing, shelter, safety, and health. Some individuals, such as those born with profound mental retardation, are never legally competent. Healthcare decisions for these individuals are generally made by parents when the individual is a minor and by court-appointed guardians after the individual reaches adulthood. Competent individuals may experience temporary or permanent loss of competence as a result of injury or illness. How healthcare decisions are made in these situations depends on whether an individual executed an advance directive such as a DPOA-HCD while he or she was still competent.

When a competent adult refuses consent to lifesaving medical treatment, two competing sets of interests arise. The first is the individual's well-established interest in privacy, due process, and self-determination. The second is the government's compelling interest in protecting and preserving human life, which has also been established through years of case law. While both interests are strong, the interests of a competent individual usually outweigh the interests of the government.

In the Matter of Robert Quackenbush demonstrates how the two sets of interests are balanced. The case involved a 72-year-old patient who, because of his previous refusal to seek medical care for arteriosclerosis, had such advanced gangrene in his legs that one foot was literally dangling, about to fall off. Without amputating both legs, doctors expected the patient to die within three weeks. The patient, who had refused medical care for over 40 years, was described by doctors as a "conscientious objector to medical therapy." He refused to consent to the operation because he simply wanted to return home and "live out his life." Based on the apparent irrationality of the patient's decision and the belief that infection was cognitively impairing the patient, the hospital petitioned the court to appoint a guardian who would consent to the amputation on behalf of the patient. In hearing the case, the first issue that the court addressed was whether the patient was a competent adult. The following is a summary of the evidence presented regarding competency:

- A physician who evaluated the patient on January 6th concluded that the patient was not competent to make an informed medical decision because he was disoriented as to his location, confused about who was around him, responded to questions inappropriately, and suffered visual hallucinations. The physician acknowledged that the patient's confusion could have stemmed from septicemia, which was treatable with antibiotics.

- A physician who evaluated the patient on January 11th found some fluctuations in mental lucidity, but not to such a degree that the patient was mentally incompetent. The patient and the physician thoroughly discussed his condition and the ramifications of having the operation. The physician determined that the patient had the mental capacity to make an informed choice regarding the operation. (At that point, the septicemia was better controlled, which reduced the patient's confusion.)

- The judge, who interviewed the patient on January 12, found him to be responsive and reasonably alert. The patient again expressed his wishes to forgo the surgery but left open the possibility of changing his mind if he began to experience pain (*In the Matter of Robert Quackenbush*, 1978).

Based on the evidence as a whole, the court found the patient to be mentally competent. However, the finding of competence did not end the court's inquiry—the court still needed to balance the patient's interests against the interest of the state. The hospital equated the patient's decision to refuse treatment with suicide and argued that allowing a patient to commit suicide was inconsistent with the state's compelling interest in preserving life. The court did not directly address whether the patient was committing suicide, but instead acknowledged that the "... State's interest weakens and the individual's right to privacy grows as the degree of bodily invasion increases and the prognosis dims, until the ultimate point when the individual's rights overcome the State's interest in preserving life."

The court went on to hold that "the extensive bodily invasion involved here—the amputation of both legs above the knee and possibly the amputation of both legs entirely—is sufficient to make the State's interest in the preservation of life give way to [the patient's] right of privacy to decide his own future regardless of the absence of a dim prognosis ... No decision of this nature is easily made. Always present is the predominant interest in the preservation of life. But constitutional and decisional law invest [the patient] with rights that overcome that interest. [The patient], therefore, as a mentally competent individual, has the right to make his informed choice concerning the operation and I will not interfere with that choice."

In the Quackenbush case, the hospital's main argument was that the patient was committing suicide by refusing treatment and that permitting a patient to commit suicide was inconsistent with the state's interest in preserving life. When faced with this argument, courts typically distinguish between refusal of consent and suicide. The distinction is that suicide involves an act, whereas refusal of consent involves the withholding or revocation of an act. The state has a strong interest in prohibiting affirmative acts that will lead to death, such as intentionally administering a drug that will end the patient's life. However, the state's interest is not as strong when it is the patient's refusal to act (the refusal or revocation of consent) at issue. Again, the right to refuse consent is rooted in the long-standing principles of personal autonomy and self-determination.

Whenever an individual refuses consent or withdraws his or her consent, providers should clearly document that the risks, benefits, and alternatives of not administering treatment or withdrawing consent were explained to the patient. They should also obtain the individual's written acknowledgement that the risks, benefits, and alternatives of withdrawing consent were explained, and that the patient is still electing to do so.

Incompetent Adults

If an individual is no longer competent due to an illness or an injury, then that individual cannot be expected to provide informed consent for nonemergency medical treatment. An individual's incompetence may arise from a temporary problem, such as acute impairment stemming from the use of alcohol or drugs, or it may arise from a long-term or chronic condition, such as Alzheimer's disease or brain injury. Contrary to common belief, not all states have "surrogate consent" laws that automatically permit spouses or adult children and siblings to provide legal consent on behalf of an incompetent individual. Therefore, absent any advance directive, it may be necessary to appoint a guardian for the individual, especially when incompetence is likely to be long-term.

Guardianship proceedings are typically initiated by a healthcare provider or family member involved in the incompetent individual's care. At the guardianship proceeding, evidence regarding the individual's alleged incompetence is presented by qualified healthcare providers. The court will also hear testimony from a guardian ad litem, which is a lawyer appointed by the court to represent the interests of the incompetent individual during the guardianship proceedings. It may also hear evidence from other sources, such as social workers appointed to evaluate the appropriateness of a proposed guardian. After hearing the evidence, a court may appoint the spouse, adult child, or sibling as an individual's guardian or it may choose to appoint some other qualified person. Healthcare providers involved in the treatment of an individual are not usually appointed as guardians. Courts are concerned that appointing a treatment provider as a patient's guardian could give rise to a conflict of interest. For example, the treatment provider may have incentive to make consent decisions based on economic factors rather than what is in the patient's best interest. Once appointed, guardians are required to make regular reports to the court on the status of the ward (the patient).

The extent of the guardian's ability to consent to medical treatment on behalf of the incompetent individual varies from state to state (KS Stat. Ann. 59-3075). Typically, guardians have statutory authority to consent or refuse to consent to medical interventions in accordance with what is in the best interest of the ward (incompetent individual). However, states often limit a guardian's power to consent to certain interventions, unless those interventions have been approved by the court. For example, nonemergency interventions involving psychosurgery, organ removal, amputation, sterilization, and experimental treatments must be approved by a court in advance.

Cases involving incompetent adults can be divided into three broad categories:

- Adults who were once competent and executed an advance directive
- Adults who were once competent but did not execute an advance directive
- Adults who never had competence

From a legal standpoint, the first category is the most straightforward. When an individual has properly executed an advance directive, then treatment decisions are generally made in accordance with that advance directive. Conflicts do not usually arise unless there is disagreement about whether the agent is acting in the principal's best interest or making decisions that are inconsistent with the principal's previously expressed wishes.

As mentioned earlier, many adults have preemptively expressed their wishes regarding medical treatment through advance directives. Many others simply have occasional end-of-life discussions with family and friends, where they informally express their desires (that is, not to be maintained in a persistent vegetative state, or PVS). However, the absence of a formal advance directive can raise complex consent-to-treatment issues. How do healthcare providers know what treatment options an individual would consent to if he or she still had competence? Some states address this issue through surrogate consent laws that permit spouses, adult children, parents, siblings, and so on, to consent on behalf of an incompetent adult. Consent decisions are made by the person who is highest in the hierarchy specified by the law. For example, if the hierarchy is spouse, adult child, adult siblings, parents, then an incapacitated individual's spouse would first provide consent on the individual's behalf. If no spouse were available, then consent decisions would be made by the individual's adult children. If there were no adult children, then any adult siblings would make consent decisions, and if no adult siblings, consent would default to parents. If the individual has no family that fit into the surrogate consent hierarchy, then a court would most likely appoint a guardian to make consent decisions on behalf of the individual.

Surrogate consent laws may or may not provide a framework for addressing disagreement about consent decisions among individuals at the same hierarchal level (such as adult children or adult siblings). If conflict over treatment options exists, a hearing is held before a court. Further, surrogate consent laws often limit the kind of consent choices that can be made by surrogates in the hierarchy. For example, the law may prohibit surrogates from making consent decisions relating to mental health treatment, pregnancy care, or withdrawal of life-sustaining treatment. The Uniform Health-Care Decisions Act, a model for state-adopted surrogate consent laws, is discussed later in this chapter.

If no surrogate consent law exists or the proposed medical intervention is outside the scope of the surrogate consent law, then the treatment decision is usually made by a court-appointed guardian. Once appointed, the guardian is obligated to step into the shoes of the incapacitated individual and must attempt to make treatment decisions in accordance with what the individual would want if he or she were still competent. However, when treatment decisions by guardians involve end-of-life decisions, the courts may step in.

The first major case to deal with this kind of issue was *In re Quinlan* (1976). The case involved a young woman who had suffered severe brain damage and entered a PVS. Her father, who was her legally appointed guardian, petitioned the court to approve the disconnection of Quinlan's respirator after her providers refused to terminate her life support. The court held that, even while incompetent, Quinlan had a constitutional right of privacy to terminate treatment. The only practical way to exercise this right was to allow her guardian and family to decide whether Quinlan would exercise her right to refuse treatment under the circumstances.

After Quinlan, courts grappled with the question of how much evidence is necessary to prove an incompetent individual's intent to consent to the withdrawal of life-sustaining treatment after he or she has become permanently incompetent. The seminal case addressing this question was *Cruzan v. Director, Missouri Department of Health* (1990). Like Quinlan, Cruzan was a young woman who had entered a PVS. Cruzan had been in a PVS for several years when her parents, as guardians, asked that her artificial nutrition and hydration be removed. Hospital staff refused to remove the artificial nutrition and hydration because doing so would cause Cruzan's death. A state trial court authorized the withdrawal based upon the constitutional right to direct or refuse the withdrawal of life-sustaining treatment. The trial court found that a prior statement by Cruzan to her housemate that she would not wish to continue her life if sick or injured unless she could live "at least halfway normally" was sufficient evidence that Cruzan would not consent to artificial nutrition and hydration. The state supreme court reversed the decision of the trial court, finding that Cruzan's statements to her housemate were unreliable for the purpose of determining her intent.

The court went on to hold that where no advance directive exists, no person can assume an end-of-life choice on behalf of an incompetent person unless there is "clear and convincing" evidence that the person would refuse consent to life-sustaining treatment under the circumstances. Cruzan's parents appealed the decision of the state supreme court to the United States Supreme Court. The US Supreme Court affirmed the decision of the state supreme court and held that a state may require evidence of an incompetent individual's wishes as to the withdrawal of life-sustaining treatment be proved by clear and convincing evidence. After the Supreme Court decision, additional evidence of Cruzan's wishes surfaced and a new hearing was held regarding the termination of her artificial nutrition and hydration. The trial court found that the additional evidence met the "clear and convincing" standard set by the Supreme Court and ordered the withdrawal of her artificial nutrition and hydration. No legal challenges succeeded against the order and Cruzan's artificial nutrition and hydration were ultimately removed.

A more recent and by far the most highly publicized and politically charged end-of-life case involved that of Terri Schiavo. Ms. Schiavo was a 26-year-old woman who collapsed in 1990, suffering cardiac

Table 8.1 Key differences among the three end-of-life cases

Case	Quinlan	Cruzan	Schiavo
Issue	Removal of respirator	Removal of nutrition/hydration	Removal of nutrition/hydration
Key conflict	Conflict among family members and provider(s)	Conflict among family members and provider(s)	Conflict among family members

and respiratory failure that sent her into a PVS. Eight years later, Michael Schiavo, her husband and legal guardian, sought intervention through the Florida court system (where Ms. Schiavo resided and which had jurisdiction over the case) to have her feeding tube removed. The court ordered the removal of the feeding tube in 2000, finding that testimony provided by Mr. Schiavo and other in-laws of Ms. Schiavo's constituted "clear and convincing evidence" that Ms. Schiavo would not have wished to receive life-prolonging measures given her current condition (Pinellas County Probate Court, Florida 1990).

The removal was opposed by Ms. Schiavo's parents. Years of legal battles culminated in 2005 with numerous motions and petitions filed with the courts and a media frenzy that fueled the "right-to-life" versus "right-to-die" debate. Both the Florida legislature and the US Congress had passed laws that would have had the effect of precluding the removal of Ms. Schiavo's feeding tube, thus creating a seesaw effect between legislative and judicial powers and calling into question the legal authority of legislative bodies to intervene in judicial matters such as this. The legal battle came to an end on March 18, 2005, when Ms. Schiavo's feeding tube was removed per the local court's order. She died on March 31, 2005, at the age of 41 years (Law Center 2005). One positive outcome of the Schiavo case was the interest it generated in the concept of advance directives and the renewed desire for individuals to memorialize their own end-of-life wishes through these documents. See table 8.1 for a comparison of the Quinlan, Cruzan, and Schiavo cases.

The clear and convincing evidence standard set forth by the Supreme Court applies to determining the wishes of a formerly competent individual. However, the standard does not apply well to circumstances where an individual has never had competence. *In Re Storar* involved a profoundly retarded 52-year-old man who had been diagnosed with bladder cancer. Part of his treatment included periodic blood transfusions, which were necessary to prolong his life. His mother, who was also his legal guardian, refused consent to the transfusions because she believed that they caused Storar too much distress. The New York Court of Appeals noted that where an individual has never been competent, "it is unrealistic to attempt to determine whether he would want to continue potentially life-prolonging treatment if he were competent" (*In Re Storar*, 1981). After hearing evidence about the transfusions, the court concluded that it should not "allow an incompetent patient to bleed to death because someone, even someone as close as a parent or sibling, feels that this is best for one with an incurable disease" (*In Re Storar*, 1981). Instead, the court applied a "best interest" standard and determined that continued transfusions were in the best interest of Storar. The transfusions did not involve excessive pain and without them, Storar's mental and physical abilities would deteriorate. Therefore, the court concluded that it was in Storar's best interest to continue the transfusions.

Uniform Health-Care Decisions Act

As the preceding discussion indicates, there has been much more attention and legislation focused on incapacitated individuals who are dying than on incapacitated individuals who are seeking recovery. As a result, the Uniform Law Commissioners of the National Conference of Commissioners on Uniform

State Laws created in 1993 the **Uniform Health-Care Decisions Act** (UHCDA), a model law that several states have adopted. "Leaping over" state DPOA-HCD and living will legislation, it provides an additional option to the creation of these documents. Specifically, it provides that an individual who is an "adult with capacity or emancipated minor [described later in this chapter] may give an oral or written instruction to a health-care provider, which remains in force even after the individual loses capacity." Advance directives that comply with the UHCDA continue to be honored in states that have adopted the UHCDA.

In the absence of an advance directive (which entails the appointment of an agent) or a court-appointed guardian, a surrogate that has been identified for the healthcare provider by the individual may make healthcare decisions on behalf of that individual. Absent the selection of a surrogate by the individual, a person related to the individual may assume that authority. Any person who acts as a surrogate must follow the individual's instructions regarding his or her healthcare or, without instructions, act in the individual's best interests. Under the model law, healthcare providers who decline to comply with a surrogate must make reasonable efforts to transfer the individual to a provider who will comply. A healthcare provider's good faith compliance with the surrogate's instructions shields the provider from civil and criminal liability.

The Uniform Health-Care Decisions Act suggests that decision-making priority for an individual's next of kin be as follows, but state laws may tailor the order differently:

- Spouse
- Adult child
- Parent
- Adult sibling
- If no one is available who is so related to the individual, authority may be granted to "an adult who has exhibited special care and concern for the individual, who is familiar with the patient's personal values, and who is willing and able to make a health-care decision for the patient."
- Absent an unrelated adult who exhibits the above characteristics, a healthcare provider may seek appointment of a decision-maker by the court having jurisdiction (Uniform Law Commissioners 2002).

Minors

Although the general rule is that an individual must be a competent adult to consent to medical treatment, state laws allow minors to provide their own consent in certain situations. A **minor** is generally defined (varies by state) as an individual who is under 18 years of age and who has not been legally emancipated (declared to be an adult) by a court. By virtue of their age, minors are generally considered legally incompetent and unable to consent to their own treatment. Therefore, the consent of a parent or other legal guardian, if applicable, is sought before treatment is provided. However, some special situations and exceptions related to the consent of treatment for minors are discussed below. The National District Attorney Association's (2013) also provides a list of consent to medical treatment laws for minors. As noted previously in this chapter, emergency situations are an exception to the consent requirement whether the patient is an adult or a minor.

Emancipated and Mature Minors

As stated previously, **emancipated minors** are those who have been afforded legal status as an adult, generally by a situational change such as marriage. Depending on the state, statutes or judicial decisions define the parameters for emancipation. They may provide that the minor and his or her parents agree to the emancipation and the minor is self-supporting and living independently. With respect to medical treatment, parental consent should first be attempted in the absence of documentation proving emancipation. If this cannot be accomplished and a minor claims to be emancipated without supporting documentation, advice from legal counsel should be sought. It is noted that this situation applies to nonemergency situations. As described earlier in this chapter, emergencies provide an exception to the consent requirement for minors as well as adults.

Mature minors are those who meet age limits and, in some cases, other factors provided by state law that enable them to consent to their own treatment in certain situations. Many of the state laws that provide for minors to consent to their own treatment are based on public policy; that is, it is deemed more desirable for a minor to consent to his or her own treatment than to forgo that treatment because the minor does not want parents to have knowledge of a specific health condition. Such conditions, including sexually transmitted diseases and substance abuse, are detailed later.

Separated and Divorced Parents of a Minor

When parents of a minor are legally separated or divorced, issues can arise regarding the authority of either parent to consent to treatment. As with children in intact families, the consent of only one parent is generally required. However, do both parents have equal legal standing when only one of them is the custodial parent? State law should be consulted regarding the relative rights of custodial and noncustodial parents. As a matter of policy, healthcare providers may first seek consent from the custodial parent. However, care should be taken not to violate state laws that, absent a court order to the contrary, afford both parents equal legal standing regarding the medical treatment of their minor child. If a healthcare provider has reason to believe that a court has not given a parent full legal rights with respect to his or her child, documentation from the court should be required prior to honoring that parent's consent to treatment of the minor in nonemergency situations.

Treatment for Sexually Transmitted Diseases

State laws generally allow minors to seek medical interventions for the diagnosis and treatment of sexually transmitted diseases (STDs) without requiring parental consent. Therefore, providers may diagnose and treat minors for STDs without having to inform a minor's parents or guardians, and cannot be held liable for failing to obtain parental or guardian consent. The policy behind these laws is based on the presumption that many minors would not seek diagnosis and treatment of STDs if they thought their parents or guardians would find out. As a result of not seeking treatment, a minor could suffer medical complications as well as spread the STD to others. An excerpt of one such law, from Kansas, is provided here:

> Any physician, upon consultation by any person under eighteen (18) years of age as a patient, may, with the consent of such person who is hereby granted the right of giving such consent, make a diagnostic examination for venereal disease and prescribe for and treat such person for venereal disease including prophylactic treatment for exposure to venereal disease whenever such person is suspected of having a venereal disease or contact with anyone having a venereal disease. All such examinations and treatment may be performed without the consent of, or notification to, the parent, parents, guardian or any other person having custody of such person. (KS Stat. Ann. 65-2892)

Treatment for Drug or Alcohol Conditions

States generally have laws permitting minors to consent on their own behalf to the diagnosis and treatment of substance abuse and related problems. The policy behind these laws is similar to that for permitting minors to consent to the diagnosis and treatment of STDs. The concern is that minors would refuse to seek medical treatment for alcohol or drug problems if they thought that their parents or guardians would be told about the treatment. By not seeking treatment, a minor is not only endangering himself or herself, but also may place others in danger while under the influence. Therefore, states do not want to create barriers (such as parental consent) to minors seeking necessary diagnosis and treatment. An excerpt of a law allowing minors to consent to drug abuse or misuse or addiction is provided here:

> Any physician licensed to practice the healing arts in Kansas, upon consultation with any minor as a patient, may examine and treat such minor for drug abuse, misuse or addiction if such physician has secured the prior consent of such minor to the examination and treatment. All such examinations and treatment may be performed without the consent of any parent, guardian or other person having custody of such minor, and all minors are hereby granted the right to give consent to such examination and treatment (KS Stat. Ann. 65-2892a).

Induced Termination of Pregnancy (Abortion)

State laws generally prohibit providers from performing abortions on minors unless certain conditions are satisfied. For example, if a minor is legally emancipated or has written consent of at least one parent or guardian, then a state may permit the abortion to be performed. Otherwise, states have varying laws that may allow a minor to petition the court for an order or permission to consent to the abortion without parental or guardian consent or knowledge. For example, in Missouri, to substitute judicial consent for parental or guardian consent for a minor's abortion, a court must determine that judicial consent is in the best interests of the minor and that the minor has been fully informed of the risks and medical consequences of an abortion (MO Rev. Stat. 188.028).

Prenatal Care

State laws may provide for a minor to receive prenatal care without her parents' consent. Such laws further the public policy purpose of promoting the health of the mother, her unborn child, and, later, her infant. It follows, then, that the consent of the parent, even if that parent is a minor, must be secured prior to treating the minor's child.

Check Your Understanding 8.3

Instructions: Indicate whether the following statements are true or false (T or F).

1. A competent adult's right to refuse consent to medical treatment applies even when the treatment is lifesaving.
2. A healthcare organization can confidently follow the wishes expressed in a properly executed advance directive, even if the patient (who is competent) has changed his or her mind.
3. In right-to-die cases, courts will balance an individual's right to self-determination against the interest of the state.
4. An emancipated minor is one who has not been afforded legal status as an adult.
5. State laws generally allow minors to seek medical treatment for sexually transmitted diseases without parental consent.

Challenges to Consents

Much of this chapter has discussed challenges to consent brought before the proposed intervention is actually performed. For example, in the *Quackenbush* case, the patient was challenging a doctor's opinion that he should consent to the amputation of his legs. The challenge was made before the amputation actually occurred. However, sometimes challenges to consent are brought after an intervention has already been performed. They are usually based on a total lack of consent or a lack of fully informed consent.

Lack of Consent

If an individual alleges that he or she never gave consent to an intervention that was actually performed, then the basis of the claim is usually battery. As discussed in chapter 6, battery consists of the intentional and nonconsensual contact with the plaintiff's person. In *Duncan v. Scottsdale Medical Imaging*, the plaintiff alleged that she informed defendants that she was allergic to certain medications and specifically stated that she only consented to the injection of morphine or Demerol. According to the plaintiff, the defendants injected her with fentanyl despite telling her that the proper medication was being used. The plaintiff further claimed that the administration of fentanyl caused severe headache, projectile vomiting, breathing difficulties, posttraumatic stress disorder, and vocal cord dysfunction. She sued the defendants for battery.

In analyzing the case, the court stated that "the battery theory should be reserved for those circumstances when a doctor performs an operation to which the patient has not consented. When the patient gives permission to perform one type of treatment and the doctor performs another, the requisite element of deliberate intent to deviate from the consent given is present" (*Duncan v. Scottsdale Medical Imaging*, 2003). The defendant argued that administering the injection did not constitute battery because the plaintiff had in fact consented to an injection, even if that injection was fentanyl. However, the court noted that the plaintiff "explicitly conditioned her consent on the use of morphine or Demerol and rejected the use of any other drug. Conduct involving the use of a sedative other than morphine or Demerol, contrary to explicit instruction and understanding, cannot be viewed as consensual." The court went on to state, "The relevant inquiry here is not whether the patient consented to an injection; the issue is whether the patient consented to receive the specific drug that was administered. Duncan could have given broad consent to the administration of any painkiller, but she gave specific instructions that she would accept only morphine or Demerol and nothing else. We hold that when a patient gives limited or conditional consent, a healthcare provider has committed a battery if the evidence shows the provider acted with willful disregard of the consent given."

Lack of Fully Informed Consent

Sometimes an individual consents to a procedure but later alleges that he or she was not fully informed of the risks, benefits, and alternatives associated with that procedure. Under these circumstances, a negligence claim specifically based on lack of informed consent is most appropriate. To be successful, the plaintiff must first prove that the defendant fell below the applicable standard of care. The standard of care is usually determined through expert testimony and can vary somewhat from state to state. For example, in *Hamilton v. Ashton*, the plaintiff experienced permanent facial paralysis after undergoing an ear surgery. She sued the defendant on multiple theories, including malpractice and lack of informed consent. With respect to the standard of care, the court stated, "Under the doctrine of informed consent, a doctor must disclose the facts and risks of a treatment which a reasonably prudent physician would be expected to disclose under like circumstances and which a reasonable person would want to know. This is separate and apart from the doctor's duty to 'exercise that degree of care, skill, and proficiency exercised by reasonably careful, skillful, and prudent practitioners in the same class to which he belongs, acting under the same or similar circumstances'" (*Hamilton v. Ashton*, 2006).

In *Acuna v. Turkish*, the court stated, "A physician's duty of disclosure in the typical malpractice case is measured by the 'prudent patient' or 'materiality of risk' standard. The standard relates to the patient's needs, not the physician's judgment. '[A] physician must disclose to a patient all material information that a 'prudent patient' might find significant for a determination whether to undergo the proposed [medical procedure].' This standard is objective. 'The test for determining whether a particular risk must be disclosed is its materiality to the patient's decision, i.e., all risks potentially affecting the decision must be divulged.'"

Even if it is determined that the defendant fell below the applicable standard of care, the plaintiff must also prove that the defendant's failure to meet the standard actually caused the plaintiff's injury. In other words, the plaintiff must show that he or she would have made a different treatment decision if there had been full disclosure. The specific standard for establishing causation varies from state to state but usually involves the application of an objective reasonable or prudent person standard. The standard asks what a reasonable person, in the plaintiff's situation, would have done if he or she had been fully informed. For example, in *Wilson v. Merritt*, the plaintiff was a paraplegic who suffered a torn rotator cuff and a fractured shoulder during a manipulation under anesthesia procedure performed by a chiropractor. The plaintiff claimed that he would not have consented to the surgery if he had been aware that there were risks of a bone fracture or a torn rotator cuff. In applying the objective standard for causation, the court stated, "[the plaintiff] must show that a reasonable, prudent paraplegic, who had been largely paralyzed by a prior surgery and was dependent upon the use of his arms and shoulders for any mobility at all, and who, at that point, had already achieved about a 20 percent improvement in his adhesive capsulitis condition based on physical therapy alone, would have declined the procedure if informed that it could result in a torn rotator cuff and a fractured bone" (*Wilson v. Merritt*, 2006). The court went on to note, "there was sufficient evidence for a jury to conclude that, under the circumstances, a reasonable, prudent paraplegic would indeed have passed up the opportunity" (*Wilson v. Merritt*, 2006).

Documenting Consent

As a general rule, obtaining consent is a non-delegable duty. In other words, it is the responsibility of the treating provider to obtain informed consent, and it may not be delegated to some other person. When individuals enter a hospital, they are often provided with a general consent form as part of their initial paperwork. This form covers routine diagnostic procedures and medical treatment by hospital staff, as well as other activities, such as release of information for treatment purposes and disposal of human tissue and body fluids. General consent from an individual can be obtained by a staff member of the organization providing the healthcare services. However, if the patient is having a specific type of surgery (for example, open heart surgery), the surgeon is responsible for obtaining informed consent specifically for that surgery. For both general consent and informed consent, organizational policy may provide for staff members to check for the presence of signed consent forms on patient records.

Whether consent is written or oral, it should be documented in the individual's health record. Written consent is typically provided on a separate document signed by the individual. Especially when consent is provided orally, documentation should describe the risks, benefits, and alternatives discussed by the patient and provider and reflect that patient questions were adequately answered. In certain situations, consent must be obtained in writing. For example, the Common Rule requires the written consent of research subjects, unless the consent requirement has been waived or altered by an IRB (National

Institutes of Health 2006). Various state laws also provide that certain medical interventions require written consent. Those interventions often pertain to the following:

- Sterilization
- Hysterectomy
- Breast cancer treatment
- Prostate cancer treatment
- Gynecological cancer treatment
- Psychosurgery
- Electroconvulsive therapy (Foundation for Taxpayer and Consumer Rights n.d.)

CMS and other insurers also require written consent for specific procedures. Their requirement may include a specific form or language to be used when documenting the consent process.

Types of Consent Forms

There are three main types of consent forms: general (or blanket), short form, and long form.

General

Typically, a general consent form is used when individuals are admitted to a hospital or outpatient facility. By signing this form, an individual consents to whatever procedures, interventions, or other routine services (as compared to invasive services that require informed consent) a provider may determine to be medically necessary (Pozgar 2015). Other types of general consent forms may allow school nurses, sports coaches, and camp counselors to consent to nonmedical treatment in place of a minor's parent or guardian. These consents are limited in scope and are temporary.

Short Form

In the human subjects research context, a **short form** is a written document stating that the elements of informed consent required by the Common Rule have been orally presented to and understood by the subject or the subject's legally authorized representative. When the short form is used, there must be a witness to the fact that subjects were orally provided with the requirements for informed consent. The witness must sign the short form (along with the subject) as well as a copy of an IRB-approved written summary of what was said to the subject or the subject's representative (45 CFR 46.117(b)(2)).

The same standards for a short form consent may also be applied in a nonresearch context. Providers may orally explain risks, benefits, and alternatives and have the individual sign a document acknowledging that such an explanation was provided and understood. In such cases, it is advisable for the provider to also have a witness sign the short form and acknowledge the information that was explained.

Long Form

Again, in the human subjects research context, a **long form** is a consent form that includes all of the informed consent requirements included in the Common Rule (see previous section on informed consent requirements). Outside of research, long consent forms should be used when a proposed medical intervention is particularly high risk, invasive, or experimental.

Check Your Understanding 8.4

Instructions: Indicate whether the following statements are true or false (T or F).

1. Battery is the usual basis of a claim for which an individual did not give consent for a procedure that was performed.

2. The basis for a lack of informed consent claim is generally negligence.

3. General consent allows healthcare providers to provide routine noninvasive services.

4. The use of short consent forms generally requires the signature of a witness to the explanation of risks, benefits, and alternatives.

5. So-called long consent forms are only associated with human subjects research.

Scenario 8

Mr. Jones is a 92-year-old gentleman with acute congestive heart failure. He has a long list of comorbidities, and his prognosis is guarded. Upon discussion with Mr. Jones' family members present, the medical resident documents a "do not resuscitate decision" in the electronic record on day one of hospitalization. On day three of hospitalization, Mr. Jones' daughter, named as agent in Mr. Jones' durable medical power of attorney, arrives from out of town and speaks to the attending physician, asking him to cancel the DNR order and resuscitate, if necessary. This is handwritten in the progress notes, which are scanned into the electronic record, but the electronic field where DNR orders are documented is not changed. In addition, in the daily progress notes entered by the medical resident, the day one discussion resulting in the DNR order continues to be copied and pasted into the record each day, making it appear that the DNR order is still in force. Mr. Jones' son disagrees with the daughter's decision and feels it was uninformed; he complains that he (as a registered nurse) was in a better position to make the correct decision. Unfortunately, on day 5 of hospitalization, Mr. Jones' condition deteriorates and he has a cardiac arrest. Code Blue is called by the nurse on duty, and the team arrives to begin resuscitation. Shortly after they begin, the unit clerk enters the room and tells the team that "this patient is DNR." Resuscitation is canceled and Mr. Jones dies.

1. Who had authority to decide whether Mr. Jones should be resuscitated? Is any information that is necessary to answer this question missing from the scenario? If so, what else must be known to decide this question?

2. Who should be responsible for documenting DNR decisions?

3. What should happen if a record reflects conflicting documentation?

4. Are there circumstances in which family members should NOT be allowed to make DNR decisions on behalf of a patient?

5. How did the format and capabilities of the electronic record contribute to the confusion in this case? What could be done to address those problems?

References

American College of Surgeons. 2014. Statement on advance directives by patients: "Do not resuscitate" in the operating room. *Bulletin of the American College of Surgeons* 99(1):42–43.

American Medical Association Council on Ethical and Judicial Affairs. 2006. CEJA report 2-A-06: Withholding information from patients (therapeutic privilege). http://www.ama-assn.org.

American Medical Association. n.d. Patient physician relationship topics: Informed consent. http://www.ama-assn.org.

Arizona Secretary of State. 2015. Arizona Advance Directive Registry. http://www.azsos.gov.

Department of Health and Human Services. 2015. Organ donation statistics. https://www.organdonor.gov/statistics-stories/statistics.html#glance.

The Foundation for Taxpayer and Consumer Rights. n.d. The California patient's guide: Your health care rights and remedies. http://www.calpatientguide.org.

General Accountability Office. 1995. Patient Self-Determination Act: Providers offer information on advance directives but effectiveness uncertain (Letter Report GAO/HEHS-95-135). http://www.gao.gov.

General Accountability Office. 2015. Advance directives: Information on federal oversight, provider implementation and prevalence. (GAO-15-416). http://www.gao.gov.

Illinois Department of Public Health. 2010. Uniform do-not-resuscitate (DNR) advance directive. Guidance for individuals. http://www.dph.illinois.gov/.

Kansas Legal Services. 2016. Living wills and durable powers of attorney. http://www.kansaslegalservices.org/.

Law Center. 2005. Terri Schiavo has died. http://www.cnn.com.

Missouri Bar. 2014. Living wills and other advance directives. http://www.mobar.org.

National Cancer Institute. n.d.a. Research on human specimens. http://www.cancerdiagnosis.nci.nih.gov.

National Cancer Institute. n.d.b. Dictionary of cancer terms. DNR order. http://www.cancer.gov.

National District Attorneys Association. 2013. Minor consent to medical treatment laws. http://www.ndaa.org.

National Institutes of Health, Office of Human Subjects Research. 1979. The Belmont report: Ethical principles and guidelines for the protection of human subjects of research.

National Institutes of Health. Office of Human Subjects Research 2006 (Dec. 28). Sheet 6—Guidelines for writing informed consent documents. http://ohsr.od.nih.gov.

Ohio Hospice & Palliative Care Organization. 2004. Choices: Living Well at the End of Life. Advance Directives Packet. https://www.daybar.org/_files/Advance_Directives.pdf.

Oregon Department of Motor Vehicles. n.d. Suspensions and revocations. http://www.oregon.gov.

Pinellas County Probate Court, Florida. 1990. In re: The Guardianship of Theresa Marie Schiavo, Incapacitated. File No. 90-2908GD-003. http://abstractappeal.com.

Pozgar, G. 2015. *Legal Aspects of Health Care Administration*, 12th ed. Sudbury, MA: Jones and Bartlett.

State of California Emergency Medical Services Authority. 2013. Do not resuscitate (DNR) and other patient-designated directives. http://emsa.ca.gov.

Tennessee Department of Health. n.d.a. Advance directives. http://www.tn.gov/health.

Tennessee Department of Health. n.d.b. Advance directives for health care decision making. http://www.tn.gov/health.

The Conversation Project. (2016). http://theconversationproject.org/.

Uniform Law Commission. 2002. Uniform Health-Care Decisions Act. http://www.uniformlaws.org.

Uniform Law Commission. 2009. Revised Uniform Anatomical Gift Act (2006) (Last Revised or Amended in 2009). http://www.uniformlaws.org/shared/docs/anatomical_gift/uaga_final_aug09.pdf.

Cases, Statutes, and Regulations Cited

Acuna v. Turkish, 384 NJ Super. 395 (App. Div. 2006).

Cruzan v. Director, Missouri Department of Health, 497 US 261; 110 Sect. 2841 (1990).

Duncan v. Scottsdale Medical Imaging, Ltd., 70 P.3d 435; 415 AZ Adv. Rep. 43 (2003).

Hamilton v. Ashton, 846 N.E.2d 309 (IN Ct. App. 2006).

In the Matter of Robert Quackenbush, 156 NJ Super. 282; 382 A.2d 785 (1978).

In Re Quinlan, 70 NJ 10. 355 A.2d 647 (1976).

In Re Storar, 52 NY 2d 363; 420 N.E.2d 64; 52 NY 2d 382; 420 N.E.2d 73 (1981).

Schloendorff v. Society of New York Hospital, 211 NY 125; 105 N.E. 92 (1914).

Union Pacific R. Co. v. Botsford, 141 US 250; 11 Sect. 1000 (1891).

Wilson v. Merritt, 142 Cal. App. 4th 1125, 48 CA Rptr. 3d 630 (2006).

Pub. L. No. 93-348: National Research Act (1974).

21 CFR Parts 50 and 56: Prisoners, reporting and recordkeeping requirements, research, safety. 1991.

45 CFR 46(a): Basic HHS Policy for Protection of Human Research Subjects. 2005.

45 CFR 46.101–46.112: Protection of human subjects. 2005.

45 CFR 46.107: Protection of human subjects: IRB membership. 2006.

45 CFR 46.116: Protection of human subjects: General requirements for informed consent. 2006.

45 CFR 46.117(b)(2): Documentation of informed consent. 2010.

KS Stat. Ann. 22-3302: Competency of dependent to stand trial. 1992.

KS Stat. Ann. 58-625: Powers and letters of attorney. 1989.

KS Stat. Ann. 59-2953, 2954: Care and treatment of mentally ill persons. 1998.

KS Stat. Ann. 59-2966: Order for treatment dismissal. 1998.

KS Stat. Ann. 59-3075: Guardian duties, responsibilities, power, authorities. 2002.

KS Stat. Ann. 65-1734: Order of priority of persons authorized to dispose of decedents' remains; immunity of funeral directors, funeral establishments and crematories. 2011.

KS Stat. Ann. 65-2892: Examination and treatment of persons under 18 for venereal disease, liability. 1972.

KS Stat. Ann. 65-2892a: Examination and treatment of minors for drug abuse, misuse or addiction; liability. 2009.

KS Stat. Ann. 65-6009: Persons arrested or convicted; disclosure of test results; costs of counseling and testing. 2001.

MO Rev. Stat. 188.028: Minors, abortion requirements and procedures. 2007.

MO Rev. Stat. 510.040: Court order physical and mental exams. 2007.

MO Rev. Stat. 522.030: Pleadings and proceedings. 2007.

MO Rev. Stat. 537.037: Emergency care (Good Samaritan Law). 2007.

Legal Health Record: Maintenance, Content, Documentation, and Disposition

Laurie A. Rinehart-Thompson, JD, RHIA, CHP, FAHIMA

Learning Objectives

- Compare the purposes of the health record
- Examine the potential components of the legal health record and the challenges associated with their inclusion
- Examine the differences between a paper health record and an electronic health record
- Differentiate the entities that establish documentation and maintenance standards for the health record
- Create policies that support legally sound documentation principles
- Examine the elements of a legally defensible health record
- Develop procedures for the identification, retention, and disposition of health records

Key Terms

- Abbreviations
- Accuracy
- Active records
- Addendum
- Amendment
- Attestation
- Authentication
- Authenticity
- Authorship
- Auto-attestation
- Auto-authentication
- Batch signing
- Business record
- Cloning
- Completeness
- Conditions of Participation (CoP)
- Countersignature

- Custodian
- Cut, copy, paste
- Data governance
- Deletion
- Designated record set (DRS)
- Destruction
- Deterministic algorithm
- Digital signature
- Digitized signature
- Disposition
- Documentation templates
- Electronic health record (EHR)
- Electronic signature
- Enterprise master patient index (EMPI)
- Handwritten signature
- Hybrid health records
- Inactive records

- Information governance
- Initials
- Joint Commission
- Late entry
- Legal health record (LHR)
- Legibility
- Master patient index (MPI)
- Medical plagiarism
- Metadata
- Patient matching
- Personal health record (PHR)
- Physician order
- Retention
- Retention schedule
- Retraction
- Retrieval
- Revisions
- Rubber signature stamps

- Scribe
- Standalone PHR
- Statistical/mathematical algorithm
- Tethered PHR
- Timeliness
- Transfer of health records
- Uniform Electronic Transactions Act (UETA)
- Uniform Photographic Copies of Business and Public Records as Evidence Act (UPA)
- Version management

Health records have existed for as long as there has been a need to deliver healthcare and communicate information about patient treatment. Patient health records are maintained by myriad health organizations to provide documentation of services and care provided. Health record content varies by type of organization, but records must be maintained to meet patient care needs and to comply with ever-evolving licensure and accreditation standards, as well as other relevant laws. Further, health records are transforming rapidly from paper to electronic, creating new challenges related to confidentiality, privacy, and security.

Healthcare organizations maintain health records using paper or electronic formats or a combination of both. Data captured in the health record are from source systems such as administrative, financial, and clinical information systems. The bulk of the record is usually composed of electronically stored information from numerous clinical information systems such as laboratory, pharmacy, radiology, nursing, and other ancillary systems, along with paper documents. The data may be handwritten, direct voice entry captured in a word processing system, or from provider mobile wireless devices such as handheld personal computers (Amatayakul 2013). Those responsible for managing patient health records must define the legal health record and establish a legally sound health record in whatever format it is maintained.

This chapter discusses the purposes of the health record and the concept of defining a legal health record. It also discusses the principles and guidelines related to the maintenance, content, and documentation necessary to support a legally sound health record, whether that record is paper or electronic. It discusses concepts associated with a legally defensible record and concludes with a discussion of the life cycle of the health record, from creation and retention to eventual disposition.

Purposes of the Health Record

Patient health records serve several purposes, as outlined in figure 9.1. The most important purpose is to document patient treatment and continuity of care. A health record describes the reasons for a patient's encounter, background facts, observations, treatment, and care. Regardless of its format, the health record provides a place for the healthcare team to record information that can be used to make healthcare decisions. A team member can review the patient's status and actions taken by other team members. Thus, the health record is the healthcare team's primary reference and communication tool.

Another purpose of the health record is to provide proof of services rendered for reimbursement. Insurance companies, managed care organizations, and government programs such as Medicare require that specific information be documented in the health record to support the bill and to prove that the care provided was medically necessary. Documentation in the health record is also used to prove the quality and effectiveness of care rendered by the healthcare provider, including information necessary for internal and external review and data required for a healthcare organization to achieve accreditation, certification, and/or licensure.

Health records support medical research by providing information used to investigate medical conditions, treatment modalities, and prevention and control procedures, and to monitor disease trends. The health record supports the education and training of a variety of health professionals and consumers. Healthcare consumers may use personal health records (discussed later in this chapter) for health and wellness initiatives and to assume responsibility for their healthcare.

Figure 9.1 Purposes of the health record

- Facilitate the ongoing care and treatment of individual patients
- Support clinical decision making and communication among clinicians
- Document the services provided to patients in support of reimbursement
- Provide information for the evaluation of the quality and efficacy of the care provided
- Provide information in support of medical research and education
- Help facilitate the operational management of the facility
- Provide evidence in legal cases and information as required by local and national laws and regulations

From an organizational standpoint, information from health records supports operational activities. For example, information gathered from health records may provide data on the use of services, provider patterns, and other important issues for benchmarking and strategic planning. Operationally, information in the health record also facilitates managerial decision making to improve the quality of patient care.

Finally, the health record serves as a legal document. It is a legal business record of the organization and serves as evidence in lawsuits or other legal actions, as discussed in chapter 5. In medical malpractice cases, the record may be used by either the plaintiff or the defendant to prove or disprove a patient's case regarding treatment provided. It may also be used in personal injury lawsuits, workers' compensation hearings, and criminal prosecutions where the health record of a victim of a violent crime is introduced into evidence. It may provide details that witness testimony cannot.

The Legal Health Record

A **business record** is made and kept in the usual course of business at or near the time of a recorded event. Because information recorded in conjunction with business practices is presumed to be trustworthy and have potential evidentiary value, a business record is generally admissible as evidence in legal proceedings. Likewise, the health record is a legal business record of an organization and serves as evidence in lawsuits or other legal actions. Thus, the health record serves as an organization's **legal health record (LHR)**. It is used for legal purposes and is the record released upon a valid request. The contents of an organization's LHR vary depending on how the organization defines it.

To contextually understand today's LHR, it is important to also understand its evolution. Although the LHR has always been an organization's official health record of each patient, it has changed dramatically over time. Historically, the definition of the LHR focused on the paper record and radiologic images. This began to change during the 1980s and 1990s as new technologies emerged that enabled collection, storage, retrieval, and generation of information electronically. Automated registration systems replaced the paper-based Master Patient Index, incorporating information from those systems into the LHR. The advent of imaged paper documents, ancillary systems such as laboratory and pharmacy, and importation of transcribed documents further changed the composition of the LHR. In the 21st century, systems have become further integrated through **electronic health record (EHR)** development. Now, virtually all documentation is online, tests results are interfaced, and EHRs host features such as computerized provider order entry (CPOE), clinical decision support tools such as alerts and reminders, patient portals that enhance consumer engagement and lead to patient-generated content, and the capability to mine data and conduct analytics. Further, mobile devices provide the means for communications about diagnosis and treatment between providers as well as between providers and patients, and clinical wearable devices such as blood sugar monitors and heart monitors feed information into the EHR (Dunagan 2016). Information from these devices may be stored in a variety of places. Because the LHR is the record that is released upon valid request and represents the organization's official health record of a patient, an organization must be certain that it can produce these components before it commits to their inclusion in the LHR. Most organizations have **hybrid health records**, which are a combination of paper (which often includes documents such as consents and advance directives) and electronic components, making the definition of an LHR even more complex.

The content of the LHR must be identified and managed by first listing all source systems (clinical, administrative, and financial) that contribute to the record. A master list should then be created that contains documents, data, images, and reports. These can number in the thousands (McLendon 2012). There is no one-size-fits-all definition of the LHR, because laws and regulations governing the maintenance, content, and documentation requirements of a health record vary by practice setting, state and federal laws and regulations, and accrediting body standards (AHIMA 2011a). However, the American Health Information Management Association (AHIMA) suggests that the following common principles be considered, taking into account both paper and electronic information, when defining the LHR and therefore determining what is to be disclosed upon request:

- Decide what documents and data make up the legal health record, then inventory them. Should information in formats other than paper documents, such as radiologic images, videos and photos, and e-mails, be an official part of the legal health record? Once these are determined, organizational policy should clearly state what the official legal health record is.
- Use records management software to carry out records declaration and records life cycle management, especially for messages such as e-mails and instant messages that are part of the legal health record.
- Clinicians should be involved in identifying information from outside the organization that is used in patient care. Plans should be made to include this information (both paper and electronic) in the patient's record. The organization should consider, in both paper and electronic records, filing or indexing information from outside the organization under a separate tab. Organizations should be familiar with state statutes that require information from the outside to be included in the health record.
- Policies and procedures should limit personnel who can request information from the outside the organization and place it in patients' records. They should also address clinicians' use of information from outside the organization and staff redisclosure of health information.
- Any health information that has not been requested or used by the organization should be returned promptly to the patient or disposed of per the organization's destruction procedures (AHIMA 2011a).

Given the complexities of a paper- and electronic-based record environment, AHIMA (2011a) identifies documents and data that must be evaluated to determine whether they will be included in or excluded from the LHR and designated record set (DRS). These are listed in figure 9.2.

Another important consideration when defining an LHR is an organization's **designated record set** (DRS). A DRS refers to a HIPAA covered entity's health records and records involved in billing, insurance enrollment and coverage, and other documents "used, in whole or in part … to make decisions about individuals" (45 CFR 164.501). It includes records in all formats and records from other providers that are used to make decisions about an individual, including e-mail communications between a patient and a provider. The DRS encompasses more information than what is normally considered part of an LHR. Thus, a healthcare organization will need to determine which elements of the DRS will be part of its LHR and which will not.

Defining the LHR is important to an organization's business and legal processes. Also important is ensuring that the record is legally sound or defensible. Many principles and guidelines that support maintaining a legally sound health record, whether paper or electronic, are discussed in the remainder of this chapter.

Paper versus Electronic Health Records

For decades, the paper health record retained a relatively consistent appearance and format across many types of healthcare organizations. A provider who practiced in different types of healthcare organizations could generally pick up a paper health record and understand its organization and content. Now, with the implementation of EHRs, many healthcare organizations function with a hybrid health record. This results

Figure 9.2 Documents and data to be evaluated for the LHR and DRS

- Administrative data or documents: Patient-identifiable data used for administrative, regulatory, healthcare operations, and payment (financial) purposes.

- Annotations (sticky notes): Additional information that is added as a layer on top of the note. The annotation or sticky note may be suppressed when viewing or printing. These may be considered part of the health record. This documentation may become a permanent part of the record and is maintained in a manner similar to any other information contained within the health record.

- Clinical decision support systems: A subcategory of clinical information systems that is designed to help healthcare professionals make knowledge-based clinical decisions. Currently there are no generally accepted rules on including decision support such as system-generated notifications, prompts, and alerts as part of the health record. Alerts, reminders, pop-ups, and similar tools are used as aides in the clinical decision-making process. The tools themselves are usually not considered part of the legal health record; however, associated documentation is considered a component. At a minimum, the EHR should include documentation of the clinician's actions in response to decision support. This documentation is evidence of the clinician's decision to follow or disregard decision support. The organization should define the extent of exception documentation required (for example, what no documentation means). When an organization decides to include the decision support trigger as part of the health record, the organization will need to define if all triggers will be part of the record or just the clinical decision support triggers. For example, alerts for patient appointment reminders may not be considered part of the legal health record, but alerts for drug–drug interaction may be.

- Coding queries: A routine communication and education tool used to advocate complete and compliant documentation. Retention of the query varies by healthcare organization. First, an organization must determine if the query will be part of the health record. If the query is not part of the health record, then the organization must decide if the query is kept as part of the business record or only the outcome of the query is maintained in a database.

- Continuing care records: Records received from another healthcare provider. Historically, these records were generally not considered part of the legal health record unless they were used in the provision of patient care. In the EHR it may be difficult to determine if information was viewed or used in delivering healthcare. It may be necessary to define such information as part of the legal health record. Policies should reflect the proper disposition of health records from external sources (for example, other healthcare providers) if they are not integrated into the electronic and legal health record.

- Data or documents: Documentation of patient care that took place in the ordinary course of business by all healthcare providers.

- Data from source systems: Written results of tests. Data from which interpretations, summaries, notes, flowcharts, and such are derived.

- Discrete structured data: Laboratory orders/refills, orders/medication orders/MARs, online charting and documentation, and any detailed charges.

- Document completion (lockdown): Organizations must determine when users can no longer create or make changes to electronic documentation. Organizations with several source systems should consider locking down documents at some determined time after a patient encounter. There may be limitations with how the EHR handles this function, which organizations will need to factor into their policies.

- External records and reports: Healthcare records that are created by providers outside of the organization that are received by the organization for patient care. The decision of which category external records and reports fall into depends on the applicability of HIPAA privacy rules, state law or regulation, source of the request, and type of request. If external records and reports are used to make decisions about an individual, they become part of the designated record set. If those decisions are care decisions, in most cases those same records and reports will also be included in the provider's legal health record, especially if they are created pursuant to a contract.

- Personal health records (PHRs): Copies of PHRs that are created, owned, and managed by the patient and are provided to a healthcare organization(s) may be considered part of the health record if so defined by the organization.

- Research records: Organizational policy should differentiate whether research records are part of the health record and how these records will be kept.

Figure 9.2	Documents and data to be evaluated for the LHR and DRS (Continued)

- Version control: Organizations must decide whether all versions of a document or ancillary report will be displayed or just the final version.
- Diagnostic image data: CT, MRI, ultrasound, nuclear medicine, and others.
- Signal tracing data: EKG, EEG, fetal monitoring signal tracings, and such.
- Audio data: Heart sounds, voice dictations, annotations, and others.
- Video data: Ultrasound, cardiac catheterization examinations, and others.
- Text data: Radiology reports, transcribed reports, UBS, itemized bills, and such.
- Original analog document/document image data: Signed patient consent forms, handwritten notes, drawings, and others.

Source: AHIMA 2011a Appendix C.

Figure 9.3	Six key characteristics of electronic records

1. Large volume and ease of duplication: Thousands of electronic documents can be created each day; copies can be made by forwarding, saving, and backing up.
2. Persistence: Electronic documents are difficult to dispose of; deleted data may remain.
3. Attached to tracking information: Metadata (data about data) can track creation and authorship, edits, access, and printing of data.
4. Updated automatically: Electronic data is dynamic and changeable, updated either by users or through system changes that may not be apparent to users.
5. Obsolescence: Electronic data may become incomprehensible or unavailable when the application or program on which it runs is updated or removed.
6. Searchable and capable of being stored in multiple locations: Electronic records can be searched quickly, and specific pieces of information can be located readily. They can also be stored simultaneously in multiple locations, either in identical or modified versions that include collaborative software.

Source: The Sedona Conference 2016.

in health records with very different appearances from one organization to another. The boundaries of the health record have expanded to include a compilation of information from a variety of media sources (paper, databases, images, text, tracings, pictures, and so forth) created both inside and outside the healthcare organization. In addition, electronic records differ from paper records in six key areas as summarized in figure 9.3. The differences among paper health records, hybrid health records, and EHRs add to the challenge of ensuring that an organization's health records are legally sound or defensible if called into question.

The **Uniform Photographic Copies of Business and Public Records as Evidence Act (UPA)** (28 USC 1732), of which there are both federal and state versions, states that the reproduction of any record retained in the regular course of business and kept by a process that accurately reproduces the original in any medium is just as admissible as the original when submitted as evidence in judicial and administrative proceedings. This act is important because it supports the transition from paper to electronic storage of information. It is imperative that the method used to electronically store information be reliable and able to accurately reproduce an exact copy of the original record. Healthcare organizations must consider preservation requirements of electronically stored information, including any migration of the record from one system or medium to another. Requirements of discovery and retention, as outlined in chapter 4, define these expectations in greater detail.

Instructions: Indicate whether the following statements are true or false (T or F).

1. The most important purpose of the health record is to provide proof of services for reimbursement.
2. Health records using a combination of paper and electronic formats are hybrid records.
3. The health record is not a business record of an organization.
4. Paper records are persistent, but electronic records are not.
5. There are both federal and state versions of the Uniform Photographic Copies of Business and Public Records as Evidence Act.

Health Record Maintenance, Content, and Documentation

Standards for record maintenance, content, and documentation have been established by a number of sources, including state and federal laws, accrediting bodies, and professional standard-setting organizations. State licensure requirements must be met in order for specific healthcare organizations to remain licensed, and they may include specific requirements for the content, format, retention, and use of patient records. Statutes and their resulting regulations are usually under the jurisdiction of state health departments. The requirements may be specific or broad depending on the type of organization and the state. Most healthcare organizations defer to the record maintenance, content, and documentation requirements set forth by the Department of Health and Human Services (HHS), the Centers for Medicare and Medicaid Services (CMS), The Joint Commission, or other accrediting bodies. The health information management and informatics professional, as the record **custodian**, is responsible for complying with these requirements.

Federally, CMS is responsible for developing and enforcing regulations regarding the participation of healthcare providers in Medicare and Medicaid programs, which provide healthcare services to qualified individuals. CMS sets forth health record maintenance, content, and documentation requirements in the **Conditions of Participation (CoP)** for hospitals, as well as in the Conditions of Participation for a variety of healthcare settings, such as psychiatric hospitals and ambulatory surgical centers. The Conditions of Participation for hospitals, for example, require that a health record be maintained for every inpatient or outpatient (42 CFR 482.24(b)). In addition, the Conditions of Participation for hospitals specifically require that health records "contain information to justify admission and continued hospitalization, support the diagnosis, and describe the patient's progress and response to medications and services" (42 CFR 482.24(c)).

The Joint Commission, which accredits many types of healthcare organizations, also requires that health records be maintained and that content and documentation standards be followed. The Joint Commission *Comprehensive Accreditation Manual for Hospitals* (CAMH) has standards dedicated to defining the components of a complete health record. *CAMH* includes guidance for developing policies and procedures for the compilation, completion, authentication, retention, and release of health records. The Joint Commission's standards include specific content requirements pertaining to the health record, such as demographic information, discharge summary, history and physical, operative report, and anesthesia record (Joint Commission 2016a, RC.01.01.01, RC02.01.01, RC02.01.03, RC.02.04.01). AHIMA also addresses maintenance, content, and documentation issues as a component of its professional practice standards.

In addition to external standards, an organization's medical staff bylaws (detailed in chapter 19) and internal policies may also delineate requirements for the maintenance and content of health records, as well as documentation and completion standards. Approved by an organization's board of trustees or governing body, bylaws usually delineate the content of health records, identify personnel permitted to document in the health record, describe time limits for record completion, and restate applicable health record requirements, such as Medicare Conditions of Participation, Joint Commission standards, and state regulations and penalties for noncompliance. State, federal, and/or Joint Commission surveyors routinely review health records, regardless of the record format or type of organization, to ensure that regulations, standards, and internal requirements as described in the bylaws are being followed (Joint Commission 2016a, MS.01.01.01). Figure 9.4 provides a listing of standard health record content. For readers not familiar with health record content or the way the health record is compiled, the student workbook for chapter 9 contains a detailed listing of documents typically found in a health record and information specific to various types of healthcare organizations and providers who contribute to the health record.

Just as important as complying with standards for the maintenance and content of the health record is establishing and enforcing documentation principles that not only facilitate quality patient care and patient safety but also provide a legally sound document. Many documentation guidelines that have historically applied to paper health records also apply to documentation in EHRs. The following sections address documentation principles for health record entries that relate to language used, who may document in the health record, gaps and omissions; orders, documentation pertaining to hostile patients, staff disagreements, documentation of injuries resulting from criminal activity, and liability for improper entries.

Figure 9.4   Content of the health record

Health record summary sheet (face sheet)	Medication administration records (MARs)
Administrative and demographic information	Ancillary reports
Registration data	Laboratory reports
Consent to treatment	Radiology reports
Consent to use or disclose protected health information	EKGs
Consent to special procedures	EEGs
Advance directives	MRIs or CT scans
Acknowledgment of receipt of patient's rights statement	Surgical services
Property and valuables list	Anesthesia records
Birth and death certificates	Operative report
Clinical data	Pathology report
Medical history	Discharge summary
Physical examination	Discharge plan
Diagnostic and therapeutic orders	Specialized documents
Special orders	Obstetrical care
Discharge orders	Neonatal care
Clinical observations	Emergency care
Progress notes	Ambulatory/outpatient care
Consultation reports	Home health care
Ancillary notes	Behavioral health care
Nursing services	Hospice care
Assessment	Rehabilitation care
Care plan	Long-term care
Flow sheet	

Language

Regardless of the medium in which a health record entry resides (that is, electronic, imaged, paper, or hybrid), fundamental documentation principles apply to ensure the quality of a health record entry and reduce the risk of liability. Health record content should be specific, objective, and factual (what is known versus what is thought or presumed) and should contain complete information. Examples of generalizations and vague words that should be avoided include "patient doing well," "appears to be," "confused," "anxious," "status quo," "stable," and "as usual." If an author must speculate, the documentation must state that it is speculation. If the record documents what can be seen, heard, touched, tasted, and smelled, the entries will be specific and objective. Signs and symptoms should be described, and quotation marks should be used when quoting the patient's exact words.

A patient's treatment and response to treatment are documented. Deviations from standard treatment, including the reason for the deviations, must also be documented. Situations that generate incident reports (described in chapters 5 and 17) should also be described objectively in the health record, with care taken not to assign blame or identify failures. For example, a patient fall must be recorded in the health record. However, the health record is not the appropriate place to identify the fall as being the result of "the janitor's consistent failure to put up 'wet floor' signs."

Individuals Who May Document

A governing body or board of trustees has ultimate legal responsibility for the quality of care rendered in a healthcare organization, except in organizations owned by individuals or the government. An organization's medical staff bylaws set rules for record content and who may document in the health record. Once the bylaws have been established, however, ultimate responsibility for the quality of documentation is delegated to individual providers who create and authenticate entries in the health record. The categories of individuals permitted to document in the health record will vary depending on the type of entry. Providers are permitted to create progress notes relative to their specific discipline and generally include physicians, nurses, therapists, social workers, case managers, dietitians, nurse anesthetists, pharmacists, radiology technologists, and others providing direct treatment or consultation.

Each person authorized to enter documentation into the progress notes must create his or her own note, authenticate it, provide a complete date (month, day, year) and time, and indicate authorship by signing his or her full name and title. (Authentication, attestation, and authorship are discussed in greater detail later in the chapter.) Charting for a block of time (for example, 7 a.m. to 4 p.m.) is not recommended. First, the information is likely to be less accurate because the documenting provider's memory becomes less clear over the course of time. Second, it becomes extremely difficult to correlate occurrences to the specific times they took place. Documentation must be created and authenticated by the person responsible for examinations, procedures, interpretations, and other similar types of treatments. Special rules govern orders, which are discussed later.

Gaps and Omissions

A health record must reflect the chronology of the patient's care. Gaps (spaces between entries) and omissions (missing entries) detract from a chronology and do not contribute to quality patient care, leaving a healthcare organization susceptible to liability. There are two types of gaps.

First, gaps are spaces left between entries in the paper health record. Although physical gaps do not necessarily indicate that documentation has been omitted, the spaces allow subsequent entries to be made in a space previous to an already-existing entry. This can create confusion and hamper a patient's care. If the document is the subject of a lawsuit, misplaced entries can create suspicion or evidence of wrongdoing. Individuals who document in paper health records must avoid leaving blank spaces between entries to prevent information from being added out of sequence. EHR systems do not allow for gaps in the health record since all entries are timed and dated by the EHR system.

In addition to gaps in physical documentation, gaps and omissions can also occur in time. Long periods of time without documentation can also hamper patient care when necessary information is either entered late or not entered at all, particularly when the information could have already proved useful to patient care or may no longer be completely reliable due to the passage of time. Gaps and omissions in time negatively impact the timeliness of the health record, a requirement that will be discussed later in the chapter.

Orders

One of the most important pieces of documentation within the health record is the **physician order**. Physicians give orders for medical interventions such as treatments, ancillary medical services, tests and procedures, medications, and seclusion and restraint. The accuracy of medication orders, which specify a particular drug, dosage, frequency, duration, and route (for example, orally or intravenously), is extremely important. However, medication orders are often a source of treatment errors. For example, the wrong dosage or frequency may be ordered, or a medication may erroneously be ordered for a patient who is allergic to it. Orders for the administration of medications such as narcotics and sedatives have time limits or stop orders, which automatically discontinue the medication unless the physician gives a specific order to continue.

Legibility has historically been problematic in paper records; this issue is being resolved through the implementation of computerized provider order-entry (CPOE) systems that eliminate handwritten orders and reduce the risk of illegible handwriting and its associated liability. Physicians were historically the only class of healthcare professionals permitted by law to give orders, but this is changing as states grant physician assistants and nurse practitioners the ability to give orders and prescribe medications. Medical staff bylaws delineate which providers in an organization are authorized to give orders and the scope of practice for which they are authorized to give orders.

There are two types of orders, written and verbal. Verbal orders are of two types. They may be communicated in person or over the telephone to individuals authorized to receive them. The person receiving the order should sign his or her name, give his or her credential (for example, RN, PT, or LPN), and record the date and time the order was received. Because of the risks associated with miscommunication, verbal orders are strongly discouraged and are not permitted in certain healthcare organizations for treatments or procedures that might put the patient at risk. When a provider is physically present, it is suggested that he or she document the order instead of dictating it to another individual. However, the Joint Commission has required a process that mandates staff to "read back" to the dictating provider what was written before action could be taken on the order. This reduced verbal order errors. Joint Commission standards require that the hospital identify, in writing, staff who are authorized to receive and record verbal orders (Joint Commission 2016a, RC.02.03.07).

Medical staff bylaws must state the categories of personnel authorized to accept orders. Verbal orders for medication are usually required to be given to, and to be accepted only by, nursing or pharmacy personnel. Some categories of personnel that may accept verbal orders for services within their area of practice include physical therapists, registered nurse anesthetists, dietitians, and medical laboratory professionals.

All orders must be authenticated (verified) by the provider who gave the order or who is responsible for the patient's care. Verbal orders should be authenticated as soon as possible after they are given. Although time requirements for authentication of orders are governed by state law, accreditation standards and organizational policies are also factors for determining time frames for the authentication of verbal orders. Medicare regulations state that in the absence of state law, authentication shall occur promptly. Organizations may require the ordering provider to authenticate orders within as few as 24 hours.

Some hospitals perform retrospective post-discharge reviews and analyses, in which personnel indicate orders that are lacking signatures. The responsible provider can then individually authenticate them after patient discharge. However, because retrospective reviews do not affect the patient's care process, a more effective system is the review of orders while the patient is in the hospital. This is also known as concurrent or open-record review. Through these reviews, orders can be authenticated in a timely manner, and providers with patterns of unsigned orders can be detected. A comparison of orders with laboratory reports, other ancillary reports, and nursing documentation also ensures that orders were carried out correctly and that the reports are included in the health record. In a paper system or a system where records are imaged after patient discharge, concurrent reviews ensure that documents are in the correct patient record. Concurrent reviews are also used for progress notes and other documents that require authentication.

One of the most recent issues associated with orders is text messaging. With evidence of high acceptance levels of health text messaging among teens and young adults, patient preference for texting is expanding (HHS 2014). Originally prohibited by accrediting bodies such as the Joint Commission, orders may now be transmitted through text messaging if they are transmitted through a secure text messaging platform and include features such as secure sign-on and date and time stamps (Joint Commission 2016b). Previously existing requirements for orders must also continue to be met.

Hostile Patients

When entries in the health record reflect a patient who is particularly hostile or irritable, general documentation principles apply, such as charting objective facts and avoiding the use of personal opinions, particularly those that are critical of the patient. These general principles are especially important because a disagreeable patient may cause a provider to use more expressive and inappropriate language. Further, a hostile patient may be more likely to file legal action in the future if the hostility is a personal attribute and not simply a manifestation of his or her medical condition.

Staff Disagreements

Professionals working in the healthcare field will not always agree on a patient's course of treatment and may need to communicate these differing professional opinions to one another. One's professional standards may require him or her to question another's decisions if one believes those decisions will harm the patient. However, documentation of staff disagreements in the health record heightens the risk of liability for both the healthcare organization and those involved in the disagreement. Documentation in the health record should not highlight disagreements and raise suspicion of negligence that will result in the record becoming the centerpiece of litigation. For example, identifying a colleague in the record as "mistaken" or "negligent" or otherwise using inflammatory language provides a basis for liability and does not promote quality patient care. Although the professional conclusions of each practitioner may be inconsistent, and each conclusion should be present in the record, drawing attention to those differences or the emotions associated with a disagreement is best left to conversations outside the health record.

Organizational policy should outline the parameters for staff disagreements that align with the principles just discussed. General documentation principles, introduced earlier in this chapter, should be followed to ensure an objective and factual record.

Documentation of Injuries Resulting from Criminal Activity

Healthcare providers may encounter and treat individuals whom they believe to be the victims of abuse, which may constitute criminal activity. As described in chapter 16, most states require healthcare personnel to report suspected abuse of specified vulnerable classes such as children, the elderly, and individuals with developmental disabilities. Many of these statutes also provide immunity to individuals who report their suspicions in good faith. Healthcare providers may also encounter victims of criminal activities such as gunshot wounds and stabbings. Objective and factual documentation in the health record should accompany reports made to authorities. Documentation should include statements made by the suspected victim, the identification of injuries, a thorough description of injuries, and photographs of the injuries.

Liability for Improper Entries

As described throughout this section, inappropriate documentation may lead to **liability** for an organization and its personnel and can make the health record the focal point of legal action. Missing or incomplete information in the health record may lead a court to instruct the jury that it may infer provider negligence. Further, documentation that is present can be equally damaging if it is biased, is critical of a patient or another provider, or includes personal opinions instead of medically relevant facts. Healthcare providers must be trained to document appropriately to achieve quality patient care and minimize the risk of legal liability.

Check Your Understanding   9.2

Instructions: Indicate whether the following statements are true or false (T or F).

1. A jury may be permitted to infer provider negligence based on missing or incomplete information in the health record.
2. Concurrent reviews of unsigned orders lead to timelier authentication.
3. "Patient appears to be anxious" is an example of good documentation in the health record.
4. Charting for a block of time is recommended because it saves time.
5. Professional conclusions of individual practitioners should be documented in the health record so that they agree with one another.

Maintaining a Legally Defensible Health Record

The integrity of a health record—the accuracy and completeness of documentation—is critical to its defensibility in a court of law. It includes data governance and information governance, patient identification, assurance of authorship, changes to the record, and documentation validity for reimbursement purposes (AHIMA Work Group 2013). **Data governance** is the "enterprise authority that ensures control and accountability for enterprise data" (Johns 2015). Data governance is often linked to data creation; thus, it emphasizes accuracy and integrity. **Information governance** emphasizes the safeguarding of information, including use and disclosure, after it has been created. In essence, the difference between data governance and information governance is the time period involved. Although both emphasize stewardship and accountability, data governance is concerned with the time period during which data is created (thus, its accuracy and integrity), whereas information governance is concerned with the time period after information has been created (thus, its protection).

Documentation guidelines are similar for both paper records and EHRs; however, there are additional issues exclusive to ensuring the integrity of electronic records, including the electronic capture, storage, and retrieval of health information. Many elements contribute to a health record's integrity and, ultimately, to patient safety: authentication and attestation, accuracy, authorship, use of abbreviations, legibility, transparent changes to the record, timeliness, completeness, and the appropriate use of the print function. All of these contribute to the accuracy and legal soundness of the health record, whether paper or electronic.

Authentication and Attestation

As introduced in chapters 4 and 5, **authenticity** refers to the genuineness of a record that it is what it purports to be. This includes accurate recording of information as well as freedom from tampering and corruption. Establishing the authenticity of documentation is critical because individuals who work with or otherwise rely on health records must be assured that the information has not been altered either intentionally or accidentally. The Federal Rules of Evidence allow records of regularly conducted activity, kept as a regular practice of the activity (that is, business records) to be admitted into evidence (Federal Rules of Evidence (803(6)). As mentioned earlier, the Copies of Business and Public Records as Evidence Act allows for the admissibility of a reproduced business record without the original as long as it accurately reflects the original. This uniform act has been adopted by over 30 states.

Authenticity is especially important with EHRs because of the perception that electronic documentation can be manipulated and altered. Authenticity pertains not only to the information created but also to the system used to create and store the information. System reliability and perception of the system's uptime (versus downtime) are important to support the information's authenticity. Controlled access to the application itself is another crucial component of ensuring authenticity. Inappropriate handling of information, from a purely technical standpoint, may invalidate the information or lead one to question whether users rely on it in the normal course of business.

Related to the concept of authenticity are authentication and attestation. These terms are often used interchangeably by regulatory and accrediting bodies, but their definitions have evolved with the use of electronic signatures. (Thus far in this chapter, only the term *authentication* has been used.) **Authentication** is a security process that verifies one's identity and authorizes system access. It assigns responsibility to a system user "for entries he or she creates, modifies, or views." **Attestation** is applying a signature to documentation, thus showing authorship (Downing 2013). With these evolving definitions, the terms continue to be used interchangeably by various sources, and there is no distinction between the two when dealing with paper records. Authentication and attestation can be accomplished in several ways, although state statutes and regulations should be consulted regarding the legality of each.

The Medicare Conditions of Participation for hospitals contain two references to health record authentication. Section 482.24(b) states that "the hospital must use a system of author identification and record maintenance that ensures the integrity of the authentication and protects the security of all record entries." Section 482.24(c)(1) states that "all patient medical record entries must be legible, complete, dated, timed, and authenticated in written or electronic form by the person responsible for providing or evaluating the service provided …" Section (c) also requires that "the author of each entry must be identified and must authenticate his or her entry; and authentication may include signatures, written initials or computer entry." These are described later in this section. The Conditions of Participation for settings other than hospitals require that all entries in the record be signed but do not include details about methods of authentication.

Attestation of paper records includes handwritten signature, initials, and rubber signature stamps. EHR attestation methods include electronic signatures that can take different forms (Downing 2013). Attestation of an imaged document can follow paper or electronic guidelines. Joint Commission standards also permit the above conventions (Joint Commission 2016a, RC 01.02.01). The following sections discuss attestation of paper records; attestation of electronic records; and issues associated with the attestation process.

Attestation of Paper Records

Handwritten signatures completed in ink are the most common method of attesting to paper health records. Identifying information in addition to the name, such as the author's title, discipline (for example, physical therapy) or credential provides more robust documentation.

In lieu of a full signature, **initials** (that is, letters indicating an individual's first and last names, and perhaps the middle name) may be permitted as long as they are readily identifiable as the author's through a signature legend on the same document. Although initials are more practical than full signatures on documents with limited space such as flow sheets, they should be avoided on entries such as narrative notes and may not be used if a signature is legally required. An organization may prohibit them altogether. **Rubber signature stamps,** which contain an individual's signature and can be pressed on an ink pad prior to affixing the inked signature to a document, are acceptable if allowed by state and federal law, and by payers. CMS does not permit stamp signatures on medical documentation (HHS 2008). Organizations must determine if they will allow signature stamps, even if payers do permit them. Using both external rules and internal considerations, organizational policies should define the situations when rubber stamp signatures are acceptable, if at all. As with initials, a list of signatures should be maintained to cross-reference each signature to an individual author when rubber signature stamps are used. According to the Joint Commission, the individual identified by the signature stamp is the only individual who uses it (Joint Commission 2016a, RC.01.02.01).

Attestation of Electronic Records

Thus far, the discussion has focused on paper records or imaged (scanned) records that were attested to when they existed in paper form. The EHR presents a separate set of issues. Without a single governing standard for e-signatures, organizations should consult those created by established standards setting organizations such as HL7 (Health Level Seven International), ASTM (American Society for Testing and Materials), and ISO (International Organization for Standardization) (Downing 2013). For example, the HL7 EHR-System Records Management and Evidentiary Support Functional Profile Standard "identifies system functionality and conformance criteria" for authentication and attestation (Downing 2013).

An **electronic signature** (e-signature) is a general term that refers to all the ways an electronic record can be signed, or attested to. It includes digitized images of signatures, buttons, personal identification numbers (PINs), biometric identifiers, tokens, or digital signatures. The e-signature serves three main purposes:

- **Intent:** A symbol of confirmation and approval of content; authorship

| Figure 9.5 | Levels of EHR signature security |

Level 1. A digitized signature can be captured in real time or from a previously saved image. It is the weakest type of EHR signature, because a previously saved image can be obtained and used to forge a document.

Level 2. Button, PIN, biometric identifier, or token. At the completion of documentation, the user attests by clicking a button or entering a PIN, biometric scan (such as fingerprint or palm print), or using a token (such as an identification badge with a bar code) that he or she carries. This can be used in addition to a digitized signature, or more than one Level 2 method can be used to enhance security.

Level 3. A digital signature, unlike a digitized signature, does not produce an electronic version of a handwritten signature. It is the strongest signature because it uses a tamperproof seal that is broken when the content is altered.

Source: Downing 2013.

- **Identity:** Identification of the person signing the document or entry
- **Integrity:** Protection against alteration and repudiation (claim by the signer that the documentation is invalid) (Downing 2013)

The Joint Commission requires that, for electronic authentication, only the individual identified by the e-signature mechanism (such as personal identification number or code) should use it (Joint Commission 2016a RC 01.02.01). Strong policies on secure use of PINs, tokens, and passwords are critical to ensure data integrity. Thus, users should be required to sign statements attesting that only they will use and control them.

There are three common EHR signature methods, listed in figure 9.5, from the weakest to the strongest security. A **digitized signature** is an image of a handwritten signature created by signature pads, scanning, or digital photography. A **digital signature** is a cryptographic signature (represented by a code) that uses a digital key to authenticate the user by linking the code to the user; it also links the user with a document in a database.

Laws associated with e-signatures have been passed to promote e-commerce. The **Uniform Electronic Transactions Act (UETA)** (1999) makes electronic records and signatures legally equivalent to paper records and handwritten signatures. This act removes barriers to e-commerce and increases the level of trust associated with electronic business transactions. It is subject to adoption by each state.

In 2000, Congress passed the **Electronic Signatures in Global and National Commerce Act (E-SIGN)** (15 USC 7001, et seq.). It too validates electronic records and signatures and provides that they are generally to be legally recognized for interstate and foreign commerce. With the goal of facilitating e-commerce and addressing some of the legal barriers to electronic transactions, it provides that a signature or record may not be denied legal effect solely because it was created electronically. E-SIGN also provides guidance on how records may be stored and retained electronically. If a document is required by law to be retained, an electronic version is acceptable if the document is accessible, accurately reflects the information in the record, and can accurately be reproduced for later reference. No specific technology is required, thereby allowing other federal and state agencies to establish more specific standards. Inconsistencies regarding the acceptability of e-signatures from state to state can create an issue, particularly for those organizations whose facilities span state lines.

The most recent laws, per state, can be obtained at www.alllaw.com/state_resources (AHIMA 2013b). Because e-signature requirements vary among states, it is important to verify the relevant state's regulations before adopting an e-signature process.

Attestation Issues

Several attestation issues exist whether a record is paper, imaged, electronic, or hybrid. It is imperative that the author of each entry in a health record be identified and all entries in the health record be attested to. Therefore, the following issues must be addressed to ensure appropriate attestation: countersignatures, multiple attestations, attestations on behalf of another person, auto-attestation, batch signing, and the use of scribes.

Countersignatures

A **countersignature** is attestation by a second provider that signifies review and evaluation of the actions and documentation, including attestation, of a first provider. Entries of individuals who are required to practice under the direct supervision of another professional should be countersigned by someone with authority to evaluate the entry. This is particularly necessary in teaching hospitals, where the attending physician who is responsible for a resident physician must also be involved in the patient's care. Once countersigned, the entry is legally adopted by the supervising professional as his or her own. For example, an attending physician may be required to countersign a medical student's or resident physician's entries or dictated reports. The use of countersignatures is generally dictated by state licensing or certification statutes related to the professional scope of practice. Their uses are also typically outlined in medical staff bylaws and other healthcare organization policies. The CMS Interpretive Guidelines for Hospitals (482.24(c)(1)) require that medical staff rules and regulations address countersignature requirements by attending and supervisory medical staff if either state law or hospital policy requires countersignatures of entries created by residents or non-physicians.

Multiple Attestations

Several staff members complete documents such as assessments at different times, requiring multiple attestations. At a minimum, a signature area at the end of the document should exist for staff to sign and date. Staff completing sections of the assessment should indicate the sections they completed at the signature line or initial the sections they completed. EHRs must allow for the capture of each person's identity, and all signatures should be clearly identified, retained, and date and time-stamped (Downing 2013).

Attestation on Behalf of Another

At times, authors can no longer attest to documentation they have created because of circumstances such as resignation or death. To close a record, qualified alternate signers must be identified who are familiar with the case and who can validate the accuracy of the documentations. If a qualified signer cannot be located, documentation should be provided to explain why the documentation is not attested to (Downing 2013).

Auto-Attestation

Auto-attestation (auto-authentication) occurs when failure of an author to review and actively approve or disapprove an entry in an EHR within a specified time period results in attestation. For example, an organization's policy may allow a physician or other provider to state in advance that dictated and transcribed reports may be considered approved and signed if the provider does not make corrections within a certain period of time. The Uniform Electronic Transactions Act, Medicare Conditions of Participation, and Joint Commission do not permit auto-attestation because they require specific action to verify and attest to a document or entry (Downing 2013). Processes should be in place to ensure that authors review and attest to dictated documents after they are transcribed.

Batch Signing

Batch signing involves attesting to multiple entries or orders at one time. This is acceptable if all of the entries or orders can be viewed; each can be acted upon individually (such as editing content); and each can be removed from the batch (Downing 2013). It is not acceptable for a provider to sign the list of entries or orders without reviewing them.

Scribes

A **scribe** is a person who documents in the health record for the provider. Entries created by scribes must be uniquely identified in the EHR. Further, the provider must review and attest to the entries (Downing 2013).

Integrity of Electronic Record Content

The integrity of information produced within an EHR can be validated through the use of metadata. **Metadata,** which is data about data, provides background information including how data was created, who created it, when it was created, when it was revised, when it was accessed, and where on the network it was created. Verbal testimony from the record custodian will most likely not be sufficient to attest to an EHR's reliability. However, an audit trail can demonstrate the actions of every individual who affected or accessed the record, confirming its reliability. It is important for organizations to know what metadata their EHRs collect.

Documentation templates are functionalities in EHRs that already have some phrases in place, but allow for the standardized collection of specific data through features such as drop-down menus that providers can select from to describe a patient's condition, or to describe or order treatment. Although documentation templates increase efficiency and allow narrative data to become searchable because of their structured format, they also create integrity issues. If the options available in a template do not match a patient's condition or treatment provided, the documentation will be inaccurate or inexact. Templates may not capture information that is necessary for complete documentation, thus compromising patient care and potentially creating liability (AHIMA Work Group 2013).

Check Your Understanding 9.3

Instructions: Indicate whether the following statements are true or false (T or F).

1. Auto-attestation is favored by the Joint Commission because it is an efficient attestation tool.
2. Author initials are universally prohibited as an attestation mechanism in a health record.
3. Metadata provides information about an entry's content, including date and time of creation.
4. A digitized signature is a handwritten signature that is converted into an electronic image.
5. A countersignature signifies review and evaluation of the actions and documentation of another provider.

Accuracy

Accuracy is the degree to which information in the record correctly reflects what actually happened. The author is responsible for the accuracy of his or her health record entries. EHRs pose accuracy challenges because they may contain data from multiple databases and sources. Also, EHR features such as drop-down menus may force users to select from options that don't accurately depict a patient's condition or treatment. Training providers about appropriate data entry and system use, as well as checks and balances in the system that include audits, is necessary. Some EHR systems automatically audit data with rules-based tools that compare the data being entered with data that have already been entered. While this can be cumbersome to the user, it contributes to the accuracy of the information. An audit plan should be developed to ensure health record accuracy.

Authorship and Cut, Copy, Paste

Authorship is the creation of recorded information attributed to a specific individual or entity. The Joint Commission requires that organizations permit only authorized individuals to document in the health record, regardless of whether the record is paper, electronic, or hybrid. Those who are authorized must be identified by organizational policy and medical staff bylaws.

The cut, copy, paste function (also referred to as cloning) that may exist in an EHR can weaken the integrity of documentation and raises authorship questions. Although similar functions were available in paper records through methods such as photocopying, gluing, and cropping, they were not widely used because they were cumbersome to accomplish and easily observed. These barriers have been removed in the EHR, creating significant legal challenges related to record integrity. The risks are significant. **Cut, copy, paste (cloning)** includes placing information on the wrong encounter or wrong patient, entering information that does not reflect the current situation and failing to customize it to the appropriate patient, omitting the identity of the original author of the information, and using information without the original author's knowledge or permission (**medical plagiarism**). If these actions result in documentation of services not provided, it is also healthcare fraud. To minimize risk, policies and procedures should define the appropriate use of cut, copy, and paste; who can do it; and how the system tracks the original author and changes that were made.

In addition to integrity, there are other concerns that accompany the cut, copy, paste function. Duplication of information leads to unnecessarily voluminous records that can stress storage systems and create expensive bills for individuals requesting copies of records. Further, when the same information is copied and pasted, it produces redundant documentation that one must read through prior to locating relevant and important patient updates. This can be a hindrance to patient care.

Abbreviations

Historically used in health record documentation, **abbreviations** compromise patient safety because they can have duplicate meanings and be misunderstood. Organizations should have a list of approved terminology and definitions as well as approved and prohibited abbreviations, acronyms, symbols, and dose designations (Joint Commission 2016a, IM.02.02.01). The Joint Commission has established a list of prohibited abbreviations, acronyms, symbols, and dose designations that must be included in written hospital policy (Joint Commission 2016a, IM.02.02.01). They are available at https://www.jointcommission.org. Concurrent and retrospective analyses of records should ensure that abbreviations, acronyms, and symbols used in documentation have been approved by the medical staff and have only one meaning. Because EHR systems can be designed to either deny entered abbreviations or convert them into complete words, abbreviations should be eliminated as a documentation option as EHRs become the predominant type of health record.

Legibility

The quality of provider entries includes **legibility**, which is a focus area of accreditation and licensure bodies. The Joint Commission requires ongoing health record reviews at the point of care for several indicators, including legibility (Joint Commission 2016a, RC 01.04.01). Illegibility creates liability, because providers may not act correctly based on documentation they cannot read. If an entry cannot be read, it must be assumed that it cannot be or was not used in the patient care process, or was not used safely if there was speculation about its content. Entries that cannot be read should be rewritten on the next available line, refer back to the original documentation, explain the reason for the duplicate entry, and be written legibly. The rewritten entry must be the same as the original. A long-standing problem with paper health records, illegibility has been reduced through the presence of EHRs. However, readability of images or scans can still be negatively affected by the use of color (for example, to indicate test results), low resolution, and poorly imaged documents in a document management system.

Changes to the Health Record

Documentation within the health record may need to be changed or added for many reasons. Foremost are entries that contain erroneous information or are incomplete. While changes may be necessary to ensure record integrity, the manner in which the changes occur can, in fact, diminish its integrity and subject it to legal scrutiny. Because of this, policies and procedures should define the process for making changes and the time period in which changes can be made, along with retention of previous versions (version management is discussed later in this chapter). Changes to entries in the health record can be used against a healthcare organization as evidence of negligence or a consciousness of guilt if they are not completed appropriately and with transparency. Changes can be referred to by many terms, such as amendments, additions, addenda, late entries, corrections, alterations, modifications, deletions, and retractions. For the purposes of this chapter, changes are categorized as follows and are addressed in the following sections: revisions (also referred to as corrections or alterations); additions (late entries, amendments, or addenda); removal (deletions or retractions); and version management. The AHIMA "Amendments in the Electronic Health Record Toolkit" (2012a) provides a comprehensive overview of changes to the EHR.

Revisions to the Health Record

Revisions to health record entries generally involve replacing inaccurate information with accurate information after the documentation has been attested to or otherwise deemed complete. Revisions should be completed in a manner that ensures the original entry is preserved and future readers can rely on it. Corrections in paper records should be completed by drawing a line through the erroneous information so the original information remains legible, and marking it as an error. A notation of the date, time, and signature of the individual making the correction should accompany the correct information.

Errors in EHRs should be handled in a similar manner. Recommendations for standards on appropriate methods to correct information in the EHR can be found in the HL7 functional model (Health Level Seven International 2016). Information should not be deleted in paper records (for example, erasing, obliterating, or whiting out) or EHRs; however, corrections in the EHR may not be visible like they are on paper. Because of this, the ability to track changes in an EHR (for example, the person who made the change, and the date and time of the change) is critical for evidentiary purposes. The person making the correction should enter the correct information and reference the incorrect information. A notation or flag should be visible with the new information to indicate a change occurred, along with a link to the original incorrect information. Otherwise, there is no clear distinction between original and new text.

Individuals who document in paper or electronic records must be educated about organizational policies and procedures for making appropriate document revisions, as well as sanctions for doing so inappropriately. Alterations that intentionally change the content or character of health information for nefarious purposes such as concealing wrongdoing, are referred to as tampering. Such alterations may constitute criminal conduct such as fraud, and policies and procedures should be in place to prevent such occurrences.

Additions to the Health Record

A **late entry** is documented in the health record when a pertinent entry was missed or was not written in a timely manner. Late entries should be documented as follows:

- Identify the new entry as a late entry.
- Enter the current date and time. Do not try to give the appearance that the entry was made on a previous date or time.
- Identify or refer to the date and incident for which the late entry is written.
- If the late entry is used to document an omission, validate the source of additional information as much as possible (for example, where the information was obtained to write the late entry).
- When using late entries, document as soon as possible; the more time that passes, the less reliable the entry becomes. Organizations should specify in their policies and procedures how the late entry process is to occur in the EHR. If an EHR does not allow for late entries, it will show as an addendum (described next) (AHIMA 2012a).

An **amendment** is a type of late entry in which information is added to support or clarify a previous entry. Often, more space is required and the amendment cannot be documented in the same location as the original entry.

In addition to a change made by a provider, a patient may also request an amendment to his or her health record, as defined by the HIPAA Privacy Rule (45 CFR 164.526), which will be discussed in more detail in chapter 11.

An **addendum** is new documentation that is added to an original entry after attestation has occurred (Wiedemann 2011). A specific policy and procedure for addenda should be present (AHIMA 2012a).

The process for creating an addendum should include

- Documenting the date and time of the addendum
- Writing "addendum" and stating the reason for the addendum, referring back to the original or parent document or entry
- Entering an addendum as soon as possible after the original entry
- Linking the addendum to the original entry in the EHR

Removal from the Health Record

Organizational policy should define the rare occasions when documentation may be deleted or retracted from a health record. **Deletion** is the permanent elimination of information from a document. Most

EHRs do not permit deletion (AHIMA 2012a). Deletion of documentation should not occur except in very specific circumstances (for example, documentation is entered in the wrong patient record and is discovered immediately after it is entered). In this case, a special procedure may allow for the removal of the incorrect information before anyone else has had a chance to view it.

In an electronic environment, appropriate deletion may be referred to as a **retraction**, where the information is no longer available for viewing but is available behind the scenes or through an administrative record view. For example, in an EHR the incorrect information would remain attached to the record in the background, but no indication of an error would be present (AHIMA 2012a). Information may be retracted to preserve confidentiality. In adoptions, references to the birth mother's identity may be deleted from the record. A flag or other marker would indicate the information had been deleted, and only authorized individuals would have access to it in another location. The retracted information would not be released with the record unless permitted by state law. Each organization should evaluate situations where deletion or retraction is appropriate and develop policies and procedures to address them.

Version Management

It is acceptable for a draft of a dictated and transcribed note or report to be changed before attestation unless there is a reason to believe the changes are suspect, would not reflect actual events or action, or it has been relied upon for patient care. For this reason, there may be more than one version of a document. **Version management** refers to how an organization handles the numerous versions of a document or collection of data that may exist as a result of changes to the health record. If the information has been used for patient care, whether it was attested to or not, it must be retained and managed. A decision must be made as to which version or versions of the document or information will be displayed, who will have access to the versions, and how they will be flagged in the record.

Organizational policy should clearly differentiate preliminary (draft) documents from final signed (attested) documents. It should also specify how long a document will remain as a draft. After that time period or after a document has been attested to, any changes should follow the organization's late entry or amendment procedures (AHIMA 2012a). The original document must be maintained along with the new revised document.

Timeliness and Completeness

The final elements that contribute to the legally defensible health record are **timeliness,** which is promptness of documentation; **completeness,** which is comprehensiveness of documentation; and appropriate use of the print function.

Timeliness and completeness are the responsibility of the author. If all documentation is performed in a timely manner, the health record will ultimately be complete within the time lines established by legal and accreditation standards and by organizational policy and medical staff bylaws.

Licensure and accrediting bodies mandate timeliness of entries, but timeliness is also important from an evidentiary and admissibility standpoint. Entries should be made in the health record as soon as possible after an event or observation. As described earlier, the complete date and time for each entry in a paper record must be recorded to show when the entry occurred. This will also provide the chronology of care provided to the patient. EHR users do not need to enter the date and time because the system will do this automatically (AHIMA 2012a). However, the date and time for late entries should be manually entered in an EHR to reflect when the entry should have been made. The manually entered information will exist in addition to the system's automatic time and date stamp for when the entry was made.

The health record is not complete until all its parts are compiled and the appropriate documents are attested to. EHR settings can facilitate documentation completeness by requiring that certain pieces of data be captured before the user can move on to the next field or exit the system. Medical staff bylaws must include time limits for health record completion. Completion of a health record may be ensured by concurrent analysis (record review by HIM staff during the patient's stay in a healthcare organization to determine whether signatures or other pertinent information are missing). If documentation is missing, healthcare providers are reminded to complete and attest to items in the record before the patient is discharged. Another form of record analysis is discharge analysis, which occurs after patient discharge. The patient's record is reviewed by HIM staff to ensure the record is complete and all information is in the correct patient record. Analysis can be greatly streamlined in EHR systems that automatically check for missing documents and signatures.

EHRs offer unique issues for determining completeness. EHR users could potentially make changes or additions to the health record at any point in time. Organizational policy should determine the point at which no additional changes can be made. System functionality needs to support organizational policy to ensure and demonstrate health record integrity, although exceptions should be permitted where new information or a correction needs to be made for the sake of accuracy.

Printing

Printing can create legal challenges for healthcare organizations with an EHR system if clinicians print from the EHR and then document on printouts rather than in the system. Reliance on both paper and electronic documentation will also complicate the e-discovery process, which was presented in chapter 4. Organizations must establish strict printing policies, including justification for printing paper internally, who has authority to print, how printing will be tracked in an audit trail, and the format and version of documents that may be printed. Organizations may also discourage printing from the EHR solely for the purpose of having a paper copy by creating cumbersome and time-consuming printing processes (for example, requiring a separate print command for each page that is printed) and generating copies with formats that cannot be read easily. It has been suggested that EHRs should provide a functionality that creates views based on requestor type and use (for example, one view for attorneys and their needs, but a separate view for patients seeking an overview of their medical information) (Carey and Beahan 2016). For evidentiary purposes, the printout of a record from an EHR should approximate the record as viewed on a computer screen, so as not to give the impression that there are two separate records for the same patient and that the printout is not the LHR.

The problem of duplicate copies is not unique to EHRs. Photocopies of original paper documents can also create problems when providers document on them. Although the original paper document is ordinarily considered the "source of truth," this is questioned when a photocopy contains additional and updated information. Whether printed from an electronic system or photocopied from a paper original, multiple copies also heighten the risk of privacy breaches. The creation, use, and disposal of additional copies must be monitored closely, regardless of the type of health record used.

Personal Health Records

The personal health record (PHR) offers unique challenges to health information management and informatics professionals in the management of the LHR. The PHR, also known as a consumer health record or patient health record, is created, maintained, and managed by the individual or patient to whom the information pertains. Like health records maintained by healthcare providers, PHRs can be paper or electronic. There are two types of PHRs. The first type is the **standalone PHR**, which consists of information provided by the patient and which is present either on paper, on the patient's computer or thumb drive, or in an Internet repository of the patient's choosing. The second type, the **tethered PHR**, is connected via a secure electronic portal to an organization's information system, such as a healthcare provider's EHR (Lester et al. 2016). Despite the Center for Medicare and Medicaid Services' Stage 2 meaningful use criteria (addressed further in chapter 14) that incentivize providers to encourage patient engagement through online access to patient portals and secure patient-provider messaging, one study has shown that 87 percent of patients still use paper-based PHRs instead of electronic PHRs (Wang and Dolezel 2016).

There are legal issues associated with deciding whether to integrate a PHR into the LHR. There is concern that a PHR does not qualify as a business record and should not be included in the LHR, even though it may affect treatment decisions. However, as information created by patients continues to proliferate through multiple sources, including personal wearable fitness devices, health information management and informatics professionals must consider the role of the PHR relative to the LHR and how it will be maintained. Increasingly, information collected and provided by the patient is becoming relevant to treatment that the patient receives. At the same time, however, an organization must decide the degree to which it can accept information generated by the patient as being reliable and sufficiently trustworthy to be included in the LHR.

The most obvious mechanism for a PHR to become integrated into an organization's LHR is via a formal request to amend the health record. The amendment request process is outlined in the HIPAA Privacy Rule provisions (chapter 11) and may be outlined in state statutes. Health information management and informatics professionals must be prepared for questions about how the organization may incorporate information from their PHRs. In provider-sponsored patient portals where patients can enter health information into a system that the provider owns and controls, there are many policy decisions to be made, such as whether the PHR becomes part of the facility's LHR and who may access, amend, and disclose information from the PHR. Guidance from a health information management and informatics professional is important. Several standards development initiatives have begun to focus on PHRs. The HL7 PHR-S FM standard focuses on the consumer's right to edit information that feeds into the PHR from an EHR and to maintain a longitudinal view of his or her health history (Health Level Seven International 2016).

Non–provider-sponsored PHR repositories have historically been at risk because no legislation protected them; however, the American Recovery and Reinvestment Act of 2009 (ARRA) extended protections to PHRs held by entities not covered by HIPAA. (More information about ARRA is included in chapter 10.) Many in the healthcare industry are calling for the creation of a PHR liaison, personal health information custodian, or patient information coordinator to assist patients or consumers in managing their personal health information. This role would include consumer education regarding privacy and security issues associated with the creation of a PHR.

Check Your Understanding 9.4

Instructions: Indicate whether the following statements are true or false (T or F).

1. Illegibility has been reduced through the presence of EHRs.
2. A Joint Commission–accredited organization may use any abbreviation in a health record as long as it is explained in a facility-wide key or legend.
3. Incorrect information in the health record should be obliterated so that it cannot be confused with the updated, corrected information placed in the record.
4. EHR cut, copy, and paste functions strengthen documentation integrity.
5. A late entry in the health record should not be identified as such because it may lead to negligence liability.

Health Record Identification, Retention, and Disposition

Sound policies and procedures for the identification, retention, and disposition of health records are vital to information integrity when information is at the heart of litigation, regardless of record format. An organization must know where its information is housed, how long it should be retained, and when and whether it may be destroyed. It is important for retention policies and procedures to address the LHR, but they should also address backup tapes, voice mail, word processing drafts, and shadow records (that is, duplicate records or copies). When an organization is ready to replace or upgrade either an EHR or a paper record system, it must consider its policies on the accessibility, retention, and destruction of information. This section discusses the legal issues associated with the creation and identification of health records, retention (including storage and retrieval), and disposition (destruction, transfer, or loss). The term *maintenance* broadly refers to the life cycle of the health record, from the time of creation through disposition.

Health Record Identification

Upon a patient's first encounter with a healthcare organization, a unique identifier is assigned to the patient, and a health record is created with the collection of admission or registration information, as well as clinical information.

Depending on the size of an organization and the number of patients treated, the patient is usually assigned a unique identification number or other form of identification, which is essential for future record retrieval purposes. This initial information becomes part of the facility's **master patient index** (MPI) or patient-identifying directory. The MPI serves as a link to the patient record and facilitates patient identification. Because it contains master data that is the key to proper patient identification, the MPI is critical for patient safety and quality care (Kloss 2015). The first and most immediate goal of an MPI is **patient matching**, which is accurately connecting a patient to his or her medical information. The long-term goal of an MPI is to assist in maintaining a longitudinal patient health record from birth to death. The MPI can be maintained in a variety of ways, although most providers use electronic systems.

Ensuring the correct identification of patients and ensuring that one (and only one) patient is assigned a particular identifier, whether it is a number or patient name, are ongoing challenges. For example, patients may not remember previous admissions or episodes of outpatient care, or they may have been admitted under a different name or a different spelling of their name; additionally, incorrect information may have been entered. Each of these situations can result in an incorrect number being assigned to the patient at subsequent encounters. Any of these issues may hinder the retrieval of information for patient care. Even worse, however, is the potential for the wrong patient information to be retrieved and used to treat a patient, resulting in dangerous treatment mistakes.

The complexities of patient matching have become more pronounced as the **enterprise master patient index** (EMPI) becomes more commonplace. Because an organization's healthcare services are often no longer confined to one location, the EMPI is needed to track patients in integrated healthcare systems that increasingly consist of multiple care sites and a variety of information systems (Dooling et al. 2016).

Beyond the criticality of patient matching in the EMPI are initiatives, nationwide, to adopt interoperable health information exchanges (HIEs). These HIEs, by facilitating the sharing of information among healthcare organizations, aim to "improve the efficiency, safety, and quality of the delivery of healthcare" (Lusk et al. 2014). As the evolution from the MPI to the EMPI has heightened the need for more sophisticated patient matching techniques, so has the HIE environment created the need for patient matching that spans regions, states, and the country. Two types of algorithms are typically used to match patient records. The **deterministic algorithm** compares values in various database fields (for example, date of birth, race, marital status) to detect exact or partial matches. The **statistical/mathematical algorithm** assigns weights to data that nearly match, determining the probability that two records are those of the same patient (Lusk et al. 2014). Both methods can nonetheless result in false negatives (that is, non-matches), so that returning patients are treated as new patients and duplicate health records are created; or false positives (that is, incorrect matches) that match patients to wrong numbers and result in a comingling of information that belongs to more than one patient. Both false negatives and false positives create patient safety risks (Kloss 2015).

To facilitate accurate and timely retrieval of patient health records both within an organization and nationally, the concept of a universal identifier unique to each patient (similar to the concept of a Social Security number) has been debated extensively among government, public, and private groups. Although AHIMA has promoted the patient identifier concept in an effort to reduce patient identification errors (AHIMA 2016), particularly in light of the increasing use of health information exchanges, patient confidentiality concerns have stalled adoption of an identifier on a national level.

Health Record Retention

The **retention** of health records in any format involves storing the records, providing for timely retrieval, and establishing lengths of times that various types of records will be retained by the healthcare organization. This section addresses storage and retrieval of health records, factors that influence health record retention periods, record retention schedules, and retention of electronic health records.

Storage and Retrieval

Healthcare organizations need policies that address the storage of health records. Although storage and retention are closely linked (retention and factors that affect retention periods are discussed in detail later), storage considerations for paper records include the amount of physical space available and, in the absence of policies providing for record destruction, the cost and feasibility of storing records off-site or converting them to another medium. Storage considerations for electronic records differ because a much greater volume can be stored in a smaller space. Organizations with EHRs may choose to add more storage capacity because advancements in storage technology have grown at an exceptional rate and a reasonable price, thus providing a variety of options for data retention.

Mobile devices, including smartphones, tablets, and laptop computers, are ubiquitous in provider settings and can contain massive amounts of information. However, associated privacy and security risks such as loss, theft, and compromised confidentiality during transmission must be addressed. Organizational policies and procedures should address users' rules of behavior; password requirements; lock-out features; rules regarding texting, camera, and video; use of sensitive information on mobile devices; and ability of the organization to examine the system for compliance and to investigate incidents (AHIMA 2012b). Storage decisions must also be made in conjunction with retention decisions and factors that affect those decisions.

Retrieval is quickly locating requested records and information needed for patient care or other uses. When a patient's record cannot be located, a provider cannot access prior medical information, and the patient's care may be compromised because of duplicate or improper treatment. Retrieval of paper health records involves checking out records from a filing area and tracking those that are not returned within a specified period. A software system may be used to track patient records. Retrieval of EHRs includes automatic access or approval of a request and placement of the record in a work queue or work list for the requestor to access.

Factors That Influence Retention Periods

Because the health record is a multifaceted document with demands placed on it by many diverse interests, policies establishing retention schedules are critical to the record management process. In addition to federal and state laws including statutes of limitations, as well as other legal issues, healthcare organizations must take into account requirements of external organizations such as the Joint Commission and other applicable accrediting bodies (which generally require the existence of policies and otherwise defer to state law) and the Department of Health and Human Services Office of Inspector General, and recommended retention standards published by AHIMA. Internal operational factors include emerging EHR technology, patient populations (for example, severity and readmission rates), institutional medical practice, research activity, educational needs, access to new technology, storage constraints or capabilities, cost, and disaster recovery plans. These external and internal factors, discussed in greater detail in this section, require the availability of a patient's health record for varying periods of time. Thus, a record retention policy that meets an organization's needs must be developed. Record retention policies are developed around the concept of active and inactive records. **Active records** are those that are used or consulted routinely, generally because patient encounters are still taking place. **Inactive records** are those that are not used often, generally because patient encounters have ceased because of death or other factors, but must be retained either as a reference or because they have not reached the required retention period (AHIMA 2013a).

Federal and State Laws

All applicable state and federal statutes and regulations must frequently be reviewed and compared with one another to ensure that health records are retained for the time period required. Medicare requires records to be maintained for at least five years (42 CFR 482.24(b)), including radiologist records (printouts, films, scans, and other images), home health agency records, long-term care records, laboratory records, and any other records that document information about claims for reimbursement. When state laws or licensing standards require a longer retention period, the longer requirement must be followed. Many states recommend that patient health records be retained for 10 years following patient discharge or death. Special requirements for minor patients are discussed in detail later. Some types of records, such as mammograms, may have retention periods up to 20 or 30 years.

Source data records (for example, fetal monitoring strips, EEGs, EKGs, videotapes, treadmill tests, magnetic tapes, and other images that are interpreted and/or summarized into final transcribed reports) can be incorporated into the EHR or maintained in the department where they originated. They must be retained for the legally required maintenance period. Fetal monitoring strips are considered part of the mother's record; however, because they relate to the newborn, they should be maintained for the same period of time that the newborn's record is maintained. State and federal agencies may also have retention requirements relative to specific types of applicable health records. For example, the Occupational Safety and Health Administration (OSHA) requires that most health records of employees be maintained for the duration of employment plus 30 years (AHIMA 2013a).

Statutes of Limitations

Applicable statutes of limitations (discussed in chapter 6), which are the time periods in which a lawsuit may be filed, must be considered when establishing a retention schedule. There is no one statute of limitations that must be considered, as they vary by state and by the type of action being brought (for example, torts, contracts, and specific periods for professional malpractice lawsuits). Although it must be given primary consideration, the statute of limitations for the types of lawsuits that concern a healthcare organization ordinarily will be much shorter than the retention periods mandated by Medicare, patient care needs, and many of the organization's other operational needs.

There are exceptions:

Minors: The statute of limitations for minors, which generally includes those who are younger than 18 years of age, may exceed the time for which health records are ordinarily retained. Whereas a minor may file a lawsuit on his or her own behalf upon reaching the age of majority, the statute of limitations does not begin to run until the minor reaches the age of majority (generally age 18 years). If the statute of limitations for the lawsuit being brought is two years, the minor would be able to bring legal action until he or she is 20 years old. If the lawsuit related to alleged medical malpractice when the child was 2 years old, the retention period—in order to comply with the statute of limitations—would be 18 years (from the time the child was 2 years old until he or she reached 20 years of age). This can create operational burdens for a healthcare organization and must be factored into its record retention policy.

Incompetent Individuals: A state's statute of limitations may also be extended for incompetent individuals, who are those deemed by a court to have a mental disability that renders them unable to act on their own behalf to handle their affairs or represent themselves legally. Because a person's incompetence may never be lifted (for example, an individual with a developmental disability), thus enabling a lawsuit to be filed at any time, an organization's record retention policy should specify that the records of these individuals should never be destroyed.

Accreditation Standards

There are several entities that accredit healthcare organizations. Because of its long-standing existence and its predominance in the acute care setting, however, the Joint Commission is often used as a representative example of accrediting bodies. The Joint Commission defers to applicable statutes, regulations, patient care purposes, and an organization's operational and legal needs for determining appropriate record retention periods. In the chapter, "Record of Care," in *Comprehensive Accreditation Manual for Hospitals: The Official Handbook*, the Joint Commission states that the retention period of the original or legally reproduced health record is also determined by its use and hospital policy (Joint Commission 2016a, RC.01.05.01). The Joint Commission surveys organizations to ensure that they comply with legal requirements and their own health record retention policies. The Joint Commission's record retention standards are similar to those of other accrediting bodies.

AHIMA Recommendations

Although they do not have the force and effect of law, professional practice guidelines are valuable in making operational decisions. AHIMA has established health record retention recommendations that guide practice in many healthcare organizations. Figure 9.6 displays the AHIMA-recommended retention standards (AHIMA 2011a).

Figure 9.6 AHIMA's recommended retention standards

Health Information	Recommended Retention Period
Diagnostic images (such as x-ray film)	5 years
Disease index	10 years
Fetal heart monitor records	10 years after the infant reaches the age of majority
Master patient/person index	Permanently
Operative index	10 years
Patient health records (adults)	10 years after the most recent encounter
Patient health records (minors)	10 years after the most recent encounter
Physician index	10 years
Register of births	Permanently
Register of deaths	Permanently
Register of surgical procedures	Permanently

Source: AHIMA 2011c, Appendix D.

Operational Needs

AHIMA recommends that healthcare organizations develop health record retention schedules that meet the organization's operational needs (AHIMA 2013a). The paramount need is patient care, but operational needs may also include other uses by patients, physicians, non-physician providers, researchers, and staff or patient educators. An organization, depending on its specific needs, may have many legitimate uses that necessitate extending retention periods. These include research, cost of retention, education, and the inconvenience of purging.

Record Retention Schedules

A healthcare organization must consider the previously mentioned factors when developing its health record **retention schedule**. Organizations may also decide to retain records for different periods of time based on the media types on which they reside. A retention schedule should specify what information should be retained, the time period for which it should be retained, and the storage medium (that is, format) on which it is to be retained. Retention schedules should address the transfer of health records from one medium to another (for example, from paper to scanned images). This is discussed later in the chapter. It should also include destruction policies and procedures (AHIMA 2013a). For a list of federal and accrediting body record retention requirements, see the AHIMA publication "Retention and Destruction of Health Information" (AHIMA 2013a).

EHR Retention

Many decisions pertaining to health record retention are determined by the organization's existing record formats. Retention of electronic information is a complex task. In addition to retention guidelines that govern paper records, policies and procedures should specifically outline retention of the myriad electronic media types that exist, many in portable form (for example, images, optical disks, computer disks, CDs, and DVDs). In addition to health information, data inherent to EHR systems, such as metadata, alerts, and reminders, should be addressed in a retention policy. This information will be important for certifying the integrity of the record for business and legal purposes. Organizational retention requirements should be part of the selection and management of an EHR system. Purging involves separating active records from inactive records in either a filing system or an electronic database (AHIMA 2013a).

An organization must also consider record permanence in its retention policies. The life cycle of a software system is limited once implemented due to rapid advances in technology. Thus, information maintained in an EHR system is subject to technology changes or obsolescence that will impact its permanence and ability to be accessed. Procedures to protect data integrity during system conversions must be implemented and documented. A retention policy must factor in the projected life of the current systems software. Older information will need to be made accessible after the original system has been upgraded or technology has changed. This can occur by continuing to maintain the older system, migrating records to the new system, or maintaining records in some other format that is independent of either the old or new system (for example, a document management system).

Other factors that should be considered when creating retention policies for electronic information are scanned images and fetal monitoring strips. Scanned images that have been directly fed into a document management system (and are available to physicians and other providers) are not always of diagnostic quality. In these cases, retention policies should state that the ancillary departments that created the information should maintain the information for the appropriate retention period. Also, because fetal monitoring strips are often not compatible with scanning systems, specific computer software that digitally stores fetal monitoring tracings may need to be installed within the labor and delivery area so that retention requirements can be met.

Check Your Understanding | 9.5

Instructions: Indicate whether the following statements are true or false (T or F).

1. A patient's PHR is a business record.
2. Statutes of limitations may not be considered when establishing a health record retention schedule.
3. Printing of paper copies from electronic health records should be encouraged because it allows more providers to access the information.
4. A master patient index is a directory of patient-identifying information.
5. When establishing a health record retention schedule, an organization must retain all records for the same period of time.

Health Record Disposition

Disposition involves the removal of records from a record storage system, either paper or electronic. Removal may occur for many reasons but is often the result of a record becoming inactive due to the cessation of patient encounters (for example, a live patient has not returned within a specified period of time or a patient has died) or achievement of the maximum retention period. Disposition can include destruction, or transfer to another medium or custodian. Although a healthcare organization may not retain paper health records indefinitely, for reasons such as cost and storage capabilities, organizations with EHRs may also develop disposition procedures because the benefit of retaining older records may not outweigh their usefulness in treating the patient or fulfilling other organizational needs. Establishing policies that incorporate state and federal laws and other standards is part of the disposition process.

AHIMA recommends taking all of the following factors into consideration when determining the appropriate disposition of health records:

- State laws regarding record retention and disposal, record preservation for historic purposes, and statutes of limitations
- State licensing standards
- Medicare and Medicaid requirements
- Federal laws governing treatment for alcohol and drug abuse (if applicable)
- Guidelines issued by professional organizations
- The needs and wishes of patients, physicians, other providers, and public health organizations for follow-up and research needs
- Organizational policies (AHIMA 2011b)

This section addresses several facets of health record disposition: health record destruction, the transfer of health records, and liability associated with the loss or unauthorized destruction of records.

Destruction of Health Records

Not every piece of data or information needs to be kept permanently. **Destruction**, which is the removal of health records from existence, should be carried out according to federal and state law and pursuant to an approved retention schedule and destruction policy. For example, providers that offer alcohol or drug abuse services such as education, training, treatment, rehabilitation, or research, must dispose of records as required by federal law (AHIMA 2011b).

A good retention plan includes instructions and guidelines for information destruction. The plan is included in an organization's policies and procedures to ensure that record destruction is part of the normal course of business and that no one particular record or group of records is singled out for destruction. Where organizations fail to apply destruction policies uniformly or where destruction is contrary to policy, a court may allow a jury to infer in a negligence suit that, had the record been available, it would have shown that the organization acted improperly in treating the patient.

Even if they are otherwise scheduled for destruction, records involved in an open investigation, audit or litigation should not be destroyed. Such destruction, or spoliation of evidence, would subject the organization to greater liability for failure to retain information. Appropriate safeguards should be implemented within electronic systems to prevent inappropriate destruction of information. (For example, a legal hold, as discussed in chapter 5, should be initiated.)

Destruction policies and procedures must ensure that paper records are destroyed so that protected health information (PHI) is not revealed and cannot be re-created. AHIMA recommends burning, shredding, pulping, or pulverizing (AHIMA 2013a). The HIPAA Privacy Rule mandates that agreements with shredding companies and other destruction companies include language ensuring that information will not be further disclosed (45 CFR 164.504(e)(2)). Destruction that is outsourced should be documented with a certificate of destruction once the process is complete. The certificate should include, or be accompanied by, a list of the specific documents destroyed and a description of the manner of destruction. AHIMA recommends that organizations maintain destruction documents permanently, because they may be required as evidence that records were destroyed in the regular course of business. Figure 9.7 provides a list of recommendations from AHIMA regarding the destruction of records (AHIMA 2013a).

EHR destruction policies should include specific instructions about how the information will be destroyed. Deleting information from its original location or file folder does not prevent it from being

Figure 9.7	AHIMA recommendations for destruction of records

AHIMA recommends that destruction should be documented, including:

- Date of destruction
- Method of destruction
- Description of the disposed record series of numbers or items
- Inclusive dates covered
- A statement that the records were destroyed in the normal course of business
- The signatures of the individuals supervising and witnessing the destruction

If destruction services are to be contracted, the contract should:

- Specify the method of destruction
- Specify the time that will elapse between acquisition and destruction of data
- Establish safeguards against breaches in confidentiality
- Indemnify the healthcare facility from loss due to unauthorized disclosure
- Provide proof of destruction

Source: AHIMA 2013a.

accessed from the hard drive or storage media. Several methods are available to permanently remove the information (AHIMA 2013a). Physically destroying the storage media, rendering it unusable, is the most secure means of destruction. CDs and DVDs should be destroyed by shredding or cutting. Laser discs can be destroyed by pulverizing. Overwriting of hard drives utilizing Department of Defense–accepted software replaces previously stored information with a pattern of meaningless information that renders the original information unrecoverable. Hard drives may be neutralized with a magnetic field (degaussing) to erase data. Magnetic tapes can be destroyed by demagnetizing. Whichever methods are chosen, the organization must ensure that they allow no possibility for reconstruction (AHIMA 2013a). Two types of electronic information that are produced in vast quantities by healthcare organizations and which must specifically be managed are e-mails and text messages. Because they contain highly sensitive information, not only must they be appropriately maintained and safeguarded for confidentiality and integrity purposes, but destruction must be methodical and in accordance with applicable laws. E-mails and text messages are particularly challenging because, even though they are deleted by the user and from the server, they may still be in circulation.

Transfer of Health Records

The **transfer of health records** can include moving a record from one medium to another (for example, from paper to a document management/imaging system) or to another records custodian. Because the transfer of records from one medium to another often does not include a custodial change, fewer legal implications apply. Many circumstances can lead to the transfer of health records. Transfers can frequently pertain to smaller businesses such as physician practices, but they are also occurring with greater frequency in larger healthcare organizations through mergers, acquisitions, and sales. The transfer of health records may be associated with ownership changes (sale of a business to a new owner or a buyout by co-providers when another provider leaves, retires, or dies) or closure of a healthcare organization due to retirement, cessation of practice, or death of a provider.

The HIPAA Privacy Rule (chapters 10 and 11) does not require the patient's authorization to carry out healthcare operations, even if an activity uses health information that identifies a patient. The transfer of records through activities such as sales and transfers are within the HIPAA definition of healthcare operations (45 CFR 164.501) and are further specifically exempted from the patient authorization requirement. However, healthcare organizations must also refer to applicable state laws and other federal laws to determine whether requirements exist that are more stringent than HIPAA requirements before record transfer occurs. The following sections address various causes of health record transfer, including ownership changes, departure of providers, and organizational closures.

Ownership Change

An ownership change may occur when a healthcare organization is sold. In physician or other provider practices where the providers have a shared ownership, an ownership change can also occur when one of the providers retires, dies, or otherwise relinquishes his or her interest in a practice. In these cases, health records are considered assets and are most likely to be transferred to successors who purchased or assumed responsibility for the organization. However, in physician practices, patients should be given the choice to transfer their records to the succeeding physician in the practice or to another physician. This position is supported by the American Medical Association (AMA) Code of Medical Ethics Opinion 3.3.1 (n.d.).

Departing Providers

Sometimes a provider leaves a practice and goes elsewhere, but an ownership change does not occur. When a physician goes to another practice, patients should be given the choice to move with the physician and transfer their records or have their care and their records transferred to another provider in the current group. If the situation does not allow the patient to continue with the same physician, the patient should be encouraged to find a new physician. Once they sign an authorization, the records should be made available to the new physician (AMA Code of Medical Ethics Opinion 3.3.1 n.d.).

Although noncompete contracts may be in place to limit a physician's ability to treat patients within a certain geographical area upon his or her departure and relocation, this contractual limitation is not imposed on the patient. As a result, the patient must be given his or her own information to take wherever he or she chooses. Because contracts may specify that health records are owned by the provider group, the practice from which a provider is departing may only be obligated to provide copies of the record rather than the original. Applicable state and federal laws should be consulted for the handling of records when an ownership change occurs.

Closure

Many of the same circumstances that lead to a change in ownership can also cause a healthcare organization to close if a successor is not identified. Although this may occur most commonly in smaller provider practices, it can also take place in larger healthcare organizations when a hospital closes as the result of financial distress or as part of corporate restructuring. The integrity, accessibility, and continued confidentiality of patient information following closure are extremely important. Guidance can often be obtained from the state health department or the state agency that licenses the organization that is closing. Applicable state laws should be consulted for handling records when closure occurs, because state legal requirements may vary. They may mandate that records be transferred to another healthcare organization, permit storage in a secure warehouse, require that the state licensing agency simply be notified of the disposition that will occur (destruction or transfer of the records to a new location), or require delivery of the records directly to the licensing agency. If the facility that is closing maintains paper documentation, that information must be routed appropriately to the new location (Lail et al. 2016). Transfer of records to another provider is optimal; however, when this cannot be accomplished in the face of a closure, AHIMA recommends that other storage options be considered, such as archival with a reputable commercial storage firm (AHIMA 2011b). Such a firm should be considered only if it

- Has experience in handling confidential patient information
- Has experience handling various media types (for example, paper, electronic, CDs)
- Guarantees the security and confidentiality of the records
- Ensures that patients and other legitimate requestors will have access to the information
- Has a climate-controlled environment in which to maintain the records

If a storage firm is used, specific provisions should be negotiated and included in the written agreement. These provisions include

- Agreement to keep all information confidential, disclosing only to authorized representatives of the provider or with written authorization from the patient/legal representative
- Upon the provider's request, prompt return of all confidential information without retaining copies
- Prohibition against selling, sharing, discussing, assigning, transferring, or disclosing confidential information in any other manner with any other individuals or business entities
- Prohibition against use of confidential information for any purpose other than providing mutually agreed-upon services
- Agreement to protect information against theft, loss, unauthorized destruction, or other unauthorized access
- Return or destruction of information at the end of the mutually agreed upon retention period
- Assurance that providers, patients, and other legitimate users will have access to the information (AHIMA 2011b)

When transfer is not feasible and destruction must occur as a last resort, it must be done appropriately, as described earlier in this chapter.

Whether the ultimate fate of health records belonging to an organization that is closing its doors is transfer or destruction, there must be a plan to provide a patient access to his or her own information either at the new location or prior to destruction. If a record is being transferred to a new location, only copies should be given to a patient if the required record retention period has not expired. For both transfers and destruction of their health records, patients should be individually notified. If this is not possible, information about the organization's closure and the ultimate disposition of its health records should be published for distribution to the general population. Records involved in a closure can be either paper or electronic. Their format must be taken into consideration in the transfer or destruction process. An organization's malpractice insurance carrier should also be apprised of the disposition status of the organization's health records.

Record retention laws that govern the organization must be followed for transferred records. As with health records maintained by continuously operating organizations, appropriate record retention schedules should be followed to allow destruction to occur as legally required for health records of organizations that have closed. For a list by state of laws and other guidelines pertaining to facility closure, see the AHIMA practice brief, "Protecting Patient Information after a Facility Closure" (AHIMA 2011b).

Liability Associated with Loss or Destruction of Records

A healthcare organization is responsible for maintaining health records in its custody according to applicable laws and organizational policies. When an organization cannot produce a health record, its risk of liability increases, particularly when the record is needed for patient care or evidence in a legal action. If a healthcare organization fails to produce a health record, the burden of proof shifts to that organization to prove that the loss was unintentional and that there was no negligent treatment. As discussed earlier, however, a court may instruct a jury or conclude that failure of a healthcare organization to produce evidence in the form of a health record creates an inference of negligence or a consciousness of guilt. Although failure to produce a health record most often conjures up images of a lost paper record, data can also be lost in electronic and document management systems, resulting in the same liability risks. Mechanisms ensuring that health information can be located will differ depending on the record format, but a carefully designed records management program is critical in all settings and will lessen the possibility of misplaced records in whatever formats they exist.

Check Your Understanding | 9.6

Instructions: Indicate whether the following statements are true or false (T or F).

1. Health record disposition includes transferring records from paper to a document management/imaging system.
2. The most secure way to destroy electronic information is to destroy the medium that the information is stored on.
3. When a physician closes a practice, all health records should be destroyed immediately to protect the privacy of patient information.
4. Data in a health record should be kept permanently.
5. When an e-mail message is deleted, it is eliminated from an organization's electronic system.

Scenario 9

Elizabeth Mullins was a patient in Mercy Hospital. During her hospital stay, a medication administration error occurred, resulting in permanent harm. She sued Mercy Hospital, the hospitalist, and several members of the nursing staff and the pharmacy staff. During the discovery process, her attorney obtained her authorization and requested a copy of her health record. Per its procedure, the HIM department at Mercy Hospital produced a paper copy from the patient's electronic health record. Elizabeth's attorney then requested to review her electronic health record on the EHR system. He was granted access after Elizabeth signed an authorization and a time was arranged for him to review the EHR in the HIM department. The attorney reviewed the paper record and found that the progress notes were voluminous and identical from one day to the next, reflecting no change in Elizabeth's status. This made him angry because the copied record was quite expensive, yet information was redundant and appeared not to have been updated from one day to the next. Further, in three progress notes, he found references to a patient named "Theresa" who had a different diagnosis. When the attorney compared the paper record and the record that he reviewed on the screen, they looked very dissimilar (although references to "Theresa" were also present in the electronic record). He also was unable to locate any e-mails or text messages in either the paper or electronic version of the record, although Elizabeth produced several between her and her physician from

Scenario 9 (Continued)

her mobile phone. When the attorney requested a list of the components of Mercy Hospital's legal health record policy, he found that its list of components included e-mail and text communications between providers and patients, as well as those among providers.

1. What legal problems will Mercy Hospital encounter regarding its legal health record?
2. What operational problems does Mercy Hospital need to address regarding its legal health record?
3. Who should be included on a team to address the previously identified problems?

References

AHIMA. 2011a. Fundamentals of the legal health record and designated record set. *Journal of AHIMA* 82(2): expanded online version. bok.ahima.org.

AHIMA. 2011b. Protecting patient information after a facility closure (updated August 2011). *Journal of AHIMA*: Web extra. bok.ahima.org.

AHIMA. 2011c. Retention and destruction of health information. Appendix D: AHIMA's recommended retention standards (updated August 2011). bok.ahima.org.

AHIMA. 2012a. Amendments in the electronic health record toolkit. bok.ahima.org.

AHIMA. 2012b. Mobile device security. *Journal of AHIMA* 83(4):50–55. bok.ahima.org.

AHIMA. 2013a. Retention and destruction of health information (Updated October 2013). bok.ahima.org.

AHIMA. 2013b. Electronic signature, attestation, and authorship. Appendix B: Laws, regulations, and electronic signature acts. (October). bok.ahima.org.

AHIMA. 2016. AHIMA's advocacy and policy efforts. www.ahima.org/myhealthid

AHIMA Work Group. 2013. Integrity of the healthcare record: Best practices for EHR documentation. *Journal of AHIMA* 84(8): 58–62 [extended web version]. bok.ahima.org.

Amatayakul, M. 2013. *Electronic Health Records: A Practical Guide for Professionals and Organizations*, 5th ed, revised reprint. Chicago: AHIMA.

American Medical Association Code of Medical Ethics. n.d. http://www.ama-assn.org/about-us/code-medical-ethics.

Carey, S. and S. Beahan. 2016. Pain at the printer: How to stop HIM's addiction to print records from the EHR. *Journal of AHIMA* 87(9):20–23. bok.ahima.org.

Dooling, J., L. Fernandes, A. Kirby, L. Kadlec, G. Landsbach, K. Lusk, M. Munns, N. Noreen, and O'Connor, M. 2016. Losing the match game: Study reveals gaps in HIM's patient identity integrity practices. *Journal of AHIMA* 87(10):39–47.

Downing, K. 2013. Electronic signature, attestation, and authorship (AHIMA Practice Brief, October 2013). bok.ahima.org.

Dunagan, B. 2016. Legal medical record definition and emerging technologies: Can they co-exist? AHIMA Convention and Exhibit. Baltimore, MD (October 18).

Health Level Seven International. 2016. HL7 Electronic Health Record-System (EHR-S) Functional Model, Release 1. www.hl7.org.

Johns, M. 2015. *Enterprise Health Information Management and Data Governance*. Chicago: American Health Information Management Association.

Joint Commission. 2016a. *Comprehensive Accreditation Manual for Hospitals*. Oakbrook Terrace, IL: Joint Commission.

Joint Commission. 2016b. The Joint Commission Perspectives (May). 36:5.

Kloss, L. 2015. *Implementing Health Information Governance.* Chicago: AHIMA.

Lail, P.J., S. Laird, K. McCall, J. Naretto, and A. York. 2016. Facility closure: How to get in, get out, and get what is important. *Perspectives in Health Information Management* (Fall):1–11. perspectives.ahima.org.

Lester, M., S. Boateng, J. Studeny, and A. Coustasse. 2016. Personal health records: Beneficial or burdensome for patients and healthcare providers? *Perspectives in Health Information Management* (April). perspectives.ahima.org.

Lusk, K., N. Noreen, G. Okafor, K. Peterson, and E. Pupo. 2014. Patient matching in health information exchanges. *Perspectives in Health Information Management.* perspectives.ahima.org.

McLendon, K. 2012. Creating a legal health record definition. *Journal of AHIMA* 83(1):46–47. bok.ahima.org.

The Sedona Conference. 2016. Introduction. https://thesedonaconference.org.

U.S. Department of Health and Human Services, Center for Medicare & Medicaid Services. 2008. Pub 100-08 Medicare Program Integrity. Transmittal 284. www.cms.gov.

Wang, T. and D. Dolezel. 2016. Usability of web-based personal health records: An analysis of consumer's perspectives. *Perspectives in Health Information Management* (Spring). perspectives.ahima.org.

Wiedemann, L.A. 2011. Amendment, corrections and deletions technical paper. 2011 AHIMA Convention Proceedings, October 2011. bok.ahima.org.

Cases, Statutes, and Regulations Cited

42 CFR 482.24(b): Form and retention of record. 2012.

42 CFR 482.24(c): Content of record. 2012.

45 CFR 164.501: Privacy of individually identifiable health information: Definitions. 2006.

45 CFR 164.504(e)(2): Implementation specifications: business associate contracts. 2006.

45 CFR 164.526: Amendment of protected health information. 2006.

15 USC 700l, et seq.: Electronic Signatures in Global National Commerce Act. 2000.

28 USC 1732: Uniform Photographic Copies of Business and Public Records as Evidence Act. 1977.

American Recovery and Reinvestment Act of 2009. Public Law 111-5.

HIPAA Privacy Rule: Part I

Laurie A. Rinehart-Thompson, JD, RHIA, CHP, FAHIMA

Learning Objectives

- Identify the purpose and goals of the HIPAA Privacy Rule
- Compare the applicability of the HIPAA Privacy Rule to that of other laws that protect patient information
- Analyze HIPAA Privacy Rule application to entities and information
- Define HIPAA terms of art
- Compare and contrast the HIPAA notice of privacy practices, consent, and authorization
- Evaluate when written authorization is and is not required for uses and disclosures
- Examine the restrictions that the HIPAA Privacy Rule places on the use of protected health information for commercial purposes
- Distinguish situations when the minimum necessary requirement does and does not apply

Key Terms

- Administrative simplification
- Affiliated covered entity
- American Recovery and Reinvestment Act (ARRA)
- Authorization
- Business associate (BA)
- Business associate agreement (BAA)
- Comprehensive Alcohol Abuse and Alcoholism Prevention, Treatment, and Rehabilitation Act of 1970
- Conditions of Participation
- Consent

- Covered entity (CE)
- Deidentified information
- Designated record set (DRS)
- Disclosure
- Drug Abuse Prevention, Treatment, and Rehabilitation Act of 1972
- Facility directory
- Freedom of Information Act of 1967 (FOIA)
- Fundraising
- Health Information Technology for Economic and Clinical Health (HITECH) Act

- Health Insurance Portability and Accountability Act of 1996 (HIPAA)
- Hybrid entity
- Incidental uses and disclosures
- Individual
- Limited data set
- Marketing
- Minimum necessary
- Notice of Privacy Practices (NPP)
- Organized healthcare arrangement (OHCA)

- Personal representative
- Privacy Act of 1974
- Privacy Rule
- Protected health information (PHI)
- Psychotherapy notes
- Redisclosure
- Request
- Safe Harbor method
- Treatment, payment, and operations (TPO)
- Use
- Workforce

April 14, 2003, marked the effective date of a law heralded by some as the most dramatic change to healthcare since the implementation of Medicare and Medicaid. The healthcare industry ushered in the portion of the Health Insurance Portability and Accountability Act (HIPAA) known as the Privacy Rule. The Privacy Rule's purpose is consistent with a central value of the health informatics and information professional, which is the protection of patient information. Since the HIPAA Privacy Rule, which is federal law, first went into effect on April 14, 2003, those affected by its requirements have worked to uphold the spirit of the law. The HIPAA Privacy Rule is addressed in chapters 10 and 11. This chapter discusses the composition of the HIPAA Privacy Rule; how it compares to other laws and standards that protect patient information; the entities, individuals, and types of information it applies to; terms of art; key privacy rule documents; rules surrounding the use and disclosure of patient information for both noncommercial and commercial purposes; and the minimum necessary requirement.

HIPAA and Other Patient Privacy Laws

The HIPAA **Privacy Rule** is a key federal law governing the privacy and confidentiality of patient information. The law's first goal is to protect the privacy of one's health information, which includes limiting access by others. The law's second goal is to provide an individual with greater rights with respect to his or her health information. While navigating the Privacy Rule's terms of art, concepts, and many exceptions, remember that the rule was written to accomplish these two goals.

Source of HIPAA

The **Health Insurance Portability and Accountability Act of 1996 (HIPAA),** from which the HIPAA Privacy Rule was created, was enacted by Congress on August 21, 1996, and became federal statutory law. As described later under Scope and Anatomy of HIPAA Privacy, HIPAA is expansive and covers a broad array of issues. From the statutory requirements of the privacy portion of HIPAA, the Department of Health and Human Services (HHS) created an administrative rule that became effective April 14, 2003. The final rule was influenced by feedback from stakeholders. The federal government published the Standards for Privacy of Individually Identifiable Health Information, more commonly referred to as the HIPAA Privacy Rule (the final rule) in the Federal Register on December 28, 2000 (HHS 2000). With amendments, the final modified Privacy Rule was published August 14, 2002 (HHS 2002). Although available from many sources, including the HHS website, the rule is officially available in the Code of Federal Regulations (45 CFR 160 and 164). The American Recovery and Reinvestment Act, passed by Congress in 2009, contained changes to the HIPAA Privacy Rule as delineated in the HITECH Act. These acts are described in greater detail later in this chapter.

Scope and Anatomy of HIPAA Privacy

HIPAA immediately connotes privacy because that aspect of the law has been so highly publicized. However, privacy is only one portion of the entire law, albeit an extremely important aspect in the management of health information. HIPAA consists of five broad sections (titles), most of which do not specifically address the protection of patient information. HIPAA also amended three pieces of existing federal legislation: the Internal Revenue Code of 1986 (26 USC), the Employee Retirement Income Security Act of 1986 (ERISA) (29 USC 1001 et seq.), and the Public Health Service Act (42 USC 6A).

As shown in figure 10.1, HIPAA contains five titles and addresses more than the privacy of patient information. Title I protects individuals and their dependents from losing their health insurance when leaving or changing jobs by providing insurance continuity (portability). It also prohibits discrimination based on a person's status or that of his or her dependents in the enrollment in health insurance plans and the amount of premiums charged. Titles III, IV, and V contain tax-related provisions relevant to the Internal Revenue Code and requirements for group health plans. In particular, Title III provides certain deductions for medical insurance, and Title IV specifies group health plan coverage for individuals with pre-existing conditions and income tax requirements for specific groups (45 CFR 165.512(e), Pub. L. 104-191).

Title II is the most relevant title to the management of health information, containing provisions relating to the prevention of healthcare fraud and abuse, medical liability (medical malpractice) reform, and administrative simplification. The Privacy Rule resides in the administrative simplification provision

Figure 10.1 HIPAA components

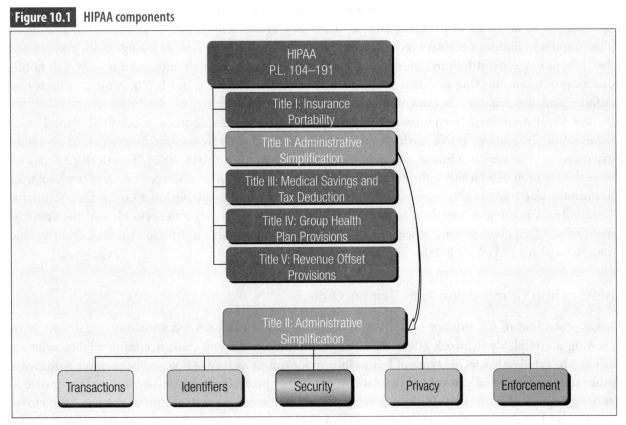

Source: Walsh 2011.

of Title II along with the HIPAA security regulations (which relate to safeguards—often technical in nature—that protect the privacy of electronic patient information and are covered in chapter 12); transactions and code set standardization requirements; unique national provider identifiers; and the enforcement rule. Because the complexity of HIPAA is well known, the term **administrative simplification** seems counterintuitive. However, this term refers to HIPAA's attempt to streamline and standardize the healthcare industry's non-uniform and inefficient business practices, such as billing. A significant part of this simplification process is the creation of standards for the electronic transmission of data. This was the original intent of HIPAA. The privacy and security rules were created thereafter.

American Recovery and Reinvestment Act of 2009

On February 17, 2009, President Barack Obama signed the **American Recovery and Reinvestment Act (ARRA)** into law. This multifaceted statute, which included significant funding for health information technology and other stimulus funding, also provided for significant changes to the HIPAA Privacy Rule. These changes are located in the **Health Information Technology for Economic and Clinical Health (HITECH) Act**, a statute within ARRA. Varying timelines for federal rule drafting resulted in multiple compliance deadlines. Two interim final rules relating to breach notification and enforcement (an update to a pre-HITECH 2006 final enforcement rule) were published in 2009. On July 14, 2010, and May 31, 2011, HHS issued proposed rules with suggested modifications to the HITECH Act. The January 2013 final rule, "Modifications to the HIPAA Privacy, Security, Enforcement, and Breach Notification Rules," finalized the two interim final rules and provisions in the July 2010 proposed rule (AHIMA 2013a). Part of the May 2011 proposed rule is still pending. Major revisions, which are addressed in this chapter, included changes to requirements relating to business associates and their subcontractors; protected health information of deceased individuals; Notice of Privacy Practices; the sale of information; provisions affecting the minimum necessary requirement; individual rights (access, accounting of disclosures, and the right to request restrictions); student immunization records; research authorizations; breach notification; provisions affecting personal health record vendors; marketing and fundraising; and increased enforcement and penalties for noncompliance.

ARRA also codified (recognized per statute) the Office of the National Coordinator for Health Information Technology (ONC), which was previously established by an executive order, to give it an expanded role in health information technology implementation (HHS 2009). Practical implications were the creation of a Health Information Technology (HIT) Policy Committee to address technologies to promote electronic health record (EHR) privacy and security; the establishment of an HIT Standards Committee consisting of members with expertise in healthcare privacy and security; and the appointment of an ONC chief privacy officer to advise on electronic health information privacy, security, and data stewardship (AHIMA 2009).

History and Comparison with Existing Laws

Legal protection of the privacy of patient information historically resided with individual state laws, creating a complex patchwork effect. Some states broadly addressed patient confidentiality, whereas others protected only specific types of health information such as HIV/AIDS and behavioral health. Still other states were virtually devoid of patient confidentiality protections. Inconsistent state laws provided varying degrees of protection. With increasing demand for access to patient information and the movement toward electronic billing transactions and an EHR, public concern about threats to health information privacy gained momentum and resulted in federal legislation directed specifically toward the privacy of patient information.

Several bills designed to create a national law protecting the privacy of patient information were unsuccessfully introduced during the 1990s. Many years passed before federal legislation was eventually passed by Congress in the form of HIPAA. Further, limited federal laws (discussed later) existed to protect only certain types of health information (for example, drug and alcohol abuse records) or information held only by certain entities (for example, agencies of the federal government). Limited and inconsistent federal and state laws left many types of health information, especially those not deemed to be of a highly sensitive nature, unprotected by any statute. Often, the only recourse that individuals had if their confidentiality was breached was through the court system, which is often an expensive, time-consuming, and emotionally exhausting experience with no guaranteed outcome. Under the HIPAA Privacy Rule, however, all types of health information are treated equally, regardless of their nature. Further, HIPAA violations result in sanctions outside the judicial system. Overall, the Privacy Rule is designed to increase privacy and confidentiality of patient information and to provide a less cumbersome recourse.

Because of the broad impact of the HIPAA Privacy Rule, the privacy of patient information is a priority as individuals and organizations affected by it strive to comply with its requirements. It has also created a number of challenges for the healthcare industry and to health information management (HIM) departments in particular.

The HIPAA Privacy Rule (hereafter referred to as "the Privacy Rule") transformed the landscape of patient information by expanding the breadth of privacy protection and protecting the confidentiality of a widely defined scope of medical and personal information. The following discussion of federal laws in effect prior to the implementation of the Privacy Rule demonstrates their limited application and authority.

Freedom of Information Act of 1967

The underlying purpose of the federal **Freedom of Information Act of 1967** (5 USC 552), commonly referred to as FOIA, is not the privacy of information but, instead, the right of disclosure to and access by the public regarding federal agency records. The rationale for such openness is government accountability to its citizens and ultimately its taxpayers. Although the public's right to inspect the documents and the work of its government is compelling, the sensitive and private nature of certain documents rises above the public's right to know. This legislation provides exceptions for documents such as medical records (if the reasons for disclosure do not outweigh the exception), to preserve the privacy of the individuals about whom they are written. This law has a narrow application to the healthcare system because most healthcare organizations are not federal. One significant exception is the Department of Veterans Affairs, through its operation of federal inpatient and outpatient healthcare facilities.

Privacy Act of 1974

In 1974, a federal law was passed to protect privacy. In part, the **Privacy Act of 1974** (5 USC 552a) provides individuals with privacy rights by requiring federal agencies that hold personally identifiable records to safeguard the information. Individuals also have the right to access and request amendments to their records (Rinehart-Thompson 2013). Although the purpose of the legislation is nondisclosure, as opposed to FOIA's focus on disclosure, this act is also narrow because it only applies to information collected by the federal government (for example, Veterans Affairs facilities); further, it is not tailored to protect health information. As a result, its impact on the protection of patient information is extremely limited.

Federal Drug and Alcohol Laws

The **Drug Abuse Prevention, Treatment, and Rehabilitation Act of 1972** (42 USC 4541–4594; 42 CFR 2.1–2.67; orig. 21 USC 1101–1800) and the **Comprehensive Alcohol Abuse and Alcoholism Prevention, Treatment, and Rehabilitation Act of 1970** (42 USC 4582 to 209dd-3) are federal statutes that provide specific and highly particularized safeguards to protect information relating to the diagnosis, treatment, or referral for treatment of conditions relating to drug abuse or other substance abuse. Although these acts are more global than the Privacy Act of 1974 (because they apply to all federally assisted alcohol and drug abuse treatment programs, not just federal providers), they still only apply to a niche population of patients rather than to the protection of patient information generally. These laws will be discussed more extensively in chapter 15.

Medicare Conditions of Participation

The requirements that govern providers receiving Medicare and Medicaid reimbursement include confidentiality provisions (Rinehart-Thompson 2013). As with the laws discussed earlier, however, the **Conditions of Participation** regulate only providers and, narrower still, only those receiving funds from the Medicare and Medicaid programs. While this includes a vast number of providers, the Conditions of Participation are inapplicable to nonproviders holding confidential patient information and do not apply to patients insured by other payers or those who are uninsured.

State Laws

As noted earlier, laws protecting the privacy of patient information and governing access, use, and disclosure largely resided with individual states and varied considerably. Although many states passed laws to protect highly sensitive health records such as behavioral health and HIV/AIDS, not all states possessed laws that protected health information generally. With the passage of the Privacy Rule, a minimum amount of protection (that is, a floor) was achieved uniformly across all the states through the establishment of a consistent set of requirements that affected providers, healthcare clearinghouses, and health plans.

Professional Ethical Standards and Codes of Conduct

Ethical standards and codes of conduct govern a variety of healthcare professionals, including health information management (HIM) and informatics professionals, and provide guidance regarding privacy protection of patient information. In particular, the American Health Information Management Association (AHIMA) Code of Ethics states that HIM professionals "preserve, protect, and secure personal health information in any form or medium and hold in the highest regards health information and other information of a confidential nature…" Although the AHIMA Code of Ethics does not have the force of law, it nonetheless provides ethical principles that guide the profession and bind individuals who are members of AHIMA and who hold an AHIMA credential (AHIMA 2011a).

Check Your Understanding 10.1

Instructions: Indicate whether the following statements are true or false (T or F).

1. Drug and alcohol abuse treatment records receive special protection under federal law.
2. The Privacy Rule resides in the administrative simplification provision of Title II of HIPAA.
3. The HITECH Act of ARRA of 2009 made minimal changes to the HIPAA Privacy Rule.
4. FOIA was enacted to address the privacy of health information.
5. The Conditions of Participation regulate all providers, including those who receive funds from the Medicare and Medicaid programs.

HIPAA Applicability

The HIPAA Privacy Rule applies to specific individuals and organizations and protects specific types of information. The first element, *who*, consists of covered entities and their business associates. The second element, *what*, protects health information.

Covered Entities

The Privacy Rule defines a covered entity (CE) as one or more of the following:

- A healthcare provider who transmits any health information pertaining to certain transactions (financial or administrative in nature) in electronic form
- A health plan, which is an individual or group plan that provides or pays the costs of medical care
- A healthcare clearinghouse, an entity that processes billing transactions between a healthcare provider and a health plan (45 CFR 160.103(3))

These categories are broad. Healthcare providers—as providers of medical or health services, or any other person or organization who furnishes, bills, or is paid for healthcare—range from individual practitioners (such as physicians, dentists, and chiropractors) to healthcare organizations (such as pharmacies, hospitals, and long-term care facilities). Additionally, CEs are responsible for their **workforce**, consisting of employees, volunteers, student interns, and trainees (45 CFR 160.103). A workforce encompasses those who work under the direct control of the CE and is not limited to those who receive wages. With this in mind, a CE should consider even employees of outsourced vendors who routinely work on-site in the CE's facility to be workforce members.

Transactions, referred to in the previous paragraph, that are affected by the Privacy Rule are those that relate to

- Health claims and encounter information
- Health plan enrollment and disenrollment (termination)
- Eligibility for a health plan
- Healthcare payment and remittance advice
- Health plan premium payments
- Health claim status
- Referral certification and authorization
- Coordination of benefits
- First report of injury
- Health claims attachments
- Other transactions as prescribed by the Secretary of HHS (45 CFR 160.103).

Business Associates

A **business associate (BA)** is a person or organization other than a member of a CE's workforce that performs functions or activities on behalf of or affecting a CE that involve the use or disclosure of individually identifiable health information (45 CFR 160.103(1)), which will be discussed later in this chapter. Per HITECH, the BA definition specifically includes patient safety organizations (PSOs), which receive and analyze patient safety issues; health information exchanges (HIEs) and health information organizations (HIOs), which share health information among providers electronically; e-prescribing gateways, which facilitate the prescribing process between physicians and pharmacies; other persons who facilitate data transmissions; and personal health record (PHR) vendors that, by contract, enable CEs to offer PHRs to their patients as part of the CE's EHR (HHS 2010, 40872). Per HITECH, a BA's subcontractors are BAs under HIPAA if they require access to an individual's protected health information, regardless of whether a business associate agreement has actually been signed (HHS 2010, 40873).

Once a CE identifies a person or organization as a BA, the CE is obligated to initiate a **business associate agreement (BAA)** to legally protect information handled outside the CE. Through this written and signed contract, CEs may lawfully disclose protected health information (PHI) to BAs such as consultants, billing companies, accounting firms, or others that may perform services for the provider. In the BAA, the BA agrees to comply with the CE's requirements to protect the information. In other words, the BA must agree not to use or disclose the PHI in ways the provider would not permit and must agree to protect patient information from unauthorized access or disclosure. Under HITECH, a BA's workforce, as with CEs, includes paid and unpaid individuals working under the BA's direct control (HHS 2010, 40874). At a minimum, the agreement between a CE and a BA should contain the requirements specified in figure 10.2, which includes the BA requirements instituted by HITECH.

Figure 10.2 BA contract specifics

The requirements placed on business associates under HIPAA and ensuing HITECH legislation have heightened the importance of business associate agreements. Covered entities cannot disclose PHI to business associates unless the two have entered into a written contract that meets HIPAA and HITECH requirements. Under HITECH, privacy, security, and breach notification requirements apply to business associates.

Such a contract would include provisions that:

- Prohibit the business associate from using or disclosing the PHI for any purpose other than that stated in the contract, and pursuant to the Privacy Rule and minimum necessary standard

- Prohibit the business associate from using or disclosing the PHI in a manner that would violate the requirements of the HIPAA Privacy Rule

- Require the business associate to maintain safeguards, as necessary, to ensure that the PHI is not used or disclosed except as provided by the contract

- Require the business associate to report to the covered entity any use or disclosure of the PHI that is not provided for in the contract

- Clarify that the business associate is responsible to report breaches of unsecured PHI

- Clarify that the business associate must adhere to policy and procedure, and documentation requirements imposed by the HIPAA Security Rule

- Establish how the covered entity would provide access to PHI to the individual whom the information is about when the business associate has made any material alterations to the information

- Require the business associate to make available its internal practices, books, and records relating to the use and disclosure of PHI received from the covered entity to the Department of Health and Human Services or its agents

- Establish how the entity would provide access to PHI to the individual whom the information is about in circumstances where the business associate holds the information and the covered entity does not

- Require the business associate to incorporate any amendments or corrections to the PHI when notified by the covered entity that the information is inaccurate or incomplete

- At termination of the contract, require the business associate to return or destroy all PHI received from the covered entity that it still maintains and prohibit the associate from retaining it

- State that individuals who are the subject of disclosed PHI are intended third-party beneficiaries of the contract

- Authorize the covered entity to terminate the contract when it determines that the business associate has repeatedly violated a term required in the contract

- State the business associate is subject to the HIPAA Security Rule, including implementation of administrative, technical and procedural safeguards, and procedural and documentation requirements

- State that the business associate will receive satisfactory assurances from its subcontractors that the subcontractors will appropriately safeguard protected health information

- State that subcontractors of the business associate are responsible for complying with HIPAA, and are directly liable for HIPAA violations, as is the business associate, even if the business associate has not entered into a contractual agreement with the subcontractor

- Clarify that the business associate is responsible to take action, possibly including termination, against a subcontractor if it violates HIPAA or provisions of the BAA

- Clarify that the business associate is subject to civil monetary penalties for violation of the Privacy Rule or the Security Rule

Source: Adapted from Cassidy 2000; updated 2010 per ARRA/HITECH requirements (NPRM 40872–40874).

Under HIPAA as originally written, a BA was bound to the law to virtue of its association (via contract) with a CE. HITECH changed this by directly requiring organizations or individuals meeting the definition of BA to comply with certain provisions of HIPAA, including breach notification and restrictions on the sale of health information, and subjecting them to the same civil and criminal penalties that CEs face for violating the law (AHIMA 2009). This is the case even if a BA has not entered into a BAA with a CE. BAs must also comply with the administrative, physical, and technical safeguards of the HIPAA security regulations, along with the policies, procedures, and documentation requirements imposed by the HIPAA security regulations (discussed in chapter 12) (AHIMA 2009). Additional requirements, as explained throughout the chapter, will be addressed as being applicable to BAs. BAs are now much more vulnerable if they violate HIPAA. CEs were historically required to respond to BA noncompliance, but HITECH also requires BAs to respond to CE noncompliance by requiring corrective action or severing the relationship with the CE.

Protected Health Information (PHI)

The Privacy Rule safeguards a category of information called **protected health information (PHI)**. To be PHI, it must pass a three-part test. It first must be deemed individually identifiable by meeting the first part of the test:

1. It must either identify the person or provide a reasonable basis to believe the person could be identified from the information given (including demographic information).

2. It must then also meet the second and third parts of the test to be PHI:

3. It must relate to one's past, present, or future physical or mental health condition; the provision of healthcare; or payment for the provision of healthcare.

4. It must be held or transmitted by a CE or its BA in any form or medium, including electronic, paper, and oral forms. (45 CFR 160.103).

Figure 10.3 outlines the test for determining whether the information meets the definition of PHI.

Under HITECH, individually identifiable health information of persons deceased for more than 50 years is no longer PHI and loses its Privacy Rule protection (HHS 2010, 40874). Further, genetic information has been specifically identified as PHI if it is individually identifiable and is held or transmitted by a CE or BA.

Figure 10.3 Test for determining whether information is PHI

Individually identifiable health information in any form or medium (paper, imaged, electronic, oral) that:

1. Identifies the person or provides a reasonable basis to believe the person could be identified from the information given

AND

2. Relates to one's health condition (physical or mental health; past, present, OR future), provision of healthcare, OR payment for provision of healthcare

AND

3. Is held or transmitted by a covered entity or (via a business associate agreement) its business associate

Source: 45 CFR 160.103

Deidentified Information

Key to defining PHI is the first part of the previously mentioned test, which requires information to either identify an individual or provide a reasonable basis to believe the person could be identified from the information given. This definition does not include deidentified information, which fails the first part of the test and therefore does not receive Privacy Rule protection (see figure 10.3).

Deidentified information is information from which personal characteristics about the individual or the individual's relatives, employers, or household members have been removed and that, as a result, neither identifies nor provides a reasonable basis to believe it could identify an individual. Deidentified information cannot later be constituted or combined to reidentify an individual. Deidentified information is commonly used in research, in decision support, and for other purposes.

Because of the power of current information technologies in assisting with the collection and analysis of data, it is possible to identify individuals by combining specific data. Therefore, the Privacy Rule requires the CE to do one of the following things to ensure deidentification of information:

- The CE can remove certain elements to ensure that the patient's information is truly deidentified. This is the **Safe Harbor method**. These 18 elements are listed in figure 10.4 (45 CFR 164.514(b)).

Figure 10.4 Data elements to be removed for deidentification of information

The following 18 identifiers pertain not only to the individual but also to relatives, employers, and the individual's household members, and they must be removed:

1. Names
2. Geographic subdivisions smaller than a state, including street address, city, county, precinct, and zip code, if that geographic unit contains fewer than 20,000 people. The initial three digits of such zip code may be changed to 000, or zip codes with the same three initial digits may be combined to form a unit of more than 20,000 people.
3. All elements of dates, except the year, directly related to an individual, including birth, admission, discharge, and death dates. In addition, all ages over 89 and all elements of dates (including the year) that would identify such age cannot be used. However, individuals over 89 can be aggregated into a single category of 90 or over.
4. Telephone numbers
5. Fax numbers
6. E-mail addresses
7. Social Security numbers
8. Medical record numbers
9. Health plan beneficiary numbers
10. Account numbers
11. Certificate/license numbers
12. Vehicle identifiers and serial numbers, including license plate numbers
13. Device identifiers and serial numbers
14. Web universal resource locators (URLs)
15. Internet protocol (IP) address numbers
16. Biometric identifiers, including fingerprints and voice prints
17. Full-face photographic images and any comparable images
18. Any other unique identification number, characteristic, or code, except for permissible reidentification

Source: 45 CFR 164.514(b) (2) (i).

- The CE can have an expert apply generally accepted statistical and scientific principles and methods to minimize the risk that the information might be used to identify an individual.

What if the CE needs to reidentify information that has been stripped of individual identifiers? In other words, how might the entity match information back to the person it identifies? The Privacy Rule allows an entity to assign a code to deidentified information to allow for reidentification. However, in doing so, the entity must ensure that the code assigned is not derived from or related to the information about the patient and cannot be translated to his or her identity. It also has to ensure that the code is not used for any other purpose and does not disclose the mechanism for reidentification in any way.

Health Information in Personnel and Educational Records

Although a person or organization may be subject to the Privacy Rule, not all information that the person or organization holds or comes into contact with is protected by the Privacy Rule. For example, the Privacy Rule specifically excludes employment records held by the CE in its capacity as employer (45 CFR 160.103). Under this exclusion, employee physical examination reports contained within personnel files are specifically exempted from the rule. Education records, including student grades and disciplinary records, but also health records created or collected by the school, are covered by the Federal Educational Records Privacy Act (FERPA) (20 USC 1232(g)) and are also excluded from the Privacy Rule's definition of PHI.

Check Your Understanding | 10.2

Instructions: Indicate whether the following statements are true or false (T or F).

1. A hospital employee's pre-employment physical examination is in his personnel file in Human Resources; this report is PHI.
2. A CE need only consider its employees when evaluating HIPAA compliance within the organization.
3. Deidentified information receives Privacy Rule protections.
4. In part, information must be individually identifiable to meet the definition of PHI.
5. A BA is anyone who might have access to a CE's PHI.

HIPAA Terminology

In addition to understanding who and what the HIPAA Privacy Rule applies to, there are additional terms of art that further explain the rule's applicability. These include individuals; personal representatives; the designated record set; disclosure, use, and request; treatment, payment, and operations; and types of organizations recognized by HIPAA.

Individual

The Privacy Rule refers to an **individual** rather than a *patient* or *client*. An individual is the person who is the subject of the PHI (45 CFR 160.103).

Personal Representative

The Privacy Rule also addresses a **personal representative** (45 CFR 164.502(g)) by clarifying that persons with legal authority to act on behalf of another adult, an emancipated minor, an unemancipated minor, or a deceased individual shall be treated as a personal representative under the Privacy Rule. A personal representative must be treated the same as the individual regarding the use and disclosure of the individual's PHI. Although parents are generally the personal representatives of their minor children, with legal authority to exercise all the individual rights in the Privacy Rule (including access to the minor's record), parents, guardians, or others acting *in loco parentis* of a minor are not treated as personal representatives if the minor has consented to his or her own treatment. Personal representative rights may be denied if one is suspected of abusing or neglecting the individual, and granting rights could endanger the individual.

Designated Record Set

The Privacy Rule (45 CFR 164.524; 45 CFR 164.526) allows individuals to inspect, obtain a copy of, and amend information in their designated record set, including information that exists in paper, imaged, and electronic forms.

A **designated record set** (DRS) is a group of records maintained by or for a CE that is:

- The medical records and billing records about individuals maintained by or for a covered healthcare provider;
- The enrollment, payment, claims adjudication, and case or medical management record systems maintained by or for a health plan; or
- Used in whole or in part by or for the CE to make decisions about individuals (45 CFR 164.501)

The DRS includes records held by a CE's BA, if they meet the DRS definition. Shadow records are included in the DRS. The DRS concept is important because information outside of its definition (such as an appointment schedule) is not subject to HIPAA.

Figure 10.5 provides a comparison between the DRS and the legal health record (which was discussed in chapter 9).

Disclosure, Use, and Request

With the twin goals of giving individuals greater control over their PHI and restricting access by others, the Privacy Rule affects three types of situations in which PHI is handled: disclosure, use, and request. **Disclosure** of PHI is divulging, releasing, or disseminating information about an identifiable person by a CE or a BA to another entity or person outside the entity holding the information (45 CFR 160.103). While disclosure is often emphasized, the Privacy Rule is equally concerned with the appropriate degree of **use**, which is the sharing, employment, application, utilization, examination, or analysis of individually identifiable health information within an entity that maintains such information (45 CFR 160.103). CEs must also comply with the Privacy Rule when they request PHI. A **request** for PHI is made by a CE or its BA. Of the three, the Privacy Rule emphasizes disclosure and use.

Treatment, Payment, and Operations

Treatment, payment, and operations (45 CFR 164.501), collectively and hereafter referred to as **TPO**, are functions of a CE that are necessary for the CE to successfully conduct business. It is not the intent of the Privacy Rule to impose onerous rules that hinder CE's functions. Thus, some of the Privacy Rule's requirements are relaxed or removed where PHI is needed for TPO purposes.

Figure 10.5 Comparison of the designated record set and legal health record

Designated Record Set versus the Legal Health Record

This side-by-side comparison of the designated record set and the legal health record demonstrates the differences between the two sets of information, as well as their purposes.

	Designated Record Set	Legal Health Record
Definition	A group of records maintained by or for a covered entity that is the medical and billing records about individuals; enrollment, payment, claims adjudication, and case or medical management record systems maintained by or for a health plan; information used in whole or in part by or for the HIPAA covered entity to make decisions about individuals.	The business record generated at or for a health-care organization. It is the record that would be released upon receipt of a request. The legal health record is the officially declared record of healthcare services provided to an individual delivered by a provider.
Purpose	Used to clarify the access and amendment standards in the HIPAA Privacy Rule, which provide that individuals generally have the right to inspect and obtain a copy of protected health information in the designated record set.	The official business record of healthcare services delivered by the entity for regulatory and disclosure purposes.
Content	Defined in organizational policy and required by the HIPAA Privacy Rule. The content of the designated record set includes medical and billing records of covered providers; enrollment, payment, claims, and case information of a health plan; and information used in whole or in part by or for the covered entity to make decisions about individuals.	Defined in organizational policy and can include individually identifiable data in any medium collected and directly used in documenting healthcare services or health status. It excludes administrative, derived, and aggregate data.
Uses	Supports individual HIPAA right of access and amendment.	Provides a record of health status as well as documentation of care for reimbursement, quality management, research, and public health purposes; facilitates business decision making and education of healthcare practitioners as well as the legal needs of the healthcare organization.

Source: AHIMA 2011b.

Treatment usually means providing, coordinating, or managing healthcare or healthcare-related services by one or more healthcare providers (for example, the usual provision of care to patients admitted to the hospital or during an office appointment with a physician). Treatment in the Privacy Rule definition also covers healthcare provider consultations relating to a patient or the referral of a patient for healthcare from one provider to another.

Payment includes a broad set of activities. For example, it can refer to activities by a health plan to obtain premiums, or to activities by a healthcare provider or health plan to obtain reimbursement for care or services provided. Billing, claims management, claims collection, review of the medical necessity of care, and utilization review are all included under payment.

The Privacy Rule provides a broad list of activities that fall under the umbrella of healthcare operations: quality assessment and improvement, case management, review of healthcare professionals' qualifications, insurance contracting, legal and auditing functions, and general business management functions such as providing customer service and conducting due diligence. It is important to distinguish activities that are operations from those that are not and to include examples of operations in the Notice of Privacy Practices, discussed later in this chapter.

Organization Types

Covered entity is a term of art under the Privacy Rule and generally encompasses the neatly defined categories of healthcare providers, health plans, and healthcare clearinghouses. However, these categories are neither mutually exclusive nor all-inclusive. For example, an organization may function as a CE in one aspect of its business but not in another. Further, an organization may function as more than one type of CE. Specific examples are explored next.

A **hybrid entity** performs both covered and noncovered functions under the Privacy Rule (45 CFR 164.103). For example, a university that educates students and maintains student educational records is not covered by the Privacy Rule; however, the same university, in its operation of a medical center, is covered by the Privacy Rule as a healthcare provider.

The term **affiliated covered entity** refers to legally separate CEs affiliated by common ownership or control. For purposes of the Privacy Rule, these legally separate entities may refer to themselves as a single CE (45 CFR 164.105). Such references must be in writing.

An **organized healthcare arrangement (OHCA)** is characterized by two or more CEs who share PHI to manage and benefit their common enterprise and are recognized by the public as a single entity (45 CFR 164.103).

Finally, CEs may perform multiple covered functions (45 CFR 164.504(g)). They must operate each covered function separately and must not disclose PHI to a function not involved with the individual, remaining compliant with the Privacy Rule relative to each function they perform (Rinehart-Thompson 2013). For example, a medical facility may also be a self-insured health plan. If an employee of the medical facility is a patient but not an enrollee of the health plan, that individual's PHI may only be used by the medical facility in its capacity as a healthcare provider and may not be shared with the health plan.

Check Your Understanding │ 10.3

Instructions: Indicate whether the following statements are true or false (T or F).

1. Use is the sharing of individually identifiable health information within an entity.
2. Under the Privacy Rule, a personal representative must be treated the same as the individual regarding the use and disclosure of the individual's PHI.
3. A university with a medical center is a hybrid entity under the Privacy Rule.
4. Some of the Privacy Rule's requirements are relaxed or removed where PHI is needed for purposes of TPO.
5. By definition, a DRS excludes billing records.

Key Privacy Rule Documents

The Privacy Rule contains parameters for three key documents that inform patients and give them a measure of control over their PHI. Two of these documents, the Notice of Privacy Practices and the authorization, are required, but the consent document is optional. Each of these documents is discussed in the following sections. Additionally, table 10.1 outlines the differences among these three key documents.

	Notice of Privacy Practices	**Consent**	**Authorization**
Required?	Required by HIPAA	Optional	Required by HIPAA
Requirements re: TPO	Must explain TPO uses and disclosures, along with other types of uses and disclosures	Obtains patient permission to use or disclose PHI for TPO purposes only	Is used to obtain several types of uses and disclosures, although is not required for TPO uses and disclosures
PHI that this document addresses	Provides prospective and general information about how PHI might be used or disclosed in the future (and includes information that may not have been created yet)	Provides prospective and general information about how PHI might be used or disclosed in the future for TPO purposes (and includes information that may not have been created yet)	Obtains patient permission to use or disclose specific information that generally has already been created and for which there is a specific need
Required for treatment?	May not refuse to treat an individual because he or she declines to sign this form	May condition treatment on individual signing this form	May not refuse to treat an individual because he or she declines to sign this form
Time limit on document validity	No time limit on validity of the document	No time limit on validity of the document	Time limit on validity of document (specified by an expiration date or event)

Table 10.1 Notice of privacy practices, consent, and authorization requirements

Notice of Privacy Practices

It is important that patients have some control over—or at least knowledge of—the disclosures and uses of their health information. Ensuring that patients have knowledge about how CEs use or disclose their PHI is a key purpose of the Notice of Privacy Practices.

In general, section 164.520 of the Privacy Rule requires that, except for certain variations or exceptions for health plans and correctional facilities, an individual has the right to a notice explaining how PHI will be used and disclosed. This required document is called a **Notice of Privacy Practices (NPP)** or Notice of Health Information Practices. Further, this notice explains an individual's rights and the CE's legal duties with respect to PHI. The notice must be provided to an individual at his or her first contact with the CE (for example, first visit to a physician's office, first admission to a hospital, or first encounter at a clinic).

The requirements for the content of the NPP are listed in figure 10.6. A sample NPP is located at the end of this chapter (appendix 10.A).

Healthcare providers with a direct treatment relationship with an individual must provide the notice no later than the date of the first personal service encounter. Where services are provided by telephone, prompt mailing of the notice is required. Where services are provided electronically, automatic and simultaneous delivery of the notice is required. This requirement reminds CEs that the Privacy Rule recognizes more than just face-to-face visits as service encounters. Encounters such as telephone consultations and electronic prescribing may also necessitate a notice. Notices must be available at the site where the individual is treated and must be posted in a prominent place where the patient can reasonably be expected to read it. If a CE has a website with information about services or benefits, the notice must be prominently posted to it. In emergency situations, a CE must provide notice to the individual as soon as possible after the emergency has ended. In addition, notices must be provided to those individuals who request a copy. Finally, good faith attempts must be made to obtain a written acknowledgment from the patient stating that

Figure 10.6 Requirements for the content of the Notice of Privacy Practices

In general, the NPP must contain the following:

1. A header such as "THIS NOTICE DESCRIBES HOW INFORMATION ABOUT YOU MAY BE USED AND DISCLOSED AND HOW YOU CAN GET ACCESS TO THIS INFORMATION. PLEASE REVIEW IT CAREFULLY."

2. A description, including at least one example of the types of uses and disclosures that the CE is permitted to make for treatment, payment, and healthcare operations.

3. A description of each of the other purposes for which the CE is permitted or required to use or disclose PHI without the individual's written consent or authorization.

4. A statement that other uses and disclosures will be made only with the individual's written authorization, and a notation that the individual may revoke such authorization at any time.

5. When applicable, separate statements that the CE may contact the individual to provide appointment reminders or information about treatment alternatives and other health-related benefits and services that may be of interest to the individual.

6. A statement indicating that most uses and disclosures of psychotherapy notes (where appropriate), uses and disclosures of protected health information for marketing purposes, and disclosures that constitute a sale of protected health information require authorization.

   a. CEs that do not record or maintain psychotherapy notes are not required to include a statement in their NPPs about the authorization requirement for uses and disclosures of psychotherapy notes.

7. A statement in the NPP regarding fundraising communications and an individual's right to opt out of receiving such communications, if a CE intends to contact an individual to raise funds for the CE.

   Note: If a CE does not make fundraising communications then this statement does not need to be included on the NPP.

   a. The mechanism of the opt-out does not have to be included in the NPP because individuals will be provided the opportunity to opt out of fundraising communications with each solicitation.

8. For health plans that perform underwriting activities only, a statement must be included in the NPP indicating the health plan is prohibited from using or disclosing genetic information for underwriting purposes.

9. A statement of the individual's rights with respect to PHI and a brief description of how the individual may exercise these rights, with certain exceptions, including:

   a. The right to request restrictions on certain uses and disclosures as provided by 45 CFR 164.522(a), including a statement that the CE is not required to agree to a requested restriction

   b. For healthcare providers only, a statement indicating the right to restrict certain disclosures of PHI to a health plan when the individual pays out of pocket in full for the healthcare item or service

   c. The right to receive confidential communications of PHI

   d. The right to access, inspect, and receive a copy of PHI on paper, including the right to have electronic copies if kept in electronic form

   e. The right to request electronic copies of PHI be forwarded to a third party

   f. The right to request an amendment of PHI

   g. The right to receive an accounting of disclosures

   h. The right to be notified of the CE's privacy practices

   i. The right to control PHI use for marketing, sales, and research

   j. The right to be notified of a breach to PHI

   k. The right to file complaints with the Office for Civil Rights

10. A statement that the CE is required by law to maintain the privacy of PHI and to provide individuals with a notice of its legal duties and privacy practices with respect to PHI.

11. A statement that the CE is required to abide by the terms of the notice currently in effect.

12. A statement that the CE reserves the right to change the terms of its notice and to make the new notice provisions effective for all PHI that it maintains.

Figure 10.6 Requirements for the content of the Notice of Privacy Practices (Continued)

13. A statement describing how the CE will provide individuals with a revised notice.

14. A statement that individuals may complain to the CE and to the Secretary of Health and Human Services if an individual believes their privacy rights have been violated; a brief description of how to file a complaint with the CE; and a statement that the individual will not be retaliated against for filing a complaint.

15. The name or title and the telephone number of a person or office to contact for further information.

16. An effective date, which may not be earlier than the date on which the notice is printed or otherwise published.

A covered healthcare provider with a direct treatment relationship with an individual must:

- Provide the notice no later than the date of the first service delivery, including service delivered electronically, or in an emergency treatment situation, as soon as reasonably practicable after the emergency situation.

- Have the notice available at the service delivery site for individuals to request and take with them; this availability does not include requiring the patient to ask for the NPP. It should be prominently displayed and made available within waiting rooms and waiting areas.

- Post the notice in a clear and prominent location where it is reasonable to expect individuals seeking service from the covered healthcare provider to be able to easily locate and read the notice.

- When e-mailing the notice, provide a paper copy if the transmission fails.

- The NPP must be posted on the CE's website, if one is maintained.

- Except in emergency situations, make a good faith effort to obtain written acknowledgment of receipt and, as appropriate, document good faith efforts and reasons why the acknowledgment could not be obtained.

- If providing notices electronically, capture the individual's acknowledgment of receipt electronically in response to that transmission.

Source: McLendon and Dinh-Rose 2013.

the notice was received. Failure to obtain the acknowledgment, whether it is due to patient refusal or non-compliance or failure by the covered healthcare provider, must be documented (45 CFR 164.520(c)(2)).

Consent to Use or Disclose PHI

Under the Privacy Rule, healthcare providers are not required to obtain the patient's signed **consent** to use or disclose personally identifiable information for TPO purposes (45 CFR 164.506(b)). However, some providers may choose to obtain consent as a matter of policy. The Department of Health and Human Services makes clear that covered entities electing to obtain patient consent have "complete discretion to design a process" that works the best for them (HHS 2016). In such cases (except for the special circumstances discussed later), consent would be obtained at the time that healthcare services are provided. Because the consent for use and disclosure has no expiration date, in most cases it is indefinite unless specifically revoked by the individual. Further, consent cannot be used where an authorization would otherwise be required under the Privacy Rule (45 CFR 164.506(b)(2)).

Several situations exist in which obtaining consent may be difficult or impossible. One would be an emergency treatment situation where there are substantial barriers to communicating with the individual. Another example would be when the healthcare provider is required by law to treat the individual but is unable to obtain consent. In such circumstances, the provider should document its attempt to obtain consent and the reason it was unable to do so. In emergency treatment situations, the provider should obtain consent as soon as reasonably possible after the delivery of treatment. A sample consent form is located at the end of this chapter (appendix 10.B).

Authorization

An **authorization** is written permission for a specific disclosure. The Privacy Rule provides specific requirements for patient authorization forms, including elements an authorization for release of information (disclosure) must contain. Although these required core elements do not differ significantly from the elements historically recommended by AHIMA as professional best practice, they now have the force and effect of federal law. Under the Privacy Rule, a valid authorization must be written in plain language and contain at least the elements listed in figure 10.7. An authorization is invalid (defective) when any one of the following occurs:

- The expiration date has passed or the expiration event is known by the CE to have occurred.
- The authorization has not been filled out completely with respect to a required element or lacks a required element.
- The authorization is known by the CE to have been revoked. (Note: An individual may revoke an authorization at any time if it is done in writing, but the revocation does not apply when the CE has already acted on the authorization.)
- The authorization violates the compound authorization requirements, if applicable. (A compound authorization combines an individual's authorization for the disclosure of health information with informed consent for the performance of medical treatment.)
- Any material information in the authorization is known by the CE to be false.
- Completion of an authorization is required for an individual to be eligible for treatment, payment, or enrollment in a health plan, or to be eligible for benefits on an authorization (with certain exceptions to this rule delineated in 45 CFR 164.508(b)(4)). (45 CFR 164.508(b) 2–4)

Because of their unique nature, HIPAA specifically addresses psychotherapy notes. **Psychotherapy notes** are behavioral health notes recorded by a mental health professional who documents or analyzes contents and impressions of conversations that are part of private counseling sessions. Psychotherapy notes are not part of the health record and do not contain information such as diagnoses, prescriptions, treatment modalities, or test results (45 CFR 164.501). Authorizations are always required for the use or disclosure of psychotherapy notes except to carry out TPO or to fulfill one of the following purposes:

- Use by the originator of the psychotherapy notes for treatment
- Use or disclosure by the CE in training programs for students, trainees, or practitioners in mental health
- Use or disclosure by the CE to defend a legal action or other proceeding brought by the individual
- Use or disclosure that is required or permitted with respect to the oversight of the originator of the psychotherapy notes (45 CFR 164.508(a)(2))

Use and Disclosure When Authorization Is Not Required

The Privacy Rule is specific about uses and disclosures that require a patient's **authorization** and those that do not (45 CFR 164.502; 45 CFR 164.508; 45 CFR 164.510; 45 CFR 164.512). The following general rule provides a starting point to the Privacy Rule's intricate authorization requirements and exceptions:

General rule: Patient authorization is required for the use or disclosure of PHI unless it meets an exception where authorization is not required.

Figure 10.7 Privacy Rule requirements for a valid authorization

Description of Information

This description must identify the information to be used or disclosed in a specific and meaningful fashion. For example, the request should specify what is wanted, such as "the discharge summary and the operative report," rather than asking for "any and all information." Providing the time frame for the information that is to be released (for example, hospitalization from 6/1/16 to 6/5/16) also provides a more specific description of the desired information.

Name of Person or Entity Authorized to Use or Disclose

The authorization must include the name or other specific identification of the person(s) or class of persons authorized to use or disclose the information. For example, the name of a hospital that is disclosing a patient's health information must be included.

Recipient of Information

The Privacy Rule requires that the authorization include the specific person(s) or class of persons (by name or other specific identification) to whom the covered entity may make the disclosure, such as an insurance company. This information should be verified by checking the patient demographic information that is collected on admission. If the insurance company information does not match, the patient should be contacted for clarification.

Purpose of Disclosure

Although the Privacy Rule requires that this element be present on authorizations, the patient is not required to provide a statement of purpose, and "at the request of the individual" is sufficient per the Privacy Rule.

Expiration

The Privacy Rule requires that an expiration date or expiration event (for example, "at the end of the research study" or "none") that relates to the individual or the purpose of the use or disclosure be included on the authorization.

Signature and Date

The patient must sign and date the authorization. It is essential that the signature be compared with one already existing in the medical record for validation purposes. A patient's personal representative may sign the authorization in lieu of the patient provided that a statement is included that describes that person's authority to act for the patient.

Although it is best practice for an authorization to be completed and dated after the date of the service (so that information is not created after the authorization was signed), the Privacy Rule does not prohibit predated authorizations as long as the authorization encompasses the category of information that is later created and the authorization has not expired or been revoked. In summation, "the covered entity may use or disclose PHI that has been identified in the authorization regardless of when the information was created" (HHS 2007).

Statement of Right to Revoke

An authorization must contain a statement of the individual's right to revoke the authorization in writing and the exceptions to the right to revoke, together with a description of how the individual may revoke it.

Statement of Redisclosure

An authorization must include a statement that information used or disclosed pursuant to the authorization may be subject to redisclosure by the recipient and, subsequently, would no longer be protected by the Privacy Rule.

Statement of Eligibility

A statement in the authorization must specify that treatment, payment, enrollment, or eligibility for benefits cannot be denied because an individual declines to sign the authorization.

Copy Provided

A copy of the signed authorization is provided to the individual when authorization for use or disclosure is sought by the covered entity.

Source: Adapted from 45 CFR 164.508(c)(1–4).

Stated another way, unless the Privacy Rule specifically mentions circumstances that do not require an authorization for use or disclosure (outlined later in this chapter and listed in figure 10.8), all other uses and disclosures require an individual's authorization. Because PHI may be requested for medical, legal, personal, and myriad other purposes, CEs must be familiar with the Privacy Rule so that each type of disclosure and use can be assessed to determine whether an authorization is required, how much information can be used or disclosed (discussed in the section entitled Minimum Necessary Requirement, later in this chapter), and how to handle each type of situation appropriately. CEs must consider not only the authorization requirements of the HIPAA Privacy Rule but also the authorization requirements that govern use and disclosure in the CE's particular state (see chapter 15).

When Use or Disclosure is *Required*, Even Without Authorization

One of the Privacy Rule's goals is to provide greater privacy protections for one's health information by limiting access by others. This includes both use and disclosure. As figure 10.8 shows, PHI may not be used or disclosed by a CE without patient authorization unless the Privacy Rule *requires or permits* such use or disclosure. The Privacy Rule *requires* use or disclosure, even without authorization, in only two situations:

- When the individual or the individual's personal representative requests access to PHI or an accounting of disclosures of the PHI
- When the HHS conducts an investigation, review, or enforcement action

Figure 10.8 lists these two situations where use and disclosure are required.

When Use or Disclosure is *Permitted* Without Authorization

In addition to the two situations where use or disclosure is required, even without the individual's authorization (see also figure 10.8), there are many situations where the Privacy Rule *permits* a CE to use or disclose PHI without an individual's authorization (Rinehart-Thompson 2013). These situations are also listed in figure 10.8. This significant number of exceptions to the patient authorization requirement leads critics to argue that the Privacy Rule diminishes the privacy of patient information rather than improving it. However, the Privacy Rule is only *permissive* in this respect. Its exceptions may be subject to stricter state laws or organizational policies that provide greater privacy protections. In other words, CEs may be required by state law or may choose to obtain patient authorization, even if the Privacy Rule permits use or disclosure without it.

The following two examples illustrate this point, where the HIPAA Privacy Rule relaxes the authorization requirement, but CEs may adhere to more stringent practices.

Example 1: A hospital (CE), under the Privacy Rule, is not required to obtain a patient's authorization before sending records from the patient's hospital stay to a physician who is following up with that patient (treatment purposes). While many hospitals, in accordance with prior policy, will continue to require an authorization in a situation such as this, the Privacy Rule has removed that requirement. Note: The minimum necessary requirement (discussed later in this chapter) does not apply when PHI is disclosed for treatment purposes, although CEs should exercise caution.

Example 2: A healthcare provider (CE), under the Privacy Rule, is not required to obtain a patient's authorization before sending records from a patient encounter to the patient's health insurance company for payment purposes. Again, many providers will continue to require

Figure 10.8 Authorization requirements for use and disclosure of PHI

I. Patient Authorization Required:

All situations except those listed in Part II

II. Patient Authorization Not Required:

A. When use or disclosure is required, even without patient authorization

- When the individual or the individual's personal representative requests access or accounting of disclosures (with exceptions)
- Dept. of HHS investigation, review, or enforcement action

B. When use or disclosure is permitted, even without patient authorization

- Patient has opportunity to informally agree or object
  - Facility directory
  - Notification of relatives and friends
- Patient does not have opportunity to agree or object
  - Public interest and benefit (12 types)
    1. As required by law
    2. For public health activities
    3. To disclose PHI regarding victims of abuse, neglect, or domestic violence
    4. For health oversight activities
    5. For judicial and administrative proceedings
    6. For law enforcement purposes (six specific situations)
    7. Regarding decedents
    8. For cadaveric organ, eye, or tissue donation
    9. For research, with limitations
    10. To prevent or lessen serious threat to health or safety
    11. For essential government functions
    12. For workers' compensation
  - TPO
  - To the individual/patient
  - Incidental uses and disclosures
  - Limited data set

an authorization in accordance with their prior policies; however, it is not required per the Privacy Rule. The minimum necessary requirement does apply to disclosures made for payment purposes.

Uses and Disclosures that Require an Opportunity to Agree or Object

Section 45 CFR 164.510 of the Privacy Rule lists two circumstances in which PHI can be used without the individual's written authorization, but the individual must be informed in advance and given an opportunity to agree, prohibit (object to), or restrict the use or disclosure. These are also illustrated in figure 10.8. The CE may inform the individual in a verbal communication and obtain his or her verbal agreement or objection rather than obtaining a written authorization.

First, a healthcare facility may maintain a **facility directory** of patients being treated. Once the individual has verbally agreed, the Privacy Rule makes provisions for the facility to maintain in its directory the following information about an individual: name, location in the facility, condition described in general terms, and religious affiliation. This information may be disclosed to persons who ask for the individual by name, with the exception of an individual's religious affiliation, which can be disclosed only to clergy members of the individual's religion. The CE must inform the patient of the information to be included in the directory and the people to whom the information may be disclosed. The individual must be given the opportunity to restrict or prohibit some or all of the uses or disclosures.

In an emergency situation, if it is impractical or impossible to inform the patient and obtain agreement, the facility can use and disclose PHI, but it must be consistent with the prior expressed preference of the patient, or the facility must determine that it is in the patient's best interest to do so. When it becomes possible after the emergency, the healthcare facility must inform patients and give them the opportunity to object to such use and disclosure.

Second, the Privacy Rule allows a CE, exercising its professional judgment, to disclose PHI to a family member or a close friend if it is directly relevant to his or her involvement with the individual's care or payment, if the individual is not present. This includes allowing a person acting on behalf of the individual to pick up prescriptions and medical supplies. Likewise, a CE may disclose PHI, including the individual's location, general condition, or death, to notify or assist in the notification of a family member, personal representative, or some other person responsible for the patient's care (45 CFR 164.510(b)).

However, if the individual is present and otherwise able to make healthcare decisions, the CE may only use or disclose the PHI in the previous situations if it has done one of the following:

- Obtained the individual's agreement
- Provided the individual with the opportunity to object to the disclosure and the patient has not objected
- Reasonably inferred from the circumstances that the individual does not object to the disclosure (45 CFR 164.510(b)(2))

As provided for by guidance issued by the Office for Civil Rights in 2014, parameters for sharing information with family members also apply to mental health information, which is treated the same by HIPAA as other types of information (HHS 2014).

The CE may also use or disclose PHI to a public or private entity authorized by law or by its charter to assist in disaster relief efforts.

Uses and Disclosures for Which Authorization or Opportunity to Agree or Object Is Not Required

There are 16 circumstances (see figure 10.8) in which PHI can be used or disclosed without the individual's written authorization and for which the individual does not have the opportunity to agree or object. Section 45 CFR 164.512 of the Privacy Rule, titled "Uses and disclosures for which an authorization or opportunity to agree or object is not required," lists the first 12 circumstances (public interest and benefit activities), which have been identified as activities that serve national priority purposes (see figure 10.8). There are four remaining uses and disclosures for which authorization and the opportunity to agree or object are not required (denoted by the four line items at the bottom of figure 10.8); however, they are not listed in section 164.512 of the Privacy Rule. They are TPO, disclosure to the subject individual, incidental disclosures, and limited data sets (discussed later).

The Privacy Rule *permits* uses and disclosures without an individual's authorization in the 12 public interest and benefit circumstances; however, if such a use or authorization would violate a state law that otherwise protects the information more than the Privacy Rule (that is, the state law is "more stringent"), then the information cannot be legally used or disclosed.

Oftentimes, a disclosure may meet more than one of the following 12 public interest and benefit situations, as outlined in the Privacy Rule (45 CFR 164.512):

1. **As required by law:** Disclosures are permitted when required by laws that meet the public interest requirements of disclosures relating to victims of abuse, neglect, or domestic violence; judicial and administrative proceedings; and law enforcement purposes. These three areas are detailed more fully later.

2. **Public health activities:** Use or disclosure of PHI for public health activities serves such purposes as preventing or controlling diseases, injuries, and disabilities; reporting disease, injury (such as child abuse), and vital events such as births and deaths; and public health surveillance, investigation, or interventions.

   Examples include the reporting of adverse events or product defects to comply with Food and Drug Administration regulations and, when authorized by law, reporting a person who may have been exposed to a communicable disease and might be at risk for contracting or spreading it. Per HITECH, disclosure of student immunization records also constitutes a public health activity.

3. **Victims of abuse, neglect, or domestic violence:** An example is the reporting of a situation to authorities, such as Adult Protective Services, who are authorized by law to receive information about abuse or neglect. (Note: Child abuse reporting is contained within public health activities above.)

   Although disclosures for the purpose of reporting abuse, neglect, or domestic violence do not require an authorization, the Privacy Rule does require the CE to promptly inform the individual that such a report has been or will be made, unless it believes that doing so would place the individual at risk of serious harm if the CE would be informing the personal representative, whom it reasonably believes is responsible for the abuse, neglect, or other injury.

4. **Healthcare oversight activities:** An authorized health oversight agency may receive PHI under the Privacy Rule for activities authorized by law, such as audits, civil or criminal investigations, licensure, and other inspections.

5. **Judicial and administrative proceedings:** Disclosures for judicial and administrative proceedings are permitted in response to an order of a court or an administrative tribunal, provided that the CE discloses only the PHI expressly authorized by such an order or in response to a subpoena, discovery request, or other lawful process. With regard to subpoenas and discovery requests, the party seeking the PHI must assure the CE that it has made reasonable efforts to make the request known to the individual who is the subject of the PHI. In this situation, the entity must also be assured that the time for the individual to raise objections to the court or administrative tribunal has elapsed and that no objections were filed, all objections have been resolved, or a qualified protective order has been secured.

6. **Law enforcement purposes:** Are disclosures of PHI to law enforcement officers allowable? The Privacy Rule specifies six instances in which disclosures to law enforcement do not require patient authorization or the opportunity to agree or object:

   a. Pursuant to legal process or otherwise required by law. Examples of legal process include a court order, court-ordered warrant, subpoena, or summons issued by a judicial officer. Relative to the "as required by law" situation, for example, a law may exist that requires the reporting of certain types of wounds or other physical injuries to law enforcement.

   b. In response to a law enforcement official's request for the purpose of identifying or locating a suspect, fugitive, material witness, or missing person. In such cases, only the following information may be disclosed:

      - Name and address
      - Date and place of birth
      - Social Security number
      - ABO blood type and Rh factor
      - Type of injury
      - Date and time of treatment
      - Date and time of death, if applicable
      - Description of distinguishing physical characteristics, including height, weight, gender, race, hair and eye color, and presence or absence of facial scars or tattoos

   c. In response to a law enforcement official's request about an individual who is or is suspected to be a victim of a crime (when the individual agrees to the disclosure or when the CE is unable to obtain the individual's agreement because of incapacity or other emergency circumstance). The law enforcement official must represent that such information is needed to determine whether a violation of law has occurred, that immediate law enforcement activity depends on the disclosure, and that disclosure is in the best interest of the individual as determined by the CE.

   d. About a deceased individual when the CE suspects that the death may have resulted from criminal conduct.

   e. To a law enforcement official when the CE believes in good faith that the information constitutes evidence of criminal conduct that occurred on the CE's premises.

   f. To a law enforcement official in response to a medical emergency when the CE believes that disclosure is necessary to alert law enforcement to the commission and nature of a crime; the location or victims of such a crime; and the identity, description, and location of the perpetrator of such a crime. Further, it is permitted when the CE believes the medical emergency was the result of abuse, neglect, or domestic violence.

      (Again, the Privacy Rule is permissive in this respect, and state law can prohibit or restrict such use or disclosure.)

7. **Decedents:** HIPAA's privacy protections survive an individual's death for 50 years; nonetheless, disclosures to a coroner or medical examiner are permitted in order to identify a deceased person, determine a cause of death, or accomplish other purposes as required by law.

In accordance with applicable law, disclosures to funeral directors are permitted as necessary to allow them to carry out their duties with respect to the decedent. This type of information may also be disclosed in reasonable anticipation of an individual's death.

8. **Cadaveric organ, eye, or tissue donation:** PHI may be disclosed to organ procurement agencies or other entities to facilitate the procurement, banking, or transplantation of cadaveric organs, eyes, or tissue.

9. **Research:** The Privacy Rule permits a CE to use or disclose PHI for research if an approved authorization waiver or alteration or other exceptions are met. Research is described more fully later in chapter 11.

10. **Threat to health and safety:** Disclosures are allowed in circumstances where the CE believes the use or disclosure of information is necessary to prevent or lessen a serious and imminent threat to the health or safety of an individual or the public. In such cases, disclosure must be made to a person who can reasonably prevent or lessen the threat. Disclosures are also permissible when it is necessary for law enforcement officials to apprehend an individual who may have caused harm to the victim or when it appears that the individual has escaped from a correctional institution or lawful custody.

11. **Essential (specialized) government functions:** There are a number of instances with regard to specialized government functions where uses and disclosures are permitted without authorization or the opportunity to agree or object. Primarily, these include circumstances involving release of information regarding armed forces personnel for military and veterans activities, for purposes of national security and intelligence activities, for protective services for the president of the United States and others, and for public benefits and medical suitability determinations.

Disclosure of an inmate's PHI to correctional institutions or to a law enforcement official who has lawful custody is permitted by the Privacy Rule, provided that the correctional institution states that the information is necessary to provide continuing healthcare; to secure the health and safety of the individual or other inmates, officers, employees, transportation personnel, or law enforcement on the premises; or to ensure the administration and maintenance of the institution's safety, security, and good order.

12. **Workers' compensation:** The Privacy Rule permits the disclosure of PHI relating to work-related illness or injury, or workplace-related medical surveillance to the extent such disclosure complies with workers' compensation laws.

In addition to the 12 public interest and benefit situations, specifically categorized in the Privacy Rule as "uses and disclosures for which authorization or opportunity to agree or object is not required," the following four types of uses and disclosures also do not require patient authorization or an opportunity for the patient to agree or object (see the four line items at the bottom of figure 10.8); however, they have not been categorized as such in the Privacy Rule. They are

1. TPO

2. Disclosure to the subject individual/patient

3. Incidental uses and disclosures

4. Limited data set

The first two have been discussed at length in this chapter; the latter two will be examined here.

Incidental uses and disclosures occur as part of a permitted use or disclosure (45 CFR 164.502(a)(1)(iii)) and are a component of doing business. For example, calling out patients' names in a physician's office is an incidental disclosure because it occurs as part of the office operations. As long as the information disclosed is the minimum necessary (for example, the patient's name with no diagnostic information), this is permissible under the Privacy Rule without the patient's authorization or opportunity to agree or object.

A **limited data set** is PHI that excludes most direct identifiers of the individual and the individual's relatives, employers, and household members (45 CFR 164.514(e)(2)) but does not deidentify the information. Such PHI may be used or disclosed without the patient's authorization or the opportunity to agree or object, provided it is used or disclosed only for research, public health, or healthcare operations.

Redisclosure

Patient information is often created by a healthcare provider and assimilated into another healthcare provider's records. Examples include copies of reports sent by a physician to a hospital upon patient admission or a patient's hospital records sent to a nursing facility for the patient's follow-up care. **Redisclosure** is disclosure by a healthcare organization of information that was created by and received from another entity. Providers need to balance requests for patient information, which are necessary for continuity of care, with the appropriateness of redisclosing this information. Federal laws specifically protect substance abuse records from routine redisclosure and strictly limit other disclosures without patient authorization, but what about information that is not highly sensitive in nature?

The HHS Office for Civil Rights (OCR) provides guidance stating that it is permissible for "a provider who is a CE to disclose a complete medical record, including portions that were created by another provider, assuming that the disclosure is for a purpose permitted by the Privacy Rule, such as treatment" (HHS 2007). State laws that address the issue of redisclosure must also be read with the Privacy Rule, as discussed in the preemption section in the next chapter. In the interest of patient care, health records from other facilities should be made part of the DRS at the current facility if that information is needed for diagnosis or treatment, and if state law does not otherwise prohibit it. If conflicts of law do occur, legal counsel should be consulted. Further, facility policies and procedures must be developed regarding redisclosure, including mechanisms to identify situations where redisclosure is and is not appropriate. Appropriate redisclosures include those that

- Facilitate patient care
- Are disclosed only after a patient has been encouraged to first attempt to obtain records from the originating facility
- Are disclosed to comply with legal process
- Include only information contained within the DRS

Further, when testifying as to the authenticity of redisclosed health information, it is necessary to state that the information was received from another organization via usual business practices, that the information was received in good faith, and that testimony regarding the record keeping practices at the organization that created the records is not possible (AHIMA 2013b).

Check Your Understanding 10.4

Instructions: Indicate whether the following statements are true or false (T or F).

1. One of the 12 public interest and benefit exceptions to the authorization requirements is disclosure to organ procurement agencies.

2. The HIPAA consent explains an individual's rights and the CE's legal duties with respect to PHI.

3. Per the HIPAA Privacy Rule, patient authorization is required for the use or disclosure of PHI unless it meets an exception whereby authorization is not required.

4. Incidental disclosures require an individual's written authorization.

5. Although an individual must verbally agree to be included in a facility directory, written authorization is not required.

Commercial Uses and Disclosures of PHI

Protected health information is a valuable resource for commercial, or money-making, purposes. Because of the potential for unethical and even criminal uses and disclosures for financial gain, the Privacy Rule has established requirements and prohibitions around marketing, fundraising, and the sale of PHI.

Marketing

The Privacy Rule defines **marketing** as communication about a product or service that encourages the recipient to purchase or use that product or service (45 CFR 164.501). Generally, the Privacy Rule requires that an individual's authorization be obtained prior to using his or her PHI for marketing. However, marketing has posed some difficulty since the Privacy Rule's inception, because CEs at times have classified a marketing activity as a healthcare operation, thus eliminating the need (in the CE's mind) to obtain an individual's authorization. HITECH clarifies that communications are considered to be marketing *unless* they

- Describe a health-related product or service (or payment for the product or service) provided by or included in the benefit plan of the CE making the communication, including communications about participants in the health provider's or health plan's network
- Describe replacements or enhancements to a health plan
- Describe available health-related products or services that are of value, although not part of a benefit plan
- Are for treatment of the individual
- Are for case management or care coordination for the individual, or to direct or recommend alternative treatments, therapies, healthcare providers, or settings of care (45 CFR 164.501)

Therefore, although the communications just listed look like marketing, by definition they have been exempted. Rather, they are considered to be healthcare treatment or operations, and no authorization is required.

Common communications that meet the definition of marketing, on the other hand, but also do not require authorization are those that

- Occur face-to-face between the CE and the individual
- Concern a promotional gift of nominal value provided by the CE (45 CFR 164.508(a)(3))

A CE must obtain patient authorization to send communications about *non–health-related* products or services, or to give or sell the individual's PHI to third parties for CE marketing. However, concerns exist regarding the ability of CEs to sell individuals' PHI so that third parties can market their own *health-related* products or services. Under HITECH, the ability of CEs to categorize health-related communications as healthcare operations (which exempts them from marketing requirements) is limited. If a CE is to make a communication in exchange for financial remuneration, prior authorization (clearly stating that the CE is being paid for the communication) is required before the CE (or BA) makes the communication. Exceptions include communications describing currently prescribed drugs and, per HITECH, refill reminders as long as the amount of remuneration received by the CE is reasonable.

Per HITECH, subsidized communications require individual authorization, even if they look like healthcare operations. A CE's NPP must specify the CE's intent to send subsidized communications and the individual's ability to opt out. The communication itself must disclose the remuneration and reiterate the ability to opt out (HHS 2010, 40884–40887).

Fundraising

For **fundraising** activities that benefit the CE, 45 CFR 164.514(f) permits the CE to use or disclose to a BA or an institutionally related foundation, without authorization, demographic information and dates of healthcare provided to an individual. The CE must inform individuals in its NPP that PHI may be used for this purpose. The CE must include instructions either before the first solicitation or as part of the fundraising materials about how to opt out of receiving materials in the future. Reasonable efforts must be made to ensure the individual's wishes are honored. If a fundraising activity targets individuals based on diagnosis (for example, patients with kidney disease are targeted to raise funds for a new kidney dialysis center), prior authorization is required. Per HITECH, fundraising communications that use or disclose PHI are healthcare operations and must clearly and conspicuously provide the recipient the opportunity to opt-out of the communications. This opt-out is considered a revocation of authorization (AHIMA 2009). Under HITECH, an opt-out may be applied to the current campaign only or to all future fundraising campaigns (HHS 2010, 40896–40897).

Sale of PHI

HITECH prohibits both CEs and BAs from selling PHI without patient authorization. In the authorization, the patient must declare whether the recipient of the PHI can exchange it further for payment. Exceptions to this prohibition include public health and research data; treatment and healthcare operations (including, for example, the sale or merger of a CE); a BA pursuant to a BAA; an individual who is receiving a copy of his or her own PHI; and for other exchanges deemed by the Secretary of HHS to be permissible (AHIMA 2009). Under HITECH, disclosures are permitted in exchange for reasonable remuneration, without patient authorization, for other reasons including payment, accounting of disclosures, and as required by law (HHS 2010, 40890–40891).

Minimum Necessary Requirement

The Privacy Rule introduced the standard of **minimum necessary**, a "need to know" filter that is applied to limit access to a patient's PHI (45 CFR 164.502(b)(1)) and to limit the amount of PHI used, disclosed, and requested. Essentially, this means that healthcare providers and other CEs must limit uses, disclosures, and requests to only the amount needed to accomplish the intended purpose, with individuals having access only to information to which they are entitled and that they need to conduct business. For example, for payment purposes, only the minimum amount of information that is necessary to substantiate a claim for payment should be disclosed. HIM professionals have always followed policies and procedures to release the minimum amount of information requested for the specific purpose, but the Privacy Rule reinforces this traditional practice.

With respect to individuals working for a CE, the minimum necessary standard must be carefully applied to the use of information by the workforce. For example, policies and procedures should identify persons or classes of persons working for the CE who need to access PHI to perform their duties. In addition, categories of PHI that each person or class of persons can access and use should be identified. For example, employees working in the dietary department would not have the same level of access to PHI as a nurse working in critical care.

There are certain circumstances where the minimum necessary requirement does not apply, such as

- To healthcare providers for treatment
- To the individual or the individual's personal representative
- Pursuant to the individual's authorization
- To the Secretary of HHS for investigations, compliance review, or enforcement
- As required by law
- To meet other Privacy Rule compliance requirements (45 CFR 164.502(b)(2))

TPO as a whole is not exempted; rather, only treatment is exempted from the minimum necessary requirement. Use and disclosure of PHI for payment and operations purposes must still adhere to the requirement.

Because "minimum necessary" has been somewhat unclear depending on who is making the determination, HITECH has sought to provide clarification via guidance from the Secretary of HHS. Clarification is still pending. Until a final determination is made, CEs are to use the limited data set (that is, PHI with certain specified direct identifiers removed) as a guideline for using or disclosing only the minimum necessary information, while reverting to the "amount needed to accomplish the intended purpose" definition when the limited data set definition is inadequate (AHIMA 2009). As per the January 2013 final rule, the minimum necessary standard now also applies to BAs.

Check Your Understanding 10.5

Instructions: Indicate whether the following statements are true or false (T or F).

1. All communications that meet the definition of marketing require an authorization.
2. Fundraising may not target an individual based on diagnosis without prior authorization.
3. Sale of PHI as part of a merger is exempt from the authorization requirement.
4. The minimum necessary requirement does not pertain to disclosures for payment purposes.
5. The minimum necessary amount of information needed by individuals to do their jobs can vary across the workforce.

Scenario 10

Staff at Community Hospital, a 200-bed facility, has been busy with HIPAA Privacy Rule issues recently. Community Hospital is regularly surveyed by the city safety department for compliance with local codes related to issues such as fire and water safety. Community Hospital's privacy officer has issued an unsigned business associate agreement to the department of health, instructing the chief of its survey office to sign it because its surveyors, who may come into contact with Community Hospital's PHI, function as business associates.

Recently, the hospital's emergency room staff has informed the privacy officer that patients' family members have been bringing cameras into the emergency room to photograph treatment as it is occurring. The privacy officer instructs emergency room staff to log the names of individuals who are taking the pictures. He then sends letters to the family members, notifying them that they have committed a HIPAA violation and their names may be turned over to the Office for Civil Rights for investigation.

Elderly patients are frequently discharged from the hospital to local nursing homes for skilled rehabilitation following orthopedic issues such as hip fractures and many types of surgeries. Staff on the units from which patients have been discharged have routinely copied the entire patient chart to accompany the patient to the nursing home, but the privacy officer informed them that this is a violation of the HIPAA Privacy Rule.

1. Identify the HIPAA Privacy Rule concept that is at issue in each paragraph of this scenario.

2. Has Community Hospital's privacy officer correctly interpreted the Privacy Rule requirements in each situation?

3. For each, analyze and explain why or why not.

References

AHIMA. 2009. Analysis of health care confidentiality, privacy, and security provisions of the American Recovery and Reinvestment Act of 2009, Public Law 111-5. Chicago: AHIMA.

AHIMA. 2011a. *Code of Ethics.* http://www.ahima.org.

AHIMA. 2011b. Fundamentals of the legal health record and designated record set. *Journal of AHIMA* 82, no. 2 (February 2011): expanded online version. http://www.ahima.org.

AHIMA. 2013a. Analysis of Modifications to the HIPAA Privacy, Security, Enforcement, and Breach Notification Rules Under the Health Information Technology for Economic and Clinical Health Act and the Genetic Information Nondiscrimination Act; Other Modifications to the HIPAA Rules. http://www.ahima.org.

AHIMA. 2013b. Practice Brief. Redisclosure of patient health information (Updated). http://www.ahima.org.

Department of Health and Human Services. 2000. Standards for privacy of individually identifiable health information. 45 CFR Parts 160 and 164. *Federal Register* 65(250):82461–82510.

Department of Health and Human Services. 2002. Standards for privacy of individually identifiable health information; Final rule. 45 CFR Parts 160 and 164. *Federal Register* 67(157):53181–53273.

Department of Health and Human Services. 2007. Office for Civil Rights. HIPAA medical privacy: National standards to protect the privacy of personal health information. http://www.hhs.gov/ocr/hipaa/.

Department of Health and Human Services. 2009. HIPAA administrative simplification enforcement. 45 CFR Part 160. *Federal Register* 74(209):56123–56131.

Department of Health and Human Services. 2010. Modifications to the HIPAA Privacy, Security, and Enforcement Rules under the Health Information Technology for Economic and Clinical Health Act; Proposed Rule. 45 CFR Parts 160 and 164. *Federal Register* 75(134):40868–40924.

Department of Health and Human Services. 2014. HIPAA Privacy Rule and sharing information related to mental health. http://www.hhs.gov/ocr/.

Department of Health and Human Services. 2016. What is the difference between "consent" and "authorization" under the HIPAA Privacy Rule? www.hhs.gov/hipaa/.

McLendon, K. and A.D. Rose. Notice of Privacy Practices (2013 update). AHIMA Practice Brief, October 2013.

Rinehart-Thompson, L. 2013. *Introduction to Health Information Privacy and Security.* Chicago: AHIMA.

Walsh, T. 2011. AHIMA Practice Brief: Security risk analysis and management: An overview (updated). *Journal of AHIMA.* http://library.ahima.org/doc?oid=103659

Statutes and Regulations Cited

45 CFR 160.103: General administrative requirements: General Provisions: Definitions. 2006.

45 CFR 164.103: Security and privacy: General provisions: Definitions. 2006.

45 CFR 164.105: Security and privacy: General provisions: Organizational requirements. 2006.

45 CFR 164.501: Privacy of individually identifiable health information: Definitions 2006.

45 CFR 164.502: Uses and disclosures of protected health information (general rules) 2006.

45 CFR 164.504: Uses and disclosures: Organizational requirements. 2006.

45 CFR 164.506: Uses and disclosures to carry out treatment, payment, and healthcare operations 2006.

45 CFR 164.508: Uses and disclosures for which authorization is required. 2006.

45 CFR 164.510: Uses and disclosures requiring an opportunity for the individual to agree or to object. 2006.

45 CFR 164.512: Uses and disclosures for which an authorization or opportunity to agree or object is not required. 2006.

45 CFR 164.514: Other requirements relating to uses and disclosures of protected health information. 2006.

45 CFR 164.520: Notice of privacy practices for protected health information. 2006.

45 CFR 164.522: Rights to request privacy protection for protected health information. 2006.

45 CFR 164.524: Access of individuals to protected health information. 2006.

45 CFR 164.526: Amendment of protected health information. 2006.

45 CFR 164.528: Accounting of disclosures of protected health information. 2006.

45 CFR 165.512(e): HIPAA. 1996.

5 USC 552: Freedom of Information Act of 1967.

5 USC 552a (App. 3 sec. (6)(a)(4)): The Privacy Act of 1974.

20 USC 1232(g): Federal educational records privacy act (FERPA). 1974.

26 USC: Internal Revenue Code. 1986.

29 USC 1001 et seq.: Employee Retirement Income Security Act of 1986 (ERISA).

42 USC 6A: Public Health Service Act. 1944.

42 USC 4541–4594; 42 CFR 2.1–2.67: Drug Abuse Prevention, Treatment, and Rehabilitation Act of 1972 (orig. 21 USC 1101–1800).

42 USC 4582 to 290dd-3: Comprehensive Alcohol Abuse and Alcoholism Prevention, Treatment, and Rehabilitation Act of 1970.

American Recovery and Reinvestment Act of 2009, Title XIII—Health Information Technology, Subtitle D Sections 13400, 13402.

Cases, Statutes, and Regulations Resources

Health Insurance Portability and Accountability Act of 1996. Public Law 104-191. Available online from http://www.gpo.gov/.

Appendix 10.A

Sample Notice of Privacy Practices

This Notice Describes How Information About You May Be Used And Disclosed And How You Can Get Access To This Information. Please Review It Carefully.

Our Pledge Regarding Medical Information

We understand that medical information about you and your health is personal. We are committed to protecting medical information about you. We create a record of the care and services you receive at the Provider. We need this record to provide you with quality care and to comply with certain legal requirements. This Notice applies to all the records of your care and records related to payment for that care, generated or maintained by the Provider, whether made by Provider personnel or your personal doctor.

This Notice will tell you about the ways in which we may use and disclose medical information about you. We also will describe your rights and certain obligations we have regarding the use and disclosure of medical information.

We are required by law to:

- Make sure that medical information that identifies you is kept private
- Give you this Notice of our legal duties and privacy practices with respect to medical information about you

How We May Use and Disclose Medical Information about You

The following categories describe different ways that we use and disclose medical information. For each category of uses or disclosures we will explain what we mean and try to give some examples. Not every use or disclosure in a category will be listed. However, all of the ways we are permitted to use and disclose information will fall within one of the categories.

- Treatment. We may use medical information about you to provide you with medical treatment or services. We may disclose medical information about you to doctors, nurses, technicians, healthcare students, or other Provider personnel who are involved in taking care of you at the Provider. For example, a doctor treating you for a broken leg may need to know if you have diabetes because diabetes may slow the healing process. In addition, the doctor may need to tell the dietitian if you have diabetes so that we can arrange for appropriate meals. Different departments of the Provider also may share medical information about you in order to coordinate the different services you need, such as prescriptions, lab work, x-rays and clergy. We also may disclose medical information about you to people outside the Provider involved in your medical care upon discharge from Provider, such as family members or other healthcare professionals.

- Payment. We might use and disclose medical information about you so that the treatment and services you receive at the Provider can be billed properly, whether payment is collected from you, an insurance company, or a third party. For example, we might need to give your health plan information about a surgery you underwent at Provider so your health plan will reimburse you or us for the cost of the procedure. We also may tell your health plan about a treatment you are going to receive to obtain prior approval or to determine whether your plan will cover the treatment.

- Healthcare Operations. We may use and disclose medical information about you for Provider operations, and they are necessary to make sure that all of our patients receive quality care. For example, we may use medical information to review our treatments and services and to evaluate the performance of our staff in caring for you. We also might combine medical information about many of the Provider's patients to decide what additional services the Provider should offer, what services are not needed, and whether certain new treatments are effective. We also might disclose information to doctors, nurses, technicians, healthcare students, and other Provider personnel for review and learning purposes. We also may combine the medical information we have with medical information from other providers to compare how we are doing and see where we can make improvements in our care and service. We might remove information that identifies you from this set of medical information so others can use it to study healthcare and healthcare delivery without learning a patient's identity.

- Appointment Reminders. We may use and disclose medical information to contact you as a reminder that you have an appointment for treatment or medical care at the Provider.

- **Treatment Alternatives.** We may use and disclose medical information to tell you about or recommend possible treatment options or alternatives that may be of interest to you.

- **Health & Related Benefits and Services.** We may use and disclose medical information to tell you about health and related benefits or services that could be of interest to you.

- **Fundraising Activities.** If we intend to use your medical information for fund-raising purposes, we will inform you of such intent and let you know that you have the right to opt out of receiving fundraising communications. We might use such information to contact you in an effort to raise money for the Provider and its operations. We may disclose information to a foundation related to the Provider so that the foundation may contact you about raising money for the Provider. We would only release contact information, such as your name, address, phone number and the dates you received treatment or services at the Provider. If you do not want the Provider to contact you for fundraising efforts, you must notify us in writing and you will be given the opportunity to opt-out of these communications.

- **Authorizations Required.** We will not use your PHI for any purposes not specifically allowed by federal or state laws or regulations without your written authorization. Specifically, the following types of uses and disclosures of your medical information require an authorization: 1) disclosure of psychotherapy notes; 2) disclosures for marketing purposes; and 3) disclosures that constitute a sale of PHI. Other uses and disclosures not described in the NPP will not be made unless an individual provides an authorization and that authorization may be revoked prospectively at any time by written revocation.

- **Emergencies.** We may use or disclose your medical information if you need emergency treatment or if we are required by law to treat you but are unable to obtain your consent.

- **Communication Barriers.** We may use and disclose your health information if we are unable to obtain your consent because of substantial communication barriers and we believe you would want us to treat you if we could communicate with you.

- **Provider Directory.** We may include certain limited information about you in Provider's directory while you are a patient here. This information may include your name, location, general condition (e.g., fair, stable, etc.) and religious affiliation. The directory information, except for your religious affiliation, also may be released to people who ask for you by name. Your religious affiliation may be given to a member of the clergy, such as a priest or rabbi, even if they do not ask for you by name. This is so your family, friends and clergy can visit and generally know how you are doing.

- **Individuals Involved in Your Care or Payment for Your Care.** We may release medical information about you to a friend or family member who is involved in your medical care and we also may give information to someone who helps pay for your care, unless you object and ask us not to provide this information to specific individuals, in writing. In addition, we may disclose medical information about you to an entity assisting in a disaster relief effort so that your family can be notified about your condition, status, and location.

- **Research.** Under certain circumstances, we may use and disclose medical information about you for research purposes. For example, a research project could involve comparing the health and recovery of all patients who received one medication to those who received another, for the same condition. All research projects, however, are subject to a special approval process. This process evaluates a proposed research project and its use of medical information, trying to balance the research needs with patients' need for privacy of their medical information. All research projects are subject to an approval process involving an Institutional Review Board (IRB). The IRB evaluates proposed research projects and their use of PHI, balancing research needs and a patients' right to privacy. We may disclose PHI about you to people preparing to conduct a research project in order to help identify patients with specific medical needs. PHI disclosed during this process never leaves our control. We might ask for specific permission from you if the researcher will have access to your name, address or other information that reveals who you are, or will be involved in your care at the Provider.

- **As Required By Law.** We will disclose medical information about you when required to do so by federal, state, or local law.

- **To Avert a Serious Threat to Health or Safety.** We may use and disclose your medical information when necessary to prevent a serious threat to the health and safety of the public or another person.

- **E-mail Use** E-mail will only be used for communications in accordance with this organization's current policies and practices and with your permission. The use of secured, encrypted e-mail is encouraged.

Special Situations

- **Organ and Tissue Donation.** If you are an organ donor, we may release medical information to organizations that handle organ, eye, and tissue procurement as necessary to facilitate donation and transplantation.

- **Military and Veterans.** If you are a member of the armed forces, we may release medical information about you as required by military command authorities. We also might release medical information about foreign military personnel to the appropriate foreign military authority.

- **Workers' Compensation.** We may release medical information about you for workers' compensation or similar programs.

- **Public Health Risks.** We may disclose medical information about you for public health activities. These activities generally include the following:
  - To prevent or control disease, injury or disability
  - To report births and deaths
  - To report child abuse or neglect
  - To report reactions to medications or problems with products
  - To notify people of recalls of products they may be using
  - To notify a person who may have been exposed to a disease or may be at risk for contracting or spreading a disease or condition
  - To notify the appropriate government authority if we believe a patient has been the victim of abuse, neglect, or domestic violence. We will only make this disclosure if you agree or when required or authorized by law.

- **Health Oversight Activities.** We may disclose medical information to a health oversight agency for activities authorized by law. These oversight activities include, for example, audits, investigations, inspections, and licensure. These activities are necessary for the government to monitor the health care system, government programs, and compliance with civil rights laws.

- **Lawsuits and Disputes.** If you are involved in a lawsuit or a dispute, we may disclose medical information about you in response to a court or administrative order. We may also disclose medical information about you in response to a subpoena, discovery request, or other lawful process by someone else involved in the dispute, but only if efforts have been made to tell you about the request or to obtain an order protecting the information requested.

- **Law Enforcement.** We may release medical information if asked to do so by a law enforcement official:
  - In response to a court order, subpoena, warrant, summons or similar process
  - To identify or locate a suspect, fugitive, material witness, or missing person
  - About the victim of a crime if, under certain limited circumstances, we are unable to obtain the person's agreement
  - About a death we believe may be the result of criminal conduct
  - About criminal conduct at Provider
  - In emergency circumstances, to report a crime; the location of the crime or victims; or the identity, description or location of the person who committed the crime

- **Coroners, Medical Examiners and Funeral Directors.** We may release medical information to a coroner or medical examiner. This may be necessary, for example, to identify a deceased person or determine the cause of death. We also may release medical information about Provider patients to funeral directors as necessary to carry out their duties.

- **National Security and Intelligence Activities.** We may release medical information about you to authorized federal officials for intelligence, counterintelligence, and other national security activities authorized by law.

- **Protective Services for the President and Others.** We may disclose medical information about you to authorized federal officials so they may provide protection to the President, foreign heads of state, or other authorized persons to conduct special investigations.

- **Inmates.** If you are an inmate of a correctional institution or under the custody of a law enforcement official, we may release medical information about you to the correctional institution or law enforcement official. This release would be necessary for the correctional institution to provide you with healthcare, to protect your health and safety or the health and safety of others, as well as for the safety of the institution itself.

Your Rights Regarding Medical Information About You

You have the following rights regarding medical information we maintain about you:

- Right to Access, Inspect, and Copy. You have the right to access, inspect, and copy the medical information that may be used to make decisions about your care, with a few exceptions. Usually, this includes medical and billing records, but may not include psychotherapy notes.

- If we maintain your information electronically you may request a copy of your records via a mutually agreed upon electronic format. If we fail to agree upon an electronic format for delivery of electronic copies we will provide you with a paper copy for your records. If you request a copy of the information in either paper or electronic format, we may charge a fee for the costs of copying, mailing or other supplies associated with your request.

- We may deny your request to inspect and copy medical information in certain very limited circumstances. If you are denied access to medical information, in some cases, you may request that the denial be reviewed. Another licensed health care professional chosen by Provider will review your request and the denial. The person conducting the review will not be the person who denied your request. We will comply with the outcome of the review.

- Right to Amend. If you feel that medical information we have about you is incorrect or incomplete, you may request that we amend the information. You have the right to request an amendment for as long as the information is kept by or for the Provider. In addition, you must provide a reason that supports your request.

- We may deny your request for an amendment if it is not in writing or does not include a reason to support the request or for other reasons. Typical reasons for denial of an amendment request include if you ask us to amend information that:

  o Was not created by us, unless the person or entity that created the information is no longer available to make the amendment

  o Is not part of the medical information kept by or for Provider

  o Is not part of the information which you would be permitted to inspect and copy

  o Is accurate and complete

- Right to an Accounting of Disclosures. You have the right to request an "Accounting of Disclosures.". This is a list of the disclosures we made of medical information about you. Your request must state a time period which may not be longer than six years. Your request should indicate in what form you want the list (for example, on paper or electronically, if available). The first list you request within a 12-month period will be complimentary. For additional lists, we may charge you for the costs of providing the list. We will notify you of the cost involved and you may choose to withdraw or modify your request at that time before any costs are incurred.

- Right to Request Restrictions. You have the right to request a restriction or limitation on the medical information we use or disclose about you for payment or healthcare operations. We require that any requests for use or disclosure of medical information be made in writing. In some cases we are not required to agree to these types of requests, however, if we do agree to them we will abide by these restrictions. We will always notify you of our decisions regarding restriction requests in writing. We will not comply with any requests to restrict use or access of your medical information for treatment purposes.

  You have the right to request, in writing, a limit on the medical information we disclose about you to someone who is involved in your care or the payment for your care, such as a family member or friend. For example, you could ask that we not use or disclose information about a surgery you had to your spouse. In your request, you must tell us what information you want to limit, whether you want to limit our use, disclosure or both, and to whom you want the limits to apply.

  You have the right to request a restriction on the use and disclosure of your medical information about a service or item to your health plan. This right only applies to request for restrictions to a health plan and cannot be denied. The service or item requested for restriction from the health plan must be paid in full and out of pocket by you before the restriction will be applied. We are not required to accept your request for this type of restriction until you have completely paid your bill (zero balance) for the item or service. It is your responsibility to notify other healthcare providers of these types of restrictions. We are not required to do so.

- Right to Receive Notice of a Breach. We are required to notify you by first class mail or by e-mail (if we offered and you have indicated a preference to receive information by e-mail), of any breaches of Unsecured Protected Health Information as soon as possible, but in any event, no later than 60 days following the discovery of the breach. "Unsecured Protected Health Information" is information that is not secured via a methodology identified by the Secretary of the U.S. Department of Health and Human Services (HHS) that renders the protected health information unusable, unreadable, and indecipherable to unauthorized users. The notice is required to include the following information:

- o A brief description of the breach, including the date of the breach and the date of its discovery, if known
- o A description of the type of Unsecured Protected Health Information involved in the breach
- o Steps you should take to protect yourself from potential harm resulting from the breach
- o A brief description of actions we are taking to investigate the breach, mitigate losses, and protect against further breaches
- o Contact information, including a toll-free telephone number, e-mail address, website, or postal address where you can ask questions or obtain additional information.

- In the event the breach involves 10 or more patients whose contact information is out of date, we will post a notice on the home page of our website or in a major print or broadcast media. If the breach involves more than 500 patients in the state or jurisdiction, we will send notices to prominent media outlets. If the breach involves more than 500 patients, we are required to immediately notify the Secretary. We also are required to submit an annual report to the Secretary detailing a list of breaches that involve more than 500 patients during the year and maintain a written log of breaches involving less than 500 patients.

- Right to Request Confidential Communications. You have the right to request that we communicate with you about medical matters in a certain way or at a certain location. For example, you can ask that we only contact you at work or hard copy or e-mail. We will not ask you the reason for your request, but will accommodate all reasonable requests. Your request must specify how or where you wish to be contacted. Right to a Paper Copy of This Notice. You have the right to a paper copy of this Notice. You may ask us to give you a copy of this Notice at any time. Even if you have agreed to receive this Notice electronically, you are still entitled to a paper copy. You may obtain a copy of this Notice at our website. <Insert website link, if appropriate>. To exercise the above rights, please contact <Insert appropriate contact information> to obtain a copy of the relevant form you will need to complete to make your request.

Changes To This Notice

- We reserve the right to change this Notice. We reserve the right to make the revised or changed Notice effective for medical information we already have about you as well as any information we receive in the future. We will post a copy of the current Notice in our organization as well as on our website. In addition, each time you register, are admitted, or receive inpatient or outpatient services from a Provider, we will offer you a copy of the most current Notice.

Complaints

- If you believe your privacy rights have been violated, you may file a complaint with Provider or with the Secretary of the Department of Health and Human Services; http://www.hhs.gov/ocr/privacy/hipaa/complaints/index.html

- To file a complaint with the Provider, contact the individual listed on the first page of this Notice. All complaints must be submitted in writing. You will not be penalized for filing a complaint.

Other Uses of Medical Information

- Other uses and disclosures of medical information not covered by this Notice or the laws that apply to you will be made only with your written permission. If you provide us permission to use or disclose medical information about you, you may revoke that permission, in writing, at any time. If you revoke your permission, we will no longer use or disclose medical information about you for the reasons covered by your written authorization. You understand that we are unable to take back any disclosures we have already made with your permission, and that we are required to retain our records of the care that we provided to you.

Organized Healthcare Arrangement (OHCA)

- The Provider, the independent contractor members of its ,medical staff (including your physician), and other healthcare providers affiliated with the provider have agreed, as permitted by law, to share your health information among themselves for purposes of treatment, payment, or healthcare operations, enabling us to better address your healthcare needs. Providers participating in an Organized Healthcare Arrangement may share the same NPP.

Source: McLendon and Dinh-Rose, 2013.

Appendix 10.B

Sample Authorization to Use or Disclose Health Information

Patient Name: _____

Health Record Number: _____

Date of Birth: _____

1. I authorize the use or disclosure of the above named individual's health information as described below.

2. The following individual(s) or organization(s) are authorized to make the disclosure:

3. The type of information to be used or disclosed is as follows (check the appropriate boxes and include other information where indicated):

   ❑ problem list

   ❑ medication list

   ❑ list of allergies

   ❑ immunization records

   ❑ most recent history

   ❑ most recent discharge summary

   ❑ lab results (please describe the dates or types of lab tests you would like disclosed): _____
   _____

   ❑ x-ray and imaging reports (please describe the dates or types of x-rays or images you would like disclosed):
   _____

   ❑ consultation reports from (please supply doctors' names): _____
   _____

   ❑ entire record

   ❑ other (please describe): _____
   _____

4. I understand that the information in my health record may include information relating to sexually transmitted disease, acquired immunodeficiency syndrome (AIDS), or human immunodeficiency virus (HIV). It may also include information about behavioral or mental health services, and treatment for alcohol and drug abuse.

5. The information identified above may be used by or disclosed to the following individuals or organization(s):

   Name: _____

   Address: _____

   Name: _____

   Address: _____

Source: Hughes, G. 2002 (October). Practice brief: Required content for authorizations to disclose. *Journal of AHIMA.*

6. This information for which I am authorizing disclosure will be used for the following purpose:

   ❑ my personal records

   ❑ sharing with other healthcare providers as needed

   ❑ other (please describe): _____
   _____

7. I understand that I have a right to revoke this authorization at any time. I understand that if I revoke this authorization, I must do so in writing and present my written revocation to the health information management department. I understand that the revocation will not apply to information that has already been released in response to this authorization. I understand that the revocation will not apply to my insurance company when the law provides my insurer with the right to contest a claim under my policy.

8. This authorization will expire (insert date or event): _____
   _____

   If I fail to specify an expiration date or event, this authorization will expire six months from the date on which it was signed.

9. I understand that once the above information is disclosed, it may be redisclosed by the recipient and the information may not be protected by federal privacy laws or regulations.

10. I understand authorizing the use or disclosure of the information identified above is voluntary. I need not sign this form to ensure healthcare treatment. _____
   _____

Signature of Patient or Legal Representative   Date

If signed by legal representative, relationship to patient

_____

_____

_____

Signature of Witness Date

Distribution: Original to provider; copy to patient; copy to accompany use or disclosure

Note: The types of documents listed on the authorization form may need to be modified depending on the particular health care setting. Authorizations for marketing need to disclose whether remuneration was received by the covered entity. This form was developed by AHIMA for discussion purposes only. It should not be used without review by your organization's legal counsel to ensure compliance with other federal and state laws and regulations.

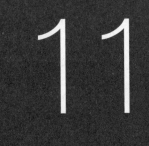

Chapter 11

HIPAA Privacy Rule: Part II

Laurie A. Rinehart-Thompson, JD, RHIA, CHP, FAHIMA

Learning Objectives

- Demonstrate the individual rights granted by the HIPAA Privacy Rule through examples
- Determine whether an unauthorized use or disclosure constitutes a breach, and apply the breach notification process when applicable
- Examine the restrictions that the HIPAA Privacy Rule places on the use of protected health information for research
- Conduct preemption analyses by examining conflicts and determine prevailing law between the HIPAA Privacy Rule and state law
- Analyze administrative requirements and penalties for noncompliance imposed by the HIPAA Privacy Rule
- Explain enforcement of the Privacy Rule and apply appropriate penalties based on the nature of violations
- Explain privacy advocacy initiatives of the American Health Information Management Association

Key Terms

- Access
- Access report
- Accounting of disclosures
- Altered authorization
- Amendment request
- Breach
- Breach notification
- Civil monetary penalties (CMPs)

- Clinical Laboratory Improvement Amendments of 1988 (CLIA)
- Compound authorization
- Conditioned authorization
- Confidential communications
- Data use agreement
- Enforcement Rule

- Federal Policy for the Protection of Human Subjects
- Institutional review board (IRB)
- Mitigation
- National Research Act of 1974
- Preemption
- Privacy board
- Privacy officer

- Request restrictions
- Resolution agreements
- Retaliation and waiver
- Search and retrieval fees
- Stand-alone authorization
- Unconditioned authorization
- Waived authorization

As introduced in chapter 10, the Health Insurance Portability and Accountability Act (HIPAA) Privacy Rule protects patient information. It also ensures the rights of individuals about whom patient information exists and imposes obligations on those responsible for that information. This chapter, which exists in conjunction with chapter 10, is part II of the HIPAA Privacy Rule. It focuses on individual rights; breaches and breach notification; requirements pertaining to researchers using patient information; preemption, which is the interplay between federal and state law; administrative requirements imposed on those who are subject to the HIPAA Privacy Rule; and privacy advocacy by the American Health Information Management Association.

Individual Rights

The Privacy Rule provides patients with significant rights that allow them some measure of control over their health information. Those rights include right of access, right to request amendment of protected health information (PHI), right to an accounting of disclosures, right to request confidential communications, right to request restrictions of PHI, and right to complain of Privacy Rule violations. These rights are described next. A chart that details all individual rights except the right to complain of Privacy Rule violations is located at the end of this chapter (appendix 11).

Access

Section 164.524 of the Privacy Rule states that an individual has a right of **access** to inspect and obtain a copy of his or her own PHI that is contained in a designated record set (DRS), such as a health record (45 CFR 164.524). The individual's right extends for the same period that the PHI is maintained.

Access to information may be denied in some situations because it is specifically exempted from access by the Privacy Rule or it is not part of the DRS. The Privacy Rule preamble makes clear that individuals do not have a right of access to

- Psychotherapy notes
- Information compiled in reasonable anticipation of, or for use in, a civil, criminal, or administrative action or proceeding
- PHI held by clinical laboratories if the **Clinical Laboratory Improvement Amendments of 1988 (CLIA)** (42 CFR 493) prohibit such access (Note: CLIA regulations aim to ensure quality laboratory testing.)
- PHI held by certain research laboratories that are exempt from the CLIA regulations (45 CFR 164.524)

Why is it so important that individuals be able to access (with exceptions) their own PHI? Although the physical health record belongs to the organization that created it, the patient has an interest (or ownership) in the information about him or her that is contained within the record. To provide no specific right of access allows providers and others the ability to deny access. For example, Ohio Revised Code 3701.74 at one time required only hospitals to provide patients with copies of their health records, thus exempting physicians and other healthcare providers (as well as other CEs that are now subject to the Privacy Rule). Thus, physicians and others could deny or ignore patients requesting their own information because there was no statute compelling them to respond. Fortunately, Ohio law subsequently changed in the face of the Privacy Rule's implementation, and patients are now dually given the right of access through Ohio law and the HIPAA Privacy Rule. Nonetheless, this law is an important reminder of the need for a federal law that protects patients' rights with respect to their own health information.

Grounds for Denial of Access

According to the Privacy Rule, a covered entity (CE) can at times deny individuals' access to PHI without providing them an opportunity to review or appeal the denial. This is an unreviewable denial and is important, particularly in the release of information.

Denials that are not subject to an appeals process include

- Requests for access to PHI contained in psychotherapy notes
- PHI held by CEs that are correctional institutions or by providers acting under the direction of correctional institutions, if it jeopardizes safety (the inmate still has the right to inspect his or her PHI)
- PHI created or obtained as part of the DRS by a covered healthcare provider in the course of research that includes treatment, and the individual in the research study agrees to suspend his or

her right to access PHI while the study is in progress. This is usually for protection of the integrity of the research study.

- PHI obtained from someone other than a healthcare provider under a promise of confidentiality, and access would be reasonably likely to reveal the source of the information
- PHI contained in records that are subject to the federal Privacy Act (5 USC 552a) if the denial of access under the Privacy Act would meet the requirements of that law

Individuals do have a right to review a denial of access in situations where a licensed healthcare professional determines that access to PHI would be reasonably likely to

- Endanger the life or physical safety of the individual or another person
- Cause substantial harm to another person (not a healthcare provider) mentioned in the PHI
- Cause substantial harm to the individual or another person if the individual's personal representative requests access

According to the Privacy Rule, when a denial subject to review is made, the CE must write the denial in plain language and include a reason. It must explain that the individual has the right to request a review of the denial and describe how the individual can complain to the CE, including the name or title and phone number of the person or office to contact. Finally, it must explain how the individual can lodge a complaint with the Secretary of the Department of Health and Human Services (HHS). When access to PHI is denied on the grounds mentioned earlier, the individual has the right to have the denial reviewed by a licensed healthcare professional who did not participate in the original denial and who is designated by the CE to act as the reviewing official. The CE must then grant or deny access in accordance with the reviewing official's decision.

Requesting Access to One's Own PHI

The Privacy Rule specifies that the CE may require individuals to make their requests in writing, provided it has informed them of such a requirement. Timely response is important. A CE must act on an individual's request for review of PHI no later than 30 days after the request is made, extending the response by no more than 30 days if within the 30-day period it gives the reason for the delay and the date by which it will respond. The CE may extend the time for action on a request for access only once.

In responding to an individual's request for access to his or her PHI, the CE must arrange a convenient time and place of inspection with the individual or mail a copy of the PHI at the individual's request. Per HITECH, CEs with EHRs must provide individuals with PHI electronically or, if the individual requests, send PHI to a designated person or entity electronically (Rinehart-Thompson 2013).

The issue of fees was addressed in the January 2013 final rule (AHIMA 2013). In early 2016, the Office for Civil Rights (OCR) issued further guidance on the individual right of access and fees. It emphasized that, while individuals may be charged a reasonable cost-based fee, it is to be limited to the cost of

- Certain labor
- Supplies
- Postage (if the individual requested that the PHI be mailed)
- Preparing an explanation or summary, if agreed to by the individual

Labor is clarified as excluding costs associated with reviewing requests, or searching for and retrieving PHI (such as locating and reviewing the PHI in the record, and segregating and preparing the requested PHI).

Search and retrieval fees are expressly prohibited for requests by individuals for their own records, although permitted for requests by other.

OCR clarifies that fee limits apply whether PHI is sent to the individual or whether the individual directs that it be sent to any third party. Both are access requests by the individual, whether submitted by the individual or forwarded to the CE by the third party on behalf of the individual. If a third party initiates a request for PHI on its own behalf, with the individual's HIPAA authorization, fee limits do not apply. Despite the permissibility of limited fees, OCR encourages providing individuals with free copies of their PHI (HHS 2016a).

When requests for access to PHI are granted, the CE must provide access to the PHI in the form or format requested if it is readily producible in such form or format. If it is not, it must be produced in a readable hard-copy form or other form or format agreed to by the CE and the individual (45 CFR 164.524(c)(2)(i)). Individuals cannot be required to purchase portable media if they prefer their PHI be mailed or e-mailed to them, and a flat $6.50 fee for electronic copies of PHI has been recommended (HHS 2016a). AHIMA has submitted its concerns regarding the HHS guidance.

Following the January 2013 final rule, HITECH makes it easier for schools to receive student immunization records where state or other law requires them prior to student admission. HITECH permits CEs to disclose a child's immunization records (considered a public health activity) to a school with the oral consent of the parent or guardian. This contrasts with the previous written authorization requirement (HHS 2010, 40895).

Request Amendment

Many states have laws or regulations that permit individuals to amend their health records. The Privacy Rule also permits individuals to request that a CE amend PHI or a record about the individual in a DRS (45 CFR 164.526). However, the CE may deny the request if it determines that the PHI or the record

- Was not created by the CE
- Is not part of the DRS
- Is not available for inspection as noted in the regulation of access (for example, psychotherapy notes, inmate of a correctional institution)
- Is accurate or complete as it stands

The CE may require the individual to make an **amendment request** in writing and provide a reason for the amendment. This requirement must be communicated in advance to the individual, usually taking place in the CE's Notice of Privacy Practices (NPP).

The Privacy Rule requires a CE to act on an individual's amendment request no later than 60 days after its receipt by either allowing the requested amendment or denying it in writing. The entity may extend its response by 30 days if it explains the reasons for the delay in writing and gives a date by which it will complete its action. There can be no additional extensions.

What must a CE do when an amendment is granted? The Privacy Rule requires it to

1. Identify the records in the DRS that are affected by the amendment and append the information through a link to the amendment's location. For example, if the diagnosis was incorrect, the amendment would have to appear and be linked to each record or report in the DRS.
2. Inform the individual that the amendment was accepted and have him or her identify the persons with whom the amendment needs to be shared and then obtain his or her agreement to notify

those persons. The CE must make reasonable efforts to provide the amendment within a reasonable amount of time to anyone who has received the PHI.

What must the CE do when it denies a requested amendment? Within the required 60 days, the CE must write a denial in plain language that contains the following information (45 CFR 164.526(d)):

- The basis for the denial
- The individual's right to submit a written statement disagreeing with the denial
- The process by which the individual can submit his or her disagreement
- A statement explaining how, if the individual does not submit a disagreement to the denial, he or she may request that both the original amendment request and the CE's denial accompany any future disclosures of the PHI that is the subject of the amendment
- A description of how the individual may complain to the CE, including the name or title and telephone number of the contact person or office

If the individual submits a disagreement, the CE can prepare a written rebuttal and it must provide a copy to the individual.

All requests for amendments, denials, the individual's disagreement, and the CE's rebuttal, if one was created, must be appended or linked to the record or PHI that is the subject of the amendment request. When any future disclosures of the information are made, this material or a summary of it must accompany them. However, if a request for amendment was denied and the individual did not write a statement of disagreement, the request for amendment and denial must only accompany future disclosures if the individual requests it.

Accounting of Disclosures

Maintaining some type of accounting procedure for monitoring and tracking PHI disclosures has been a common practice in departments that manage health information. However, the Privacy Rule has a specific standard with respect to such record keeping. Section 164.528 of the Privacy Rule, which provides for an **accounting of disclosures**, states that an individual has the right to receive an accounting of certain disclosures made by a CE.

The types of disclosures that must be included in the Privacy Rule's accounting requirement are limited, but include public interest and benefit disclosures. The May 31, 2011 proposed rule, however, proposes excluding some public and interest benefit disclosures from an accounting. Disclosures for which an accounting is not required and which are therefore exempt include the following:

- TPO disclosures (although this exception is only applicable to CEs without EHRs and will be further discussed later)
- Individuals to whom the information pertains
- Incident to an otherwise permitted or required use or disclosure
- Pursuant to an authorization
- For use in the facility's directory, to persons involved in the individual's care, or for other notification purposes
- To meet national security or intelligence requirements
- To correctional institutions or law enforcement officials
- As part of a limited data set
- Those that occurred before the compliance date for the CE

The accounting requirement includes disclosures made in writing, electronically, by telephone, or orally. Disclosures not included in this list of exemptions are permitted by the Privacy Rule; however, per the May 31, 2011 proposed rule, HITECH proposes that items to be included in an accounting be specifically listed.

A significant change to the accounting of disclosures requirement under HITECH is that CEs that use or maintain an EHR must include TPO disclosures in their accounting of disclosures. However, the May 31, 2011 proposed rule excludes both TPO and uses from the accounting requirement for paper records and EHRs (HHS 2011). Instead, it proposes a separate access report for EHRs, allowing individuals to see who has viewed their DRS in the previous three years. TPO disclosures would therefore be displayed in the **access report** rather than in the accounting of disclosures. This proposal is pending. Prior to HITECH, requesters received an accounting of disclosures made during the previous six years. Per HITECH, individuals receive an accounting including disclosures made during only the previous three years (AHIMA 2009).

To ensure that disclosures that must be tracked are not overlooked, CEs must recognize that not all of their activities meet the "healthcare operations" definition. For example, mandatory public health reporting is not part of a CE's operations. (Such reporting includes requirements by states to report births [birth certificates]; communicable diseases; and incidents of abuse or suspected abuse of children, individuals who are mentally disabled, and the elderly.) As a result, these disclosures must be included in an accounting of disclosures. For example, if a physician's office reports a patient's tuberculosis to a public health authority, that disclosure must be included if a patient requests an accounting. Additionally, if a CE provides PHI to a third-party public health authority to review, but the third party does not actually review the PHI, the mere right of access must be included in an accounting of disclosures.

Erroneous disclosures (such as a facsimile transmitted to the wrong recipient) are also subject to the accounting of disclosures requirement, regardless of whether the recipient read the information. (These may also constitute breaches, discussed later in this chapter.) Disclosure pursuant to a court order without a patient's written authorization would also be subject to an accounting of disclosures. However, disclosure pursuant to a subpoena that is accompanied by a patient's written authorization would not be subject to an accounting, because the authorization exempts the disclosure from the accounting requirement.

A CE may either account for the disclosures of its business associates (BAs) or provide for the BA to make its own accounting. Under HITECH, BAs must respond to accounting requests made directly to them (AHIMA 2009).

In some situations, the individual's right to an accounting of PHI disclosure may be suspended at the written request of a health oversight agency or law enforcement official. In these situations, the written request from the appropriate agency or law enforcement official must indicate that such an accounting would impede its activities. The oversight agency or the law enforcement official must also indicate how long such a suspension is required.

The Privacy Rule requires that certain items be included in an accounting, with HITECH to relax the specificity to some extent. The date of disclosure, the name and address (when known) of the entity or person who received the information, and a brief statement of the purpose of the disclosure or a copy of the individual's request for an accounting are required. Certain time limits also apply. A CE must act on a request no later than 60 days after its receipt with one 30-day extension, as long as it notifies the individual in writing of the reasons for the delay and when the accounting will be made available. Per the May 31, 2011 proposed rule, HITECH proposes to limit the response period to 30 days, with one 30-day extension.

The first accounting within any 12-month period must be provided without charge. For any other request within a 12-month period, the CE may charge a reasonable cost-based fee. However, the entity must inform individuals of the fee in advance and give them the opportunity to withdraw or modify the request. The Privacy Rule requires documentation to be maintained on all accounting requests, including the information in the accounting, the written accounting that was provided to the individual, and the titles of persons or offices responsible for receiving and processing requests for an accounting. Policies and procedures must be developed to ensure that PHI disclosed from all areas of an organization, especially those areas outside an HIM department, can be tracked and compiled when an accounting request is received.

Confidential Communications

Healthcare providers and health plans must give individuals the right of **confidential communications**, or the opportunity to request that communications of PHI be routed to an alternative location or by an alternative method (45 CFR 164.522(b)). Healthcare providers must honor a request without requiring a reason if the request is reasonable. Health plans must honor a request if it is reasonable and if the requesting individual states that disclosure could pose a safety risk. However, healthcare providers and health plans may refuse to accommodate requests if the individual does not provide information as to how payment will be handled or if the individual does not provide an alternative address or method by which he or she can be contacted.

An example of a request for confidential communications would be a woman who requests that billing information from her psychiatrist, from whom she is seeking treatment because of domestic violence, be sent to her work address instead of to her home.

Request Restrictions

Under the Privacy Rule, a CE must permit an individual to **request restrictions**, meaning that an individual may request the CE to restrict the uses and disclosures of PHI for carrying out TPO (45 CFR 164.522(a)). Historically, the CE has not been required to agree to these requests and may not be allowed to honor them (for example, where disclosures are required by law). When the CE does agree to a restriction, it must abide by it. The restriction can be terminated by either the individual or the CE. When the CE initiates termination of the agreement, it must inform the individual that it is doing so. However, the termination is only effective with respect to the PHI created or received after the individual has been informed (45 CFR 164.522(a)).

Although HIPAA, as noted previously, originally gave CEs discretion not to agree to restriction requests, HITECH requires they be complied with (unless otherwise required by law) if the disclosure would be made to a health plan for payment or operations (and not for treatment) and the PHI pertains solely to an item or service that has been paid for in full by other than the health plan (AHIMA 2009). The logistics of carrying out this requirement, however, can be complex.

Submit Complaints

A CE must provide a process for an individual to complain about the entity's policies and procedures, noncompliance with them, or noncompliance with the Privacy Rule. The CE's NPP must contain contact information at the CE level and inform individuals of the ability to submit complaints to the OCR. For individuals who choose not to complain to the CE or who submit complaints at both levels, the OCR maintains a complaint submission process. The CE must document all complaints it receives, along with the disposition of each complaint. As of March 31, 2016, the most frequent violations were impermissible uses and disclosures, followed by safeguard violations and violations relating to access and the minimum necessary requirement (HHS 2016b).

Check Your Understanding 11.1

Instructions: Indicate whether the following statements are true or false (T or F).

1. An individual's request for an amendment must be granted.
2. An individual has an automatic right of access to his or her psychotherapy notes.
3. A covered entity must always comply with an individual's request for restrictions.
4. Complaints about alleged Privacy Rule violations must be submitted to the covered entity.
5. Disclosures made pursuant to an authorization may be excluded from an accounting of disclosures.

Breaches and Breach Notification

One of the most significant changes presented by HITECH was the addition of the breach notification requirement. **Breach notification** imposes obligations on entities when PHI in their custody has been wrongfully used or disclosed. These requirements are significant because they place organizations on the radar of regulatory agencies and in the media spotlight when PHI is handled inappropriately. Further, they extend consequences to entities not previously bound by HIPAA.

HITECH defines a **breach** as an "unauthorized acquisition, access, use or disclosure of PHI which compromises the security or privacy of such information" (American Recovery and Reinvestment Act of 2009, Title XIII, Subtitle D Sections 13400, 13402). The January 2013 final rule states that "an impermissible use or disclosure of PHI is presumed to be a breach unless the covered entity or business associate demonstrates that there is a low probability that the PHI has been compromised." Breaches further apply only to unsecured PHI, defined as that which technology has not made unusable, unreadable, or indecipherable to unauthorized persons (AHIMA 2013). At this point in time, encryption is a technology that safeguards PHI against breaches.

There are specific exceptions to the breach definition. It does not include disclosures to unauthorized recipients if they would not reasonably be able to retain the disclosed information. Further, it does not include situations where a workforce member or individual, acting under the CE's or BA's authority, unintentionally acquires, accesses, or uses the PHI if it was in good faith, within the scope of authority, and could not be further disclosed or used in an impermissible manner. Finally, it does not include inadvertent disclosure by an individual at a CE or BA to another authorized person at a CE or BA, and the information is not further disclosed or used in an impermissible manner (Rinehart-Thompson 2013).

Breaches are deemed to have been discovered when the breach is first known or when it reasonably should have been known. Individuals whose information has been breached must be notified without unreasonable delay, and within 60 days, by first-class mail and by a faster method (such as telephone) if there is the potential for "imminent misuse." Where more than nine individuals are affected and written notice is unsuccessful, web postings or the media are recommended. A significant threshold is 500 affected people. At that point, media outlets must be used and the Secretary of HHS must be notified immediately. CEs must report all breaches using an online breach reporting system, and all breaches within a calendar year must be entered into the online system no later than 60 days of the following calendar year.

Individuals whose PHI has been breached must be provided with the following information:

- A description of what occurred (including date of breach and date that breach was discovered)

- The types of unsecured PHI that were involved (such as name, social security number, date of birth, home address, and account number)
- Steps that the individual may take to protect himself or herself
- What the entity is doing to investigate, mitigate, and prevent future occurrences
- Contact information for the individual to ask questions and receive updates (AHIMA 2009)

HIPAA CEs and BAs, which may include personal health record (PHR) vendors, are subject to HHS-issued breach notification regulations. Non-CEs and non-BAs (including non-BA PHR vendors, third-party service providers of PHR vendors, and other non-HIPAA CEs or BAs affiliated with PHR vendors) are subject to companion breach notification regulations issued by the Federal Trade Commission (FTC). Under both sets of regulations, entities must identify breaches and make appropriate notifications. In particular, entities subject to FTC regulations must notify the FTC and the individual(s) affected by the breach. Third-party PHR service providers shall notify the PHR vendor or entity of the breach. Other notification requirements, such as the content and nature of breach notices, parallel the requirements established by HHS (AHIMA 2009).

Research Uses and Disclosures of PHI

Risks associated with human subject research include violation both of an individual and his or her PHI. This section briefly discusses human subject research from an historical perspective, including past wrongdoing and laws and standards that serve to prevent future wrongdoing. Because the misuse and inappropriate disclosure of a research subject's PHI are risks associated with human subject research, the Privacy Rule has implemented requirements to prevent those from occurring.

The potential to misuse human subjects in research activities and, hence, the need to protect those subjects are historical issues. The harmful use of concentration camp prisoners by Nazi physicians for experimentation without the consent of those individuals resulted in the Nuremberg Code. Although the code did not become law in the United States, it remains a powerful statement on the ethical use of human subjects. In the United States, the US Public Health Service used male African American sharecroppers (also without their consent) for a harmful study in which treatment was often denied, in what is known as the Tuskegee Syphilis Study (1932–1972). This ultimately led to the **National Research Act of 1974** (Pub. L. 93-348), which required the Department of Health, Education, and Welfare (now the HHS) to codify its policy for the protection of human subjects into federal regulations and created a commission that generated the Belmont Report, a "statement of basic ethical principles that should assist in resolving the ethical problems that surround the conduct of research with human subjects" (NIH 1979). These studies and others demonstrate the international historical misuse of human subjects, against which protections are vital.

Today, research on human subjects is governed by the **Federal Policy for the Protection of Human Subjects** (the Common Rule), which emanated from the joint promulgation of regulations from several federal agencies and, specifically, from HHS regulations 45 CFR Part 46 (1981), based on the Belmont Report. In 1991, the portion of the HHS regulations that focused on the protection of human subjects (45 CFR 46(a)) was adopted by several federal departments and agencies involved in human subject research, either as research bodies themselves or as agencies that fund research conducted by others. The Food and Drug Administration imposes additional requirements at 21 CFR Parts 50 and 56. Requirements of the Common Rule include

- Compliance assurances by organizations conducting research
- Requirements for informed consent

- Special protections for vulnerable populations, such as prisoners, pregnant women, children, mentally disabled persons, and economically or educationally disadvantaged persons (45 CFR 46.101–46.112)

An **institutional review board (IRB)** must approve federally funded human subjects research, even if the patient has signed an informed consent (Rinehart-Thompson 2013). The HIPAA Privacy Rule provides additional protections where research places human subjects and their private information at risk. Per HIPAA, research must be approved by either an IRB or a privacy board (HHS 2016c). A **privacy board** is a group formed by a CE to review research studies where authorization waivers (discussed later) are requested and to ensure the HIPAA privacy rights of research subjects are upheld.

The Privacy Rule expands the Common Rule's requirements by regulating both privately and federally funded research, thus equalizing information privacy protections in both types of research. (HHS 2016c).

The Privacy Rule provides situations when individual HIPAA authorization is required for the use and disclosure of information for research, as well as when it is not. Authorization is not required if one of the following applies:

- An IRB or privacy board has approved the study pursuant to **waived authorization** (no authorization) or **altered authorization** (authorization is required, but one or more standard authorization elements may be omitted). Waiver is only permitted if the use or disclosure provides only a minimal risk to individuals' privacy; the research could not practicably be conducted unless a waiver or alteration was granted; and the research could not be practicably conducted unless access to and use of the PHI was granted.
- The use or disclosure of PHI is solely preparatory to research, and the researcher will not remove PHI from the covered entity; and further, the PHI is necessary for the proposed research. Researcher assurance of this is required.
- The use or disclosure of PHI will only be for research on decedents' PHI and it is necessary for research. Researcher assurance of this is required.
- The covered entity and the researcher will enter into a **data use agreement** that provides the researcher will receive only a limited data set for research, public health, or healthcare operations (HHS 2016c). Under a limited data set, 16 of the 18 identifiers listed in figure 10.4 (located in chapter 10) must be removed. The only data elements permitted are items 3 (dates) and 18 (unique code for reidentification) (45 CFR 164.514(e)). Researcher assurance of this is required (HHS 2016c).

Additionally, the Privacy Rule (45 CFR 164.508(b)(4)) has authorization requirements relevant to research uses and disclosures. The **stand-alone authorization** includes the core elements of a valid authorization (45 CFR 164.508). The **compound authorization,** which combines consent to participate in a research study with authorization to use or disclose PHI, is permitted, although this type of authorization is generally prohibited otherwise. As opposed to the **unconditioned authorization,** the Privacy Rule has generally prohibited the **conditioned authorization,** in which CEs condition treatment, payment, and health plan enrollment or benefit eligibility on an authorization (HHS 2016c). This is to discourage coercing individuals to sign authorizations to receive services. However, they are permitted for covered entities to condition the provision of research-related treatment on an authorization. Further, combined conditioned and unconditioned authorizations (adopted in the January 2013 final rule) are permitted for research if the form clearly distinguishes between the two components and provides individuals with the ability to opt in to the unconditioned research activities (HHS 2010, 40892–40893). This change eliminated problems for researchers who were previously prohibited from using a single authorization for research studies combining treatment with the collection and storage of biospecimens and related PHI for future studies.

Table 11.1 provides a detailed analysis of the responsibilities of both the IRB and the researcher under the Privacy Rule requirements.

Table 11.1 Actions required by HIPAA for use of PHI in research

Type of Information	IRB	Researcher	Research Subject (Patient or Decedent)
PHI preparatory to research	None*	Representation that use is solely and necessary for research and will not be removed from covered entity	None
Deidentified health information	None*	Removal of safe-harbor data or statistical assurance of deidentification	None
Limited data set	None*	Removal of direct identifiers and data use agreement	None
Individually identifiable health information on decedents	None*	Representation that use is solely and necessary for research on decedents and documentation of death upon request of covered entity	None
PHI of human subjects (whether research is interventional or record review)	Waive authorization requirement if determined that risk to privacy is minimal	Representation that: 1. Privacy risk is minimal based on: • Plan to protect identifiers • Plan to destroy identifiers unless there is a health or research reason to retain • Written assurance that PHI will not be reused or redisclosed 2. Research requires use of specifically described PHI 3. Justify the waiver 4. Obtain IRB approval under normal or expedited review procedures	None
	Approve alteration of authorization (such as, to restrict patient's access during study) if determined that risk to privacy is minimal	Same as above	Sign altered authorization form
	Approve research protocol ensuring that there is an authorization for use either combined with consent for and disclosure of PHI research or separate		Sign authorization combined with consent for research or sign standard authorization for use and disclosure of PHI for research as described in authorization

*The IRB may impose requirements, but HIPAA does not.
Source: Amatayakul 2003.

The issue of preemption will be discussed in the following section, as state laws that conflict with the Privacy Rule's research requirements are relevant. Where deidentified information or a limited data set is used for research, or research disclosures pursuant to individual authorization were obtained, no accounting of disclosures is required.

Check Your Understanding | 11.2

Instructions: Indicate whether the following statements are true or false (T or F).

1. The breach notification requirement was implemented under HITECH.
2. The threshold for required media notification in the event of a privacy breach is 300 affected individuals.
3. A waived authorization may be permitted by HIPAA in certain situations.
4. If encrypted PHI is disclosed without authorization, this is automatically a breach.
5. A compound authorization combines consent to participate in a research study with authorization to use or disclose PHI.

Preemption: HIPAA vs. State Law

The legal doctrine of **preemption** applies to the Privacy Rule (45 CFR 160.203). Although CEs are legally obligated to comply with both state and federal privacy laws, sometimes it is impossible to follow both. To address this conflict, preemption requires a CE to comply with federal law when federal and state laws conflict (that is, federal law preempts contrary state law). A state law is contrary when

- It would be impossible for a CE to follow both the federal and state laws or;
- Following the state law would hinder the purpose of HIPAA (45 CFR 160.202)

However, the federal Privacy Rule provides only a floor, or minimum, of privacy requirements. As a result, it does not preempt or supersede stricter (more stringent) state statutes, which are those that

- Provide individuals with greater privacy protections
- Give individuals greater rights with respect to their PHI

However, more stringent state laws are not the only ones that create an exception to preemption. If a state law is less stringent (that is, it provides less protection or fewer individual rights than HIPAA), but it serves a public policy that is recognized by HIPAA as justifying less protection or fewer rights, then state law will prevail. Following is a list of those public policy purposes that, if a state law supports it, HIPAA will recognize it and allow it to operate (that is, it will not be preempted by HIPAA):

A. The state law is determined by the Secretary of Health and Human Services as necessary to

1. Prevent healthcare fraud and abuse
2. Ensure appropriate regulation of insurance and health plans to the extent authorized by law
3. Complete state reporting on healthcare delivery or costs
4. Serve a compelling need related to public health, safety, or welfare, and the intrusion into privacy is warranted when balanced against the need

B. The state law regulates the manufacture, registration, distribution, or dispensing of any controlled substance as identified by state law, or

C. The state law provides for the reporting of disease or injury, child abuse, birth, or death, or for the conduct of public health surveillance, investigation, or intervention; or

D. The state law requires a health plan to report or provide access to information for management or financial audits, program monitoring and evaluation, or licensure or certification of facilities or individuals. (45 CFR 160.203)

It is important to review state legal requirements and determine which law prevails. Because state laws vary in the level of protection they afford patient information, a preemption analysis (which compares federal and state law to determine which one prevails) in one state may yield a different outcome than one performed in another state. Such analyses and determinations are conducted by legal professionals, but they do not have the force of law. If an interested party believes a state law should be preempted by HIPAA, then a lawsuit may be filed to challenge the state law.

Administrative Requirements

The HIPAA Privacy Rule imposes administrative requirements that govern actual implementation of the Rule. Among other mandates, the administrative requirements include policy and procedure development, designated personnel, training, and document retention. These are outlined next.

The Privacy Rule provides several important standards regarding administrative requirements, including

- Standards for policies and procedures and changes to policies and procedures
- Designation of a privacy officer and a contact person for receiving complaints
- Requirements for privacy training
- Mitigation of wrongful use and disclosure
- Requirements for establishing data safeguards
- Prohibition against retaliation and waiver
- Requirements for documentation retention

Individuals who manage health information are likely to find that their responsibilities include essential elements of the Privacy Rule.

Policies and Procedures

A CE must implement policies and procedures to ensure compliance with all standards, implementation specifications, and other requirements of the Privacy Rule. This includes conducting an ongoing review of privacy policies and procedures and ensuring that all policy changes are consistent with changes in the privacy and security regulations. Any regulatory changes that materially affect the CE's NPP, including those introduced by HITECH, must be updated in the NPP. Too, revisions must be indicated in the organization's policies and procedures.

Current topics that must be addressed include policies and procedures associated with high-risk areas where PHI may be captured or stored, but not easily controlled by a CE. These include mobile devices such as cellular phones and tablets, which may or may not be in the custody of a CE's or BA's workforce; social media such as Facebook and Twitter; the use of camera phones by staff, patients and visitors; and the use of body-worn cameras by law enforcement officers. Although the latter two involve privacy intrusions by individuals not bound by the CE (and are thus not privacy violations), they do present privacy and security concerns that must nonetheless be addressed by the organization.

Health information professionals are ideally qualified for developing and overseeing policies and procedures associated with actions by their workforce as well as by others who might infringe on patient privacy. Because of their background in privacy and security issues, they possess the expertise to address these issues.

Privacy Officer and Contact Person

The Privacy Rule requires CEs to designate an individual known as a **privacy officer** to be responsible for developing and implementing privacy policies and procedures. This position is ideally suited to the background, knowledge, and skills of individuals with expertise in health information management.

In addition to a privacy officer, the CE must designate a person as the responsible party for receiving complaints. This individual must be able to provide further information about matters covered by the entity's NPP.

Workforce Training and Management

Every member of the CE's workforce must be trained in PHI policies and procedures. New members must be trained within a reasonable period after joining the workforce. In addition, whenever material changes are made to policies or procedures regarding privacy, the workforce must receive additional training. A CE should be comprehensive in its workforce training, including even less apparent workforce members who do not work directly with PHI but could access it (for example, janitorial staff and outsourced vendors' employees who work routinely on the CE's premises). Under HITECH, there are heightened consequences for BAs that violate the Privacy Rule. Therefore, BAs should train their own workforce members (Rinehart-Thompson 2013).

CEs and BAs and, now, individual members of their workforces (per HITECH) are subject to the Privacy Rule and the penalties that accompany violations. It is important for CEs and BAs to document all steps that have been taken to ensure compliance to the extent possible by its workforce. CEs must maintain documentation showing that privacy training has occurred. BAs should also ensure that training is documented. Although not required, a signed statement of training by each workforce member is helpful to document compliance. Workforce members should also complete nondisclosure agreements stating their commitment to protecting the privacy of patient information and compliance with the Privacy Rule to further affirm their understanding and the voluntary nature of this commitment.

Mitigation

The Privacy Rule (45 CFR 164.530(f)) requires CEs to mitigate, as much as possible, harmful effects that result from the wrongful use and disclosure of PHI. Because **mitigation** requires the lessening of the effects of a wrongful use or disclosure, it is contingent upon the CE to determine possible courses of action. Although HITECH requires one type of mitigation, which is breach notification, other types of mitigation may assuage the individual, including

- Apology
- Disciplinary action against the responsible employee or employees (although such results will not be able to be shared with the wronged individual)
- Repair of the process that resulted in the breach
- Payment of a bill or financial loss that resulted from the infraction
- Gestures of goodwill and good public relations (such as awarding gift certificates)

Mitigation may occur following discovery of a breach by the CE or BA, or subsequent to a complaint that an individual has filed with the organization, the OCR, or both. Determining what constitutes a breach (which must be reported to both HHS and the individual), as well as determining the appropriate mitigation, are steps an organization must take and should be outlined in the organization's policies and procedures.

Data Safeguards

CEs are required to have in place appropriate administrative, technical, and physical safeguards to protect the privacy of PHI from either intentional or unintentional uses or disclosures that violate the rule. These safeguards must limit incidental uses and disclosures (45 CFR 164.530(c)). They may include the shredding of paper documents containing PHI (Rinehart-Thompson 2013), and limiting access to areas containing PHI through the use of devices such as keycards, passwords, or locks.

Retaliation and Waiver

To ensure an individual's right to complain about alleged Privacy Rule violations, CEs are expressly prohibited from **retaliation and waiver.** First, CEs may not retaliate against anyone who exercises his or her rights under the Privacy Rule, assists in an investigation by the HHS or other appropriate investigative authority, or opposes an act or practice that the person believes is a violation of the Privacy Rule (45 CFR 164.530(g)). Further, individuals cannot be required to waive the rights they hold under the Privacy Rule in order to obtain treatment, payment, or enrollment/benefits eligibility (45 CFR 164.530(h)).

Documentation and Record Retention

The Privacy Rule uses six years as the period for which Privacy Rule–related documents must be retained. The six-year time frame refers to the latter of the following: the date the document was created or the last effective date of the document (45 CFR 164.530(j)). Relevant documents include policies and procedures, the NPP, complaint dispositions, and other actions, activities, and designations that must be documented per Privacy Rule requirements.

Enforcement and Penalties for Noncompliance

HITECH introduced several notable changes to enforcement and penalty provisions for HIPAA violations. Overall, there is a notable movement away from a collaborative approach focusing on corrective action to a more punitive stance.

The OCR enforces the Privacy Rule. Complaints are filed with the OCR and includes an online complaint portal option. Although compliance with the Privacy Rule has historically been monitored through a complaint-driven process (and enforcement efforts have subsequently been criticized as lacking teeth), HITECH requires the HHS to conduct audits of CEs and BAs—not unlike those used by state licensure organizations. A pilot audit program was conducted in 2011 and 2012, which assessed 115 covered entities. Phase 2 of the audit, beginning in 2016, focuses on both CEs and BAs. The first set, desk audits, addresses CEs. The second set, also desk audits, addresses BAs. The third set consists of on-site audits. All sets focus on the privacy, security, and breach notification rules (HHS 2016d).

Because complaints will also continue to initiate investigations, however, CEs and BAs should minimize situations that lead to disgruntled patients (AHIMA 2009). This includes demonstrating compliance in ways that are visible to patients and visitors, such as posting signs that require individuals in line to stand back from a patient registration counter to prevent them from overhearing PHI that is being shared.

HITECH grants state attorneys general the ability to bring civil actions in federal district court on behalf of residents believed to have been negatively affected by a HIPAA violation. Further, whereas legal responsibility for HIPAA violations was previously limited to CEs, employees or other individuals can now be individually prosecuted. Civil and criminal penalties may also now apply to BAs. Further, a method for compensating individuals harmed under HIPAA and HITECH provisions was to be recommended to the Secretary of HHS, but this is pending.

The Final HIPAA **Enforcement Rule** contains provisions for compliance, investigations, civil monetary penalties, and procedures related to hearings (HHS 2016e). Per the HHS OCR website, as of February 28, 2017, 147,826 (98 percent) of 150,507 complaints had been resolved, with 2,681 (2 percent) remaining open. Of the 36,048 complaints investigated, corrective action was achieved in 24,879 cases (69 percent) and no violations were found in 11,169 cases (31 percent) (HHS 2017). As of April 24, 2017, the OCR had signed nearly 50 **resolution agreements** with CEs and BAs, which are settlements compelling them to perform obligations per the agreements (often including payments) and to submit reports to HHS for three years. If a resolution cannot be reached through compliance or corrective actions provided by a resolution agreement (in other words, a settlement cannot be reached), then the OCR will resort to **civil monetary penalties (CMPs)**, which are fines imposed on a CE or BA because of a HIPAA violation. Civil monetary penalties have been assessed against two covered entities (HHS 2016e). Figure 11.1 provides a flow chart from OCR that outlines the complaint process for the HIPAA Privacy and Security Rules.

HITECH has increased civil monetary penalties based on levels, or tiers, of intent and neglect. The nature and extent of both the violation and the harm are used to determine the amount assessed within each range. Currently, penalties for violations range as follows, with a cap of $1,500,000 for identical violations within each violation category (HHS 2009):

- $100–$50,000 per violation for unknowing violations (would not have known a violation was committed, even with reasonable diligence)
- $1,000–$50,000 per violation if due to reasonable cause (CE or BA knew or would have known with reasonable diligence), but not willful neglect
- $10,000–$50,000 per violation if due to willful neglect and corrected within 30 days of discovery
- $50,000 or more per violation if due to willful neglect and not corrected as required

The OCR may choose to pursue corrective action without assessing penalties for unknowing violations, but penalties are mandatory in all other categories. These provisions differ greatly from pre-HITECH penalties that prohibited CMPs due to reasonable cause if correction occurred within 30 days of when the CE knew or should have known of the violation (AHIMA 2009). Penalty monies collected will support further enforcement efforts (AHIMA 2013).

Figure 11.1 HIPAA privacy and security rules complaint process

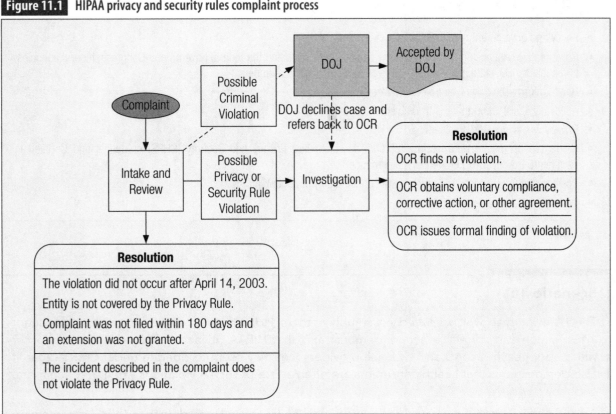

Source: HHS 2016e.

Privacy Advocacy

As the privacy of patient information becomes more transparent to the public, privacy advocates have sprung up to support patient privacy efforts and to strengthen public awareness. Other organizations also exist that more broadly address the issue of privacy (for example, protection of financial information). The American Health Information Management Association (AHIMA) is proactive both internally and externally, educating its members on privacy issues and shaping public policy and federal law to further one of the profession's central values: protecting the privacy of patient information. AHIMA serves as an instrumental privacy advocate through the functions and entities listed in figure 11.2.

Check Your Understanding   11.3

Instructions: Indicate whether the following statements are true or false (T or F).

1. Enforcement of the Privacy Rule will continue to operate exclusively on a complaint-based system.

2. The Privacy Rule provides a floor, or minimum, of privacy requirements.

3. Breach notification is one type of mitigation under the Privacy Rule.

4. To simplify processes, individuals may be required to waive their rights under the Privacy Rule to obtain treatment or benefits eligibility.

5. Under HITECH, state attorneys general may bring civil actions in federal district court on behalf of residents believed to have been negatively affected by a HIPAA violation.

Figure 11.2 AHIMA advocacy agenda for the confidentiality, privacy, and security of health information

- Policy and government relations staff
- Collaborative relationships with key privacy stakeholders, including the federal government (Congress, federal agencies, and subsidiaries), state governments, HIT vendors, and AHIMA members
- Health Information Privacy and Security Week
- Advocacy Assistant on the AHIMA Web site
- Privacy workshops and seminars
- Credentials in privacy and security (Certified in Healthcare Privacy and Security [CHPS] credential and Certified in Healthcare Privacy [CHP] credential maintenance)
- Position statements regarding privacy and confidentiality of patient information
- Privacy and Security Practice Council

Source: AHIMA

Scenario 11

The following case, which resulted in a complaint to the HHS Office for Civil Rights with a subsequent investigation and corrective action, demonstrates that HIPAA privacy violations can readily occur with paper health records and by small providers that may seem to operate under OCR's radar. It also demonstrates that health consumers are often aware of HIPAA violations when they see them, and they do take action.

A dental office was in the practice of flagging some of its medical records with red stickers containing the word "AIDS" on the outside cover. Further, office staff handled the records in a manner such that other patients and staff could read the stickers, even though they had no reason to know about the patients' diagnoses.

1. What HIPAA violation(s) can be identified in this scenario?
2. Is there a way to identify records of AIDS patients to safeguard staff, while also maintaining the privacy of the patients?
3. As a representative of the Office for Civil Rights, what corrective action steps would you require the dental practice to make?
4. What other types of mitigation could the dental practice employ?
5. Presume that this office had electronic health records instead of paper records. Would the risk of a privacy violation be as great? How could records of AIDS patients be identified to safeguard staff, while also maintaining the privacy of the patients?

References

AHIMA. 2009. Analysis of health care confidentiality, privacy, and security provisions of the American Recovery and Reinvestment Act of 2009, Public Law 111-5. Chicago: AHIMA.

AHIMA. 2013. Analysis of Modifications to the HIPAA Privacy, Security, Enforcement, and Breach Notification Rules Under the Health Information Technology for Economic and Clinical Health Act and the Genetic Information Nondiscrimination Act; Other Modifications to the HIPAA Rules. http://www.ahima.org.

Amatayakul, M. 2001. HIPAA on the job: Managing individual rights requirements under HIPAA privacy. *Journal of AHIMA* 72(6): 16A–16D.

Amatayakul, M. 2003. Another layer of regulations: Research under HIPAA. *HIPAA on the Job* series. *Journal of AHIMA* 74(1):16A–16D.

Department of Health and Human Services. 2009. HIPAA Administrative Simplification Enforcement. 45 CFR Parts 160. *Federal Register* 74(209):56123–56131.

Department of Health and Human Services. 2010. Modifications to the HIPAA Privacy, Security, and Enforcement Rules under the Health Information Technology for Economic and Clinical Health Act; Proposed Rule. 45 CFR Parts 160 and 164. *Federal Register* 75(134):40868–40924.

Department of Health and Human Services. 2011. HIPAA Privacy Rule Accounting of Disclosures Under the Health Information Technology for Economic and Clinical Health Act. 45 CFR Part 164. *Federal Register* 75 (134): 40868–40924.

Department of Health and Human Services. 2016a. Individuals' right under HIPAA to access their health information. 45 CFR 164.524. http://www.hhs.gov/ocr/.

Department of Health and Human Services. 2016b. Office for Civil Rights. Health information privacy: numbers at a glance. http://www.hhs.gov/ocr/.

Department of Health and Human Services. 2016c. Research. http://www.hhs.gov/ocr/.

Department of Health and Human Services. 2016d. HIPAA Privacy, Security, and Breach Notification Audit Program. http://www.hhs.gov/ocr/.

Department of Health and Human Services. 2016e. The HIPAA Enforcement Rule. http://www.hhs.gov/ocr/.

Department of Health and Human Services. 2017. Numbers at a Glance. http://www.hhs.gov/ocr/.

National Institutes of Health, Office of Human Subjects Research. 1979. The Belmont report: Ethical principles and guidelines for the protection of human subjects of research.

Rinehart-Thompson, L. 2013. *Introduction to Health Information Privacy and Security.* Chicago: AHIMA.

Statutes and Regulations Cited

21 CFR Parts 50 and 56: Prisoners, Reporting and recordkeeping requirements, Research, Safety. 1991.

42 CFR 493: Clinical Laboratory Improvement Amendments (CLIA). 1988.

45 CFR 46(a): Basic HHS Policy for Protection of Human Research Subjects. 2005.

45 CFR 46.101–46.112: Protection of Human Subjects. 2005.

45 CFR 160.202: General administrative requirements: Preemption of state law: Definitions. 2006.

45 CFR 160.203: General administrative requirements: Preemption of state law: General rule and exceptions. 2006.

45 CFR 164.508: Uses and disclosures for which authorization is required. 2006.

45 CFR 164.514: Other requirements relating to uses and disclosures of protected health information. 2006.

45 CFR 164.522: Rights to request privacy protection for protected health information. 2006.

45 CFR 164.524: Access of individuals to protected health information. 2006.

45 CFR 164.526: Amendment of protected health information. 2006.

45 CFR 164.528: Accounting of disclosures of protected health information. 2006.

45 CFR 164.530: Administrative requirements. 2006.

5 USC 552a (App. 3 sec. (6)(a)(4)): The Privacy Act of 1974.

American Recovery and Reinvestment Act of 2009, Title XIII—Health Information Technology, Subtitle D Sections 13400, 13402.

National Research Act of 1974 (Pub. L. 93-348).

OH Rev. Code 3701.74: Patient or patient's representative to submit request to examine or obtain copy of medical record. 2007.

Cases, Statutes, and Regulations Resources

Health Insurance Portability and Accountability Act of 1996. Public Law 104-191. Available online from http://www.gpo.gov/.

Appendix 11

Individual Rights under the HIPAA Privacy Rule

Patient Rights at a Glance

Right	Request	Acceptance	Termination	Timeliness	Fee	Denial	Review
Right to request restriction of uses and disclosures	Provider must permit request, but does not have to be in writing.	Provider generally not required to agree, but if accepted, must not violate restriction except for emergency care. However, requests must be complied with (unless otherwise required by law) if disclosure would be to a health plan for payment or operations purposes and has been paid for the service or item completely out of pocket.	Provider may terminate if individual agrees or requests in writing, or oral agreement is documented. Termination only applies to information created or received after the individual has been informed. Restrictions cannot be terminated relative to disclosures to a health plan if the item or service has been paid for in full other than by the health plan out of pocket.	There is no provision for addressing timeliness.	There is no provision for a fee.	There are no requirements associated with denying restriction.	Not applicable
Right to receive confidential communications	Provider may require written request for receiving communications by alternative means or locations.	Provider must accommodate reasonable requests and may condition how payment will be handled but may not require explanation.	There is no provision for termination.	There is no provision for addressing timeliness.	There is no provision for a fee.	Not applicable	Not applicable
Right of access to information	Provider must permit request for copying and inspection and may, upon notice, require requests in writing. Provider may supply a summary or explanation of information, instead, if individual agrees in advance. Covered entities with EHRs must make information available electronically or must send it electronically upon the individual's request.	Provider may deny access without opportunity for review if information is: psychotherapy notes, compiled for legal proceeding, subject to CLIA, about inmate and could cause harm, subject of research to which denial of access has been agreed, subject to Privacy Act, or obtained from someone else in confidence. Provider may deny access with opportunity to review if licensed professional determines access may endanger life or safety, there is reference to another person and access could cause harm, or request made by personal representative who may cause harm. The covered entity must provide the individual with access to PHI in the form and format requested, if readily producible as such; if not readily available, must be provided in readable hard copy or other form and format agreed upon by the covered entity and the individual. The individual may direct the covered entity to transmit an electronic copy of their information to an other entity or person. Covered entities must ensure reasonable safeguards are in place to protect the ePHI in transit.	Individuals have right of access for as long as information is maintained in designated record set.	Provider must act upon a request within 30 days. If information is not maintained on site, provider may extend by no more than 30 days if individual is notified of reasons for delay and given date for access.	Provider may impose reasonable, cost-based fee for copying, postage, and preparing an explanation or summary.	If access is denied, provider must provide timely written explanation in plain language, containing basis for denial, review rights if applicable, description of how to file a complaint, and source of information not maintained by provider if known. Provider must also give individual access to any part of information not covered under grounds for denial.	An individual may request a review of a denial by a different healthcare professional.

Right to amend information	Provider must permit requests to amend a designated record set and may, upon notice, require request in writing and a reason.	If amendment is accepted, provider must append or link to record set and obtain and document identification and agreement to have provider notify relevant persons with which amendment needs to be shared. Provider may deny amendment if information was not created by the provider unless individual provides reasonable basis that originator is no longer available to act on request, is not part of designated record set, would not be available for access, or is accurate and complete.	Amendment applies for as long as information is maintained in designated record set.	Provider must act upon a request within 60 days of receipt. If unable to act on request within 60 days, provider may extend time by no more than 30 days provided individual is notified of reasons for delay and given date to amend.	There is no provision for a fee.	If amendment is denied, provider must provide timely written explanation in plain language, containing basis for denial, right to submit written statement of disagreement, right to request provider include request and denial with any future disclosures of information that is subject of amendment, and description of how to file a complaint.	Provider must accept written statement of disagreement (of limited length). Provider may prepare written rebuttal and must copy individual. Provider must append or link request, denial, disagreement, and rebuttal to record and include such or accurate summary with any subsequent disclosure. If no written disagreement, provider must include request and denial, or summary, in subsequent disclosures only if individual has requested such action.
Right to accounting of disclosures (subject to revision if "access report" is made final)	Provider must provide individual with written accounting including date of disclosure, name and address of recipient, description of information disclosed, purpose of disclosure or copy of individual's written authorization or other request for disclosure.	Provider must provide accounting and retain documentation of written accounting of disclosures of PHI made in three years prior to date of request, except for disclosures (1) to carry out treatment, payment, and healthcare operations (this exception will not apply to covered entities with EHRs); (2) to the individuals themselves; (3) incident to a use or disclosure otherwise permitted or required; (4) pursuant to an authorization; (5) for the facility's directory or to persons involved in the individual's care or other notification purposes; (6) for national security or intelligence purposes; (7) to correctional institutions or law enforcement as permitted; (8) as part of a limited data set; or (9) that occurred prior to the compliance date for the covered entity. As proposed in May 2011 (HHS 2011), uses and TPO disclosures would be excluded from an accounting. Instead, an access report would be available from covered entities with EHRs. This report would allow individuals to see a record of every person who viewed the individual's DRS during the previous three years. This is pending.	Not applicable.	Provider must act upon request within 60 days of receipt. If unable to provide accounting, provider may extend time by no more than 30 days provided individual is notified of reasons for delay. (A 30-day response period, with one 30-day extension, is proposed per HITECH.)	First accounting in any 12-month period must be provided without charge. A reasonable, cost-based fee may be charged for subsequent accountings in 12-month period if individual is notified in advance.	Provider must temporarily suspend right to receive an accounting of disclosures to health oversight agency or law enforcement official if agency or official provides written statement that accounting would impede their activities.	There is no provision for review of temporary suspension.

Source: Adapted from Amatayakul 2001 and AHIMA 2009.

The HIPAA Security Rule

Rebecca B. Reynolds, EdD, MHA, RHIA, CHPS, FAHIMA;
Melanie S. Brodnik, PhD, RHIA, FAHIMA

Learning Objectives

- Describe the purposes of the HIPAA Security Rule
- Summarize the components of the Security Rule
- Recognize security components for risk management

Key Terms

- Addressable specification
- American Recovery and Reinvestment Act of 2009 (ARRA)
- Automatic log-off
- Business associates (BAs)
- Chief security officer
- Confidentiality
- Covered entities (CE)
- Electronic protected health information (ePHI)
- Encryption
- Health Insurance Portability and Accountability Act (HIPAA) of 1996
- Health Information Technology for Economic and Clinical Health (HITECH)
- Integrity
- Person or entity authentication
- Physical safeguards
- Required specification
- Scalability
- Security officer
- Technical safeguards
- Technology neutral

The **Health Insurance Portability and Accountability Act** (HIPAA), signed into law April 21, 1996, requires the use of standards for electronic transactions containing healthcare data and information as a way to improve the efficiency and effectiveness of the healthcare system. Title II of the law was designed to protect not only the privacy of healthcare data and information but also the security of the data and information. **Security** refers to protecting information from loss, unauthorized access, or misuse, and also keeping it confidential. This chapter introduces the HIPAA Security Rule, which closely aligns with the Privacy Rule. Although the rules complement each other, the Privacy Rule governs the privacy of protected health information (PHI) regardless of the medium in which the information resides, whereas the Security Rule governs PHI that is transmitted by or maintained in some form of electronic media (that is, **electronic protected health information**, or **ePHI**). ePHI is all "individually identifiable health information: held or transmitted by a covered entity (CE) or business associate (BA), in any form or media, whether electronic, paper, or oral" (HHS 2014). The Privacy Rule calls this information "PHI". The chapter begins with a discussion of the purposes of the rule, its source of law, scope, and to whom the law applies. The chapter suggests a process for complying with the rule and outlines the five key components of the rule. Where appropriate, the chapter also discusses changes to the Security Rule as a result of the **Health Information Technology for Economic and Clinical Health (HITECH)** provisions of the **American Recovery and Reinvestment Act of 2009 (ARRA)**. The HITECH Act was passed to promote the adoption and meaningful use of health information technology. Subtitle D addresses privacy and security and strengthens the civil and criminal enforcement of the HIPAA rules. It concludes with a discussion of the role of a security officer, how the rule is enforced, and the penalties for noncompliance with the rule.

Purposes of the HIPAA Security Rule

The security standards in HIPAA were developed for two primary purposes: to implement appropriate security safeguards and protect electronic healthcare information that may be at risk, and to protect an individual's health information while permitting appropriate access and use of that information. The standards ultimately promote the use of electronic health information in the industry, which is an important goal of HIPAA (HHS 2007a). The HIPAA Security Rule requires covered entities (CEs) to ensure the integrity and confidentiality of information, to protect against any reasonably anticipated threats or risks to the security and integrity of information, and to protect against unauthorized uses or disclosures of information. As a reminder, CEs are the individuals and organizations that must comply with HIPAA, as discussed later in the section, Applicability. The Security Rule defines **integrity** as data or information that has not been altered or destroyed in an unauthorized manner, and it defines **confidentiality** as data or information that is not made available or disclosed to unauthorized persons or processes (45 CFR 164.304). Ultimately, the Security Rule seeks to ensure that CEs implement basic safeguards to protect ePHI from unauthorized access, alteration, deletion, and transmission, while also ensuring that data or information is accessible and usable on demand by authorized individuals.

Source of Law

As discussed in chapter 10, HIPAA (of which security is only one piece) was enacted by Congress in 1996 and became federal statutory law. The Department of Health and Human Services (HHS) published the final Security Rule in the *Federal Register*, Health Insurance Reform, Security Standards, Final Rule (45 CFR Parts 160, 162, 164(a), and 164(c)) on February 20, 2003 (HHS 2003). The rule established security standards to protect ePHI. CEs were expected to be in compliance with the rule by April 20, 2005, and small health plans by April 20, 2006. Changes to the HIPAA Privacy and Security Rules were passed in February 2009 as part of the HITECH Act of the ARRA Act of 2009 (ARRA 2009). The HITECH Act was designed to promote widespread adoption of electronic health records (EHRs) and electronic health information exchanges (HIEs) to improve patient care and reduce healthcare costs. To achieve these goals, HITECH identified requirements to strengthen the privacy and security protections under HIPAA to ensure patients and healthcare providers that their electronic health information is kept private and secure. In July 2010 and May 2011, HHS published proposed rules to implement some of the HITECH provisions and modify other HIPAA requirements (HHS 2010a). The 2010 proposed rule went into effect with publication of the January 2013 final rule titled "Modifications to the HIPAA Privacy, Security, Enforcement, and Breach Notification Rules Under the Health Information Technology for Economic and Clinical Health Act and the Genetic Information Nondiscrimination Act; Other Modifications to the HIPAA Rules." The 2011 proposed rule is still pending (AHIMA 2013a).

Until 2009, the Centers for Medicare and Medicaid Services (CMS) were responsible for oversight and enforcement of the Security Rule, whereas the Office of Civil Rights (OCR) within HHS oversaw and enforced the Privacy Rule. In the latter half of 2009, authority for oversight and enforcement of the HIPAA Privacy and Security Rules was consolidated under the OCR (HHS 2009a). CMS continues to have authority for enforcement of administrative simplification regulations other than privacy and security (preventing healthcare fraud and abuse, and medical liability reform).

Scope and Anatomy of the Security Rule

HIPAA consists of five titles. The Security Rule is one of five administrative simplification provisions in the law (privacy, security, transaction code sets, unique national provider identifiers, and enforcement). The scope of the Security Rule is to protect individually identifiable health information that is transmitted by or maintained in any form of electronic media. The Security Rule defines electronic media to mean electronic storage media including memory devices in computer hard drives and any removable or transportable digital memory medium, such as magnetic-type storage or disk, optical disk, or digital memory card; or transmission media used to exchange information already in electronic storage media, such as the intranet, extranet, leased lines, dial-up lines, private networks, and physical, removable, transportable electronic storage media (45 CFR 160.103).

Congress published the first set of security standards for public comment in 1998. At that time, many of the public comments concluded that the rules were too prescriptive and not flexible enough. As a result, the final rule includes standards defined in general terms, focusing on what *should* be done rather than *how* it should be done. Efforts were made to make the rule **technology neutral** (this means that specific technologies are not prescribed in the rules which allows the use of the latest and appropriate technology) and flexible so that CEs could choose the security measures that best meet their technological capabilities and operational needs to comply with the standards. The flexibility and **scalability** (the concept that based on the size of the CE, the threshold of compliance varies) of the standards make it possible for any CE, regardless of size, to comply with the Rule.

The Security Rule comprises five general rules and a number of standards that encompass 1. general requirements; 2. flexibility of approach; 3. standards related to administrative, physical, and technical safeguards; organizational requirements; policies, procedures, and documentation requirements; 4. implementation specifications; and 5. maintenance of security measures (see figure 12.1), all of which will be discussed later in the chapter.

History and Comparison with Existing Laws

Until HIPAA was enacted, there were no generally accepted security standards for protecting health information. There were, however, a number of state and federal initiatives that addressed privacy, as discussed in chapter 10. With increased reliance on the use of information technology to electronically capture, store, retrieve, transmit, and exchange health information, Congress recognized the need for national security standards, resulting in the HIPAA Security Rule. The Privacy and Security Rules work in tandem to protect health information. The Privacy Rule set standards for how PHI should be controlled by establishing uses and disclosures that are authorized or required and what rights patients have in regard to their health information.

The Security Rule was written to protect ePHI and to guide how electronic health information can be accessed appropriately. There are two primary distinctions between the HIPAA Security Rule and the HIPAA Privacy Rule:

- Electronic versus paper versus oral: The Privacy Rule applies to all forms of PHI, whether electronic, written, or oral. In contrast, the narrower Security Rule covers only PHI that is in electronic form. It does not cover paper or verbal PHI.
- "Safeguard" requirement in Privacy Rule: The Privacy Rule contains provisions that require CEs to adopt administrative, physical, and technical safeguards for PHI. Although Security Rule

Figure 12.1 HIPAA title II administrative simplification—Security Rule

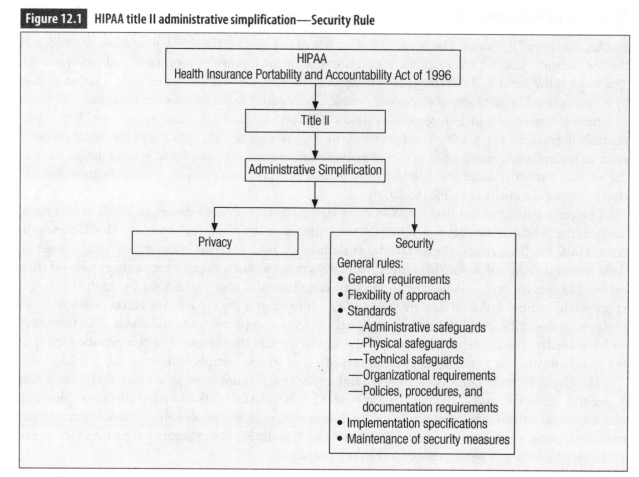

Source: Adapted from Scholl et al. 2008.

compliance was required in 2005 at the earliest, actions taken by CEs to implement the Privacy Rule may have addressed some security requirements. However, the Security Rule provides far more comprehensive and detailed security requirements (HHS 2007a, 4).

For example, to address the growing concern for the use of devices and tools that enable access to or use of ePHI outside the CE's physical purview, HHS issued a HIPAA Security Guidance report on remote access (HHS 2006a). The report lists risks of off-site use or access and possible risk management strategies for identified risks. It also contains potential security strategies for conducting business activities through 1. portable media/devices (such as USB flash drives) that store ePHI; and 2. off-site access or transport of ePHI via laptops, mobile devices, home computers, and other personal equipment. The report also encourages rigor in policy and procedure development for off-site use or access to ePHI (HHS 2006a).

Applicability

The Security Rule applies to individuals or organizations identified as CEs and, with the recent enactment of the HITECH provisions, **business associates (BAs)** and the subcontractors of BAs. The Security Rule applies to the following **covered entities (CEs):**

- Covered healthcare providers: Any provider of medical or other healthcare services or supplies that transmits any health information in electronic form in connection with a transaction for which HHS has adopted a standard
- Health plans: Any individual or group plan that provides or pays the cost of healthcare (for example, a health insurance issuer or Medicare and Medicaid programs)
- Healthcare clearinghouses: Public or private entities that process another entity's healthcare transactions from a standard format to a nonstandard format or vice versa

HITECH holds BAs to the same standards as CEs in regard to protection of health information. BAs are identified as such by the types of functions they carry out, not by contract only.

These changes are a result of HITECH which requires BAs to comply with the Security Rule provisions mandating administrative, physical, and technical safeguards, in addition to adherence to the terms of their BA agreements. They must also adhere to Privacy Rule requirements, which were discussed in chapter 10. The definition of a BA has been revised to include subcontractors of BAs, who must also follow the Security Rule or be held liable for violations. BAs must execute BA agreements with their subcontractors as well (HHS 2010a). In addition, the definition of a BA has been expanded to include entities that manage the exchange of PHI through networks, including patient locator services, e-prescribing gateways, others that provide data transmission services of PHI to a CE and require routine access to such information, or vendors that contract with CEs to offer personal health records to patients as part of the CEs' EHRs (HHS 2010a). Thus, the Security Rule now applies to a broader range of individuals and organizations (CEs, BAs, and BA subcontractors) in an effort to further protect the privacy and confidentiality of ePHI.

Ensuring Security Compliance

Security is not a one-time project but an ongoing process that requires constant analysis as the business practices of the CE and BA change, technologies advance, and new systems are implemented.

HHS has a seven-step guide to implementing a security management process:

1. Lead your culture, select your team and learn
2. Document your processes, findings and actions
3. Review existing security of ePHI (Perform Security Risk Analysis)
4. Develop an action plan
5. Manage and mitigate risks
6. Attest for Meaningful Use security-related objectives
7. Monitor, audit and update security on an ongoing basis (ONC 2015).

CEs and BAs must decide which security measures to implement, using a risk analysis to determine circumstances that leave them open to unauthorized access and disclosure of ePHI. An ongoing security analysis will assess what security measures are already in place and what measures are still necessary. Compliance with the Privacy and Security Rules should be included in the organization's compliance assurance and information governance plans and program. More information about corporate compliance programs is included in chapter 17.

Figure 12.2 Five security components for risk management

Security Component	Examples of Vulnerabilities	Examples of Security Mitigation Strategies
Administrative Safeguards	• No security officer is designated. • Workforce is not trained or is unaware of privacy and security issues. • Periodic security assessment and reassessment are not performed.	• Security officer is designated and publicized. • Workforce training begins at hire and is conducted on a regular and frequent basis. • Security risk analysis is performed periodically and when a change occurs in the practice or the technology.
Physical Safeguards	• Facility has insufficient locks and other barriers to patient data access. • Computer equipment is easily accessible by the public. • Portable devices are not tracked or not locked up when not in use.	• Building alarm systems are installed. • Offices are locked. • Screens are shielded from secondary viewers.
Technical Safeguards	• Poor controls allow inappropriate access to EHR. • Audit logs are not used enough to monitor users and other EHR activities. • No measures are in place to keep electronic patient data from improper changes. • No contingency plan exists. • Electronic exchanges of patient information are not encrypted or otherwise secured.	• Secure user IDs, passwords, and appropriate role-based access are used. • Routine audits of access and changes to EHR are conducted. • Anti-hacking and anti-malware software is installed. • Contingency plans and data backup plans are in place. • Data is encrypted.
Organizational Standards	• No breach notification and associated policies exist. • Business associate (BA) agreements have not been updated in several years.	• Regular reviews of agreements are conducted and updates made accordingly
Policies and Procedures	• Generic written policies and procedures to ensure HIPAA security compliance were purchased but not followed • The manager performs ad hoc security measures.	• Written policies and procedures are implemented and staff is trained. • Security team conducts monthly review of user activities. • Routine updates are made to document security measures.

Source: ONC 2015.

A CE or BA should also conduct a financial analysis to determine the cost of compliance, because implementing the Security Rule may be a challenge for a CE and especially for a BA who is new to the rule. Figure 12.2 provides five security components for risk management. In addition, in 2003 the Centers for Medicare and Medicaid Services (CMS) published a series of educational documents called the HIPAA Information Series to assist with the implementation of HIPAA requirements (CMS 2003). Additional educational papers specifically tailored to the Security Rule and implementation requirements were published by CMS in 2007 but now reside on the HHS ORC website (HHS n.d.). These documents continue to be useful and are supplemented by a security risk assessment tool released by HHS in 2014

(HealthIT.gov n.d.). This site contains many privacy and security resources, including a guide to privacy and security.

AHIMA has a series of information security practice briefs that contains a checklist for healthcare professionals to develop a security plan as well as guidance on policy and procedure development (AHIMA 2014).

Check Your Understanding 12.1

Instructions: Indicate whether the following statements are true or false (T or F).

1. CEs can decide to comply with only the Privacy Rule and don't have to comply with the Security Rule.
2. The goal of the Security Rule is to ensure that patient information is protected from unauthorized access, alteration, deletion, and transmission.
3. The safeguard requirements in the Privacy Rule are equivalent to compliance with the Security Rule.
4. Computers storing ePHI that are easily assessable to the public pose a vulnerability to a CE.
5. Only healthcare providers are required to comply with the Security Rule.

Components of the HIPAA Security Rule

In this section of the chapter, key components of the Security Rule are presented, including modifications to the rule as a result of the HITECH Act. The HIPAA Security Rule consists of five general rules (45 CFR 164.306) that encompass 1. general requirements, 2. flexibility of approach, 3. standards, 4. implementation specifications, and 5. maintenance of security measures. Each of the general rules will be discussed.

Section (a), General Requirements, consists of four actions that a CE and a BA must take:

- Ensure the confidentiality, integrity, and availability of all ePHI created, received, maintained, or transmitted by the CE and BA
- Protect the security or integrity of ePHI from any reasonably anticipated threats or hazards
- Protect against any reasonably anticipated uses or disclosures of ePHI not permitted or required under the Privacy Rule
- Ensure compliance with the Security Rule by its workforce

Section (b), Flexibility of Approach, allows a CE and a BA to implement the standards and their implementation specifications reasonably and appropriately. The section lists four factors to be considered when deciding on the most appropriate security measures:

- The CE's or BA's size, complexity, and capabilities
- The security capabilities of the CE's or BA's hardware and software
- The costs of security measures
- The probability and criticality of potential risks to ePHI

Section (c), Standards, requires CEs or BAs to comply with the standards as found in 45 CFR 164.308–316 and BAs to comply with all standards except 45 CFR 164.314, Organizational Requirements. The standards are divided into five categories:

- Administrative Safeguards (45 CFR 164.308)
- Physical Safeguards (45 CFR 164.310)
- Technical Safeguards (45 CFR 164.312)
- Organizational Requirements (45 CFR 164.314)
- Policies, Procedures, and Documentation (45 CFR 164.316)

The specific standards are discussed later in this chapter. The safeguards outline contains an overlap in the sections. For example, contingency plans are covered under both administrative and physical safeguards, and access controls are addressed in several standards and specifications.

Section (d), Implementation Specifications, contains detailed instructions for implementing a particular standard. Specifications are either required or addressable. Some standards include all the necessary information for implementation and are required to be implemented as published in the Security Rule. A **required specification** must be present for the CE or BA to be in compliance. Other standards are considered "addressable implementation specifications" to provide the CE or BA flexibility. The CE or BA is in compliance with an **addressable specification** if it

- Implements the addressable specification as written, or
- Implements an alternative, or
- Documents that the risk for which the addressable implementation specification was provided either does not exist in the organization or exists with a negligible probability of occurrence

The Security Rule requires CEs and BAs to evaluate their risks and vulnerabilities and implement policies and procedures to address them. Based on the risk assessment, the CE or BA must address how it plans to comply with the standards. A CE or BA may decide not to implement an addressable standard. Security protections vary based on the impact of the security measure on the individual's job and the type of healthcare organization (for example, single-entity versus multiple-hospital system). The HIPAA Security Guidance material located on the Department of Health and Human Services website includes a series of educational papers on HIPAA security guidance. This site references the National Institute of Standards and Technology (NIST) special publications as informational resources. Additionally, the HHS security risk assessment tool is useful to identify weakness in security processes and systems and to assist providers in meeting Meaningful Use incentives (HealthIT.gov, n.d.).

Section (e), Maintenance, requires a continuing review of the reasonableness and appropriateness of a CE's or BA's security measures. It requires a CE or BA to review and modify security measures if necessary and to update documentation of such measures.

Security Rule Safeguards and Requirements

The HIPAA Security Rule's third general rule, Standards, is divided into five categories. Three standards are identified as safeguards (administrative, physical, and technical); the remaining two deal with organizational requirements and policies, procedures, and documentation. An overview of the standards is presented next. Implementation specifications that are required are marked with **R**, and those that are addressable are marked with **A**.

Administrative Safeguards (614.308)

There are nine **administrative safeguard** standards (see table 12.1) (HHS 2007c):

Table 12.1 Administrative safeguards

Standard	Section	Implementation Specifications R = Required, A = Addressable	
1. Security Management Process	164.308(a)(1)	Risk Analysis	R
		Risk Management	R
		Sanction Policy	R
		Information System Activity Review	R
2. Assigned Security Responsibility	164.308(a)(2)		R
3. Workforce Security	164.308(a)(3)	Authorization and/or Supervision	A
		Workforce Clearance Procedures	A
		Termination Procedures	A
4. Information Access Management	164.308(a)(4)	Isolating Healthcare Clearinghouse Functions	R
		Access Authorization	A
		Access Establishment and Modification	A
5. Security Awareness Training	164.308(a)(5)	Security Reminders	A
		Protection from Malicious Software	A
		Log-In Monitoring	A
		Password Management	A
6. Security Incident Reporting	164.308(a)(6)	Response and Reporting	R
7. Contingency Plan	164.308(a)(7)	Data Backup Plan	R
		Disaster Recovery Plan	R
		Emergency Mode Operation Plan	R
		Testing and Revision Procedures	A
		Applications and Data Criticality Analysis	A
8. Evaluation	164.308(a)(8)		R
9. Business Associate Contracts & Other Arrangements	164.308(b)(1)	Written Contract or Other Arrangement	R

Source: HHS 2007b.

1. *Security management process (164.308 (a)(1))* requires the implementation of policies and procedures to prevent, detect, contain, and correct security violations. There are four implementation specifications in this section:

   o Risk analysis **(R)**: Must conduct an accurate and thorough assessment of potential risks and vulnerabilities to the confidentiality, integrity, and availability of ePHI

   o Risk management **(R)**: Must implement security measures that reduce risks and vulnerabilities to a reasonable and appropriate level to comply with the security standards

   o Sanction policy **(R)**: Must apply appropriate sanctions against workforce members who fail to comply with their security policies and procedures

   o Information system activity review **(R)**: Must implement procedures to regularly review records of information system activity, such as audit logs, access reports, and security incident tracking reports

2. *Assigned security responsibility (164.308 (a)(2))* requires the identification of the security official responsible for overseeing development of the organization's security policies and procedures. There are no implementation specifications with this standard (**R**).

3. *Workforce security (164.308)(a)(3))* requires the implementation of policies and procedures to ensure that all members of its workforce have appropriate access to ePHI and to prevent those workforce members who do not have access from obtaining access. There are three implementation specifications in this standard:

   ○ Authorization and/or supervision (**A**): Must have procedures for ensuring that the workforce working with ePHI has adequate authorization and/or supervision

   ○ Workforce clearance procedures (**A**): There must be a procedure to determine what access is appropriate for the workforce

   ○ Termination procedures (**A**): There must be a procedure for terminating access to ePHI when a workforce member is no longer employed or responsibilities change

4. *Information access management (164.308)(a)(4)* requires the implementation of policies and procedures for authorizing access to ePHI. There are three implementation specifications within this standard:

   ○ Isolating healthcare clearinghouse functions (**R**): May or may not apply to all healthcare organizations, but may apply to a CE or BA that is a provider and also submits claims for other providers

   ○ Access authorization (**A**): Must have policies and procedures for granting access to ePHI through a workstation, transaction, program, or other process

   ○ Access establishment and modification (**A**): Must have policies and procedures (based on the access authorization) to establish, document, review, and modify a user's right to access a workstation, transaction, program, or process

5. *Security awareness training (164.308)(a)(5)* requires the implementation of awareness and training programs for all members of its workforce:

   ○ Security reminders (**A**): Should conduct periodic security updates

   ○ Protection from malicious software (**A**): Should have procedures for guarding against, detecting, and reporting malicious software

   ○ Log-in monitoring (**A**): Should have procedures for monitoring log-in attempts and reporting discrepancies

   ○ Password management (**A**): Should have procedures for creating, changing, and safeguarding passwords

6. *Security incident reporting (164.308)(a)(6)* requires the implementation of policies and procedures to address security incidents:

   ○ Response and reporting (**R**): Identify and respond to suspect or known security incidents; mitigate, to extent practicable, harmful effects of security incidents that are known to the CE or BA; and document security incidents and their outcomes

7. *Contingency plan (164.308)(a)(7)* includes five implementation specifications:

   ○ Data backup plan (**R**): Must have procedures to create and maintain an exact retrievable copy of ePHI

- o Disaster recovery plan (**R**): Must include procedures to restore any lost data

- o Emergency mode operation plan (**R**): Must have procedures that provide for the continuation of critical business processes needed to protect ePHI while operating in emergency mode

- o Testing and revision procedures (**A**): Should have a procedure to test and modify all contingency plans periodically

- o Applications and data criticality analysis (**A**): Should assess the relative criticality of specific applications and data in support of contingency plans

8. *Evaluation (164.308)(a)(8)* requires the periodic performance of technical and nontechnical evaluations in response to environmental or operational changes affecting the security of ePHI (**R**).

9. *Business associate contracts and other arrangements (164.308)(b)*

- o CE may permit a BA to create, receive, maintain, or transmit ePHI on the CE's behalf only if the CE obtains satisfactory assurances in accordance with 164.314(a) that the BA will appropriately safeguard the information. A CE is not required to obtain such assurances from a BA that is a subcontractor.

- o BA may permit a BA that is a subcontractor to create, receive, maintain, or transmit ePHI on the BA's behalf only if the BA obtains satisfactory assurances that the subcontractor will appropriately safeguard the information.

- o Written contract or other arrangement (**R**): Must document satisfactory assurances through a written contract or other arrangement with the business associate that meets the applicable requirements of the contract

Physical Safeguards (614.310)

There are four **physical safeguard** standards (see table 12.2) (HHS 2007d):

Table 12.2 Physical safeguards

Standard	Section	Implementation Specifications R = Required, A = Addressable	
1. Facility Access Controls	164.310(a)(1)	Contingency Operations	A
		Facility Security Plan	A
		Access Control and Validation Procedures	A
		Maintenance Records	A
2. Workstation Use	164.310(b)		R
3. Workstation Security	164.310(c)		R
4. Device and Media Controls	164.310(d)(1)	Disposal	R
		Media Reuse	R
		Accountability	A
		Data Backup and Storage	A

Source: HHS 2007c.

1. *Facility access controls (164.310)(a)(1)* requires the implementation of policies and procedures to limit physical access to its electronic information systems and the facilities in which they are housed to authorized users. There are four implementation specifications within this standard:

    ○ Contingency operations (**A**): Should have procedures to allow facility access to support the restoration of lost data under the disaster recovery plan and emergency mode operations plan

    ○ Facility security plan (**A**): Must have policies and procedures to safeguard the facility and equipment from unauthorized access, tampering, and theft

    ○ Access control and validation procedures (**A**): Should have procedures to control and validate access to facilities based on users' roles or functions

    ○ Maintenance records (**A**): Should have policies and procedures to document repairs and modifications to the physical components of a facility as they relate to security

2. *Workstation use (164.310)(b)* requires the implementation of policies and procedures that specify the proper functions to be performed, the manner in which those functions are to be performed, and the physical attributes of the surroundings of a specific workstation or class of workstation that can be used to access ePHI (**R**).

3. *Workstation security (164.310)(c)* requires the implementation of physical safeguards for all workstations that are used to access ePHI and to restrict access to authorized users (**R**).

4. *Device and media controls (164.310)(d)(1)* requires the implementation of policies and procedures for the removal of hardware and electronic media that contain ePHI into and out of a facility, as well as movement within a facility. There are four implementation specifications with this standard:

    ○ Disposal (**R**): Must have policies and procedures for the final disposition of ePHI and/or hardware or electronic media on which it is stored

    ○ Media reuse (**R**): Must have procedures for removal of ePHI from electronic media before the media can be reused

    ○ Accountability (**A**): Must maintain a record of movements of hardware and electronic media and any person responsible for it

    ○ Data backup and storage (**A**): Must create a retrievable, exact copy of ePHI, when needed, before movement of equipment

Technical Safeguards (164.312)

There are five **technical safeguard** standards (see table 12.3) (HHS 2007e):

Table 12.3 Technical safeguards

Standard	Section	Implementation Specifications R = Required, A = Addressable	
1. Access Control	164.312(a)(1)	Unique User Identification	R
		Emergency Access Procedure	R
		Automatic Log-off	A
		Encryption and Decryption	A
2. Audit Controls	164.312(b)		R

(continued)

Table 12.3. Technical safeguards (continued)

Standard	Section	Implementation Specifications R = Required, A = Addressable	
3. Integrity	164.312(c)(1)	Mechanism to Authenticate Electronic Protected Health Information	A
4. Person or Entity Authentication	164.312(d)		R
5. Transmission Security	164.312(e)(1)	Integrity Controls	A
		Encryption	A

Source: HHS 2007c.

1. *Access control (164.312)(a)(1)* requires the implementation of technical policies and procedures for electronic information systems that maintain ePHI to allow access only to those persons or software programs that have been granted access rights as specified in the administrative safeguards. There are four implementation specifications with this standard:

   o Unique user identification (**R**): Must assign a unique name or number for identifying and tracking user identity

   o Emergency access procedure (**R**): Must establish procedures for obtaining necessary ePHI in an emergency

   o **Automatic log-off** (**A**): Must implement electronic processes that terminate an electronic session after a predetermined time of inactivity

   o **Encryption** and decryption (**A**): Should implement a mechanism to encrypt and decrypt ePHI as needed

2. *Audit controls (164.312)(b)* requires the implementation of hardware, software, and/or procedures that record and examine activity in the information systems that contain ePHI (**R**).

3. *Integrity (164.312)(c)(1)* requires the implementation of policies and procedures to protect ePHI from improper alteration or destruction and a corroborating electronic mechanism (**A**).

4. *Person or entity authentication (164.312)(d)* requires the implementation of procedures to verify that a person or entity seeking access to ePHI is the person or entity they claim to be (**R**).

5. *Transmission security (164.312)(e)(1)* requires the implementation of technical measures to guard against unauthorized access to ePHI that is transmitted across a network. There are two implementation specifications with this standard:

   o Integrity controls (**A**): Must implement security measures to ensure that electronically transmitted ePHI is not improperly modified without detection

   o Encryption (**A**): Should encrypt ePHI whenever it is deemed appropriate

Organizational Requirements (164.314)

Organizational requirements include two standards (see table 12.4) (HHS 2007f):

Table 12.4 Organizational requirements

Standard	Section	Implementation Specifications R = Required, A = Addressable	
1. Business Associate Contracts or Other Arrangements	164.314(a)(1)	Business Associate	R
		Other Arrangements	R
2. Group Health Plans	164.314(b)(1)	Implementation Specifications	R

Source: HHS 2007e.

1. *Business associate contracts or other arrangements (164.314)(a)(1)* as required by 164.308(b)(4) must meet the requirements of (a)(2)(i-iii) as applicable. There are three implementation specifications:

   ○ Business associate contracts (**R**): Contract must provide that BA complies with applicable requirements of subpart and ensure that subcontractors that create, receive, maintain, or transmit ePHI on behalf of BA agree to comply with the applicable requirements by entering into a contract or arrangement that complies with this section; must report to CE any security incident of which it becomes aware, including breaches of unsecured PHI

   ○ Other arrangements (**R**): CE is in compliance if it has another arrangement in place that meets requirements of 164.504(e)(3)

   ○ Business associate contracts with subcontractors (**R**): Requirements as previously required between a CE and a BA apply to the contract or arrangement between a BA and a subcontractor in the same manner

2. *Group health plans (164.314)(b)* requires the plan sponsor to reasonably and appropriately safeguard the confidentiality, integrity, and availability of ePHI. There is one implementation specification:

   Plan document (**R**): Plan documents of group health plan must require sponsor to implement administrative, physical, and technical safeguards that protect the confidentiality, integrity, and availability of ePHI that it creates, receives, maintains, or transmits on behalf of the group plan; separation of ePHI is supported by security measures; ensure that any agent to whom it provides information agrees to implement security measures to protect information and report to the health plan any security incident of which it is aware

Policies, Procedures, and Documentation (164.316)

There are two standards for policies, procedures, and documentation but no implementation specifications (see table 12.5) (HHS 2007f):

1. *Policies and procedures (164.316)(a)* requires the establishment and implementation of policies and procedures to comply with the standards, implementation specifications, and other requirements. A CE or BA may change its policies and procedures at any time, provided that those changes are documented and implemented and in compliance with the Security Rule.

Table 12.5 Policies, procedures, and documentation requirements

Standard	Section	Implementation Specifications R = Required, A = Addressable	
1. Policies and Procedures	164.316(a)	Not Applicable	
2. Documentation	164.316(b)(1)	Time Limit	R
		Availability	R
		Updates	R

Source: HHS 2007e.

2. *Documentation (164.316)(b)* requires the maintenance of the policies and procedures imple-mented to comply with the Security Rule in written form. There are three implementation specifications:

   o Time limit (**R**): Must retain the documentation for six years from the date of its creation or the date when it was last in effect, whichever is later

   o Availability (**R**): Must make the documentation available to those persons responsible for implementing the policies and procedures

   o Updates (**R**): Must review the documentation periodically and update it as needed

Security Officer Designation

The administrative safeguards of the Security Rule (45 CFR 164.308(a)(2)) contain an implementation specification that requires a single individual to be responsible for overseeing the information security program. This individual is often designated the **chief security officer**. This parallels the Privacy Rule, which requires an individual in the organization to be designated responsible for overseeing privacy policies and procedures. Generally, this person is identified as a security officer or chief security officer. The chief security officer may report to the chief information officer (CIO) or another administrator in the healthcare organization. The role of security officer may be 100 percent of an individual's job respon-sibilities or only a fraction, depending on the size of the organization and the scope of its use of health information technology and information systems. Regardless of the actual reporting structure, the chief security officer must be given authority to effectively manage the security program, apply sanctions, and influence employees. **Security officers** must periodically evaluate their organization's electronic informa-tion systems and networks for proper technical controls and processes. It is important to remember the physical security safeguards and ensure they are considered as frequently as network security, because one server room door left unlocked can cause more loss of ePHI than an external intrusion.

Enforcement and Penalties for Noncompliance

On February 16, 2006, the HHS published a final rule for imposing civil monetary penalties on CEs that violate any of the HIPAA administrative simplification requirements (HHS 2006b). As previously mentioned, oversight and enforcement of the Security Rule was the responsibility of CMS, but as of July 27, 2009, the responsibility transitioned to the OCR (HHS 2010c). Notable changes to enforcement and penalty provisions for HIPAA have occurred because of the passage of the HITECH Act, as discussed in chapter 10. These revisions are essentially the same for both the Privacy and Security Rules.

To reiterate, the HITECH Act established four categories of violations that reflect increasing levels of culpability, with corresponding tiers of penalty amounts. The nature and extent of both the violation and the harm are used to determine the amount assessed within each range. The OCR may choose to pursue corrective action without assessing penalties for unknowing violations, but penalties are mandatory in all other categories. Penalty monies collected will support further enforcement efforts (Dennis 2010).

As with the Privacy Rule, the enforcement of penalties for noncompliance begins with a complaint from a patient, some other consumer, or an employee, or by a CE or BA compliance review results. Individuals may file a formal complaint with the OCR if they believe a CE or BA has violated the Security Rule. If OCR accepts the complaint, it will investigate. If it determines that the CE or BA is not in compliance, it will work with the entity to obtain voluntary compliance, corrective action, or resolution agreement. If the entity does not act to resolve the issue, OCR may impose civil monetary penalties. If OCR believes that the actions of the entity are a violation of the criminal provision of HIPAA (42 USC 1320d-6), OCR may refer the complaint to the Department of Justice. Refer to figure 11.1 for the OCR flow chart of the Privacy and Security Rule Complaint Process. HITECH has also authorized random audits, which serve to detect noncompliance. These were discussed in chapter 10.

The HHS website provides information about the department's compliance and enforcement efforts, including HHS enforcement activities, frequency of complaint types, and corrective actions resulting from consumer complaints (HHS 2010b, 2010c). Additionally, the director of HHS OCR has the authority to issue subpoenas as part of the investigation of alleged HIPAA violations.

Currently, penalties for violations range as follows and can increase significantly for each violation, with a cap of $1.5 million for identical violations within each violation category in a calendar year:

- $100–$50,000 per violation for unknowing violations
- $1,000–$50,000 per violation if due to reasonable cause and not willful neglect
- $10,000–$50,000 per violation if due to willful neglect and corrected within 30 days of discovery
- $50,000 or more per violation if due to willful neglect and not corrected as required (HHS 2009b)

Check Your Understanding 12.2

Instructions: Indicate whether the following statements are true or false (T or F).

1. The Security Rule contains provisions that CEs can ignore.
2. Security awareness training is required every two years.
3. The Security Rule is completely technical and requires computer programmers to address.
4. The Security Rule contains both required and addressable standards.

Disaster planning and recovery

Disaster planning and recovery are components of the administrative and physical safeguard standards of the HIPAA Security Rule. The specific implementation specifications have been outlined previously in the chapter. These elements should become part of the CE and BA risk analysis. The Security Rule does not prescribe a method for the risk analysis; however, HHS published a tool to help providers with HIPAA compliance (HHS 2014). This tool contains a security risk assessment (SRA) to guide the process, as well as a report that can be provided to auditors. The SRA is a required component for compliance with HIPAA as well as for the Meaningful Use program. It is also useful to systematically identify gaps in processes, policies, or procedures. Interested parties should sign up for the alerts from the Office of the

National Coordinator as the tool and other resources are published (HHS n.d.). AHIMA has a Disaster Planning and Recovery Toolkit that outlines steps to draft a business continuity plan including communications, management, protecting health information, use and disclosure of health information, and recovery (AHIMA 2013b). The toolkit also contains a sample contingency plan, staff competency list, immediate and short-term concerns checklist and sample emergency privilege application and release form. HHS has many cybersecurity resources including a contingency planning tutorial. These resources are based on the National Institute of Standards and Technology (NIST) Framework for Improving Critical Infrastructure Cybersecurity (NIST 2014) which guides an analysis of cybersecurity risks that allow organizations to prioritize investments in managing cybersecurity risks.

Scenario 12

Acme medical center has recently acquired five large physician practices in the region, and you, as part of the team merging the system and processes into the medical center procedures, are evaluating the privacy and security concerns. During the evaluation it is discovered that the various physician practices have several different types of digital copiers that they use in the offices.

1. What potential HIPAA violation(s) can be identified in the scenario?

2. Is there a way to mitigate the risks for a potential HIPAA violation(s)?

3. What advice does the OCR have that can be utilized to guide this process?

References

AHIMA. 2013a. Analysis of Modifications to the HIPAA Privacy, Security, Enforcement, and Breach Notification Rules Under the Health Information Technology for Economic and Clinical Health Act and the Genetic Information Nondiscrimination Act; Other Modifications to the HIPAA Rules. http://www.ahima.org.

AHIMA. 2013b. *Disaster Planning and Recovery Toolkit*. Chicago: AHIMA Press

AHIMA. 2014. Information security—An overview (updated). Chicago: AHIMA. http://bok.ahima.org/doc?oid=300244#.WNAdI_krK70

Centers for Medicare and Medicaid Services. 2003. HIPAA Information Series for Providers. http://www.cms.gov/.

Dennis, J. 2010. *Privacy: The Impact of ARRA, HITECH, and Other Policy Initiatives*. Chicago: AHIMA.

Department of Health and Human Services. 2003. Health insurance reform: Security standards. Final rule. 45 CFR 160, 162, and 164. *Federal Register* 68(34):8333–8381.

Department of Health and Human Services. 2006a (December). HIPAA security guidance. Remote access. http://www.hhs.gov/ocr/.

Department of Health and Human Services. 2006b. HIPAA administrative simplification: Enforcement; Final rule. 45 CFR 160 and 164. *Federal Register* 71(32):8390–8433.

Department of Health and Human Services. 2007a. HIPAA security series. Security 101 for covered entities. 2(1). http://www.hhs.gov/ocr/.

Department of Health and Human Services. 2007b. HIPAA security series. Basics of risk analysis and risk management. 2(6). http://www.hhs.gov/ocr/.

Department of Health and Human Services. 2007c. HIPAA security series #2. Security standards: Administrative safeguards. 2(2). http://www.hhs.gov/ocr/.

Department of Health and Human Services. 2007d. HIPAA security series #3. Security standards: Physical safeguards. 2(3). http://www.hhs.gov/ocr/.

Department of Health and Human Services. 2007e. HIPAA security series #4. Security standards: Technical safeguards. 2(4). http://www.hhs.gov/ocr/.

Department of Health and Human Services. 2007f. HIPAA security series #5. Organizational, policies and procedures and documentation requirements. 2(5). http://www.hhs.gov/ocr/.

Department of Health and Human Services. 2009a. News release: HHS delegates authority for the HIPAA Security Rule to Office for Civil Rights. http://www.hhs.gov/.

Department of Health and Human Services. 2009b. HIPAA administrative simplification enforcement. 45 CFR Parts 160. *Federal Register* 74(209):56123–56131.

Department of Health and Human Services. 2010a. Modifications to the HIPAA Privacy, Security, and Enforcement Rules under the Health Information Technology for Economic and Clinical Health Act; Proposed rule. 45 CFR Parts 160 and 164. *Federal Register* 75(134):40868–40924.

Department of Health and Human Services. 2010b. Office for Civil Rights. Guidance on risk analysis requirements under the HIPAA Security Rule. http://www.hhs.gov/ocr/.

Department of Health and Human Services. 2010c. Office for Civil Rights. HIPAA Enforcement Rule. http://www.hhs.gov/ocr/.

Department of Health and Human Services. n.d. Office for Civil Rights. Security Rule guidance material. http://www.hhs.gov/ocr/.

Department of Health and Human Services. 2014. Office of the National Coordinator for Health Information Technology Security Risk Assessment (SRA) Tool. https://www.healthit.gov/sites/default/files/risk_assessment_user_guide_final_3_26_2014.pdf.

Office of the National Coordinator for Health Information Technology. 2015 (April). Guide to Privacy and Security of Electronic Health Information, version 2.0. https://www.healthit.gov/sites/default/files/pdf/privacy/privacy-and-security-guide.pdf.

HealthIT.gov. Security risk assessment. https://www.healthit.gov/providers-professionals/security-risk-assessment.

National Institute of Standards and Technology (NIST) 2014. Framework for Improving Critical Infrastructure Cybersecurity. Version 1.0. http://www.nist.gov/cyberframework/upload/cybersecurity-framework-021214.pdf.

Scholl, M., K. Stine, J. Hash, P. Bowen, A. Johnson, C. Smith, and D. Steinbery. 2008. An introductory resource guide for implementing the Health Insurance Portability and Accountability Act (HIPAA) Security Rule. Gaithersburg, MD: National Institute of Standards and Technology. http://www.hhs.gov/ocr/.

Cases, Statutes, and Regulations Cited

45 CFR 160: Definitions. 2006.

45 CFR 160.103: Definitions. 2006.

45 CFR 162: Administrative requirements. 2006.

45 CFR 164: Security and privacy. 2006.

45 CFR 164.304: Definitions. 2006.

45 CFR 164.306: General rules. 2006.

45 CFR 164.308: Administrative safeguards. 2006.

45 CFR 164.308(a)(1): Security management functions. 2006.

45 CFR 164.308(a)(2): Assigned security responsibility. 2006.

45 CFR 164.308(a)(3): Workforce security. 2006.

45 CFR 164.308(a)(4): Information access management. 2006.

45 CFR 164.308(a)(5): Security awareness and training. 2006.

45 CFR 164.308(a)(6): Security incident reporting. 2006.

45 CFR 164.308(a)(7): Contingency plan. 2006.

45 CFR 164.308(a)(8): Evaluation. 2006.

45 CFR 164.308(b)(1): Business associate contracts and other arrangements. 2006.

45 CFR 164.310: Physical safeguards. 2006.

45 CFR 164.310(a)(1): Facility access controls. 2006.

45 CFR 164.310(b): Workstation use. 2006.

45 CFR 164.310(c): Workstation security. 2006.

45 CFR 164.310(d)(1): Device and media controls. 2006.

45 CFR 164.312: Technical safeguards. 2006.

45 CFR 164.312(a)(1): Access control. 2006.

45 CFR 164.312(b): Audit controls. 2006.

45 CFR 164.312(c)(1): Integrity. 2006.

45 CFR 164.312(d): Person or entity authentication. 2006.

45 CFR 164.312(e)(1): Transmission security. 2006.

45 CFR 164.314: Organizational requirements. 2006.

45 CFR 164.314(a): Business associate contracts or other arrangements. 2006.

45 CFR 164.314(b): Group health plans. 2006.

45 CFR 164.316: Policies, procedures, and documentation. 2006.

45 CFR 164.316(a): Policies and procedures. 2006.

45 CFR 164.316(b): Documentation. 2006.

42 USC 1320d-6: Wrongful disclosure of individually identifiable health information.

American Recovery and Reinvestment Act of 2009, Title XIII—Health Information Technology, Subtitle D. Public Law 111-5.

Resources

HealthIT.gov. 2014. Health IT videos: Security risk analysis. https://www.healthit.gov/providers-professionals/video/security-risk-analysis.

Security Threats and Controls

Keith Olenik, MA, RHIA, CHP;

Rebecca B. Reynolds, EdD, MHA, CHPS, RHIA, FAHIMA

Learning Objectives

- Identify potential internal and external security threats, distinguishing human threats from natural and environmental threats and describing vulnerabilities
- List mechanisms to prevent and detect identity theft
- Identify types of medical identity theft and mechanisms to prevent, detect, and mitigate such theft
- Distinguish access controls from systems controls and provide examples of each
- Recognize the importance of contingency planning or disaster recovery planning in securing health information

Key Terms

- Audit trail
- Authentication
- Automatic log-off
- Biometric identification systems
- Context-based access control (CBAC)
- Contingency planning
- Creditor
- Cryptography
- Cyber attack
- Cybersecurity
- Data encryption
- Disaster recovery planning
- Entity authentication
- External security threat
- Fair and Accurate Credit Transactions Act (FACTA)
- Federal Information Processing Standards (FIPS)
- Firewall
- Identity and access management (IAM)
- Identity theft
- Information system
- Intentional threats
- Internal security threat
- Medical identity theft
- Password
- Phishing
- Pretty good privacy (PGP)
- Ransomware
- Red flag
- Red Flags Rule
- Role-based access control (RBAC)
- Social media
- Telehealth
- Telemedicine
- Termination of access
- Tokens
- Trojan horse
- Unintentional threats
- Unique identifier
- User-based access control (UBAC)
- Viruses
- Vulnerabilities
- Wired equivalent privacy (WEP)
- Worm

To protect the privacy and security of patient information, a healthcare organization must address threats to the information and implement ways to secure it from wrongful access. The Health Insurance Portability and Accountability Act (HIPAA) Security Rule requires that selected security safeguards be implemented to protect electronic protected health information (ePHI). Although the rule is written to be technology neutral, common controls can be employed to meet the required standards. This chapter discusses not only the threats to the security of ePHI, such as identity and medical identity theft, but also the more common mechanisms used to protect ePHI in terms of access and systems controls. Suggestions for preventing ePHI theft are offered, along with issues to consider when transmitting ePHI via fax, e-mail, internet, or other wireless devices. The importance of establishing policies and procedures for a complete security program is discussed as well as the importance of contingency or disaster recovery planning. Privacy and security of ePHI are intertwined, thus making it difficult to protect the privacy of ePHI without some form of security in place. Because of the quickly changing security and cybersecurity landscape, it is important for the health information management and informatics professional to be aware of the security resources available.

In addition to the HIPAA Privacy and Security rules, health information management and informatics professionals should be aware of the National Institute of Standards and Technology (NIST) which has several publications that are utilized for information security by business, industry and governmental agencies. The security control structure of these recommendations is similar to the HIPAA Security Rule and make of the identifiers users by NIST mirror those in the HIPAA Security Rule. This NIST publication also links to international information security standards and systems requirements that provide great reference and guidance for security compliance.

NIST has published a "Framework for Improving Critical Infrastructure Cybersecurity Version 1.0." which developed from the Executive Order 13636 "Improving Critical Infrastructure Cybersecurity" (NIST 2014). The NIST framework is neither mandatory nor healthcare specific, but is designed to protect infrastructure and, ultimately, the privacy of an individual's data, which may be compromised.

The Office of Homeland Security also has a cybersecurity program and is responsible for the National Cybersecurity Protection System, Network Security Deployment, Federal Network Resilience as promulgated by the Federal Information Security Modernization Act of 2014 (FISMA).

The **Federal Information Processing Standards (FIPS)** are issued by NIST with approval of the US Secretary of Commerce under the authority of FISMA. FIPS PUB 140-2 and 140-1 outline approved security functions, approved protection profiles, approved random number generator and approved key establishment techniques. These standards are used by non-military governmental agencies and government contractors including the National Institute of Health (NIH) (NIST 2001).

Internal and External Security Threats

In general, threats to the privacy and security of health information fall into two broad categories: human threats and natural or environmental threats. Both types can be either **internal security threats** or **external security threats**. Internal human threats are caused by individuals within the organization, such as employees, whereas external human threats are caused by individuals outside the organization. Internal natural or environmental threats include fire or water damage that originates within the organization, whereas external natural or environmental threats include flooding, lightning, and tornadoes. This section of the chapter provides an overview of human threats and natural or environmental threats. It then goes into greater detail to discuss the human threats of identity theft and medical identity theft. Criminal attacks are now the leading cause of data breach for healthcare entities (Ponemon 2015b). In the past five years there has been a shift from concern over lost or stolen devices, although this continues to be a primary cause of data breaches, **cyber attacks** are now the leading concern. A criminal or cyber attack is a deliberate and often systematic attempt to gain unauthorized access to a device or network. Although typically thought of as an outside attack, these can also be internal attacks. All healthcare organizations are subject to these breaches with small to medium sized being the most targeted (HHS 2014).

Vulnerabilities

Vulnerabilities are weaknesses that impact security of systems and networks. A vulnerability can be something physical like a server sitting in an unlocked room or it might be a software weakness. In order for the vulnerability to be exploited it must be known to others. The path that is taken to exploit the vulnerability is a threat vector. Threats vectors can be e-mails, external hardware, mobile devices, lack of patch management and any way that someone can gain access to take advantage of the vulnerability. Potential attack vectors can be a lack of proper systems configuration, unsecured connections allowing entry through an unrelated system like the HVAC which was the major attack vector from the Target network attack. Other potential sources for attack include lapses in updating operating systems and browsers and the existence of peer-to-peer programs including Bluetooth, music sharing or other sharing software on any device that is connected to the network. Identifying potential vulnerabilities is part of the risk mitigation planning. As society continues to use technology and it advances, it is challenging to identify all of the risks and work to minimize or eliminate security threats.

Human Threats

Impermissible uses and disclosures have been the number one issue in closed cases with corrective actions investigated by the OCR since 2004. However, theft continues to be the largest general cause of breaches from 2009-2012 (HHS 2014). Both of these are examples of human threats to patient information. Human threats were once individuals but now are sophisticated and organized hacking activities. Hacking takes many forms which could include disgruntled or former employees, angry patients or family members, thieves, cyber espionage and terrorists (PWC 2016).

Human threats can be unintentional or intentional. **Unintentional threats** include employee errors that may result from lack of training in proper system use. When users share their password, respond to phishing, or download information from a non-secure Internet site, for example, they create the potential for a breach in security. **Phishing** is when someone impersonates a business or other known entity to attempt to have the user provide personal information (Federal Trade Commission 2011). These may be in an e-mail, text message or a pop-up on a website. **Intentional threats** include attacks from outside the network or internal malicious actions by workforce members. Computer viruses were once the most common and virulent forms of intentional computer tampering; however, this has been replaced by large scale hacking. These attacks include embedded malware and now **ransomware** which does not require users to click or open links (HHS 2016). Ransomware is distinct from malware in that it attempts to deny access to a user's data, by encrypting the data with a key known only to the hacker. When the ransom is paid, the user is given a decryption key which allows access to the user's data (HHS 2016). They pose a serious threat to electronic patient data and healthcare applications. Intentional threats also include theft, intentional alteration of data, and intentional destruction of data. The culprit of an intentional act could be a disgruntled employee, a computer hacker, or a prankster.

Some of the more common forms of internal breaches to security across all industries are the installation or use of unauthorized software, use of the organization's computing resources for illegal or illicit communications or activities (for example, porn surfing, e-mail harassment), and the use of the organization's computing resources for personal profit. With the increased use of information technology, external security breaches are on the rise from external hackers. The Ponemon Institute (2015b) published the results of an in-depth study on actual data loss and data theft experienced by 90 healthcare organizations and 88 business associates. The results indicated that

- Data breaches were costing the industry $6 billion and provider organizations, approximately $2.1 million, with the average cost for business associates at $1 million
- Despite these numbers, half of all organizations have little or no confidence in their ability to detect all patient data loss or theft

For the first time, criminal attacks are the number one cause of data breaches in healthcare. Criminal attacks on healthcare organizations are up 125 percent compared to five years ago. In fact, 45 percent of healthcare organizations say the root cause of the data breach was a criminal attack, and 12 percent say it was due to a malicious insider. In the case of business associates, 39 percent say a criminal attacker caused the breach, and 10 percent say it was due to a malicious insider. The percentage of criminal-based security incidents is even higher; for instance, web-borne malware attacks caused security incidents for 78 percent of healthcare organizations and 82 percent for business associates. However, despite an increase in external threats, only 40 percent of healthcare organizations and 35 percent of business associates reported concern about cyber attackers (Ponemon 2015b). Unfortunately, the number of hackers and the costs to the healthcare community continue to escalate. Figure 13.1 provides an example of an internal unintentional security breach and an intentional external breach.

Natural and Environmental Threats

Natural and environmental threats, such as hurricanes, tornados, floods, fire, power surges, lightning, and water damage, can be significant factors in the loss of protected health information (PHI), whether in electronic or paper format. Healthcare providers must have a process in place for protecting and recovering

Figure 13.1 Security breach examples

Breach Due to Employee Error

In May 2014, New York-Presbyterian Hospital and Columbia University agreed to a settlement of $4.8 million for violating HIPAA Privacy and Security Rules related to the inadvertent release PHI on 6,800 patients in 2010. The breach occurred when a physician employed by Columbia University developed applications for both hospitals attempted to deactivate a personally owned computer server on the network containing information on hospital patients. Because of a lack of technical safeguards, deactivation of the server resulted in ePHI being accessible on internet search engines. The entities learned of the breach after receiving a complaint from an individual who found the ePHI of the individual's deceased partner, a former patient at NY Presbyterian, on the Internet. OCR's investigation also found that neither NY Presbyterian nor Columbia University made efforts before the breach to ensure that the server was secure and that it contained appropriate software protections. Neither entity had developed an adequate risk management plan that addressed the potential threats and hazards to the security of ePHI (HHS 2014).

Breach Due to Cyber Attack

Anthem, one of the nation's largest health insurers, discovered on January 29, 2015, that the personal information of tens of millions of its customers and employees, including its chief executive, was the subject of a "very sophisticated external cyberattack." The company worked with the Federal Bureau of Investigation (FBI) and also hired a well-known cybersecurity firm to look into vulnerabilities of its computer system. The company said it would begin notifying members in the coming weeks. In a statement, the FBI said that it was investigating the breach, and that people should alert officials to any possible instances of identity theft.

The company, through its investigation into the exact scope of the attack, was able to determine that hackers were able to breach a database that contained as many as 80 million records of current and former customers and employees. The information accessed included names, Social Security numbers, birthdays, addresses, e-mail and employment information, including income data. Anthem said no credit card information had been stolen, and it emphasized that it did not believe medical information like insurance claims or test results were compromised. It said hospital and doctor information was also not believed to have been taken.

Still, the attack, which was first reported by *The Wall Street Journal*, could be the largest breach of a healthcare company to date, and one of the largest ever of customer information. In a letter to the company's members, Joseph R. Swedish, Anthem's chief executive, said he wanted "to personally apologize" for the security breach. He said his own personal information had been accessed and emphasized that the company at the time was working around the clock to do everything possible to further secure the data." (Abelson and Goldstein 2015).

their information, not only to adhere to HIPAA and HITECH requirements but also to comply with Joint Commission standards.

Public health officials have learned many lessons from perhaps the worst public health disaster in US history in regard to protecting PHI. As a result of Hurricane Katrina, which struck New Orleans and the surrounding states in 2005, over a million people were displaced. Patient records, especially paper records, of many healthcare providers were lost, destroyed, or rendered inaccessible. Some providers that used electronic health records (EHRs), however, were able to recover patient records. Certain parts of the HIPAA Privacy Rule had to be suspended at the time to allow healthcare providers to treat displaced persons without fear of breaking the law. The disaster also brought attention to the importance of disaster recovery and contingency planning, which is now part of the HIPAA Security Rule. A more detailed discussion of contingency planning and disaster recovery planning appears later.

Identity Theft and Medical Identity Theft

Identity theft is a fast-growing crime made possible for the most part by the ease with which information can be stolen in electronic environments. Because patient demographic, financial, and healthcare information is collected, transmitted, and maintained in the course of operations of a healthcare provider, that provider has an obligation to protect such information. Employees or disgruntled former employees may be the source of patient identity theft. For example, in 2004, Richard Gibson, an employee of the Seattle Cancer Center Alliance, was convicted of using a patient's name, Social Security number, and date of birth to obtain four credit cards, which he used to purchase $9,100 worth of personal items. Gibson was convicted under the HIPAA Privacy Rule, sentenced to 16 months in prison (plus three years of supervised release), and ordered to pay more than $9,000 in restitution (Health Data Management 2004). This is the first of many cases, with increasing value of health information sold on the black market. Health information has become more valuable than stolen credit card data (NPR 2015). The World Privacy Forum (WPF) has an interactive map of the United States that shows known cases of medical identity theft by city from 2008 to 2009, as reported to the Federal Trade Commission (FTC) (WPF n.d.).

In October 1998, Congress passed the Identity Theft and Assumption Deterrence Act (18 USC 1028) (Identity Theft Act), making it a federal crime to commit an act of identity theft. The act defines identity theft as when someone "knowingly transfers or uses, without lawful authority, a means of identification of another person with the intent to commit, or aid or abet, any unlawful activity that constitutes a violation of federal law, or that constitutes a felony under any applicable state or local law" (18 USC 1028). The FTC has oversight responsibility for identity theft regulations and requires financial institutions and creditors to develop and implement written identity theft prevention programs. It is the clearinghouse for complaints related to identity theft. If a person is found guilty of identity theft, the maximum penalty is 15 years in prison and up to $250,000 in fines. Unfortunately, identity theft has not been confined to just the wrongful use of someone's identity for financial gain. In recent years, there has been an increase in medical identity theft.

Like identity theft, **medical identity theft** is a crime. It is a type of identity theft and a type of financial fraud that involves the inappropriate or unauthorized misrepresentation of one's identity. More specifically medical identity theft is defined as the fraudulent use of an individual's PHI and personally identifiable information or more simply the stealing of an individual's PHI (Gordon 2013). Studies indicate instances of medical identity theft have risen from 1.43 million to 1.85 million over a two-year period. Its victims include patients, providers, and insurers. The lion's share of medical identity theft victims can expect to pay upwards of $13,500 to resolve the crime. What's more, about 50 percent of consumers say they would find another healthcare provider if they were concerned about the security of their medical records (Ponemon 2015a).

The WPF has identified two primary types of medical identity theft (WPF n.d.). The first type is the use of a person's name and, at times, other identifiers (for example, Social Security number), without the knowledge or consent of the victim, to obtain medical services or goods. In a subset of this first type, a person's name or other identifier may be used with that individual's consent but without the individual's full understanding of the ramifications (for example, allowing an uninsured family member to use one's insurance card so that medical services will be covered). The second type is the use of a person's identity to obtain medical services by falsifying claims for medical services.

Medical identity theft can be the result of either internal or external forces. Electronic health records have improved the ability to share information, but this has also increased exposure to data making it more vulnerable. Data breaches have impacted almost 90 percent of all healthcare organizations and put patient data at risk (Ponemon 2015b). Internal medical identity theft is committed by organization insiders, such as clinical or administrative staff with access to patient information. Sophisticated crime rings may infiltrate an organization to commit internal medical identity theft, posing or functioning as staff while stealing patient-identifying information until they are either caught or exit the organization undetected. External threats are causing a greater risk for healthcare organizations due to increased threats of ransomware, malware, and denial-of-service (DOS) attacks (Ponemon 2015b). There is concern that the EHR may assist perpetrators by granting them broad access to patient information.

Implications of Medical Identity Theft

Medical identity theft is distinguished from other types of identity theft because it creates negative consequences to both the victim's financial status and medical information. Medical identity theft impacts patients, providers, and payers. A victim may face financial consequences, such as debt collection, monetary losses, damaged credit, and insurance denials (if lifetime caps are reached). Ponemon (2015a) found that 89 percent of victims said the identity theft "affected their reputation mainly because of embarrassments due to disclosure of sensitive personal health conditions." What's more, nearly 20 percent said it caused them to miss out on career opportunities (Ponemon 2015a). A victim could also receive improper medical treatment if incorrect medical information (that of the perpetrator) is inserted in the victim's health record. For example, if the medical identity theft victim is given a blood transfusion based on the different, and incompatible, blood type of a perpetrator whose medical information was wrongfully entered into the victim's health record, the result could be life-threatening.

Although many states have data breach notification laws, very few address medical information, and while financial industry regulations protect consumers against lost or stolen credit cards, no corollary exists for medical identity theft victims. HIPAA presently does not address medical identity theft. Furthermore, the right to request an accounting of disclosures does not detect the insertion of a perpetrator's medical information into a victim's health record. Under the HITECH Act as originally written, healthcare entities with EHRs would be required to provide an accounting of payment disclosures (upon patient request), which could detect disclosures to payers for services the victim did not receive (AHIMA 2013b). However, for detection to occur via either an accounting of disclosures or an access report, a victim must take the initiative to request an accounting or access report and study the disclosures and other access that occurred. In the absence of a suspicion of illicit activity involving the victim's medical account, such a request may not occur.

Of greater significance is the HITECH breach notification requirement, which requires patients to be notified if their PHI has been breached. This has the potential to inform victims of medical identity theft. Also, HITECH states personal health record vendors and third-party service providers that serve as business associates are subject to the breach notification requirement (AHIMA 2013b). In the absence of a change to accounting of disclosures the notification of a breach is much more proactive so the patient can take action to mitigate any ramifications of inappropriate access to their information.

Fair and Accurate Credit Transactions Act and the Red Flags Rule

As previously mentioned, the FTC has oversight responsibility for identity theft issues. In 2007, Identity Theft Red Flags and Address Discrepancies Rules were enacted as part of the federal **Fair and Accurate Credit Transactions Act** (FACTA) of 2003. FACTA requires financial institutions and creditors to develop and implement written identity theft programs that identify, detect, and respond to red flags that may signal the presence of identity theft. A **red flag** is defined as a "pattern, practice, or specific activity that could indicate identity theft" (Gellman and Dixon 2009, 4). Although this law does not specifically address medical identity theft, it is significant because many healthcare organizations meet the definition of **creditor,** which is anyone who regularly, and in the ordinary course of business, meets one of the following criteria:

- Obtains or uses consumer reports in connection with a credit transaction
- Furnishes information to consumer reporting agencies in connection with a credit transaction
- Advances funds to, or on behalf of, someone (except for funds for expenses that are incidental to a service provided by the creditor to that person)

The compliance date for the **Red Flags Rule** was December 31, 2010. The law consists of five categories of red flags (16 CFR Part 681), which include the following:

- Alerts, notifications, or warnings from a consumer reporting agency
- Suspicious documents
- Suspicious personally identifying information such as a suspicious address
- Unusual use of, or suspicious activity relating to, a covered account
- Notices from customers, victims of identity theft, law enforcement authorities, or other businesses about possible identity theft in connection with an account

The red flags should be used as triggers to alert an organization that an identity theft problem may exist. To assist healthcare providers that are creditors and may also be victims of medical identity theft, the World Privacy Forum recommends that providers incorporate red flags specifically related to patients and insurers into their policies and procedures for preventing, detecting, and mitigating theft. See figure 13.2 for examples of red flags for healthcare providers.

Prevention, Detection, and Mitigation of Medical Identity Theft

Healthcare organizations can be victimized by both identity theft and, more specifically, medical identity theft. As a result, they need to take appropriate steps to prevent and detect both crimes, whether committed by their employees, business partners, or others.

The following steps can be taken to proactively mitigate medical identity theft:

- Build awareness by providing education to all staff about the issue and impacts.

- Educate registration staff to watch for actions or documents that could be an indicator, such as forged documents, conflicting information, or suspicious behavior.
- Collaborate with information technology staff to educate the organization on security risks that could result in breach of patient information as a result of phishing scams, failure to use encryption, or password loss.
- Perform comprehensive pre-employment background screenings for all employees.
- Monitor business associates activities for compliance with privacy and security practices.
- Use fraud prevention measures for anomaly detection and data flagging.
- Perform proactive audits to determine if a data breach has occurred (Eramo 2016).

An additional strategy should be to provide education to consumers on the importance of protecting their medical identity just as they would their financial identity. Consideration for notifying their health insurance should be on the same list as canceling their credit cards when a wallet is lost or stolen. At a minimum, consumers should be advised to closely monitor all explanations of benefits (EOBs) that are sent to validate the services listed were provided.

To help prevent identity theft, healthcare providers should consider the following measures:

- Ensure appropriate background checks of employees and business associates who may have access to business and patient PHI.
- Minimize the use of Social Security numbers for identification; whenever possible, redact or replace some of the digits in the number; avoid displaying the entire number on any document, screen, or data collection field.
- Store patient information in a secure manner, ensuring that physical safeguards such as restricted access and locks are in place. Consider securing a release of liability from patients who refuse to use facility-provided lockboxes or other storage for personal items.
- Implement and comply with organizational policies for the appropriate disposal, destruction, and reuse of any media used to collect and store patient information.
- Implement and comply with organizational policies and procedures that provide safeguards to ensure the security and privacy of patient information collected, maintained, and transmitted electronically. At a minimum:
  - Limit access to electronic patient information to a need-to-know basis, and establish minimum necessary access controls.
  - Require unique user identification and password controls.
  - Implement encryption practices for transmitting patient information.
  - Install appropriate hardware and software protective mechanisms such as firewalls and protected networks.
  - Perform routine audits to determine appropriate access to information, including access to patient information by newly hired staff.
- Train staff on organizational policies and practices developed to provide protection and appropriate use and disclosure of patient information, as well as appropriate responses to identity theft events. (Davis et al. 2005)
- Develop a proactive identity theft response plan or policy that clearly outlines the response process and identifies the organization's obligations to report or disclose to law enforcement or government agencies information related to such crimes.

    ○ Identify federal and state laws applicable to identity theft, reporting, and disclosing.

    ○ Complete a preemption analysis addressing HIPAA's permitted disclosures to law enforcement (164.512(2)) versus state law, determining when there is a need for a court order, subpoena, or patient authorization.

To further comply with administrative safeguards, if an incident of identity theft or unintentional release of identifying information occurs, the healthcare provider should initiate a process of notification that an incident has occurred. Breach notification requirements (discussed in chapter 10) must also be followed if applicable. *The Journal of Healthcare Risk Management* has an outline and checklist of steps to take to prevent medical identify theft and what to do once it is discovered (Amori 2009).

In addition to mandated red flags, healthcare providers must take steps to prevent, detect, and mitigate both external and internal medical identity theft. Employee awareness and training, and implementation of organization-wide policies and procedures are important.

Certain types of external medical identity theft can be detected when a perpetrator presents for service or seeks to obtain benefits such as medical equipment. Providers may require a driver's license to verify a patient's identity, and registration personnel may take photographs of patients to include in their health records for future reference. More sophisticated options include biometric identifiers such as a fingerprint, a handprint, or retinal scans. Patient signatures from previous encounters may also be compared with the signature of the patient presenting for the current episode of care. All these measures, however, are dependent on valid baseline information. If the information the provider relies on is the perpetrator's signature, photograph, or biometric identifier, all future encounters will be based on fraudulent information, decreasing the chances of detecting the fraud. This may also wrongfully identify the true patient as the perpetrator when and if he or she goes to that provider for treatment (Rinehart-Thompson and Harman 2017).

Figure 13.2   **Examples of red flags for healthcare providers**

- A complaint or question from a patient based on the patient's receipt of:
  —A bill for another individual
  —A bill for a product or service that the patient denies receiving
  —A bill from a healthcare provider that the patient never patronized
  or
  —A notice of insurance benefits (or Explanation of Benefits) for health services never received
- Records showing medical treatment that is inconsistent with a physical examination or with a medical history as reported by the patient
- A complaint or question from a patient about the receipt of a collection notice from a bill collector
- A patient or insurance company report stating that coverage for legitimate hospital stays is denied because insurance benefits have been depleted or a lifetime cap has been reached
- A complaint or question from a patient about information added to a credit report by a healthcare provider or insurer
- A dispute of a bill by a patient who claims to be the victim of any type of identity theft
- A patient who has an insurance number but never produces an insurance card or other physical documentation of insurance
- A notice or inquiry from an insurance fraud investigator for a private insurance company or a law enforcement agency

Source: Gellman and Dixon 2009, 5–6.

Measures that verify patient identity are ineffective for internal medical identity theft. The AHIMA e-HIM Work Group on Medical Identity Theft has identified best practices to minimize internal medical identity theft (AHIMA e-HIM Work Group on Medical Identity Theft 2008). These include background checks for employees and business associates; minimizing the temporary hiring of individuals who are not licensed, credentialed, or bound by professional codes of ethics; minimizing Social Security numbers as patient identifiers; and avoiding Social Security numbers on any data collection field.

Other ways to protect electronic patient data include stringent application of security access and systems controls, which are discussed in more detail below. The AHIMA work group (AHIMA e-HIM Work Group on Medical Identity Theft 2008) further recommends that three areas of the HIPAA Security Rule—administrative, technical, and physical safeguards—be included in a risk analysis to identify system vulnerabilities that could subject an organization to medical identity theft. Other areas it recommends in a risk analysis include the following:

- Limiting access to the minimum necessary
- Requiring user identification and passwords
- Implementing encryption devices for transmitted data
- Installing protective hardware and software devices, including firewalls
- Eliminating open network jacks in unsecured areas
- Routinely auditing access to patient information through audit trails

When medical identity theft occurs, a response plan is necessary. An organization's compliance office is crucial in maintaining an ongoing review and revision of plans that address breach notification requirements and mitigation efforts, including the separation of intermingled health information of a victim and a perpetrator. Such plans are necessary to minimize damage. As medical identity theft continues to challenge the healthcare industry and is centered in the management of health information, effective prevention, detection, and mitigation protocols are essential (Rinehart-Thompson and Harman 2017).

Check Your Understanding 13.1

Instructions: Indicate whether the following statements are true or false (T or F).

1. Hacking is more prevalent in healthcare because of the value of patient information on the black market.
2. Internal security breaches are far more common than external breaches.
3. The Identity Theft and Assumption Deterrence Act of 1998 makes it a federal crime to commit an act of identity theft.
4. Vulnerabilities and threats are terms that can be used interchangeably.
5. Healthcare organizations are excluded from the definition of "creditor" under FACTA.
6. Red flags are used to help a healthcare provider detect medical identity theft.
7. Medical identity theft has increased because of the expansion of electronic health record utilization and the expanded availability of data.

Security Access Controls and Systems Controls

To adequately protect ePHI and prevent **security incidents**, those that breach or threaten an electronic system, an organization must employ both access controls and systems controls. This section explains the difference between the two and provides examples of each.

Access Controls

Access controls are designed to prevent unauthorized individuals from retrieving, using, or altering information. "Preventive controls try to stop harmful events from occurring, while detective controls identify if a harmful event has occurred and corrective controls are used after a harmful event to restore the system" (AHIMA 2012, 49). To prevent unauthorized access, only individuals with a "need to know" should have access to ePHI. ePHI can be easily shared through EHRs and network exchanges, so healthcare entities must establish processes that identify access rights to ePHI. Often, users of ePHI are assigned network access rights that give them the ability to use basic programs such as e-mail and other business applications. Separate application access rights must be granted based on the user's role and needed functions before they are able to access the more specific components of the systems.

As healthcare entities define what constitutes their legal health record (LHR), the time factor in electronic information systems should be considered. Best practices include systems' coordination of time and date stamps to accurately capture when an event occurred, including access, and audits to detect suspicious activity. This also becomes a compliance issue. As data sharing increases, it is important to have accurate time stamps and log files to support efficient network operations and the latest encryption and authentication standards.

Access Rights

Access to ePHI can be controlled through the use of one of the following:

- User-based access
- Role-based access
- Context-based access

Before we discuss each of these options, a brief explanation of access rights is necessary. Traditional user-based and role-based access rights have two parameters—*who* and *how*. *Who* is a list of users with rights to access electronic information. This list, called an access control list, can be organized by individual users or by groups of users. Groups are generally defined by role or job function. All coders within the health information management (HIM) department would be granted the same access rights, all RNs within a particular job classification would be granted the same access, and so on.

How specifies the ways that a user can access a resource. Examples include read, write, edit, execute, append, and print. Only so-called owners and administrators would be granted full rights so that they can modify, delete, or create new components. Clearly, owner and administrative privileges for health **information systems** should be carefully monitored.

User-based access control (UBAC) is defined as "a security mechanism used to grant users of a system access based upon the identity of the user" (HHS n.d.). With **role-based access control** (RBAC), access decisions are based on the roles individual users have as part of an organization. "With RBAC, rather than attempting to map an organization's security policy to a relatively low-level set of technical controls (typically, access control lists), each user is assigned to one or more predefined roles, each of which has been assigned the various privileges needed to perform the role" (HHS n.d.). One of the benefits of RBAC over user-based access is that, as new applications are added, privileges are more easily assigned. Discretionary assignment of access by an administrator is limited with RBAC. Users must be assigned to a specific role to be assigned access to a specific application (OWASP 2016).

Context-based access control (CBAC) is the most stringent of the three options. A CBAC scheme begins with the protection afforded by either a user-based or role-based access control design and takes it one step further. Context-based access control takes into account the person attempting to access the data, the type of data being accessed, and the *context* of the transaction in which the access attempt is made. In other words, context-based access has three parameters to consider—who, how, and in what context the data are being accessed. The following example illustrates the differences in the three types of access control.

> Mary Smith is the director of the HIM department. Under a UBAC scheme, Mary would be allowed read-only access to her hospital's laboratory information system because of her personal identity—that is, because she is Mary Smith and uses the proper log-in and password(s) to get into the system. With an RBAC scheme, Mary would be allowed read-only access to her hospital's lab system because she is part of the HIM department and all department employees have been granted read-only privileges to this system. If the hospital were to adopt a CBAC scheme, Mary might be allowed access to the lab system only from her own workstation or another workstation in the HIM department. If she attempted to log in from the emergency room or another administrative office, she might be denied access. The CBAC could also be based on time of day. Since Mary is a daytime employee, she might be denied access if she attempted to log in at night.

Most access control schemes used by healthcare organizations are a mixture of the three types—UBAC, RBAC, and CBAC. **Identity and access management (IAM)** is the security discipline that enables the right individuals to access the right resources at the right times for the right reasons. IAM addresses the mission-critical need to ensure appropriate access to resources across increasingly heterogeneous technology environments, and to meet increasingly rigorous compliance requirements. This security practice is a crucial undertaking for any enterprise. It is increasingly business-aligned, and it requires business skills, not just technical expertise. Enterprises that develop mature IAM capabilities can reduce their identity management costs and, more importantly, become significantly more agile in supporting new business initiatives (Casey 2017).

Entity Authentication

Access control mechanisms are effective in controlling what and how users access an electronic health information system, but only if there is a system for ensuring the identity of the individual attempting to gain access. **Entity authentication** is defined as "the corroboration that an entity is the one claimed" (HHS n.d.). This means the computer reads a predetermined set of criteria to determine if the user is who he or she claims to be.

To authenticate the legitimate user of ePHI, the user must be assigned a **unique identifier**. This identifier is a combination of characters and numbers assigned and maintained by the security system. It is used to track individual user activity. This identifier is commonly called the user ID or log-on ID. It is the "public" or known portion of most user log-on procedures. For example, many organizations assign a log-on identifier that is the same as the user's e-mail address, or a combination of the user's last and first names. It is generally fairly easy to identify a user by the log-on. John Doe's log-on identifier might be *doej*, for example.

Because of the public nature of the log-on ID or user ID, there is a need to authenticate the identity of the user. The three **authentication** methods are listed next (Walsh 2011).

- Something you know, such as a password or a personal identification number (PIN)
- Something you have, such as an ATM card, a secure token, a telephone number (for callbacks), or a swipe/smart card; it may also be an alert sent to a smart phone that has to be answered before being allowed network access
- Something you are, such as a biometric identifier (for example, a fingerprint, a voice scan, or an iris or retinal scan)

Combining a user name with one of the authentication methods is single-factor authentication. A combination of any two of the preceding mechanisms constitutes a two-factor system and is recommended by Walsh. Single-factor authentication that is based on what the user knows (for example, user name and password) is the least secure form of protecting information from unauthorized access.

Security methods can be used alone or in combination with other systems. Security experts often encourage layered security systems that use more than one security mechanism, even if the solutions are individually fallible.

User IDs and Passwords

The most commonly used method for controlling access to an electronic information system is through a combination of a user ID and a password or PIN. A **password** is a sequence of characters used to verify that a computer user requesting access to a system is actually that particular user. Typically, a password is made up of between 4 and 16 characters. User IDs and passwords are maintained either as part of the access control list of the network or local operating system or in a special database that is searched before the user is allowed to access the system requested. While the user ID is not secret, the password or PIN is. Although passwords are generally stored in an encrypted form, software programs exist (called password crackers) that can identify an unknown or forgotten password for legitimate purposes. Unfortunately, unauthorized persons seeking to gain access to computer systems can also use these applications. For this reason, and due to individual behaviors described below, password and PIN systems are the least secure form of entity authentication.

One common problem with passwords is that they are often simple to remember and are selected for that very reason. As a result, however, they are also simple enough for someone else to guess. To combat this, some systems automatically generate passwords that are difficult to guess or force users to select passwords that are not too easy or already in use. Unfortunately, because they are then more difficult to remember, users are more likely to write the password down or publicly display it by taping it to a workstation. A preferable strategy is to teach users to create a pass phrase that consists of eight or more words, and then use the initial letters of the words to create a password. Use uppercase for some words, such as nouns, and use lowercase letters for the rest. Substitute numbers for words where possible. Passwords created in this way are easy to remember but difficult to crack. For example, a pass phrase might be, "My mother likes to eat strawberry birthday cake," and the password developed from this might be "MMltesbc." Then add a number to the end (for example, a year), and the password becomes "MMltesbc07." The pass phrase needs to be something the user will remember.

It is essential that healthcare organizations implement clear policies on creative selection, as well as appropriate use and maintenance of passwords; employee education; and meaningful sanctions for policy violations (including prohibiting the sharing of passwords). Tips for the effective selection of passwords are included in figure 13.3.

Tokens

Tokens are devices, such as key cards, that are inserted into doors or computers or a device that uses the USB port on a device. With the increase in cloud storage, more web-based security tokens are being used. Most tokens generate a one-time password that is used along with the user ID and password to authenticate the holder. With token authentication systems, identification is based on the user's possession of the token, combined with a user name and password. The disadvantage of tokens is that they can be lost, misplaced, or stolen. When tokens are used in combination with a password or PIN, it is essential that the password or PIN not be written on the token or in a location near where the token is stored. Tokens generate a password to access the system once the user name and PIN are entered into the system. A secure token is one type of dual-factor (two-factor) authentication because the user must possess the token (something the user has) along with the user name and password (something the user knows). JSON web tokens are a secure, open-standard method of securing transmitting data and can be signed by a HMAC (hash method authentication code) algorithm or a public/private key pair using RSA.

Biometric Identification Systems

Because of the inherent weaknesses in password systems, other identification systems have been developed. **Biometric identification systems** analyze biological data about the user, such as a voiceprint, fingerprint, handprint, retinal scan, face print, or full-body scan, and are likely to play an increasing role in ePHI security. Biometric identifiers are difficult to replicate and steal and can be combined with cryptographic functions for dual-factor authentication (Chiou 2013).

Biometric devices consist of a reader or scanning device, software that converts the scanned information into digital form, and a database that stores the biometric data for comparison. IBM, Microsoft, Novell, and other computer companies are currently working on a standard for biometric devices called BioAPI. This standard will allow different manufacturers' software products to interact with one another.

Figure 13.3 Guidelines for choosing passwords

DO
- Pick a combination of letters, numbers, symbols and use upper- and lowercase letters
- Choose a word or text string that you can easily remember.
- Change your password often if not automatically prompted by your computer network.
- Use one password for e-mail and another for online accounts

DON'T
- Create a password that someone could easily guess if they know who you are—for example, your Social Security number, birthday, maiden name, pets' names, children's names, or model of your car.
- Choose a word that can be found in the dictionary. Cracker programs can rapidly try every word in the dictionary.
- Pick a word that is currently newsworthy.
- Create a password from adjacent keys on the keyboard
- Create a password that is similar to your previous password.
- Share your password with others or write it down in a visible location, such as on a sticky note on your desk.

Source: Wager, Lee, and Glaser 2009.

New methods of encryption are emerging that combine dual-factor biometric and cryptographic identification. This method provides higher security and can be combined with hardware and software applications to prevent malicious programs from stealing biometric values or posing as legitimate users (Chiou 2013).

Automatic Log-off

Automatic log-off is a security procedure that causes a computer session to end after a predetermined period of inactivity, such as 10 minutes. Multiple software products are available to allow network administrators to set automatic log-off parameters. Like other password-protected screen savers, log-off systems automatically activate after a period of inactivity. However, unlike password-protected screen savers, automatic log-off mechanisms require users to enter their network passwords to access the system. Generally, there is an installed device driver that prevents rebooting to deactivate the log-off system. Other security measures that may be included with automatic log-off products prevent users from changing the screen saver or being able to set local password options in case the user is not connected to the network. Failed log-in attempts may be recorded and reported as well as statistics on user log-ins, elapsed time, and user IDs. Generally, automatic log-off from an application session closes access to data and offers protection to the database and protection against unauthorized access. This should be differentiated from automatic timeout of the workstation, which could leave the database open and its session still running (for example, a password-protected screen saver).

Termination of Access

Healthcare organizations should safeguard themselves with policies and procedures for terminating the current level of access when an employee changes roles or terminates employment with the organization. Personnel within each organizational unit should be responsible for notifying the appropriate departments to carry out **termination of access** as it currently exists when an employee is terminated or when job responsibilities change. Failure to terminate access rights creates the potential for unauthorized access to PHI. An employee who continues with the organization but in a different capacity should be prevented from having access rights no longer needed. This can be accomplished by terminating the current level of access immediately and requesting that the user's new manager establish appropriate access for the user based on the new job responsibilities.

Audit Trails

An **audit trail** is a record that shows who has accessed a computer system, when it was accessed, and what operations were performed. Audit trails are generated by specialized software that has multiple uses in securing information systems. Audit trails can be used as either before or after access to information and may be used to identify unusual or atypical behaviors of an individual user, such as excessive printing (NIST 1995). Audit trails may be at the system, application or user levels but for HIPAA compliance user-level are required in order to determine which files and records were accessed. Tracking log-in locations of users to identify patterns of user behaviors is one method to look for deviations in user behaviors to identify cyberattacks.

The length of time that audit trails are retained is a legal factor that should be considered as part of an EHR functionality. Previous chapters that discussed the LHR and evidence established the importance of producing information that will justify one's actions or validate the integrity of the record. Audit trail information should be considered an ancillary portion of the LHR and retained according to record retention requirements. Many new requirements in the HITECH Act place greater importance on the ability to document actions for legal proceedings based on information contained in audit trails (Walsh 2014).

Employee Nondisclosure Agreements

Under HIPAA's administrative safeguards, a healthcare entity must ensure that its workforce members have appropriate access to ePHI while not having access to ePHI when it is not appropriate or necessary. Many organizations require employees to sign nondisclosure agreements. These are particularly important if employees work in remote locations or telecommute.

Security Awareness and Training

HIPAA administrative safeguards require that a covered entity (CE) implement a security awareness and training program for all its workforce members. As with other security standards, the awareness and training requirement is nonspecific, allowing the CE to design a training program to meet its particular needs. Raising awareness and subsequently changing individual behaviors about security issues is one of the single most effective tools a CE has to ensure compliance with the HIPAA Security Rule and prevent data breaches. Creating a culture of compliance with privacy and security is an essential part of an information security program. With increased implementation of EHRs, the human factor must also be supported by systems that preserve the confidentiality of information.

Because the HITECH Act extended many of the HIPAA privacy and security requirements, organizations should consider expanding their existing training programs to cover more individuals. They must also address the breach notification requirements that were outlined in the previous chapter. Training programs should continually be evaluated for effectiveness and must incorporate the most recent HIPAA/HITECH requirements. The ONCHIT incorporates HIPAA privacy and security training with meaningful use and cybersecurity training (ONC 2015). Resources are available online at HealthIT.gov which includes sample policy documents and training videos.

As a complement to workforce awareness and training, consumer education will assist in compliance with established programs. ONCHIT has consumer training on privacy and security included in the HIPAA Training and Resources.

Remote Access Control

Organizations that allow personnel to work from home or access ePHI while at home or traveling have additional security issues and must set clear guidance regarding appropriate use of organization computer resources, including hardware, software, and web access. SANS and the Centers for Medicare and Medicaid Services (CMS) have guidelines for remote access as well as the use of portable devices (laptops, mobile devices, and external hardware) and home computers to access ePHI (CMS 2014; SANS 2015). CMS offers a series of risk management strategies based on various known, universal risks (CMS 2014). Similar policies should be in place for all mobile devices.

SANS recommends the following policies be developed, implemented and enforced for remote network access. There is also a remote access policy template that can modified by CEs for compliance.

- Acceptable encryption policy
- Acceptable use policy

- Password policy
- Third-party agreement
- Hardware and software configuration standards for remote access (SANS 2015)

Each of these categories must be evaluated by the organization, and existing requirements must be considered.

Remote work may involve individuals who are traveling or routinely work from home. This requires additional security for devices that are taken off-site (for example, laptops, mobile phones, remote storage devices and other types of mobile devices) and the information they contain. Physical security of the device is the first step to ensure that information is not inappropriately released or accessed. Several tips to keep laptops more secure include avoiding the use of a computer bag, always carrying the laptop, using a physical security device such as a cable, and never leaving the laptop visible in any location (for example, a car or hotel room). Desktop firewall, antivirus, and intrusion software are other tools that can be implemented to protect not only the laptop from external threats such as viruses but also the organization's network once the laptop is reconnected. Files maintained on the laptop should be encrypted to protect them from unauthorized access or alteration.

Selection of strong passwords, as discussed previously, with a combination of more than seven alphanumeric characters should be required. Passwords should never be stored on the device or written down. All these recommendations should be considered when developing the organizational policy and education plan for remote and mobile workers. The best protection against loss of data or laptop theft is user compliance with organizational policies and procedures (Narasimman 2005).

Check Your Understanding   13.2

Instructions: Indicate whether the following statements are true or false (T or F).

1. Training is not necessary for remote workforce members as long as encryption is in place in the organization.
2. Context-based access control is less stringent than role-based access control.
3. Biometric identifiers signify something that the user knows.
4. Employee nondisclosure agreements are particularly important for employees who work in remote locations or telecommute.
5. Employee training programs are not necessary to protect the security of PHI.
6. An audit trail is a record that shows when a particular user accessed a computer system.
7. It is best practice to select a very strong password and use it for all accounts.

Systems Controls

In addition to access control mechanisms, several common administrative, physical, and technical systems controls can be used to further ensure protection of ePHI. These controls relate to systems hardware or software and functions such as transmission of ePHI via fax or e-mail. This section of the chapter addresses some of these controls.

Cybersecurity

Cybersecurity refers to "preventative methods used to protect information from being stolen, compromised or attacked. It requires an understanding of potential information threats, such as viruses and other malicious code. Cybersecurity strategies include identity management, risk management and incident management." Cybercriminal activities have become one of the major causes of data breaches according to reporting from HHS. The number of individuals impacted by hacking was over 111 million in 2015 compared to 568,358 in 2010 (Dill et al. 2016). The worldwide impact on the world economy is estimated at over $575 billion (PWC 2015). The increasing value of stolen medical information on the black market is the driving force behind this rise in attacks against healthcare organizations that are at risk due to insufficient security measures (Humer and Finkle 2014).

Healthcare organizations are being forced or required to share more information electronically as a means to increase the quality of care. This expanded sharing of information results in greater exposure to inappropriate access. Unlike the financial institutions that have locked down access to information along with fraud detection that minimizes impact to the individual data elements such as date of birth, social security numbers, and address are not able to be changed or protected from use like a credit card.

Workstation Use and Security

Workstations include both hardware and software that allow access to ePHI. Workstations should be placed in areas that are secure or monitored at all times and should be positioned so that visitors or others cannot read screens in public areas (for example, a reception area). A screen device can be placed over the workstation monitor to prevent anyone other than the person directly in front of it from reading it. Clear policies should be developed for workstation use. They should delineate, among other things, the appropriate functions to perform on the workstation and rules for sharing workstations.

Data Encryption

Data encryption ensures that data transferred from one location on a network or device to another are secure from eavesdropping data interception. This becomes particularly important when sensitive data, such as health information, are transmitted over public networks such as the Internet or across wireless networks. Secure data are data that cannot be intercepted, copied, modified, or deleted while in transit or at rest in a file system (for example, on a disk or tape).

Cryptography is the study of encryption and decryption techniques. It is a complicated science that has vast numbers of techniques associated with it. Only the basic concepts and a few current authentication technologies will be discussed in this chapter. Two common forms of encryption used in healthcare today are "pretty good privacy" and "wired equivalent privacy." The first form, **pretty good privacy (PGP)**, is used to encrypt e-mail messages and refers to encryption that uses a serial combination of hashing, data compression, symmetric-key cryptography, and public-key cryptography. **Wired equivalent privacy** is used to protect information on wireless networks. These forms of encryption are used to authenticate the sender and the receiver of messages over networks, particularly data transmission involving the Internet. To be effective, the encryption scheme should provide three things: authentication (both the sender and the recipient are known to each other), data security (data are safe from interception), and data nonrepudiation (data that were sent have arrived unchanged).

Some of the basic encryption terminology includes *plaintext, encryption algorithm, ciphertext,* and *key*. Plaintext is data before any encryption has taken place. In other words, the original data or message is recorded in the computer system as plaintext. An encryption algorithm is the computer program that converts the plaintext into an enciphered form. The ciphertext is the data after the encryption algorithm has been applied and conceals the data's original meaning and keeps it from being known or used (SANS n.d.b). The key in an encryption and decryption procedure is unique data that are needed to both create the ciphertext and decrypt the ciphertext back to the original message. The length of the key is commonly used to measure the strength of the key.

The earliest encryption systems used a single, private key. In other words, the same key (code) was needed to generate the ciphertext and to decrypt it. A problem with these systems was that they required both the sender and the receiver to have the key; in addition, the key also had to be protected from interception or tampering.

Public key cryptography addresses the basic problem with single, private key systems. A public key system has two keys, a private key and a public key. In the two-key system, data encrypted with the public key can be decrypted only by a private key, and data encrypted by the private key can be decrypted only by the public key. With public key cryptography, the encrypted data become very difficult to break. Single-key encryption is much more efficient than public-private key encryption, and thus is better suited to encrypting large text documents and files. Therefore, modern public key cryptography systems create a single-use key called a session key to encrypt the message and then send the session key and message together after encrypting again with the public key algorithm.

Public key cryptography today is used as a component of public key infrastructure (PKI), an entire system designed to make the use of public key cryptography practical. PKI is actually a combination of encryption techniques, software, and services.

A CE can adopt an in-house PKI model or contract with an application service provider (ASP) to host and manage its PKI. One potential use of PKI in healthcare is sending secure e-mail. To send a secure e-mail within the PKI environment, the sender needs to retrieve the recipient's public key from a directory within his or her organization. After obtaining the public key, the sender encrypts the e-mail message (by selecting the "encrypt" button, for example) and then sends it with the recipient's public key. When the recipient receives the e-mail, the recipient's private key will automatically decrypt the message.

Healthcare organizations should have a policy on end user protection of encryption keys to ensure that there is no compromise or disclosure of private keys.

There are other potential uses for PKI technology in healthcare, such as ensuring secure access to web-based health records or other health information systems. One example, recently reported in *Health Management Technology*, is Marconi Medical Systems, a picture archiving communications system (PACS). Marconi is integrating PKI into its web-based products to allow remote access through a standard web browser. Another example of a health-related organization using PKI is an online prescription service. PKI is expensive, and many of the systems are proprietary and will not interact with other systems. However, with HIPAA and HITECH standards demand a higher level of security for online healthcare transactions, the use of PKI technology in healthcare is likely to increase.

Mobile device encryption is essential to ensure encryption of data at rest. Mobile devices may be laptops, cell phones or tablets that contain data. Laptops should have full disk encryption with an approved software package. Data should not be stored in plain text format. Data stored on a cell phone must be saved to an encrypted file system using approved software. It should employ report wipe technology to remotely disable and delete any data stored on a lost or stolen cell phone. Healthcare organization should identify and provide software to workforce members for encryption.

Firewall Protection

A **firewall** is either a hardware or software device that examines traffic entering and leaving a network. It prevents some traffic from entering or leaving based on established rules. The term *firewall* can be used to describe the software that protects computing resources or to describe the combination of the software, hardware, and policies that protect the resources. The most common place to find a firewall is between the healthcare organization's internal network (trusted network) and the Internet (untrusted network). A firewall limits users on the Internet from accessing certain portions of the healthcare network and also limits internal users from accessing various portions of the Internet. As important as firewalls are to the overall security of health information systems, they cannot protect a system from all types of attacks. Many viruses, for example, can hide within documents that will not be stopped by a firewall.

Routers are computers that link two different networks and are responsible for routing or sending the network traffic to the correct destination. Although not as robust as firewalls, routers may be programmed to filter certain types of network traffic. Intrusion detection systems (IDS) serve as the alarm system for the network and warn of possible inappropriate attempts to access the network by examining and analyzing network traffic. Intrusion prevention systems (IPS), which identify malicious network traffic like an IDS and then apply rules to block its passage across the network like a firewall, are now available. Both an IDS and an IPS require significant human intervention to monitor the alarms and rules and check for false positives. As with all computer tools, they require people to monitor them and make sense of the messages they produce.

Virus Checking

Viruses come in many varieties. The common types are classified as the following:

- File infectors, which attach to program files so that when a program is loaded, the virus is also loaded
- System or boot-record infectors, which infect system areas of diskettes or hard disks
- Macro viruses, which infect Microsoft applications, inserting unwanted words or phrases

A **worm** is a special type of computer virus that stores and then replicates itself. Worms usually transfer from computer to computer via e-mail. A **Trojan horse** is a destructive piece of programming code that hides in another piece of programming code that looks harmless, such as a macro or an e-mail message.

Because virus attacks are very common and can cause extensive damage and loss of productivity, virus checking is an important component of a health information security program. Fortunately, there are antivirus software packages on the market that are effective as long as the virus catalog is updated frequently. Publication of defects has led to the phenomenon of "zero-day exploits." This means that a defect may be exploited to produce a virus, worm, or Trojan horse attack the same day it is published; thus, antivirus companies may not be able to stop it before it circles the globe on the Internet and does considerable harm.

Most software packages can be set to automatically obtain updated virus definitions and scan the user's computer system periodically to detect and clean any viruses found. It is important for users to also keep their workstation patch updates current, as this will enhance the security features of the operating system. Many of these operating system patches fix known and exploitable vulnerabilities in the software.

Transmission of ePHI

The ability of a healthcare provider to access all relevant healthcare information on a patient is important to the overall quality of care rendered to that patient. Electronic communications used to transmit ePHI, such as facsimiles, the Internet, electronic mail, and wireless communication devices that enable functions such as text messaging, are the business records of an organization and are therefore subject to the same storage, retention, retrieval, privacy, and security provisions as any other patient-identifiable health information (Burrington-Brown and Hughes 2003). Some commonly approved methods of transmitting ePHI, emerging technological trends such as social media, and controls necessary to ensure the privacy and security of ePHI are discussed later.

Facsimile or Faxing ePHI

A facsimile (fax) machine is a common tool used for sending either paper or electronic information over telephone lines. Fax equipment and software can enhance the quality of care by expediting the transmission of information from one provider to another, but they also increase the risk of information being misdirected or intercepted by someone other than the intended recipient. Some state laws address the topic of faxing healthcare information as related to a specific part of state code, such as faxing information pertaining to a given disease to a state health department. Many states have adopted rules based on the federal Uniform Rules of Evidence (URE) that allow business records created in the normal course of business to be considered trustworthy and admissible as evidence. The URE allows that a duplicate record such as a fax is admissible to the same extent as an original unless

- A genuine question is raised as to the authenticity or continuing effectiveness of the original, or
- In the circumstances it would be unfair to admit the duplicate in lieu of the original (National Conference of Commissioners on Uniform State Laws 2005)

Some states have also adopted the Uniform Photographic Copies of Business and Public Records as Evidence Act or the Uniform Business Records as Evidence Act, both of which address the admissibility of record reproductions, making it appropriate to accept faxes in lieu of original health records (Davis et al. 2005).

The faxing of patient information is not specifically mentioned in regulations; however, CMS addressed the faxing of physician orders to healthcare facilities in Letter No. 90-25 from the Bureau of Policy Development. The letter states that faxed copies of physician orders are permissible and do not need to be countersigned, but they should be retained as a permanent part of the patient's record. A healthcare provider should take precautions to ensure that the faxed copy of the order is legible. The HIPAA Privacy and Security Rules do not specifically address fax use, but the Department of Health and Human Services (HHS) does address it in a limited manner in its response to questions related to faxes. The guidance offered by HHS suggests that providers can use a fax to disclose PHI to another provider if safeguards are in place, such as placing the fax machine in a secure place, confirming the correct fax number between providers, and periodically auditing fax numbers in use. The guidance also indicates that a valid signed authorization for disclosure of PHI may be a copy received by fax.

Fax machines are utilized to fax between provider(s) and patient. While a fax can be an extremely convenient and efficient means of transmitting PHI, there are concerns, because fax machines are not secure means of communication. Thus, for maximum protection, whenever possible, faxing of PHI should be limited to emergency situations. It is best not to transmit highly sensitive information unless it is encrypted or transmitted only within the organization through a virtual private network.

Internet

The Internet is used in a variety of healthcare functions, such as refilling prescriptions, scheduling appointments, communicating with physicians, researching medical conditions, and performing telemedicine activities—all of which put ePHI at risk for unauthorized disclosure. Concern for Internet security depends on how the healthcare provider or patient is using the Internet and how the user is connected to it. Security risks commonly associated with Internet access are unauthorized access to the organization's information systems and networks, unauthorized disclosure of confidential patient information or the organization's proprietary information and PHI, and the introduction of computer viruses or various other threats. To address these Internet security risks, several security measures can be taken.

Electronic Mail

E-mail has become a primary means of communication for business and personal purposes. It is increasingly requested in response to litigation and is discoverable under e-discovery rules. Secure patient portals are the preferred method of transmitting e-mail to and from patients and providers. A Kaiser Permanente study found that in 2014 more than 20 million e-mails were sent via secure portals (Reed at al. 2015). The CMS Electronic Health Record Incentive Programs 2016 standards require providers to send a secure message using the electronic messaging function of the certified EHR technology (CEHRT). The certification criteria require the message to be encrypted as identified in the National Institute of Standards and Technology (NIST) approved security FIPS Publication 140-2.

Policies and procedures for the use of e-mail should be created and enforced. Healthcare organizations should develop policies that include use of company e-mail, retention, automatic forwarding, use of third party e-mail storage systems such as Google to create business communications. Information Security teams should verify compliance through periodic walk throughs, video monitoring, and internal and external audits of e-mail systems (SANS n.d.a).

Staff training regarding the risks of using e-mail, especially to communicate PHI, must be mandatory. Staff should be trained on how to use and manage e-mail and be given specific templates for e-mail content and business functions that are routinely handled through e-mail, such as scheduling appointments, communicating lab results, and providing additional treatment information. E-mail related to patient care should be incorporated into the patient medical record.

In addition, common recipients of e-mail should sign user confidentiality agreements that prohibit forwarding e-mail to multiple users and guard against such breaches as printing out multiple unauthorized copies, leaving messages onscreen for unauthorized viewing, storing messages in an unsecured file, altering the original message, and so on. Patients should also be educated regarding their responsibility for handling their information in a secure manner. They should understand the risk of using e-mail for communication and should be encouraged to maintain copies for their own personal health records. Guidelines specific to provider–patient e-mail communications are offered by the American Medical Association (AMA) and displayed in figure 13.4.

From a technical standpoint, several safeguards can be used to protect e-mail communication, such as anti-spam and antivirus software, filtering of outbound e-mail, encryption software, and archive solution and retention management programs. Anti-spam and antivirus software can be provided by an outsourced provider or installed internally on an organization's servers and desktops. Filters can be applied to detect proprietary, business, or confidential patient information that also needs to be protected with encryption. In addition to identifying e-mails that require encryption, filters can also trigger an alert if there is an inappropriate or unauthorized transmission of information. Filtering of outbound e-mail is effective only if the organization enforces the use of the tools and prevents employees from using personal e-mail, which could also contain protected or private information and bypass the network filters.

Having a process for archiving e-mail messages is important since such messages are now subject to e-discovery rules.

Figure 13.4 Summary of AMA physician–patient communication guidelines recommended for e-mail

- Establish turnaround time for messages. Exercise caution when using e-mail for urgent matters.
- Inform patient about privacy issues.
- Patients should know who besides addressee processes messages during addressee's usual business hours and during addressee's vacation or illness.
- Whenever possible and appropriate, physicians should retain electronic and/or paper copies of e-mails communications with patients.
- Establish types of transactions (prescription refill, appointment scheduling, etc.) and sensitivity of subject matter (HIV, mental health, etc.) permitted over e-mail.
- Instruct patients to put the category of transaction in the subject line of the message for filtering: prescription, appointment, medical advice, billing question.
- Request that patients put their name and patient identification number in the body of the message.
- Configure automatic reply to acknowledge receipt of messages.
- Send a new message to inform patient of completion of request.
- Request that patients use autoreply feature to acknowledge reading clinicians' message.
- Develop archival and retrieval mechanisms.
- Maintain a mailing list of patients, but do not send group mailings where recipients are visible to each other. Use blind copy feature in software.
- Avoid anger, sarcasm, harsh criticism, and libelous references to third parties in messages.
- Append a standard block of text to the end of e-mail messages to patients, which contains the physician's full name, contact information, and reminders about security and the importance of alternative forms of communication for emergencies.
- Explain to patients that their messages should be concise.
- When e-mail messages become too lengthy or the correspondence is prolonged, notify patients to come in to discuss or call them.
- Remind patients when they do not adhere to the guidelines.
- For patients who repeatedly do not adhere to the guidelines, it is acceptable to terminate the e-mail relationship.

Source: AMA 2002.

The National Archives and Records Administration (NARA) Bulletin 2013-02 has guidance on the considerations for archiving e-mail along with recordkeeping considerations and responsibilities to ensure that records are retrievable and usable and how to associate e-mails with other organizational documentation (NARA 2013). Along with an archive solution, the organization should also develop record retention policies which should be applied to all technologies and data repositories (Heinrich 2014). This should be developed as part of the information governance plan for the organization. A sample retention schedule could contain three retention periods: immediate destruction, limited retention, and archival retention. This process is complex and should be automated. NARA has guidance on managing e-mail records and recommends a role-based approach to e-mail archiving (NARA 2013). All applicable laws and regulations should be researched prior to determining which types of messages can be placed in what category. Information related to patient care should be incorporated into the patient's record and retained as stipulated by the organization's health record retention guidelines. (see chapter 9).

In addition to the HIPAA Security Rule, other federal laws and some state laws also provide protection for electronic communications. The Electronic Communications Privacy Act of 1986 (ECPA)

(18 USC 2510) was enacted by the US Congress to extend government restrictions on wiretaps from telephones to include electronic transmissions of electronic data by computer. According to the regulation, electronic communications "means any transfer of signs, signals, writing, images, sounds, data, or intelligence of any nature transmitted in whole or in part by a wire, radio, electromagnetic, photo electronic or photo optical system that affects interstate of foreign commerce" (18 USC 2510). ECPA amended Title III of the Omnibus Crime Control and Safe Streets Acts of 1968 (42 USC 3711), otherwise known as the "wiretap statute," with the intent of preventing unauthorized government access to private electronic communications. However, subsequent changes related to some provisions of the USA PATRIOT Act weakened this act.

Questions exist as to whether electronic communications are protected in temporary storage during transmission, which would apply to every electronic communication. Protection does exist for government surveillance conducted without a court order; from third parties with no legitimate access to the messages; and from the carriers of the messages, such as Internet service providers.

Medical Device Security

Medical devices pose security risks and should be included in the risk management program for compliance with the Privacy and Security Rules. The Federal Bureau of Investigation (FBI) has issued warnings about the vulnerabilities of medical devices (iHealthBeat 2014). The Food and Drug Administration (FDA) published guidance for medical device manufacturers to incorporate security control into device design (FDA 2016). The advice covers the life cycle of the medical device and calls for incorporating maintenance controls to mitigate risks. The FDA guidance recommends the 2014 NIST voluntary Framework for Improving Critical Infrastructure Cybersecurity. The 2014 NIST framework was developed based on Executive Order 13636 "Improving Critical Infrastructure Cybersecurity," which called to enhance the security of systems to assist businesses without regulatory requirements (NIST 2014). Use of the 2014 NIST framework is voluntary and is meant to evolve to ensure continuing cybersecurity protection for the nation.

Wireless networking allows a cell phone, a portable handheld device (for example, a personal digital assistant [PDA]), or a desktop, laptop, or notebook computer equipped with a network card to access the network from any location within the range of the wireless transmitter.

Organizations that allow the use of wireless communication devices that include PHI should incorporate strict guidelines as to the types of devices that may be used and installed. PDAs, smartphones, pocket PCs, tablets, and cell phones are just a few of the mobile devices healthcare providers use to create, store, and access PHI. These devices are making the practice of medicine more efficient by improving the availability of clinical information from just about any location. At a minimum, data on the devices should be encrypted and the device locked, with password access required. Users of this technology must assume an added level of responsibility to protect the device along with the information.

Some additional protection is afforded wireless communication through the Federal Communications Commission regulations (47 CFR P15.37(f)) that prohibit the manufacture or import of devices that can pick up frequencies used by cellular phones. Several federal laws (18 USC 1029, 18 USC 2511, 18 USC 2701) specifically outline sanctions for intentional interception of cordless and cellular communication. These sanctions can range from fines to imprisonment, depending on the circumstances. The Communications Assistance for Law Enforcement Act of 1994 (CALEA) requires telecommunications carriers to ensure that their equipment will comply with authorized electronic surveillance by law enforcement.

Telehealth and Telemedicine

Telemedicine is defined by the American Telemedicine Association as "the use of medical information exchanged from one site to another via electronic communications to improve patients' health status" (American Telemedicine Association n.d.). Closely associated with telemedicine is the broader term "**telehealth**," which is the use of digital technologies to deliver medical care, health education, and public health services, by connecting multiple users in separate locations (for example, video conferencing, transmission of still images, patient portals, and remote monitoring of vital signs) (Center for Connected Health Policy 2013).

Several legal issues surround the practice of telehealth and telemedicine, privacy being first and foremost, since patient information can be transmitted anywhere in the world in a matter of seconds. Telemedicine consults routinely contain PHI about the patient that is transmitted over the Internet, by e-mail, or possibly by fax, depending on the system's capability. Requirements regarding expectations for privacy and security should be incorporated into policies and procedures for telehealth/telemedicine services. Most important, appropriate technical safeguards must be put in place before any information is transmitted or received. The Internet can act as a conduit for sending information, but appropriate forms of encryption must be utilized to protect the information.

Social Media

Social media is a collection of online technologies and practices that people use to share opinions, insights, experiences, and perspectives. Tools that take the form of text, video, images, and audio expedite conversations and allow all users to participate in creating and developing content. Healthcare organizations have begun to officially adopt some of these tools as a means of marketing and communicating with consumers or patients.

Privacy and security risks are inherent with social media tools, which were not created with healthcare in mind. Organizations must evaluate the risks associated with the use of new communication tools and respond appropriately. At a minimum, organizations must develop clear policies on the appropriate use of any social media tool. Employees should be told that discussion of patient or other work-related information is strictly prohibited. The risk for inadvertent disclosures is just as great as intentional disclosures if employees do not understand the risk of posting information that does not include specific names.

The AMA has guidance to providers regarding online medical professionalism and encourages providers to separate any personal identify and professional identity in the online environment but cautions that this is a quickly changing landscape and the benefits and drawbacks of social medical must be continuously monitored (Kind 2015). Organizations must perform periodic risk analysis to ensure that information has not been posted to a social medial site. Results from the assessments should drive continued education and employee awareness. Because an organization alone cannot monitor every social media site, employees should be responsible for reporting inappropriate postings of information they discover.

Contingency Planning or Disaster Recovery Planning

Contingency planning or **disaster recovery planning** is an important component of protecting ePHI mandated by the HIPAA Security Rule. Healthcare providers need plans in the event of a power failure, disaster, or other emergency that limits or eliminates access to facilities and ePHI.

They should also implement a business continuity plan that will continue operations during and after a disaster or disruption in service (AHIMA 2013a). A business continuity plan ensures that critical business functions can withstand a variety of emergencies, whereas a contingency or disaster plan includes technical, procedural, and organizational implementation components that should be followed during and after a loss (AHIMA 2013a). A well-designed contingency or disaster plan can "protect health information from damage, minimize disruption, ensure stability, and provide for orderly recovery" (AHIMA 2013a). The plan should outline the essential components that encompass ePHI as well as other types of health information. Several key components to a contingency or disaster plan are required by the HIPAA Security Rule (45 CFR 164.308(a)(7)) and are designed to protect ePHI:

- Risk assessment and analysis
- Downtime and contingency planning
- Data backup
- Disaster recovery
- Emergency mode of operations

Risk Assessment and Analysis

A risk assessment should be performed prior to creating the business continuity plan. Requirements for the risk assessment can be found in HIPAA regulations, AHIMA Disaster Planning and Recovery Toolkit and in the NIST regulations. The organization should develop a plan to assess potential disasters that would be likely to occur in their part of the country and those of its business associates. The focus of the assessment should be on any system that supports the electronic health record and provision of patient care.

Data Backup

Information technology departments should have ongoing data backup mechanisms for all applications and systems with patient information. A variety of technical methods, including backup servers or storage media such as backup tapes, can be employed for data backup. The physical location of the backup site should be far enough from the facility that a natural disaster like flooding or hurricane would not impact both sites.

The AHIMA Disaster Planning and Recovery Toolkit recommends that a functional backup plan must go further than just the HIPAA privacy and security rules. It should include

- Processes for backing up all data on all systems and steps for recreating all components of the health information system
- Description and location of all components of the electronic, hybrid, or paper records, and the configuration of any networked device including hardware and software deployed
- Processes for recreating data tables, contracts, licenses, and policies and procedures
- Assignment of responsibility for each component which identifies backup personnel if key individuals are inaccessible or incapacitated
- An estimate of how long the organization or provider can continue to function at various stages of recovery (AHIMA 2013a)

Data Recovery

Generally, if data backup procedures are followed, the need for extensive data recovery should be minimal. However, if electronic data are damaged in a disaster, a healthcare provider might seek the services of a company that specializes in electronic data recovery. Healthcare providers or organizations may opt to contract with such a company to perform the data recovery. Standards data recovery principles include

- Provisions for reading data that were created on applications that may no longer exist by transforming the data into a human readable format prior to sunsetting a system
- Implementing data retention policies that include predetermined data destruction timetables
- Maintaining the currency of the backed up versions of policies and procedures for recreating the network environment, as outlined previously
- Developing a realistic estimate of how long the institution can go without preexisting data and creating an interim plan that realistically matches the anticipated recovery timetable

If electronic records cannot be restored, it may be necessary to reconstitute a record to the extent possible. This may involve the following:

- Uploading documents from any undamaged databases, such as admission, transcription, laboratory, and radiology databases or data backup services
- Retranscribing documents from the dictation system
- Obtaining copies from recipients of previously distributed copies, such as physicians' offices, other healthcare facilities, or the business office (AHIMA 2013a)

Emergency Mode of Operations

Another important aspect of contingency or disaster planning is to outline a set of emergency operations. These may include plans for recording clinical information in the event of a power outage. For example, how will this information be protected? If a natural disaster prevents employees from reporting to work, how will the patient information be secured? Who is responsible for ensuring the security of data and systems during an emergency? Do all employees know how to report system outages, including power, telephone, network, and others? In developing a contingency plan for securing ePHI in the event of an emergency, the healthcare organization should (AHIMA 2013a)

- List the various types of disasters that might impair the operation of the facility. For example, healthcare facilities along the coast will certainly list hurricanes; facilities in the northeast would potentially list ice storms.
- List the department (agency or organization) core processes. These processes will vary. For a large hospital health information department, core processes might include patient identification, release of information, documentation and organizational workflow (Walsh and Lucci 2015)

A specific contingency plan should be developed for each identified disaster and core process. Also, consideration should be given for temporary versus long-term effects of disasters and the ability to access the facility and perform departmental functions with and without electricity.

Figure 13.5 is a sample disaster plan development checklist. Figure 13.6 is a sample contingency plan.

Figure 13.5 Sample disaster plan development checklist

Major Function	Extended Power Outage	Fire	Flood	Hurricane	Explosion
1. MPI					
2. Assembly					
3. Deficiency analysis					
4. Coding					
5. Abstracting					
6. Release of information					
7. Transcription of dictation					
8. Chart tracking/location/provision					
9. Birth certificates					

For each plausible disaster and major function, develop a contingency plan. As plans are completed, place a check mark in the corresponding box.

Source: Walsh et al. 2009, 178.

Figure 13.6 Sample contingency plan

1. Facility name:
2. Department name:
3. Plan originator:
4. Date:
5. Major function: Maintenance of an accurate MPI
6. Disaster: Extended power outage
7. Assumptions: An ice storm has resulted in an extended power outage. The majority of the staff is able to report to work.
8. Existing process detail: The MPI contains the patient's name and medical record number. When a patient is admitted, the registration staff accesses the MPI to determine whether the patient already has a medical record number or whether a new number must be generated. HIM staff also accesses the MPI when they need a medical record number to pull medical records for a current hospitalization, to accompany a bill for payment, for continuing care, for quality monitoring or legal action, and to number documents for placement in the paper record. The MPI is generated by entries made by patient registration staff into the admission/discharge tracking system. The accuracy of the numbers assigned is verified by HIM.
9. If-then scenarios: If patient registration staff does not have access to the MPI when admitting a patient, the following might result:

   • The registration system or registrars will assign new numbers, creating duplicates that may cost $20 per set to correct
   • The registrars will issue no numbers and patient health information will have to be matched to patients using account numbers, admission or discharge dates, or birth dates. Medical record numbers will have to be assigned and entered into the database at a later date

   If HIM staff members do not have access to an MPI, records cannot be pulled for any reason or provided to anyone.

10. Interdependencies: Registration staff, patient care areas, transcription, billing, and external customers including the patient, third-party payers, attorneys, and accreditation and standards organizations have a need for the patient medical records and therefore need a functional MPI.
11. Solutions and alternatives:

Figure 13.6 Sample contingency plan (Continued)

Potential Solutions and Alternatives	Limitations	Benefits
Auxiliary power will be used to access an electronic copy of the MPI on disk.	• Will not work without auxiliary power • Cumbersome • Generation of some duplicate medical record numbers likely • Human resources to correct duplicate numbers are costly	• Admitting staff are accustomed to this process • Fewer duplicates than with no backup system • Less cumbersome than a totally manual system
Staff have to depend on a paper MPI.	Printouts will be cumbersome Printouts will probably be located in HIM Generation of duplicate or no numbers likely Manual systems to correct duplicate numbers will be costly	• Provides a mechanism to look up a patient's number and pull a chart when critical

12. Tasks to be performed for selected alternatives (before, during, and after disaster)

Activity	Responsibility
Verify availability of MPI on disk	Associate director, HIM
Implement processes where disk is updated daily	Associate director, HIM
Develop contingency plan procedures and training materials	Associate director, HIM
Train patient registration and HIM staff to use contingency plan	Associate director, HIM
Post disaster and implementation contingency plan, check accuracy of record numbers assigned during disaster and correct as needed	HIM data quality coordinator
OR	
Schedule production and delivery of paper MPI on a routine basis	Associate director, HIM
Create contingency procedures and training materials for manual system	Associate director, HIM
Train patient registration and HIM staff	Associate director, HIM
Post disaster and implementation contingency plan, check accuracy of record numbers assigned during disaster and correct as needed	HIM data quality coordinator

Implementation notification schedule

Contact	Phone number
HIM director	
HIM associate director	
HIM coordinators	
Admitting director	

Source: Walsh et al. 2009, 180–181.

Resources to Assist with Security Threats and Controls

In addition to previously mentioned access and systems controls and suggestions for addressing internal and external threats (including medical identity theft), there are other helpful security tips and cyber-security tests available from organizations. The Computer Security Resource Center of NIST provides numerous resources specifically designed to address both privacy and security issues in healthcare

(NIST n.d.). The National Cyber Security Alliance (NCSA), while not directly related to compliance with the HIPAA Security Rule, provides information that is easily understood by all individuals in an organization and includes tips about using antivirus software to help keep computers secure and using strong passwords and strong authentication technology to protect personal information (NCSA n.d.). Another source of help is the SANS Institute, which is a cooperative research and education organization and a trusted international source of information security training and certification (SANS n.d.a). SANS research is based on consensus from network administrators, security managers, and information security professionals on the best security fundamentals and technical aspects of security. It is important for security officers as well as others responsible for managing and protecting healthcare data and information to avail themselves of such resources as the reliance on health information technology continues to grow.

Check Your Understanding   13.3

Instructions: Indicate whether the following statements are true or false (T or F).

1. Data encryption ensures that data transferred from one location on a network to another are secure from eavesdropping or data interception.

2. Assignment of patient medical record numbers is one of the priorities of the HIM professional during system downtime during a disaster.

3. Facsimile machines provide a highly secure method of communication.

4. Compliance with the HIPAA Security Rule is the only standard that should be considered when developing a security plan and performing a risk assessment.

5. Disaster recovery and contingency plans related to ePHI are nice to have but not necessary.

6. An organization's firewall limits external Internet users from accessing portions of the healthcare network, but it does not limit internal users from accessing portions of the Internet.

7. E-mail related to patient care should be kept separate from the patient medical record.

Scenario 13

Town Medical Center is joining the regional health information exchange (HIE) and has formed a committee for data sharing. Many issues were discussed at the initial meeting and the group decided to develop a standard practice for dealing with medical identity theft. To move the committee along, the Chair knows background information is needed.

1. What should the chair do to prepare?

2. What resources could the Chair use to prepare?

3. What best practice recommendations should be suggested at the next meeting?

References

Abelson, R. and M. Goldstein. 2015 (February 5). Millions of anthem customers targeted in cyberattack. *New York Times.*
AHIMA. 2012. 10 security domains (updated). *Journal of AHIMA* 83(5):48–52.
AHIMA. 2013a. Disaster planning and recovery toolkit. Chicago: AHIMA.

AHIMA. 2013b (January 25). Analysis of modifications to the HIPAA Privacy, Security, Enforcement, and Breach Notification Rules under the HITECH and Genetic Information Nondiscrimination Act: Other modifications to the HIPAA Rules. Chicago: AHIMA.

AHIMA e-HIM Work Group on Medical Identity Theft. 2008. Mitigating medical identity theft. *Journal of AHIMA* 79(7):63–69.

American Medical Association. 2002. Guidelines for physician-patient electronic communications. http://www.ama-assn.org/resources/doc/code-medical-ethics/5026a.pdf.

American Telemedicine Association. n.d. Nomenclature. http://www.americantelemed.org/practice/nomenclature.

Amori G. 2009. Preventing and reporting medical identity theft. *Journal of Healthcare Risk Management* 28(2):33–42

Burrington-Brown, Jill, and Gwen Hughes. 2003. AHIMA practice brief: provider-patient e-mail security" Web extra. Chicago: AHIMA.

Casey, K. 2017. "How to get started with IAM services in the cloud." *Tech Target.* April http://searchcloudcomputing.techtarget.com/feature/How-to-get-started-with-IAM-services-in-the-cloud

Center for Connected Health Policy. 2013. What is telehealth. http://cchpca.telehealthpolicy.us/what-is-telehealth.

Center for Medicare and Medicaid Services. "Mobile Device Privacy and Security." *Guide to Privacy and Security of Electronic Health Information.* https://www.healthit.gov/providers-professionals/guide-privacy-and-security-electronic-health-information.

Chiou, S.Y. 2013. Secure method for biometric-base recognition with integrated cryptographic functions. *BioMed Research International.* https://www.hindawi.com/journals/bmri/2013/623815/

Davis, N., et al. 2006. Practice brief: Facsimile transmission of health information. Web extra. Chicago: AHIMA.

Davis, N., C. Lemery, and K. Roberts. 2005. Practice brief: Identity theft and fraud—The impact on HIM operations. *Journal of AHIMA* 76(4):64A–64D.

Department of Health and Human Services. 2011. HIPAA Privacy Rule accounting of disclosures under the Health Information Technology for Economic and Clinical Health Act. 45 CFR Part 164. *Federal Register* 76(104):31426–31449.

Department of Health and Human Services. n.d. Addendum 2: HIPAA security and electronic signature standards glossary of terms. http://www.aspe.hhs.gov/admnsimp/nprm/sec15.htm.

Department of Health and Human Services. 2014. Annual report to Congress on breaches of unsecured protected health information. https://www.hhs.gov/sites/default/files/rtc-breach-20132014.pdf.

Department of Health and Human Services. 2016. Fact Sheet: Ransomware and HIPAA. http://www.hhs.gov/sites/default/files/RansomwareFactSheet.pdf.

Dill, M.W., S. Lucci, and T. Walsh. 2016. Understanding cybersecurity: A primer for HIM professionals. *Journal of AHIMA* (87)4:46–51.

Dixon, P. 2006. Medical identity theft: The information crime that can kill you. World Privacy Forum. http://www.worldprivacyforum.org/medicalidentitytheft.html.

Dougherty, M. and R. Scichilone. 2002. Practice brief: Establishing a telecommuting or home-based employee program. *Journal of AHIMA* 73(7):72A–72L.

Eramo, L.A. Stopping thieves in their tracks: What HIM professionals can do to mitigate medical identity theft. *Journal of AHIMA* 87(8):40–43.

Federal Trade Commission. 2011. Consumer information: Phishing. https://www.consumer.ftc.gov/articles/0003-phishing.

Food and Drug Administration. 2016. *Postmarket Management of Cybersecurity in Medical Devices.* https://www.fda.gov/downloads/medicaldevices/deviceregulationandguidance/guidancedocuments/ucm482022.pdf

Gellman, R. and P. Dixon. 2009. Red Flag and address discrepancy requirements: Suggestions for health care providers. Version 2. Cardiff by the Sea, CA: World Privacy Forum. http://www.worldprivacyforum.org/pdf/WPF_RedFlagReport_09242008fs.pdf.

Gordon, G. 2013. The growing threat of medical identity fraud: A call to action. Medical Identity Fraud Alliance.

Government Accountability Office. U.S. Report to Congress. *Medical Devices* August 2012.

Health Data Management. 2004. Feds get first HIPAA conviction. http://healthdatamanagement.com/news/10101-1.html

Hackers Directly Targeting Health Care Organizations, FBI Warns." *iHealthBeat* . August 21, 2014. www.ihealthbeat .org/articles/2014/8/21/hackers-directly-targeting-health-care-organizations-fbi-warns.

Heinrich. M. 2014. "Records Management and eDiscovery Converge!" http://community.aiim.org/blogs/marty -heinrich/2014/04/17/records-management-and-ediscovery-converge

Humer, C. and J. Finkle. 2014 (September 24). Your medical record is worth more to hackers than your credit card. *Reuters.*

Kind, T. 2015. Professional guidelines for social media use: A starting point. *AMA Journal of Ethics* 17(5):441–447.

Kissel, R., ed. 2011. *Glossary of Key Information Security Terms.* NIST publication IR 7298, Revision 1. National Institute of Standards and Technology (NIST) Computer Security Resource Center. http://csrc.nist.gov.

Narasimman, R. 2005. Laptop security. http://whitepapers.hackerjournals.com.

National Archives and Records Administration. 2013 (August 29). Bulletin 2013-02. Guidance on a new approach to managing email records. https://www.archives.gov/records-mgmt/bulletins/2013/2013-02.html.

National Cyber Security Alliance. n.d. http://www.staysafeonline.org/.

National Institute of Standards and Technology. 2001. FIPS PUB 140-2. Security requirements for cryptographic modules. http://csrc.nist.gov/groups/STM/cmvp/standards.html.

National Institute of Standards and Technology. n.d. http://www.nist.gov/index.html.

National Institute of Standards and Technology. 1995. Special Publication 800-12: Introduction to computer security. The NIST Handbook. http://csrc.nist.gov/nistpubs/800-12/handbook.pdf.

National Institute of Standards and Technology. 2014. *Framework for Improving Critical Infrastructure Cybersecurity.* www.nist.gov/cyberframework/upload/cybersecurity-framework-021214-final.pdf?

NPR. 2015 (February 13). The black market for stolen health care data. Morning Edition. http://www.npr.org /sections/alltechconsidered/2015/02/13/385901377/the-black-market-for-stolen-health-care-data.

Office of the National Coordinator 2015. *Guide to Privacy and Security of Electronic Health Information.* https:// www.healthit.gov/providers-professionals/guide-privacy-and-security-electronic-health-information

Open Web Application Security Project (OWASP). 2016. Access control. The Open Web Application Security Project. https://www.owasp.org/index.php/Category:Access_Control

Ponemon Institute. 2015a. Fifth Annual Study on medical identity theft. Ponemon Institute Research Report. http:// medidfraud.org/wp-content/uploads/2015/02/2014_Medical_ID_Theft_Study1.pdf.

Ponemon Institute. 2015b. Fifth annual study on privacy and security of health data. https://media.scmagazine .com/documents/121/healthcare_privacy_security_be_30019.pdf.

PricewaterhouseCoopers. 2015. Managing cyber risks in an interconnected world: Key findings from the global state of information security survey 2015. http://www.pwc.com/gx/en/consulting-services/information-security -survey/assets/the-global-state-of-information-security-survey-2015.pdf

Reed, M., I. Graetz, N. Gordon, and V. Fung. 2015 (December 21). Patient-initiated e-mails to providers: Associations with out-of-pocket visit costs, and impact on care-seeking and health. *The American Journal of Managed Care* 21(12):e632–e639.

Rinehart-Thompson, L. and L. Harman. 2017. Privacy and Confidentiality in *Ethical Health Informatics: Challenges and Opportunities*, 3rd ed. Burlington, MA: Jones and Bartlett Learning.

SANS Institute. n.d.a http://www.sans.org.

SANS. n.d.b Glossary of security terms. https://www.sans.org/security-resources/glossary-of-terms/.

SANS. 2015. Remote access policy. https://www.sans.org/security-resources/policies/network-security/pdf /remote-access-policy

National Conference of Commissioners on Uniform State Laws. 2005. Uniform Rules of Evidence Act http://www .uniformlaws.org/shared/docs/rules%20of%20evidence/uroea_final_99%20with%2005amends.pdf

Wager, K.A., F.W. Lee, and J.P. Glaser. 2009. Health Care Information Systems: A Practical Approach for Health Care Management, 2nd ed. San Francisco: Jossey-Bass.

Walsh, T., B.C. Sher, G.A. Roselle, and S.D. Gamage. 2009. *Medical Records Disaster Planning: A Health Information Manager's Survival Guide.* Chicago: AHIMA.

Walsh, T. 2011. Practice brief: Security risk analysis and management: An overview (updated). Web extra. Chicago: AHIMA.

Walsh, T. 2014. Privacy and security audits of electronic health information. *Journal of AHIMA* 85(3):54–59.

Walsh, T. and S. Lucci. 2015. The changing face of disaster recovery. *For The Record* 27(10):15–17.

World Privacy Forum. n.d. Medical identity theft. https://www.worldprivacyforum.org/category/med-id-theft/.

Cases, Statutes, and Regulations Cited

16 CFR Part 681: Fair and Accurate Credit Transaction Act. 2003.

45 CFR 164.308(a)(7): Contingency plan. 2005.

47 CFR 15.37(f): Telecommunication radio frequency devices. 1994.

18 USC 1028: Fraud and related activities in connection with identification documents and information. 1998.

18 USC 1029: Fraud and related activity in connection with access devices. 2006.

18 USC 2510: Electronic Communications Privacy Act. 1986.

18 USC 2511: Interception and disclosure of wire, oral, or electronic communications prohibited. 2002.

18 USC 2701: Unlawful access to stored communications. 2006.

42 USC 3711: Title III Omnibus Crime Control and Safe Streets Acts. 1968.

Appendix 13

Confidentiality and Nondisclosure Agreement (for Employees)

As an employee/contracted employee affiliated with the [name of organization], I understand that I must maintain the confidentiality of any and all data and information to which I have access in the course of carrying out my work. Organizational information that may include, but is not limited to, financial, patient identifiable, employee identifiable, intellectual property, financially non-public, contractual, of a competitively advantageous nature, and is from any source or in any form (i.e., paper, magnetic or optical media, conversations, film, etc.), may be considered confidential. The value and sensitivity of information is protected by law and by the strict policies of [name of organization]. The intent of these laws and policies is to ensure that confidential information will remain confidential through its use as a necessity to accomplish the organization's mission. Special consideration is expected for all information related to personally identifiable health information accessed in the course of your work.

As a condition to receiving electronic access and allowed access to a [system, network, or files] and/or being granted authorization to access any form of confidential information identified above, I agree to comply with the following terms and conditions:

1. My computer sign-on code is equivalent to my LEGAL SIGNATURE and I will not disclose this code to anyone or allow anyone to access the system using my sign-on code and/or password.

2. I am responsible and accountable for all entries made and all retrievals accessed under my sign-on code, even if such action was made by me or by another due to my intentional or negligent act or omission. Any data available to me will be treated as confidential information.

3. I will not attempt to learn or use another's sign-on code.

4. I will not access any online computer system using a sign-on code other than my own.

5. I will not access or request any information for which I have no responsibility.

6. If I have reason to believe that the confidentiality of my user sign-on code/password has been compromised, I will immediately notify [responsible party] by calling the helpdesk at [helpdesk phone number].

7. I will not disclose any confidential information unless required to do so in the official capacity of my employment or contract. I also understand that I have no right or ownership interest in any confidential information.

8. While signed on, I will not leave a secured computer application unattended.

9. I will comply with all policies and procedures and other rules of [name of organization] relating to confidentiality of information and access procedures.

10. I understand that my use of the [name of employer or organization] system may be periodically monitored to ensure compliance with this agreement.

11. I agree not to use the information in any way detrimental to the organization and will keep all such information confidential.

12. I will not disclose protected health information or other information that is considered proprietary, sensitive, or confidential unless there is a need-to-know basis.

13. I will limit distribution of confidential information only to parties with a legitimate need in performance of the organization's mission.

14. I agree that disclosure of confidential information is prohibited indefinitely, even after termination of employment or business relationship, unless specifically waived in writing by an authorized party.

15. This agreement cannot be terminated or canceled, nor will it expire.

16. I will follow the organizational compliance plan for use of confidential information.

I further understand that if I violate any of the above terms, I will be subject to disciplinary action, including discharge, loss of privileges, termination of contract, legal action, or any other remedy available to [name of organization].

User's Name: _____

Department: _____

Adapted from the AHIMA Home Coding Community of Practice Community Resource Posting—Sample Confidentiality Policy.

This sample form was developed by AHIMA for discussion purposes only. It should not be used without review by your organization's legal counsel to ensure compliance with local and state laws.

Source: Dougherty, M. and R.A. Scichilone. 2002 (July/August). Practice brief: Establishing a telecommuting or home-based employee program. *Journal of AHIMA* 73(7):72A–72L.

Patient Rights and Responsibilities

Laurie A. Rinehart-Thompson, JD, RHIA, CHP, FAHIMA

Learning Objectives

- Distinguish the types of patient–provider relationships
- Examine the factors that determine whether a patient has the right to receive or refuse medical treatment
- Compare sources of patient rights with respect to their legal authority
- Analyze how the rights of patients with mental illnesses can be exercised, including those relating to the use of seclusion and restraints
- Differentiate various forms of patient health information rights and analyze how they benefit the patient
- Illustrate how patient responsibilities can be carried out by individuals

Key Terms

- Against medical advice (AMA)
- Billing advocates
- Community benefit standard
- Consumer Health Information Bill of Rights
- Cultural competence
- Emergency medical condition (EMC)
- Emergency Medical Treatment and Active Labor Act (EMTALA)
- Health literacy
- Hill-Burton Act
- Informative relationship
- Interpretive relationship
- Involuntary civil commitment
- Meaningful Use
- Medical screening exam (MSE)
- Paternalistic relationship
- Patient Care Partnership
- Patient-centered care
- Patient portals
- Patient rights
- Personal health records (PHRs)
- Restraint
- Seclusion

At the heart of patient rights is respect for the dignity and autonomy of a person. Patient rights are largely driven by external forces, such as social and cultural norms, as well as internal forces, such as an individual's ethical compass and sense of right and wrong. Patient rights are also externally driven by government statutes and regulations, private standards, and organizational policies. Patient rights include access to healthcare, self-determination about whether or not to receive treatment, and access to and control over one's own health information. As patients become progressively more empowered by their status as healthcare consumers, they are likely to exert their rights as they relate to existing patient rights statute and regulations. As a result, it is likely that this will become a more active area of healthcare law.

Patient Rights

At its most basic level, the term **patient rights** addresses conduct between a healthcare provider and a patient. However, it encompasses many aspects. For many, the greatest patient rights priority is the ability to receive high-quality healthcare. Even this concept, however, is multi-dimensional. High-quality care includes not only skillful care that leads to a desired clinical outcome, but also care that is respectful, compassionate, and associated with positive interpersonal experiences.

While patient rights have long emphasized the dignity of the patient, the concept has evolved into a provider-patient partnership that fosters patient empowerment by taking into account the patient's wants, needs, and preferences; to consider their families when appropriate; and to ensure patients are appropriately educated and knowledgeable about their health conditions. Individuals should receive sufficient information to make decisions about their care (Institute of Medicine 2000). Further, they should be informed about how their health information will be used and disclosed, how it will be protected, and what rights they have with respect to their information. With this knowledge, patients become empowered to exercise a degree of control–and to become the focal point of control–over their medical care.

The Patient–Provider Relationship

The patient–provider relationship can assume various forms. The most traditional is the **paternalistic relationship**, where the provider is the medical authority and the patient is the passive recipient. The provider dispenses his or her knowledge about the patient's condition and the medical options that are best for the patient. The patient is expected to defer to the provider's expertise in this "doctor-knows-best" model.

At the opposite end of the spectrum is the **informative relationship**, characterized by the provider who dispenses information, but the patient who makes the decisions. As the consumer, and by exercising the relationship in its purest sense, the patient has complete autonomy and control.

In between the paternalistic and informative relationships is the **interpretive relationship**, which involves shared decision-making. The provider supplies information to the patient, but only after knowing the patient's wishes, such as what is important to the patient and what his or her concerns are. Shared decision making emphasizes a patient's priorities. Rather than instructing a patient, as the paternalistic relationship does, or leaving the decision-making entirely up to the patient, as the informative relationship does, it involves the provider working with the patient to achieve the patient's desired goals (Gawande 2014; Emanuel and Emanuel 1992).

Right to Healthcare

From a patient perspective, one of the most important rights is the simple right to receive healthcare services. Although the United States Constitution does not provide a right to healthcare, various laws such as federal and state statutes and regulations outline circumstances where individuals have the right to receive medical treatment or to be hospitalized. However, they depend on the situation or the type of person or organization involved. For example, veterans generally have the right to be treated at federal Veterans Affairs facilities. Individuals covered by health insurance also have a right to healthcare based on the contract between a healthcare provider and their health insurer. Finally, once a physician-patient relationship is established, the right to healthcare may be established if the physician wishes to avoid claims of abandonment (Showalter 2015).

From an organizational perspective, a healthcare facility may be obligated to demonstrate that it meets the Internal Revenue Service–codified **community benefit standard** by providing a certain amount of uncompensated care and engaging in activities that benefit its community (for example, performing health screenings and participating in community health fairs). Meeting this standard is required to retain tax-exempt status. This standard, even when taking the Patient Protection and Affordable Care Act's (ACA) requirements into consideration (such as consumer protections regarding billing collection practices), doesn't specify a minimum value or dollar amount of uncompensated care, nor does it guarantee healthcare to specific individuals. It does, however, promote charity care by healthcare organizations to at least some individuals in need of healthcare services (James 2016).

Elective Treatment

In general, hospitals do not have a legal obligation to admit, and healthcare providers do not have a legal obligation to treat, nonemergency cases as long as they do not violate anti-discrimination laws, such as the Civil Rights Act of 1964, that prohibits discrimination based on race, color, religion, sex or national origin. Other factors that must be considered when making determinations about admission, in addition to emergency status and illegal discrimination, are the sufficiency of the facility to treat the patient; whether the individual's physician has medical staff privileges at the facility to treat the patient; and the patient population that the facility serves (for example, adults versus children) (Showalter 2015).

Hill-Burton Act

In 1946, Congress passed the **Hill-Burton Act**, which provided hospitals, nursing homes, and certain other healthcare facilities money for construction and modernization. As a condition of receiving Hill-Burton financial assistance, facilities had to agree, through a Community Service Assurance, to provide a reasonable volume of services to those unable to pay and make their services available to all persons residing in the area. The Hill-Burton program stopped providing funds in 1997, leaving about 150 facilities nationwide that are still obligated to provide free or reduced-cost care under the program's obligations. Application for Hill-Burton free care is required; that is, it is not automatically provided to those without sufficient financial means (HRSA n.d.). Importantly, although Hill-Burton no longer applies to many facilities, it has imbued many organizations with the mission of providing uncompensated medical care to the degree they are financially able to do so.

Specifically, Hill-Burton facilities must comply with the requirements in figure 14.1.

Figure 14.1 Hill-Burton facility obligations

Every hospital or other facility that ever gave a Community Service Assurance in exchange for Hill-Burton funds under Title VI of the Public Health Service Act must:

- Provide emergency services to any person living in its service area who cannot afford those services

- Give each person living in its service area non-emergency medical treatment at the facility no matter their race, color, national origin, creed, or any other factor unrelated to a person's ability to pay for a needed service and the facility's ability to provide the needed service

- Participate in the Medicare and Medicaid programs unless they are ineligible

- Make arrangements for reimbursement for services with principal state and local third-party payers that provide reimbursement that is not less than the actual cost of the services

- Post its community service obligations in English and Spanish, and any other language spoken by 10 percent or more of the households in the service area

- The Hill-Burton Act also applies to people working in the service area of the facility if it was funded under Title XVI of the Public Health Service Act

- The community service obligation does not require the facility to make non-emergency services available to persons unable to pay them

Source: Department of Health and Human Services n.d.

Emergency Treatment and EMTALA

In 1986, Congress enacted the **Emergency Medical Treatment and Active Labor Act (EMTALA)** as part of the Consolidated Omnibus Reconciliation Act. EMTALA was passed largely in response to many hospitals engaging in the practice of "patient-dumping," that is, transferring, discharging, or refusing to treat indigent patients in the emergency department because of their inability to pay. Although the law was passed to protect individuals unable to pay for their encounter, EMTALA's protections apply to any patient seeking care at a facility that must comply with the law. Therefore, facilities cannot discriminate against any person seeking emergency services for any reason.

Hospitals that participate in the Medicare program and that offer emergency services must comply with EMTALA. Penalties for EMTALA violations include fines and possible exclusion from the Medicare program. Per the EMTALA regulations, hospitals must follow the requirements outlined in figure 14.2. The regulations specifically refer to a **medical screening exam (MSE)**, which is an evaluation of a patient's health condition, and an **emergency medical condition (EMC)**, which is a health condition that could result in serious harm or death if not treated immediately. An EMC includes active labor.

Whenever transfer occurs without the patient having first been stabilized, copious documentation that reflects compliance with the law is essential to avoid EMTALA liability.

Right to Accept or Refuse Treatment

Competent adults have the right to consent to treatment. They also have the right to refuse treatment, a right that is reinforced by the federal Patient Self-Determination Act. As discussed in chapter 8, this act requires hospitals, nursing facilities, hospice program and home health agencies that bill Medicare or Medicaid to provide adult patients with information about advance directive options, such as living wills and Durable Powers of Attorney for Healthcare Decisions. The right to refuse treatment, because it is grounded in the principle of self-determination, exists even if that refusal may result in an individual's death. However, a court can decide that there is a compelling state interest in preserving someone's life despite a refusal, such as ensuring the welfare of a patient's minor children (Showalter 2015).

Figure 14.2 EMTALA requirements for treating and transferring patients

- Per EMTALA, if a patient presents for emergency care, a hospital must:
- Provide an appropriate medical screening exam (MSE) to anyone coming to the emergency department seeking an examination or treatment for an emergency medical condition (EMC), including active labor (CMS 2012)
- If an EMC is found, the hospital must treat and stabilize the emergency medical condition. Stabilization may not be delayed while a patient's payment status is determined (Showalter 2015).
  - The hospital may transfer an unstable patient only if at least one of following two conditions is met:
    - The patient requests transfer
    - The medical benefits of transferring the patient outweigh the risks to the patient because the hospital is not able to stabilize the patient within its capability (CMS 2012)
  - When transfer does occur, the transferring hospital must implement an appropriate transfer by providing all treatment necessary prior to the transfer to minimize risk to the patient; locating a hospital that is both willing and able to accept the patient; sending medical records with the patient to the receiving facility; and ensuring that appropriate staff and equipment are utilized to facilitate the patient's transfer (Showalter 2015).

Source: CMS 2012; Showalter 2015.

Right to Discharge

A patient is usually discharged from a hospital after a physician documents a discharge order. However, at times, a patient may wish to initiate his or her own discharge. Except in limited circumstances, competent adults have the right to discharge themselves from a hospital at any time. If a provider fails to discharge a patient, it might be considered battery or false imprisonment except in cases where a patient is determined to be a danger to self or others. This designation usually is associated with individuals who meet this definition by virtue of a contagious disease or a mental condition or illness (Showalter 2015).

When a patient discharges himself or herself before a physician has determined it to be medically appropriate, a discharge **against medical advice (AMA)** has occurred. Since AMA discharges are associated with poor outcomes such as higher readmission, morbidity and mortality rates, and increased lengths of stay on subsequent admissions, hospitals should have a discharge AMA protocol in place. This protocol could include a collaborative approach with a follow-up outpatient care team, making provisions for prescriptions to be filled, employing shared decision-making with the patient to ensure that he or she is capable of understanding the risks associated with an AMA discharge, and ensuring that not only the patient's medical needs, but also their social needs, can be met (Tummalapalli and Goodman 2016).

The circumstances surrounding a patient's AMA discharge, as well as actions taken in response to the discharge, should be documented in the patient's record. Patients leaving against medical advice should be asked to sign a form acknowledging that they understand the potential consequences of the discharge to their health and agree not to hold the healthcare facility liable for any poor outcome they experience as a result. They should also acknowledge that their insurance company may refuse to pay for their care if they leave AMA. Having the patient sign such a form after discussing the risks may strengthen protections from legal liability associated with poor outcomes related to AMA discharges, but it may not be a total shield against liability. In addition, many patients refuse to sign such a form, or leave before staff can present them with the form.

Check Your Understanding | 14.1

Instructions: Indicate whether the following statements are true or false (T or F).

1. The interpretive physician–patient relationship involves the patient as a passive recipient.
2. The United States Constitution provides a right to healthcare.
3. EMTALA was passed by Congress to combat transfer and discharge of patients, and refusal to treat, based on inability to pay.
4. Failure to discharge a patient could constitute battery or false imprisonment.
5. A court may decide that there is a compelling state interest in preserving life that overrides a patient's right to refuse treatment.

Sources of Patient Rights

The notion of patient rights stems from the broader concept that human beings have a basic right to be treated with dignity and equality, as formalized in the 1948 Universal Declaration of Human Rights (WHO n.d.). As previously mentioned, many federal and state laws address patient rights as do a number of other health-related organizations and agencies. Some common sources of patient rights, in addition to Hill-Burton and EMTALA, mentioned previously, are discussed next.

| Figure 14.3 | Patient expectations and rights per the AHA patient care partnership |

- High-quality hospital care, including the identity and professional status of your caregivers.
- A clean and safe environment.
- Involvement in your care.
- Protection of your privacy.
- Help when leaving the hospital.
- Help with your billing and insurance claims.

Source: AHA 2016.

American Hospital Association Patient Care Partnership

The American Hospital Association has developed a **Patient Care Partnership** (originally called the Patients' Bill of Rights) that helps patients understand their expectations, rights, and responsibilities when receiving hospital services (AHA 2016). The AHA clearly states what a patient should be able to expect during his or her hospital stay. These expectations are listed in figure. 14.3.

The Joint Commission Standards

As with the Medicare Conditions of Participation (CoP), The Joint Commission accreditation standards have specific requirements pertaining to patient rights. The patient rights standards center on dignity; respect; the patient's cultural and personal values, beliefs and preferences; the need for effective communication that informs the patient; privacy; right to pain management; involvement of individuals for emotional support; and prohibitions against discrimination based on age, gender, gender identity or expression, sexual orientation, race, religion, culture, ethnicity, language, disability (either physical or mental) or socioeconomic status (Joint Commission 2016). The Joint Commission requires that policies be written to address both patient rights and responsibilities. Additionally, Joint Commission standards defer to applicable statutes and regulations. The requirements of the 2016 Joint Commission Rights and Responsibilities of the Individual encompass the standards listed in figure 14.4 for all hospitals and are similar for other care settings.

Medicare Conditions of Participation

To participate in the Medicare and Medicaid programs, healthcare facilities must meet certain minimum requirements related to health and safety. Hospital requirements are found in the Medicare CoP, which are located at 42 CFR 482.13. The Medicare CoP regarding patient rights apply to all Medicare and Medicaid participating hospitals, including short-term, psychiatric, rehabilitation, long-term, children's, and alcohol and drug facilities. The following patient rights standards are required:

- Patients must be given notice of their rights and a process for bringing grievances.
- Patients must be allowed to exercise rights related to participating in their care plans, making informed decisions regarding their care, establishing advance directives, and notifying family and physicians of a hospitalization.

- Patients have the right to personal privacy, care in a safe setting, and freedom from abuse and harassment.
- Patients have the right to confidentiality of their records and to access their records in a reasonable time frame.
- Patients have the right to be free from physical or mental abuse, corporal punishment, and restraint or seclusion used for coercion, discipline, convenience, or retaliation. (Seclusion and restraint are discussed in detail later in this chapter.)
- Patients have the right to visitation privileges, and to be informed of policies and procedures that reasonably restrict or limit visitation. (42 CFR 482.13)

The Centers for Medicare and Medicaid Services publishes a booklet for consumers, "Medicare Rights & Protections," that additionally emphasizes the right to dignity and respect, protection from discrimination, access to providers, ability to receive information in an understandable and culturally sensitive manner, notice of coverage and ability to appeal coverage decisions (HHS 2014).

The Affordable Care Act (ACA)

In 2010, the ACA was passed. Challenged legally and later upheld by the United States Supreme Court, the most controversial provision of the Act was the individual mandate, which requires individuals to

Figure 14.4 Joint Commission patient rights and responsibilities of the individual (RI) standards

The hospital:
- respects, protects, and promotes patient rights.
- respects the patient's right to receive information in a manner he or she understands (to include interpretation or translation services based on language differences and/or impairments).
- respects the patient's right to participate in decisions about his or her care, treatment, and services.
- honors the patient's right to give or withhold informed consent.
- honors the patient's right to give or withhold informed consent to produce or use recordings, films, or other images of the patient for purposes other than his or her care.
- protects the patient and respects his or her rights during research, investigation, and clinical trials.
- respects the patient's right to receive information about the individuals(s) responsible for, as well as those providing, his or her care, treatment, and services.
- addresses patient decisions about care, treatment, and services received at the end of life.
- informs the patient about his or her responsibilities related to his or her care, treatment, and services (to include providing information that facilitates treatment; asking questions and acknowledging lack of understanding; following instructions, policies, rules and regulations to support quality care and a safe environment; maintain civil language and conduct with staff; and meeting financial commitments).

The patient:
- has the right to be free from neglect; exploitation; and verbal, mental, physical and sexual abuse.
- has a right to an environment that preserves dignity and contributes to a positive self-image.
- and his or her family have the right to have complaints reviewed by the hospital.
- has the right to access protective and advocacy services.

Source: The Joint Commission 2016.

purchase health insurance. The Act supports individual (patient) rights by providing individuals with a number of healthcare coverage rights and protections such as:

- Coverage of preexisting health conditions, including pregnancy
- Free preventive care
- More coverage options for young adults
- Protects choice of doctor
- Ends lifetime and yearly dollar limits on coverage of essential benefits
- Illegal to cancel a plan if individual (patient) gets sick (HealthCare.gov n.d.)

The rights and protections apply to some or all plans, depending on whether the plans are from the health insurance marketplace, individual insurance or job-based plans. Since its passage, proponents and opponents of the ACA have been quite polarized. At the time of this publication the future of the ACA is very uncertain although some patient rights, such as coverage of preexisting health conditions, appear poised to remain in effect.

State Laws

States generally provide laws that guide patient rights in hospitals and other healthcare facilities. For example, Florida law addresses both healthcare facilities and healthcare providers by including requirements for both. It provides mandates with regard to individual dignity, knowledge of health and financial information, consent to research, and knowledge of a patient's rights and responsibilities (Fla. Stat. 381.026). Illinois law states that patients have the right to care that is consistent with sound medical and nursing practice; the right to receive information relevant to his or her condition and treatment; the right to receive an explanation of his or her bill; and the right for his or her care and records of his or her care to be afforded privacy and confidentiality (410 Ill. Comp. Stat. 50/3-111 ½ par. 5403).

Organizational Patient Rights Policies

Every facility should have policies in place that identify patient rights. At a minimum, policies should meet applicable requirements such as the Medicare CoP, state law, and Joint Commission standards. However, they should also include other rights deemed appropriate by the organization and that are in keeping with its mission, vision and values. Both patients and staff must be made aware of these rights. Patients should be given notice of their rights at their first encounter or admission or as soon as reasonably possible afterward, whether they are presented as a bill of rights or as a separate policy. Staff should be trained on patient rights policies upon hire and routinely thereafter, and notified of any changes to the organization's policies.

Organizational policies must encompass concepts such as individual dignity and the protection of information. However, they should also address operational issues. For example, healthcare facilities have a general duty to respect and protect patient property. Policies should address the patient's right to retain and use their personal belongings as appropriate, and those belongings should be returned to the patient upon discharge. Policies should also address the safekeeping of property, delineating the organization's responsibility versus the patient's responsibility for safeguarding patient property, and assessing liability if patient property is lost or stolen.

Check Your Understanding 14.2

Instructions: Indicate whether the following statements are true or false (T or F).

1. The American Hospital Association's Patients' Bill of Rights is now the Patient Care Partnership, which focuses on patient expectations, rights, and responsibilities.

2. The Joint Commission standards specifically state that patients have the right to be free from neglect and exploitation.

3. The Medicare Conditions of Participation also apply to Medicaid participating hospitals.

4. The Affordable Care Act generally permits lifetime limits on health insurance benefits.

5. Safekeeping of property must always be the patient's responsibility.

Specific Patient Rights Issues

There are numerous laws and sets of guidance that provide for patient rights and, ultimately, patient protection. However, particularly vulnerable patient populations, such as those with mental illnesses, must receive special protections. Many of these special protections stem from a history of past abuses.

Rights of Patients with Mental Illnesses

Hospitalization and treatment of individuals with mental illnesses often involve the ability to institutionalize individuals against their wishes. A provider may generally avoid liability for admitting a patient or preventing discharge if the patient is deemed a danger to self or others. The "danger to self or others" designation can be assigned to patients with a mental condition or illness, particularly if they are suicidal or unable to care for themselves, or homicidal. However, this **involuntary civil commitment** of a patient is not without limits. Because they are potentially losing their freedom through involuntary confinement, individuals have the right to procedural due process, which is a hearing within a time period specified by statute.

Individuals with mental illnesses cannot be confined indefinitely based solely on a mental illness diagnosis, for custodial purposes and without a showing of being dangerous to oneself or others. Further, once committed, patients have a right to substantive constitutional rights that include adequate shelter, clothing, nutrition, medical care, and an environment that is safe. Mental illness and involuntary commitment does not equate to incompetence. Thus, unless deemed incompetent, individuals who have been admitted to a mental health facility retain their right to consent to or refuse treatment if they are not a danger to themselves or others (Showalter 2015).

Civilly committed patients with mental illnesses must be distinguished from those who have been charged with a crime. Criminally charged individuals retain their constitutional rights, but within the constraints of the criminal justice system.

Limits on Seclusion and Restraints

Of the six Medicare CoP standards listed previously, the most extensive standards apply to the use of seclusion and restraints because of the potential for their misuse and the potential for physical injury and psychological trauma among particularly vulnerable patient populations. Seclusion and restraints have historically been used, and misused, among populations with behavioral challenges. These challenges may be the result of an individual's lifelong characteristic or due to the onset of a particular condition. Populations include those with mental illnesses; developmental disabilities, either congenital or presenting later in life; and other behavioral issues, such as those that may accompany Alzheimer's disease or other forms of dementia. Children and the elderly are especially vulnerable to inappropriate use of seclusion and restraint.

Seclusion is "the involuntary confinement of a patient alone in a room or area from which the patient is physically prevented from leaving." It can only be used in response to violent or self-destructive behavior (42 CFR 482.13). **Restraint** is a device or drug that restricts a patient's freedom of movement and is not related to diagnosis or treatment, protecting a patient from falling out of bed, or permitting a patient to participate in activities without the risk of harm (42 CFR 482.13). The CoP applies limits to seclusion and restraint as outlined in figure 14.5. The CoP includes requirements regarding the reporting of injury or death related to seclusion and restraints which is discussed in more detail in chapter 16, Required Reporting and Mandatory Reporting.

Figure 14.5 Medicare CoP seclusion and restraint requirements

- Seclusion or restraint is only permissible to ensure a patient's, staff member or other person's immediate physical safety and must be discontinued as soon as possible.
- Seclusion or restraint may only be used when less restrictive mechanisms are not effective to prevent physical harm to any person.
- The type used is the least restrictive effective mechanism to prevent physical harm to any person.
- It is per a written modification to the care plan.
- It is per an order by a physician or other licensed independent practitioner responsible for the patient and authorized to order seclusion and restraint (if not ordered by the attending physician, he or she must be consulted as soon as possible).
- It may not be written as a standing order or as needed (prn).
- It is implemented according to safe and appropriate techniques per hospital policy and state law.
- Orders to manage violent or self-destructive behavior must be ordered at least every 4 hours (18+ years old); every 2 hours (9–17 years old); and every 1 hour (< 9 years old), up to a maximum of 24 hours.
- Above 24 hours, the physician or licensed independent practitioner responsible for the patient must see and assess the patient before writing a new order.
- Orders to ensure the physical safety of non-violent or non-self-destructive patients may be renewed per hospital policy.
- The condition of a secluded or restrained patient must be monitored as required by hospital policy by a physician or licensed independent practitioner who have been trained per hospital policy.
- Seclusion or restraint that is used to manage violent or self-destructive behavior that endangers the physical safety of the patient or others requires the patient to be seen in person within one hour after the intervention by a physician or other licensed independent practitioner, or a trained registered nurse or physician assistant to evaluate the patient's immediate situation; reaction to intervention; medical and behavioral status; and need to continue or terminate seclusion or restraint. An evaluating registered nurse or physician assistant must consult with the attending physician or other licensed independent practitioner responsible for the patient as soon as possible after the evaluation.
- Seclusion and restraint may only be used together if the patient is monitored in person by a trained staff member or by trained staff with both video and audio equipment, in close proximity to the patient.
- Documentation of seclusion or restraint must include: one-hour face-to-face medical and behavioral evaluation if being used to manage violent or self-destructive behavior; description of patient behavior; description of intervention; alternatives or less restrictive interventions, if attempted; patient behavior that necessitated the seclusion or restraint; patient's response to intervention; rationale for any continued use of intervention.
- Staff must be trained and demonstrate competency during orientation; before performing seclusion or restraint; and periodically thereafter per hospital policy regarding implementing seclusion; applying restraints; monitoring; assessing; and providing care for a patient in seclusion or restraint. Training must be provided by qualified staff and competency of trainees must be documented.

Figure 14.5	Medicare CoP seclusion and restraint requirements (Continued)

- Training and demonstrated knowledge by staff must include: techniques to identify behaviors and situations that trigger seclusion or restraint; use of nonphysical interventions; choosing the least restrictive intervention based on assessment of the individual; safe application and use of all types of seclusion and restraint; recognizing and responding to physical and psychological distress; identifying behavior changes that indicate seclusion or restraint is no longer necessary; monitoring the physical and psychological well-being of a secluded or restrained patient (e.g., respiration, circulation, skin integrity, vital signs, hospital requirements for the one-hour face-to-face evaluation); use of first aid techniques including cardiopulmonary resuscitation and recertification.
- Deaths occurring while in seclusion or restraint, within 24 hours after a patient has been removed from seclusion or restraint, or within 1 week after seclusion or restraint (if presumed to be related to the death) must be reported to the Centers for Medicare and Medicaid Services (CMS) no later than the close of business on the day following knowledge of the patient's death.
- If death occurs while a patient is only in soft wrist restraints (no seclusion) or within 24 hours after removal of the restraints, staff must internally log the death within seven days and include patient name, dates of birth and death, attending physician or licensed independent practitioner responsible for the patient's care, medical record number, and primary diagnosis(es).
- Documentation in the medical record must reflect date and time death was reported to CMS (where required) or logged internally.

Source: Medicare Conditions of Participation, 42 CFR 482.13.

The Children's Health Act of 2000 (Pub. L. 106-310) establishes national standards that restrict the use of restraints and seclusion in all psychiatric facilities that receive federal funds and in "non-medical community-based facilities for children and youth." In those settings, the use of restraints and seclusion is restricted to emergency safety situations and must be assessed and monitored by a trained person. This act also includes requirements regarding the reporting of injury or deaths as discussed in chapter 16.

Patient Health Information Rights

With societal changes, the tide in healthcare has shifted toward patient empowerment. This shift is significantly present in health information, where laws have been passed to give patients more rights and where information is now created, stored and retrieved electronically, enabling healthcare consumers to become more active and knowledgeable participants in their own healthcare.

Privacy and Confidentiality

A patient has the right to the social value of privacy and to the confidentiality of information that is shared with his or her healthcare provider. These longstanding rights have been mandated via regulation (for example, Medicare Conditions of Participation), through accreditation standards (for example, Joint Commission), and through professional association guidelines and best practices such as those promoted by the American Hospital Association and, specifically, the American Health Information Management Association. Although many of the concepts discussed in the following sections (for example, HIPAA and patient portals) have come to the forefront within the past two decades, the principles of privacy and confidentiality with respect to one's healthcare and health information have been pillars of medical and health information management practices since virtually their inception. As noted in figure 14.3, the American Hospital Association informs patients about what they can expect during their hospital stay. Protection of privacy is one of those elements.

HIPAA Individual Rights

As detailed in chapter 11, the HIPAA Privacy Rule provides individuals with rights related to the access and control of their protected health information (PHI). Specifically, individuals have the right to

- Access their PHI (with certain exceptions)
- Request amendments to their PHI
- Request an accounting of certain disclosures that a covered entity has made of their PHI
- Request certain restrictions regarding how their PHI is used or disclosed to carry out treatment, payment, or operations
- Request that communications of PHI be routed to an alternative location or by an alternative method

Additionally, individuals may lodge a complaint about a covered entity's alleged noncompliance with its policies and procedures or with the Privacy Rule. Individuals also have the right to receive a Notice of Privacy Practices on or before their first visit at a covered entity, which describes acceptable uses and disclosures of their PHI and also lists their rights per HIPAA.

A significant change to HIPAA occurred in 2009, when patients gained the right to be notified when their PHI is breached. Now mandatory, breach notification allows individuals a much greater awareness of where and when their information has wrongfully been accessed or disseminated. Both complaints and breach notification are outlined in chapter 11.

AHIMA Consumer Health Information Bill of Rights

The American Health Information Management Association (AHIMA) has created a **Consumer Health Information Bill of Rights** that comports with the HIPAA Privacy Rule and furthers the organization's commitment to support and protect people's rights regarding their health information. In particular, AHIMA focuses its attention on an individual's right to have health information that is "accurate, secure, and confidential." This bill of rights was created to educate people about the protection and accuracy of their personal health information, as well as the right of access and assurance of that corrective action will be taken if an individual's rights are violated (AHIMA 2015). Figure 14.6 is the AHIMA Consumer Health Information Bill of Rights.

Patient Health Information Portals

Effort to increase access to one's own health information has made significant strides. Whereas laws once provided little or no right of access, and one's own records were shielded from the patient, the HIPAA right of access was a significant move toward empowering patients with respect to their own health information. Technology has moved the dial even further. Patient engagement is encouraged as patients are now able to access their records or portions of their records through electronic health record (EHR) **patient portals**, which are provider-hosted "secure websites where patients can access their medical history and often certain information from their EHR" (ONC 2016). Patient portals can also include **personal health records (PHRs)**, which are repositories where patients can add their own health information. This information can include documentation from other healthcare organizations or information created by the patient (for example, blood pressure monitoring logs created at home).

Figure 14.6 AHIMA consumer health information bill of rights – A model for protecting Americans' health information principles

1. **The right to look at your health information or get a paper or electronic copy of it.**

   You have the right to read and review your health information. Access can be requested at any time. You have the right to get a paper or electronic copy of your health information in a timely manner according to your state or federal laws.

2. **The right to accurate and complete health information.**

   You have the right to expect that your health information is accurate and complete. The quality of the healthcare you receive depends upon accurate and complete health information. Incorrect or incomplete health information can prevent you from understanding your overall health and can keep you from receiving the care you need.

3. **The right to ask for changes to your health information.**

   You have the right to ask for changes to your health information when you think it is incorrect or incomplete. It is up to your doctor, hospital, or other healthcare provider whether or not the requested change will be made to the health record. The provider must notify you of the decision in writing. Your written or electronic request for changes will be kept with your health record.

4. **The right to know how your health information is used or shared and who has received it.**

   You have the right to a written explanation of how your health information is used. Your healthcare provider must give you a Notice of Privacy Practices that describes the possible uses and releases of your health information. You have a right to ask your provider for a list (an accounting) of those who have received your information. That list will not include information you agreed to be shared or used by those involved in the treatment, payment, or healthcare operations for your care.

5. **The right to ask for limitations on the use and release of your health information.**

   You have a right to ask for a limit on the health information your provider shares with others involved in your care or for the payment of your care. Your provider has the right to deny the request, but must provide you with a reason why. You may also ask to keep certain information hidden from your healthcare insurance company, but you must pay for that care out of your own pocket at the time of your visit.

6. **The right to expect your health information is private and secure.**

   You have the right to expect that your health information will be protected and kept secure from people who should not have it. You have the right to expect that your health information is kept secure when it is shared between your healthcare providers. You also have the right to ask that your provider contact you in the way you prefer, such as e-mail or phone.

7. **The right to be informed about privacy and security breaches to your health information.**

   You have the right to expect that organizations will hold staff responsible for any illegal access, use, or release of your health information. As required by law, you have the right to expect that any illegal use of your health information will be investigated and that you will be notified and given instructions on what to do next.

8. **The right to file a complaint or report a violation regarding your health information.**

   You have the right to file a complaint if you think your health information is not being handled correctly. You have a right to expect a timely response. The Notice of Privacy Practices must tell you how to file a complaint with the organization and with the United States Department of Health and Human Services.

Source: AHIMA 2015.

Although technology enables the use of patient portals, CMS promoted their usage through its **Meaningful Use** objectives, which required hospitals and eligible providers to meet goals to receive EHR implementation incentive payments. Patient portal objectives included patients being able to view, download, and transmit their health information; exchange secure messages with their providers; and review clinical summaries (ONC 2016). Viewing test results has become the portal feature that is used most by patients (ONC 2016). As more health information becomes available via the EHR patient portal and more functions become common activities on the patient portal, such as online scheduling, bill payment, and patient requests for prescription refills, patient engagement and control over their own healthcare will increase.

Health Literacy and Cultural Competence

The Health and Medicine Division of the National Academies of Sciences, Engineering, and Medicine, formerly known as the Institute of Medicine, has defined **health literacy** as the degree of capacity that an individual has to not only read health information, but to "obtain, process, and understand basic health information and services needed to make appropriate health decisions" (HHS 2016). Thus, access to information is often not enough. Individuals have to be able to understand the information they have access to, including the medical record, consent forms, and conversations with healthcare providers (Nielsen-Bohlman et al. 2004). This includes not only patients for whom English is a second language, but also patients with limited reading proficiency and those accustomed to dialects. To the extent the information is embedded in technology, familiarity with and proficiency in technology is also a component of health literacy.

Health literacy often relates to the issue of **cultural competence**, which is how an organization, through its policies and human behaviors and attitudes, functions effectively in cross-cultural situations (NCCC n.d.). Cultural competence also involves "understanding and appropriately responding to" all of the cultural variables that both the patient and the healthcare professional bring to treatment interactions (ASHA 2016). Cultural competence takes into consideration not only recognition of different ethnic cultures; it must acknowledge differing characteristics, values, beliefs and life experiences that form a person's individual's views. These can include a number of factors including spiritual beliefs and practices, gender and gender identity, age and generational differences, sexual orientation, and social strata, including level of education as well as individuals facing food insecurity and homelessness. Cultural competence issues specific to healthcare include different cultures' beliefs about diseases and the disease process, values and attitudes toward issues such as modesty, and caregiving interactions between individuals of opposite genders.

Health literacy and cultural competence must both be considered in the context of patient rights when taking into account language barriers and the need for interpreters, as well as educational levels and the ability of individuals to understand information that is presented to them. Both health literacy and cultural competence are also components of **patient-centered care**, which the Institute of Medicine in its landmark report, *Crossing the Quality Chasm,* identified as care that is "respectful of and responsive to individual patient preferences, needs, and values and ensuring that patient values guide all clinical decisions" (Institute of Medicine 2000).

Transparency of Healthcare Costs

Even among well-informed consumers, the cost of healthcare has historically been elusive. This is ironic given that medical bills are among the highest that many people will ever have to pay. In many other industries, consumers do not accept not knowing the cost of a service or product until after it has been delivered, particularly if they are to be charged thousands or hundreds of thousands of dollars. However, the healthcare market in the United States is different than other markets and there are several reasons for this (Hostetter and Klein 2012). First, reporting of prices has not historically been required by law. Second, an individual may not be able to price-compare because he or she doesn't know in advance what care they will require and, therefore, what services and products will need to be purchased. Further, in emergency situations, such price comparison is not feasible. Finally, prices vary widely among providers and among beneficiaries of different insurance plans. For those who are covered by health insurance, once insurance benefits are applied, the final cost to the patient does not match a listed price even if one is provided.

Many patients, even those with health insurance, have found healthcare prices to be unmanageable and exorbitant when they are billed. As a result, a new area of patient rights has emerged. **Billing advocates** are individuals who advocate on behalf of patients to negotiate and lower their medical bills (Brill 2013). Additionally, a number of states require hospital charge data to be made available to consumers. For example, Ohio requires that hospitals must inform patients of the presence of the hospital's price list and provide it free of charge to the patient upon request (ORC 3727.42). Colorado requires hospitals to inform patients of their right to see the average charges for treatments or procedures to be obtained (if they are common), prior to admission (C.R.S.A. 6-20-101).

Patient Responsibilities

Although the majority of this chapter has addressed patient rights, the patient–provider relationship is a two-way street. In addition to being protected legally and through policies, patients also have responsibilities to the providers that treat them. Most hospitals and physicians, along with organizations such as the American Medical Association (AMA), have adopted codes of patient responsibilities. These codes are meant to recognize the collaborative nature of the relationship between providers and patients. Generally speaking, patients have the responsibility to

- Provide full and honest information to providers
- Ask questions regarding information that they do not understand
- Work with providers in carrying out agreed-upon treatment plan
- Show respect for providers and other patients
- Make good-faith efforts to meet their financial obligations

The American Hospital Association's Patient Care Partnership, which enumerates patient rights and expectations and was described earlier in the chapter, also lists patient responsibilities; in other words, what is expected of the patient. They are outlined in figure 14.7.

Figure 14.7 Patient responsibilities per the AHA patient care partnership

- Ask questions
- Tell your healthcare providers of concerns about your care of if you have pain
- Inform your healthcare providers if more information is needed to make treatment decisions
- Provide complete and accurate information about your health and coverage, including previous illnesses, surgeries and hospitalizations; allergic reactions; medicines or dietary supplements being taken; health plan network or admission requirements
- Follow medication, diet, and therapy plans provided by your healthcare providers
- Share your wishes with providers and family regarding healthcare goals and values, and spiritual beliefs
- Give copies of advance directives to your doctor, family, and healthcare team
- Confirm, if you agree, your understanding of and consent to surgeries and/or experimental treatments in writing when asked
- Collect necessary information and meet other requirements to obtain health insurance coverage or assistance

Source: AHA 2016; adapted from Patient Care Partnership brochure.

Check Your Understanding   14.3

Instructions: Indicate whether the following statements are true or false (T or F).

1. A restraint is a physical device only.
2. Cultural competence deals primarily with language differences among patients.
3. Patient portals are hosted by healthcare providers.
4. Billing advocates work for healthcare providers to ensure that patients pay their medical bills in full.
5. Patients have the responsibility to work with providers in carrying out agreed-upon treatment plans.

Scenario 14

Nancy's father, Joe, is a resident in a skilled nursing facility. He has dementia and is very active, walking frequently throughout the unit and occasionally entering other residents' rooms. He is sometimes unsteady and will trip over furniture. Nancy is very concerned that the number of psychotropic drugs her father is on is leading to diminished kidney function. She is also concerned that they are being used for an improper purpose, which is to inhibit her father's mobility for the convenience of staff. The nursing facility conducted a battery of lab tests, but the facility's paper-based health record allows her–as her father's Durable Power of Attorney–to view the results only if she arranges a time with one of the nursing staff to do so, or if she requests a copy from the medical records department. Because of his condition, Joe is also a patient of a neurologist. The neurologist also conducted a battery of lab tests, and the test results were posted on the patient portal of the electronic health record. Nancy was able to view the test results, using her user ID and password, the day after the tests were conducted. In both situations, Nancy would like to discuss the results with someone who can explain them further because she has an 8th grade education and does not readily understand the test results.

1. Reviewing the health information patient rights discussed in this chapter, which ones apply to this situation?

2. Do you believe the Medicare CoP Seclusion and Restraint requirements are being violated by the nursing facility?

3. Are patient portals beneficial or detrimental to those with limited health literacy?

References

American Health Information Management Association. 2015. AHIMA Consumer Health Information Bill of Rights: A model of protecting Americans' health information principles. http://www.bok.ahima.org.

American Hospital Association. 2016. The Patient Care Partnership. http://www.aha.org.

American Speech-Language-Hearing Association (ASHA). 2016. Cultural competence. http://www.asha.org /Practice-Portal/Professional-Issues/Cultural-Competence/.

Brill, S.. 2013 (March 4). Bitter pill: Why medical bills are killing us. *Time Magazine*.

Centers for Medicare and Medicaid Services. 2012. Emergency Medical Treatment & Labor Act (EMTALA). https:// www.cms.gov/Regulations-and-Guidance/Legislation/EMTALA/.

Department of Health and Human Services. n.d. Medical treatment in Hill-Burton funded healthcare facilities. http://www.hhs.gov/civil-rights/for-individuals/hill-burton/index.html.

Department of Health and Human Services. 2016. Quick guide to health literacy. https://health.gov.

Department of Health and Human Services. 2014. Medicare rights & protections. https://www.medicare.gov/Pubs/pdf/11534.pdf.

Emanuel, E.J. and L.L. Emanuel. 1992. Four models of the physician-patient relationship. *JAMA* 267:2221–2226.

Gawande, A. 2014. Being Mortal: Medicine and What Matters in the End. New York: Henry Holt.

HealthCare.gov. n.d. Health coverage rights and protections. https://www.healthcare.gov/health-care-law-protections/.

Health Resources and Services Administration. n.d. Hill-Burton free and reduced-cost health care. http://www.hrsa.gov/gethealthcare/affordable/hillburton/.

Hostetter, M. and S. Klein. 2012 (April/May). Health care price transparency: Can it promote high-value care? Quality Matters: Innovations in Health Care Quality Management. The Commonwealth Fund. www.commonwealthfund.org.

Institute of Medicine. 2000. Crossing the quality chasm: A new health system for the 21st century. http://www.nationalacademies.org/hmd/~/media/Files/Report%20Files/2001/Crossing-the-Quality-Chasm/Quality%20Chasm%202001%20%20report%20brief.pdf.

James, J. 2016 (February 25). Health policy brief: Nonprofit hospitals' community benefit requirements. *Health Affairs.*

Joint Commission. 2016. Patient Rights and Responsibilities of the Individual. *Comprehensive Accreditation Manual for Hospitals, The Official Handbook* (CAMH). Oakbrook Terrace, IL: Joint Commission.

National Center for Cultural Competence (NCCC). n.d. Georgetown University Center for Child and Human Development. http://www.nccccurricula.info/culturalcompetence.html.

Nielsen-Bohlman, L., A. Panzer, and D. Kindig, Committee on Health Literacy, Board on Neuroscience and Behavioral Health, Institute of Medicine. 2004. Health literacy: A prescription to end confusion. http://www.nationalacademies.org/hmd/~/media/Files/Report%20Files/2004/Health-Literacy-A-Prescription-to-End-Confusion/healthliteracyfinal.pdf.

Office of the National Coordinator for Health Information Technology (ONC). 2016. ONC patient engagement playbook. www.healthit.gov/playbook/pe/.

Showalter, J.S. 2015. *The Law of Healthcare Administration*, 7th ed. Chicago: Health Administration Press.

Tummalapalli, S. and E. Goodman. 2016 (January 27). What are best practices for patients discharged against medical advice? *The Hospitalist.* http://www.the-hospitalist.org/article/what-are-best-practices-for-patients-discharged-against-medical-advice/3/.

World Health Organization. n.d. Patients' rights. http://www.who.int/genomics/public/patientrights/en/.

Cases, Statutes, and Regulations Cited

42 CFR 482.13: Condition of Participation: Patient's Rights. 2012.

410 Ill. Comp. Stat. 50/3-111 ½ par. 5403). 2015.

Children's Health Act. Pub. L. 106-310. 2000.

Civil Rights Act. Pub. L. 88-352. 1964.

Colorado Rev. Stat. Ann. 6-20-101. 2004.

Fla. Stat. 381.026. Florida Patient's Bill of Rights and Responsibilities. 2016.

Ohio Revised Code 3727.42. Price Information List. 2006.

Access, Use, and Disclosure and Release of Health Information

Melanie S. Brodnik, PhD, RHIA, FAHIMA

Learning Objectives

- Discuss the issues surrounding ownership and control of health information
- Contrast access and disclosure rights between adults, incompetent adults, and minors
- Explain the access and disclosure rights employers, employees, and other members of the workforce
- Compare access and disclosure issues related to highly sensitive health information
- Describe the access, request, and disclosure laws and concern for a variety of situations related to protecting the privacy and confidentiality of health records and information
- Summarize the issues related to managing the release of information

Key Terms

- Access
- Active record
- Adoption
- Age of majority
- Americans with Disabilities Act (ADA)
- Autopsy
- Behavioral health
- Clinical Laboratory Improvement Amendments (CLIA)
- Competent adult
- Confidentiality of Alcohol and Drug Abuse Patient Records Regulation
- Court order
- Disability determination services

- Disclosure
- Duty to warn
- Electronic Records Express (ERE)
- Emancipated minor
- Fair and Accurate Credit Transactions Act (FACTA)
- Freedom of Information Act (FOIA)
- Health information exchange (HIE)
- Health information handler (HIH)
- Homeland Security Act
- Human Genome Project
- Incompetent adult
- Inpatient
- Legal guardian

- Medical emergency
- Minor
- National Instant Criminal Background Check System (NICS)
- National Human Genome Research Institute (NHGRI)
- Next-of-kin
- Noncustodial parent
- Nondisclosure agreement
- Open records laws
- Outpatient
- Patriot Act
- Personal representative
- Primary data source
- Privilege statutes
- Psychotherapy notes
- Public records laws

- Release of information (ROI)
- Secondary data sources
- Social Security Administration (SSA)
- Subpoena
- Substance Abuse and Mental Health Services Administration (SAMHSA)
- Sunshine laws
- Syndromic surveillance
- Uniform Health-Care Decisions Act (UHCDA)
- Use

The challenge of managing data and information, especially protected health information (PHI), is to ensure access, use, and disclosure of PHI are handled according to state and federal rules and regulations. The HIPAA Privacy and Security Rules, along with HITECH provisions as discussed in chapters 10 and 11, set the bar for protecting and securing patient information. However, there are circumstances in which access, use, and disclosure of patient information with or without patient authorization are appropriate. This chapter discusses these circumstances as well as the process for managing patient information when these circumstances arise. The chapter covers who owns patient information, who can access it, how to handle highly sensitive patient information (mental health, communicable diseases, genetic information, etc.), and the special requests for PHI. As a reminder, HIPAA defines **access** as the right of an individual to inspect and obtain a copy of his or her own health information that is contained in a designated record set, while **use** is defined as the sharing, employment, application, utilization, examination, or analysis of individually identifiable health information within an entity that maintains such information. **Disclosure** is defined as "the release, transfer, provision of, access to or divulging in any other manner of information outside the entity holding the information" (45 CFR 160.103). In general, **release of information** refers to providing access to PHI to an individual or entity authorized to receive or review it (Dunn and Burton 2015, 6). Protecting the privacy and confidentiality of health information is a major priority for healthcare organizations and providers who must adhere to state and federal laws.

The chapter opens with a discussion of ownership of health information and how previously held beliefs about ownership may change as the industry increases its reliance on health information technology. Core to the issue of a patient's right to access or disclose his or her health information is the question of whether the patient is competent to make such a decision. The chapter addresses the rights of competent and incompetent adult patients as well as the rights of individuals deemed as minors. The chapter continues with an overview of workforce members who have access rights to patient information and for what reasons. Issues surrounding highly sensitive information related to behavioral health, substance abuse, HIV/AIDS, genetic information, and adoption are discussed, including their relationship to the HIPAA Privacy Rule and its recent modifications. Similarly, a number of situations involving requests for patient information are discussed. The chapter concludes with a discussion of the practical aspects of managing the process of releasing health information.

Ownership and Control of the Health Record and Health Information

Ownership of the health record has traditionally been granted to the healthcare provider who generates the record and has physical custody of it. The record as the **primary data source** contains information about the patient as documented by professionals who provided the care or services to the patient (Sharp and Madlock-Brown 2016, 170). As both a medical document and a legal document, the record provides proof of care and serves as the business record of the provider. Many state laws grant ownership of health records (whether paper or electronic) to the provider who generates the record, and also have laws that give patients access and control over their records and the information within (HealthInfoLaw.org 2015a, 2015b). On the federal level, the HIPAA Privacy Rule and HITECH provisions remain silent on the question of health record ownership but grant patients the right to access, view, copy, or amend their record(s) (45 CFR 164.524, 164.526).

Health information found within a health record is collected, stored, retrieved, and disseminated, not only by providers but also by health plans, clearinghouses, payers, technology and service vendors, researchers, employers, financial service firms, and public health agencies, all of which may use the information for purposes other than direct patient care. These **secondary data sources** are created when data are taken from a primary data source (health record) and used for purposes other than their original intended use" (Johns 2015, 232). Secondary data sources may be internal to an organization such as a hospital cancer or trauma registry. Secondary data sources can also be external, such as a statewide cancer or trauma registry or any number of local, state, and federal, agency or company data sets. Ownership of a secondary data source belongs to the entity that created or authored it, however, contract, copyright or patent laws may also affect ownership (HealthInfoLaw.org 2015a).

New forms of health records may arise as patients (consumers) generate health data which is shared through provider-based patient portals or other personal health record applications. Biometric data, generated through mobile apps and wearable fitness devices that record how a patient is doing between medical visits, poses questions of who has ownership, authority or control over such records and information (HHS n.d.c.; HealthInfoLaw.org 2015a). Providers should have policies and procedures in place as part of their overall information or data governance plans that defines provider and patient responsibilities for the generation, access, use, and disclosure of patient health information.

Access to Patient Health Information

An individual has the right to control his or her own body and the right to consent or refuse consent to medical treatment as defined by federal and state laws. Similarly, an individual has certain rights to access, use, and disclose his or her PHI as defined by state and federal laws as mentioned above. The HIPAA Privacy Rule is specific about the access, uses, and disclosures of PHI that require patient authorization and those that do not, and allowing individuals to receive an accounting of disclosures, as discussed in chapter 10 and later in this chapter (45 CFR 164.508). Prior investigation into state health record laws in 2009 revealed that few states had access provisions as extensive as those found in the HIPAA Privacy Rule (RTI 2009). However, that is no longer the case.

Today, most state statutory and regulatory provisions provide patients with the right to access their health information and offer some means of protecting the confidentiality of the information. This right may also enable a patient to request the use of an alias in place of his or her legal name as a way to provide additional patient privacy protection (Barrett et al. 2016). Use of patient aliases is acceptable as long as the healthcare provider has appropriate policies and procedures in place including electronic health records (EHR) systems features and functionality (Barrett et al. 2016). Sources for state health record laws can be found on websites such as HealthInfoLaw (2015a) or Thomson Reuters FindLaw (2016). At the federal level laws, regulations, and guidance from the Office of the National Coordinator for Information Technology (ONC) support the right of patients to "opt-in or opt-out" of sharing their health data with state **health information exchanges (HIEs)** as well as allowing patients choice in accessing and disclosing their information from exchanges that store, assemble or aggregate individually identifiable health information (HHS ONC 2015). While there are many issues related to access, use, and disclosure rights, the following discussion focuses on common situations that require oversight by those who manage the privacy and security of patient information.

Competent Adult

A **competent adult** is an individual who is mentally and physically competent to manage to his or her own affairs and has reached the **age of majority**. The age of majority in most states is 18 years or older, as discussed in chapter 8. Just as a competent adult may consent to treatment, the adult may authorize the access or disclosure of his or her health information. A competent adult may also wish to appoint another person to be his or her **personal representative**. A personal representative is legally authorized to make healthcare decisions on an individual's behalf or to act on behalf of a deceased individual or that individual's estate. A personal representative could include, for example, a spouse or next-of-kin as defined by state law, an agent, or an individual who holds a durable power of attorney (DPOA) or a durable power of attorney for healthcare decisions (DPOA-HCD) for the patient. The personal representative has the right to request and receive information about the adult's personal affairs and physical and mental health, including legal and health records.

Some states have implemented the **Uniform Health-Care Decisions Act** (UHCDA), which allows a competent adult to communicate to a supervising healthcare provider the selection of a "surrogate" (personal representative) who may make healthcare decisions for the adult (Uniform Law Commission 2016). If a surrogate has not been named, then a person related to the adult, the **next-of-kin**, can step forward and assume responsibility. The UHCDA suggests the decision-making priority order for an individual's next-of-kin, which is basically the same for decisions related to medical treatment as well. Chapter 8 has additional information on consents and a discussion of advance directives related to DPOA and DPOA-HCD. The UHCDA priority order list is as follows:

1. Spouse
2. Adult child
3. Parent
4. Adult sibling
5. If no one is available who is so related to the individual, authority may be granted to an adult who has exhibited special care and concern for the individual, who is familiar with the patient's personal values, and who is willing and able to make a healthcare decision for the patient.
6. Absent an unrelated adult who exhibits the above characteristics, a healthcare provider may seek appointment of a decision maker by the court having jurisdiction.

The adult patient or the personal representative of the adult patient has the right to request, receive, examine, copy, amend, and authorize disclosure of the patient's healthcare information. However, before disclosing any information, the healthcare organization must identify and verify that the requester is who he or she purports to be and that the requester has the authorization to access the information. If the requester is the competent adult patient, then the requester should be asked for identification. If the requester is a personal representative, this person should be asked to produce a copy of the appropriate legal documentation to verify their right to access and disclose the patient's information. This documentation should be a witnessed DPOA or DPOA-HCD. It is a good practice to require an additional statement explaining the requester's relationship to the patient and stating why the patient is unable to sign (Reynolds and Bowman 2016).

Incompetent Adult

When an individual who is at or above the age of majority becomes incapacitated due to illness or injury, either permanently or temporarily, he or she may be designated as an **incompetent adult**. When this occurs, another person should be designated to make decisions for that individual, including decisions about the use and disclosure of the individual's PHI. That person may be a parent, sibling, agent, attorney, or surrogate. Whoever serves as the incompetent adult's personal representative should, at a minimum, hold the incompetent adult's DPOA or DPOA-HCD. In the absence of an advance directive, the court system, with support from the appropriate medical community, will declare the individual incompetent. The court will then appoint a **legal guardian** to handle the matters of the incompetent adult.

The guardian may be the spouse, adult child, or sibling of the individual, or another designated person. It is important to avoid the assumption that individuals with mental illnesses are also mentally incompetent. They must be formally deemed mentally incompetent by the court. In acting for the incompetent adult, the personal representative has the right to request, receive, examine, copy, and authorize disclosure of the incompetent adult's PHI. However, as noted above, before disclosing any information, the healthcare organization should require legal documentation of the incompetent adult's legal position and the reason the adult is unable to sign the authorization, along with documentation of the personal representative's authority to access or authorize disclosure of the incompetent adult's PHI (Reynolds and Bowman 2016).

Minors

A **minor** is defined as an individual under the age of 18 who has not been legally emancipated (declared an adult) by the court. Because of their age, minors are generally deemed legally incompetent—unable to consent for their own medical treatment or to access, use, amend, or disclose their health information. However, special situations and exceptions that allow minors to do so are explained below. Because HIPAA defers to state law on the issue of minors, applicable state laws must be consulted regarding who has authorization to access, use, or disclose a minor's PHI.

Parental Authorization Required

Because minors are generally legally incompetent and unable to make decisions regarding the access, use, and disclosure of their own healthcare information, this authority usually belongs to the minor's parent(s) unless an exception applies. However, several categories of parents are recognized by laws, including the following:

- Married biological parents
- Separated or divorced biological parents
- Stepparents
- Adoptive parents
- Foster parents
- Grandparents (children living with grandparents who are not legal guardians)
- Legal guardians
- Others, such as a parent in the service or overseas who has transferred guardianship to a relative or friend with whom the child is temporarily living (Reynolds and Bowman 2016)

Generally, only one parent's signature is required to authorize the access, use, or disclosure of a minor's PHI. In some states, only the mother's signature, regardless of the mother's age, is required, and in other states it is the custodial parent (as determined by the court) who is responsible for authorizing the access, use, and disclosure of the minor patient's PHI.

Parental Authorization Not Required

Minor patients may authorize the access, use, or disclosure of their PHI without parental authorization in several situations, most of which are defined by state statutory or regulatory provisions. An **emancipated minor** is one who is under the age of majority and self-supporting with parents who have surrendered their rights of custody, care, and support. Emancipated minors generally may authorize the access, use, and disclosure of their own PHI. If the minor is married, previously married, or in the military, the minor controls his or her PHI. If the minor is under the age of 18 and is the parent of a child, the minor may authorize the access, use, and disclosure of his or her own PHI as well as that of his or her child. In this case, the minor falls under the provisions set forth for parental authorization as discussed above. If the patient is a minor at the time of treatment or hospitalization and reaches the age of majority during this period, the patient may authorize the access, use, or disclosure of his or her PHI. The fact that the parents, parents' insurance, or other third-party payer is paying the bill does not matter; the patient retains control over his or her PHI.

Many state laws allow a minor to be treated for drug or alcohol dependency, mental health, sexually transmitted diseases (STDs), or HIV/AIDS or be given contraceptives and prenatal care without prior parental or legal guardian consent or knowledge. Federal rules specific to alcohol and drug abuse further define the right of minors to authorize the access, use, or disclosure of their information and will be discussed in more detail later in the chapter. Minors may also seek judicial (court) permission for induced termination of a pregnancy in states in which it is permissible by law. In any of these situations, the minor must authorize the access, use, or disclosure of his or her PHI. However, depending on state law and the medical condition of the minor, healthcare providers may be legally permitted to notify the parent(s) or legal guardian(s) of the minor's condition or treatment. In this situation, the parent(s) or legal guardian(s) may have access to the minor's PHI since the information was disclosed by the healthcare provider.

Access and Authorization Rights of Noncustodial Parents and Others

State laws generally address situations involving the rights of divorced or separated parents as well as grandparents with respect to accessing and authorizing the use or disclosure of a minor's PHI. A **noncustodial parent** is a parent who does not have legal custody of the child. Noncustodial parents are legally endowed with parental rights, which generally allow them to access the healthcare information of their minor children subject to the situations stated above regarding minors. This right, which is explicitly stated in state laws and the HIPAA Privacy Rule, may be overridden if a court determines that denial of the parental right is in the best interests of the child. In the absence of a "best interests of the child" determination by the court, state laws should be consulted regarding the specific rights granted to noncustodial parents. For example, Tennessee law requires that a copy of the child's health records be furnished to the noncustodial parent by the treating physician or the treating hospital upon a written request by the noncustodial parent (TN Code Ann. 36-6-103).

In some states, either parent may authorize the release of information; however, best practice dictates that authorization should be first sought from the custodial parent whenever possible (Reynolds and Bowman 2016). If state law distinguishes between custodial and noncustodial parents' rights of access, persons working with health records of minors should review requests from noncustodial parents to determine that the disclosure complies with state law. It is often the duty of the parent who is holding the restriction against a noncustodial parent to make a healthcare provider aware of the restriction order. In the case of a grandparent, other family member, or friend, this individual should produce proof of guardianship to authorize the access, use, or disclosure of the minor's PHI.

Providers of pediatric services may wish to include information about the rights of minors and noncustodial parents in their Notice of Privacy Practices and on all authorizations for disclosure of information as a way of providing information to patients and custodial parents or guardians about the access rights of noncustodial parents. Obtaining information about the minor patient's custody, limitations on parental rights, or special circumstances when patients are first seen or admitted can often help providers avoid problems later (Reynolds and Bowman 2016).

Minors in Foster Care or Allegedly Abused

In some states, an authorization for the access or disclosure of the PHI of a child in a foster care system may be signed by the appropriate department of human services or children's services personnel. Some states delegate this responsibility to the department's designated representative. Depending on the state, a foster parent may authorize the access, use, or disclosure of a child's PHI; however, legal documentation of the relationship is required. Healthcare organizations and providers should not release any information to persons alleged to have abused the child, if known, regardless of the relationship of the person to the child (Reynolds and Bowman 2016).

Employer, Employee, and Other Members of the Workforce

The HIPAA Privacy Rule broadly defines "workforce" as employees, volunteers, trainees, and other persons, whether paid or not, who work for and are under the direct control of the covered entity (CE) (45 CFR 160.103). Access to and disclosure of patient information to various workforce members varies by the job and responsibility.

Employers

Employers that may or may not be HIPAA-covered healthcare entities may request patient information for several reasons, including family medical leave certification, return to work certification for work-related injuries, and information for company physicians. Patient authorization is required for such disclosures, but in some states, the patient's employer, employer's insurer, and employer's and employee's attorneys do not need patient authorization to obtain health information for workers' compensation purposes.

Employees

Employees of a HIPAA-CE are categorized as either directly involved or not directly involved in a patient's care. Although those involved directly in a patient's care (nurses, nurse's aides, case managers, physical therapists, respiratory therapists, and so on) do not require authorization to access the health record, job descriptions and procedures must document patient care responsibilities and justify an employee's need to access the information. Employees in hospital or healthcare organization departments, who are not involved directly in patient care, will vary in their need to access patient information. The HIPAA "minimum necessary" principle must be applied to determine what access employees legitimately have to PHI (45 CFR 164.502(b)). The HIPAA security regulations should also identify facility access controls on electronic PHI (45 CFR 164.310(a)(1)). As discussed in chapter 13, employees and others discussed in this section of the chapter should be required to sign a **nondisclosure agreement** relating to the confidentiality and privacy of patient information as a condition of employment.

Physicians

Physicians are classified in numerous ways and thus must be considered according to their classifications for access purposes: attending physicians, fellows, residents, interns, house staff members in the post-doctoral programs, researchers, physicians of record versus referring physicians, consulting physicians versus follow-up physicians, treating physicians versus non-treating physicians. Physicians who are on the medical staff or part of the organized healthcare arrangement and who are treating a patient should be given access to the patient's information for treatment and payment purposes following verification of their treatment relationship. Referral or follow-up physicians may also access a patient's information following verification of the treatment relationship with the patient. In each case, the patient's authorization is not required, but verification of the treatment relationship is required.

A physician should have access to patient information if he or she is treating a specific patient. The physician should not have access to patient information of individuals that he or she is not treating unless the physician is performing designated healthcare operations such as research, peer review, or quality improvement activity. Physician office staff and personnel to whom the physician or group has outsourced billing services may access patient information or records for payment purposes.

Students

Students enrolled in health related educational programs (i.e., medicine, nursing, allied health), who are involved in direct or indirect patient care should have access to patient health records and information without patient authorization as part of their training program. A contract or letter of agreement between the educational institution and healthcare provider or CE that outlines student responsibilities when accessing PHI, and patient privacy compliance should be maintained by both parties. Healthcare providers who accept students for on-site training or job shadowing purposes often require students to adhere to the same onboarding requirements used for new employees which may include background checks, proof of immunizations, and HIPAA, safety and sexual harassment training. The Office for Civil Rights has confirmed that CEs can allow healthcare students the use of and access to PHI as long as the CE has policies and procedures for minimum necessary uses and disclosures in place that permits student trainees access to PHI and patient records (HHS 2006).

Attorneys

Attorneys may or may not be employees of a healthcare organization. Those who are employed by a healthcare organization (for example, privacy officer, risk manager, compliance officer) are considered members of the workforce and do not require authorization prior to accessing a patient's healthcare information for such purposes as defending lawsuits, handling collections, and dealing with other legal issues. A nonemployee attorney who is retained to provide legal representation to a healthcare organization or provider does not require patient authorization prior to accessing patient information; however, a business associate agreement is required per the HIPAA Privacy Rule for access to occur. If a patient has hired an attorney and requests that his or her attorney receive the patient's information, then the attorney must present a signed authorization from the patient that authorizes the release of the patient's information to the attorney.

Vendors

Vendors present in a healthcare organization will often have access to patient information in the course of their work. Such vendors include consultants, those who sell equipment and supplies, those who perform release-of-information functions and transcription services, and those who provide laundry, food, or equipment repair services. If the vendor meets the definition of a business associate (that is, it is using or disclosing an individual's PHI on behalf of the healthcare organization), a business associate agreement must be signed. If a vendor is not a business associate, employees of the vendor should sign confidentiality agreements and undergo HIPAA training because of their routine contact with and exposure to patient information. Neither situation requires patient authorization.

Instructions: Indicate whether the following statements are true or false (T or F).

1. Ownership of a health record has traditionally been granted to the provider.

2. A patient must allow their health information to be shared with a health information exchange.

3. An emancipated minor may authorize for disclosure of his or her health information.

4. Employees directly involved in patient care do not require authorization to access the patient's record.

5. Attorneys have automatic access to patient information because they are officers of the court.

Highly Sensitive Health Information

There are certain types of patient information that require special handling in regard to access, requests, uses, and disclosures due to the sensitive nature of the information. Information related to such issues as behavioral healthcare, substance abuse, communicable diseases, genetic testing, and adoption birth records often requires additional protection. HIPAA affords protection to all types of health information; it does not distinguish between highly sensitive health information and other types of health information but instead defers to state laws and existing federal regulations to address specific protections. Thus, policies and procedures related to the management of sensitive health information should be a part of the organization's overall information and data governance plans.

Behavioral (Mental) Health Information

Behavioral or mental health treatment is delivered through a broad array of services provided in acute and long-term hospitals, ambulatory care clinics, publicly funded community mental health centers, and group homes. **Behavioral health** encompasses the treatment of mental disorders, and intellectual and developmental disabilities. Patient information generated through behavioral health treatment is highly sensitive. In addition to containing very private information related to personal thoughts and relationships, the very fact that an individual is receiving behavioral health treatment is associated with a powerful and unfortunate stigma that influences an individual's life. "Our society tends to develop limited, and often negative, perceptions about that individual's intellectual capabilities, educability, employability, social skills, ability to be a good neighbor, propensity for violence, and ability to lead a productive life" (Randolph and Rinehart-Thompson 2006, 465).

Patients with mental illness, mental retardation, and developmental disabilities are given access rights to their behavioral health records through the HIPAA Privacy Rule and individual state statutory and regulatory provisions (45 CFR 164.524). A caveat to this access right is if the patient's healthcare provider has restricted access by documenting such restriction in the patient's treatment plan with clear reasons as to why access should be denied. Aside from providing general access rights and restricting psychotherapy notes, HIPAA does not address behavioral health records specifically.

Psychotherapy notes are a mental health professional's documentation or analysis of conversations related to private, group, joint, or family counseling sessions. They are kept separate from the behavioral health record, which contains information related to an individual's diagnosis, prescriptions and medication monitoring, treatment modalities, and test results (45 CFR 164.501). The access, use, and disclosure of behavioral health records are mainly addressed by individual state statutes. Most state statutes identify records or reports related to a mentally ill, mentally retarded, or developmentally disabled person as confidential, requiring patient or appointed designee authorization before information is disclosed unless for treatment, payment, or healthcare operation purposes. Authorizations that could reveal an individual's behavioral health diagnosis or treatment should specifically state so in a manner that is obvious to the individual legally authorized to sign the authorization form.

Because of the highly sensitive nature of behavioral health information, state statutes generally include the identity of an individual as confidential information as well as the treatment information itself. Healthcare organizations that maintain a facility directory as designated by the HIPAA Privacy Rule must take care to develop protocols that specifically describe facility directory disclosures and explain to patients that such disclosures could result in a requester knowing an individual's status as a behavioral health patient (45 CFR 164.510(a)). An organization may omit the facility directory altogether for behavioral health patients, taking care to develop protocols so that the process of withholding information does not also breach an individual's confidentiality (Rinehart-Thompson and Randolph 2017).

Provider-patient privilege statutes exist in many states. Privilege statutes may include a variety of providers such as physicians, psychologists, psychiatric or mental health nurses, certified social workers, marital therapists, licensed counselors, pastoral therapists, and others. **Privilege statutes** legally protect confidential communications between provider and patient related to diagnosis and treatment from disclosure during civil and some criminal misdemeanor litigation. The mental health professional cannot be compelled to testify or disclose information without the authorization of the patient in a judicial situation. Exceptions to such statutes usually include the following situations:

- The patient brings up the issue of the mental or emotional condition.
- The health professional performs an examination under a court order.
- A psychiatrist in an involuntary commitment procedure recommends admission and confinement of the patient to avoid harm to the patient or others. (Reynolds and Bowman 2016)

However, there are situations where there is a legal **duty to warn,** a required disclosure of information to an intended victim when a patient threatens to harm an individually identifiable person or persons and the psychiatrist or other mental health provider believes that the patient is likely to actually harm the individual(s). The healthcare provider may warn the victim or begin commitment proceedings to ensure that the patient is admitted and receives inpatient mental health treatment. State reporting laws also require that law enforcement be informed of the situation. Most states require that all mental health providers testify in commitment hearings. These laws generally include the duty to warn.

A well-known case regarding the duty to warn is *Tarasoff v. the Regents of the University of California* (1976). A therapist was told by a patient that he wanted to kill his girlfriend, Tatiana Tarasoff. No one warned Ms. Tarasoff and the patient ultimately killed her. The court ruled that the therapist had a duty to let Tarasoff know of the threat. The case established that the duty to warn consists of three aspects: first, there is a relationship between the therapist and the client; second, the therapist has a responsibility to control the actions of the client; and third, there is an identifiable potential victim (Schlossberger and Hecker 1996). Because later rulings have somewhat limited the requirements of Tarasoff, applicable case and statutory law must be consulted to determine a state's duty to warn.

In addition to the duty to warn, the 1968 federal Gun Control Act prohibits the sale of firearms to individuals who have been involuntarily committed to a mental institution or otherwise have been determined by a lawful authority to be a danger to themselves or others (HHS 2016c). In an effort to reduce gun violence in 2016, the Department of Health and Human Services (HHS) amended the HIPAA Privacy Rule to permit but not require states and certain HIPAA CEs flexibility to disclose limited PHI about an individual to the Federal Bureau of Investigation (FBI) **National Instant Criminal Background**

Check System (NICS). The information disclosed includes only minimal identifying information and no clinical information. The law requires that licensed dealers must check the NICS to determine if a potential buyer who has been prohibited from possessing or receiving firearms has been reported to the system before they sell a firearm to the individual (Law Center to Prevent Gun Violence 2016).

With the transition of behavioral health and substance (alcohol and drug) abuse programs (discussed in more detail later) use of EHR systems, the HHS's **Substance Abuse and Mental Health Services Administration** (SAMHSA), in collaboration with the ONC, published two sets of frequently asked questions (FAQs). One was specific to releasing information to HIEs (2010), and the other related to applying substance abuse confidentiality regulations in general (2011). Both FAQs address the requirements as found in 42 CFR 2.11 Part 2, discussed later.

Substance Abuse Records

Special privacy protection is given to patients treated for substance (alcohol and drug) abuse to encourage individuals to seek treatment. Because of the highly sensitive nature of this treatment, both the identity of the patient and their treatment information are confidential. In 1987, Congress enacted the **Confidentiality of Alcohol and Drug Abuse Patient Records Regulation** to encourage individuals to seek substance abuse treatment without fear of their health information being disclosed. The regulations define facilities covered by the law as those institutions providing a federally assisted alcohol and drug program. "Program" is defined in 42 CFR 2.11 Part 2 as

1. An individual or entity (other than a general medical care facility) which holds itself out as providing and which actually provides alcohol or drug abuse diagnosis, treatment, or referral for treatment

2. An identified unit within a general medical facility which holds itself out as providing and which actually provides alcohol or drug abuse diagnosis, treatment, or referral for treatment

3. Referral or medical personnel or other staff in a general medical facility whose primary function is the provision of alcohol or drug abuse diagnosis, treatment, or referral for treatment and who are identified as such providers. A program may provide other services in addition to alcohol and drug abuse services, for example, mental health or psychiatric services, and nevertheless be an alcohol or drug abuse program within the meaning of these regulations.

Special access and disclosure procedures must be followed in handling health records that contain the identity, diagnosis, prognosis, and treatment of patients having a primary or secondary diagnosis of alcohol or drug abuse or, within the patient records of federally assisted programs, any mention of alcohol or drug abuse.

When the HIPAA Privacy and Security Rules were enacted, they did not change the current responsibility of a federally assisted program in adhering to the alcohol and drug abuse regulations regarding confidentiality and release of information. In 2004, SAMHSA published a guidance document explaining the relationship between the two sets of regulations. The guidance document states,

Substance abuse treatment programs must comply with both rules. Generally, this will mean that they will continue to follow Part 2's general rule and not disclose information unless they can obtain consent or point to an exception to that rule that specifically permits the disclosure. Programs must then make sure that the disclosure is also permissible under the Privacy Rule (SAMHSA 2004).

Because the information in the alcohol and drug abuse patient's health record is protected, disclosures from the records are prohibited without the patient's written authorization. Both HIPAA and substance abuse laws require that patients be notified of the healthcare provider's privacy practices. A healthcare provider can combine the requirements of both programs into a single notice (SAMHSA 2004, 12). See figure 15.1 for the elements required in a single notice.

SAMHSA efforts to update and modernize the substance abuse confidentiality regulations are currently underway. Significant changes in substance abuse care and along with growing reliance on the use of information technology has prompted SAMHSA to update the regulations. A Notice of Proposed Rulemaking on the Confidentiality of Substance Use Disorder Patient Records was published in February 2016 with the comment period ending in April 2016 (HHS 2016b).

Authorization for Disclosure (Release) of Information from Substance Abuse Facilities

The regulations under 42 CFR 2.11 Part 2 are specific regarding who can authorize disclosure of patient information.

> Programs may not use or disclose any information about any patient unless the patient has consented in writing (on a form that meets the requirements established by the regulations) or unless another very limited exception specified in the regulations applies. Any disclosure must be limited to the information necessary to carry out the purpose of the disclosure. (SAMHSA 2004, 5)

The Part 2 authorization form must include the elements listed below in addition to a written statement that the information cannot be redisclosed:

- Name or general designation of the program or person permitted to make the disclosure
- Name or title of the individual or name of the organization to which disclosure is to be made
- Name of the patient
- Purpose of the disclosure
- How much and what kind of information is to be disclosed
- Signature of patient (and, in some states, a parent or guardian)
- Date on which authorization is signed
- Statement that the authorization is subject to revocation at any time except to the extent that the program has already acted on it
- Date, event, or condition upon which authorization will expire if not previously revoked (SAMHSA 2004, 5)

In order for the substance abuse program authorization form to also be in compliance with the Privacy Rule, the program should include additional elements required by the Privacy Rule (45 CFR 164.508). These are listed in figure 10.7.

The patient is generally the only person who can authorize the disclosure of information. In the case of minors, the minor patient who consented to treatment must always sign the authorization for a program to disclose information even to his or her parents or guardians (SAMHSA 2004, 7). In states that require parental permission before treating a minor, both parent and minor authorization must be obtained to disclose information (42 CFR 2.14(c)(2)). In Tennessee, for example, where a minor may be treated for drug or alcohol dependency without prior parental consent, the minor must authorize the disclosure of information (TN Code Ann. 33-8-202).

| **Figure 15.1** | **Elements required for a notice of privacy practices** |

- A statement, prominently displayed, stating: "This notice describes how medical information about you may be used and disclosed and how you can get access to this information. Please review it carefully";
- A detailed description of the types of uses and disclosures that may be made without the patient's consent or authorization. For substance abuse treatment programs, these would include uses and disclosures:
  - In connection with treatment, payment or health care operations (include at least one example of each);
  - To qualified service organizations or business associates who provide services to the program's treatment, payment or health care operations;
  - In medical emergencies;
  - Authorized by court order;
  - To auditors and evaluators;
  - To researchers if the information will be protected as required by Federal regulations;
  - To report suspected child abuse or neglect; and
  - To report a crime or a threat to commit a crime on the premises or against staff
- A statement that other disclosures will be made only with the patient's written consent or authorization which can be revoked, unless the program has taken action in reliance on the consent or authorization;
- A statement that the program may contact the patient to provide appointment reminders or information about treatment alternatives or other health-related benefits and services that may be of interest to the patient;
- A statement that it is required by law to maintain the privacy of PHI and to notify patients of its legal duties and privacy practices, including any changes to its policies;
- A statement that the program must abide by the terms of the notice currently in effect; a statement that the program reserves the right to change the terms of its notice and to make the new notice provisions effective for all information it maintains; and a statement describing how it will provide patients with a revised notice of its practices;
- The name or title and telephone number of a person or office the patient can contact for further information;
- A statement of the patient's rights with respect to PHI and a brief description of how the patient may exercise those rights, including:
  - The right to request restrictions on certain uses and disclosures of PHI, including the statement that the program is not required to agree with requested restrictions;
  - The right to receive confidential communications of PHI (such as having mail and telephone calls be limited to home or office location);
  - The right to access and amend PHI;
  - The right to receive an accounting of the program's disclosures of PHI;
  - The right to complain—free from retaliation—to the program and to the Secretary of Health and Human Services (HHS) about violations of privacy rights, and information on how to file a complaint with the program; and
  - The right to obtain a paper copy of the notice upon request
- The effective date of the notice. See 45 CFR 164.520(b).

[1] The Privacy Rule also requires that the notice contain information about any more restrictive law. For example, if State law further limits disclosure of HIV-related information, that restriction should also appear in the notice.

[2] Programs often need to provide PHI to criminal justice agencies that mandate patients into treatment. Under Part 2, such disclosures may be made pursuant to a non-revocable consent that complies with 42 CFR §2.35. Under the Privacy Rule, such disclosures may be made pursuant to an authorization or pursuant to a court order. In order to comply with both rules, programs may find it helpful to ask the court in such a situation to issue an order that the program disclose necessary information to the court and other law enforcement personnel.

[3] A substance abuse treatment program engaging in these kinds of activities must be careful in contacting the patient that it does not make any patient-identifying disclosures to others. If the program does not intend to contact the patient, they do not need to include this statement.

[4] This is also voluntary. However, if this statement is not included, any changes in privacy practices described in the notice will apply only to PHI the program created or received after issuing a revised notice reflecting such changes. 45 CFR §164.520(b)(1)(v)(C).

Source: SAMHSA 2004.

Permissible Disclosures under Federal Drug and Alcohol Regulations

Situations in which information can be disclosed without the patient's written authorization include medical emergencies and scientific research, audits, and program evaluations where the individual patient is not identified. A court may authorize disclosure to avoid death or serious bodily harm to a patient or other individual.

HIV/AIDS, STDs, and Other Communicable Disease Information

Healthcare organizations must comply with applicable state laws to protect the privacy and confidentiality of patients with human immunodeficiency virus (HIV) or acquired immune deficiency syndrome (AIDS), sexually transmitted diseases (STDs), and in viral hepatitis or other communicable diseases. Because of the highly sensitive nature of these health conditions, the identity of the patient is confidential as well as the treatment information itself. However, each state has laws for the control of communicable diseases, including the reporting of certain diseases, and the isolation and quarantine of infected persons. State laws require physicians, clinics, hospitals, laboratories, penal institutions, and others who identify a patient with a diagnosis of HIV/AIDS or certain STDs and other infectious diagnoses to report these diagnoses to the state department of health or another appropriate agency. The requirement to report such diseases and viruses to state health agencies is an effort to protect third parties and curtail the spread of the disease or virus. Required reporting of these diseases is discussed further in chapter 16.

Many states have laws that specifically protect the confidentiality of HIV/AIDS, STDs, and other communicable disease information. However, HIPAA regulations do not provide specific privacy protection for patients with these conditions; thus, healthcare providers must follow the HIPAA Privacy and Security Rules as for other PHI unless preempted by state law.

Confidentiality Protections for HIV/AIDS

Most state laws have special procedures for the handling of HIV/AIDS patient information in regard to subpoenas, discovery, and search warrants. Release for epidemiological studies when the patient is not identified is generally allowable. Most state laws also require a specific written authorization that must include the purpose or need for information and a very specific description of the extent or nature of the information to be disclosed regarding HIV/AIDS patients (for example, AIDS test results or diagnosis and treatment with inclusive dates of treatment). Unauthorized disclosure of HIV/AIDS information on a patient can result in civil or criminal penalties depending on state law, especially if the individual who released the information is found to have done so maliciously. Thus, it is important for a healthcare provider to have policies and procedures in place to ensure that the HIV/AIDS information of a patient is handled appropriately.

The following discussion offers suggestions for handling HIV/AIDS information. Authorizations requesting disclosure of HIV/AIDS PHI must be valid and strictly limited to that information required to fulfill the purpose stated on the authorization. Authorizations specifying "any and all information" or other such broadly inclusive statements should not be honored, and information that is not essential to the stated purpose of the request should not be disclosed. A process should be in place that enables the healthcare provider to retain the signed authorization with notation of the specific information released, the date of release, and the signature of the individual who released the information (Carpenter 1999). Disclosure of information from the records of HIV/AIDS patients or those tested for the HIV virus must be carefully handled, since test results may appear in many sections of the health record.

Records of HIV/AIDS patients that are in a paper format should be maintained in a secure area with restrictive access; however, special handling or marks such as stickers on the record folder that indicate the patient's HIV/AIDS status are discouraged. When using an EHR, the electronic system should provide flags or warning messages related to HIV/AIDS test results or treatment as a way to protect against the release or copying of HIV/AIDS information without appropriate authorization (AHIMA e-HIM Work Group on Security of Personal Health Information 2008). It is important that screening programs provide for confidential testing and communication of test results and that specific written informed consent be obtained from the patient or authorized representative of the patient prior to voluntary testing, as specified in general consent for treatment rules and guidelines. Out of courtesy to patients, the healthcare organization may wish to establish a policy that no claim for medical benefits for patients with HIV can be submitted without first ensuring the patient is aware of the diagnosis, and that the diagnosis must be submitted for the benefit to be paid. A patient may request that his or her information not be submitted for medical benefits if he or she chose to pay for the testing or treatment out of pocket.

Criminal Liability Related to HIV

State law may impose criminal liability for knowingly infecting another with HIV and, likewise, may provide immunity from liability for informing another person of potential HIV infection. For example, Tennessee Code Annotated 68-10-115 (1993) states, "A person who has a reasonable belief that a person has knowingly exposed another to HIV may inform the potential victim without incurring any liability. A person making such disclosure is immune from liability for making disclosure of the condition to the potential victim."

Mandatory HIV Testing of Personnel and Reporting of HIV/AIDS

Additionally, many state laws provide for mandatory HIV testing for certain classes of individuals who may have been exposed to blood in a high-risk situation such as law enforcement officers, paramedics, emergency response employees, firefighters, first response workers, emergency medical technicians, and volunteers making an authorized emergency response. In Ohio, the results of such testing are confidential, but the individual who was exposed has the right to request the results, and the person who provides the results is immune from liability (OH Rev. Code 3701.24.3, 3701.243).

Healthcare providers must have processes in place to address whether HIV/AIDS information should be disclosed to patients who are treated by healthcare workers who are HIV-positive or become HIV-positive, and whether information should be released to individuals who have contracted the virus through a blood transfusion. In the first situation, the Centers for Disease Control and Prevention (CDC) offers guidelines that recommend that a healthcare worker inform a prospective patient of his or her HIV status before the patient undergoes any type of exposure-prone procedure such as surgery. If the healthcare worker learns of his or her HIV-positive status after caring for a patient, the decision to disclose information about the worker should be handled on a case-by-case basis (CDC 2006). The issue of whether to disclose information related to a donor's HIV status has not been easily resolved. Court decisions are split as to whether information should be disclosed and under what circumstances. The decision to disclose HIV/AIDS information about donors remains at the discretion of a state's judicial system (Roach et al. 2006).

Check Your Understanding 15.2

Instructions: Indicate whether the following statements are true or false (T or F).

1. HIPAA does distinguish highly sensitive health information from other types of health information.

2. Psychotherapy notes are always part of the behavioral health record.

3. The duty-to-warn obligation enables a physician to disclose information to a third party who may be the victim of harm perpetrated by a patient.

4. For a substance abuse program to be in compliance with the Privacy Rule, the authorization of disclosure of information should include specific elements required by the Privacy Rule.

5. It is best policy to provide a special mark or notice on an HIV/AIDS patient health record to ensure extra privacy precautions on the record.

Genetic Information

Genetic information provides insight into human disease and is both powerful and subject to misuse. While the term "genetic information" once referred to diseases or conditions that an individual had been diagnosed with, it now encompasses information about an individual's potential to develop a disease or condition in the future. The responsibility associated with protecting this information and using it legally and ethically is immense.

The ability to capture genetic information is the result of the **Human Genome Project** led by the **National Human Genome Research Institute** (NHGRI) of the National Institutes of Health (NIH). The project involved the identification and mapping of all human DNA:

> The Human Genome Project has given us the technology to decipher what were once an individual's most personal and intimate "family secrets"—that is, the information contained in our DNA. The instructions encrypted in our genes affect nearly every function the human body carries out, from fighting infection to thinking. Research to understand those instructions offers the promise of better health because it gives researchers and clinicians critical information to work out therapies or other strategies to prevent or treat a disease. In addition, genetic testing can alert individuals to a heightened risk of some health problems and the need to screen for them more frequently and thoroughly and to take more preventive measures. (Fuller and Hudson 2006, 424–425)

While whole genome sequencing is meant to improve healthcare concern regarding the misuse of genetic information related to healthcare insurance and employability surfaced as well as questions related to genetic testing and counseling. As a result lawmakers, scientists, and health advocacy groups worked to pass the federal Genetic Information Nondiscrimination Act (GINA) of 2008 (Asmonga 2008). GINA prohibits discrimination by health insurers and employers based on genetic information, which is defined as

> …Information about an individual's genetic tests and the genetic tests of an individual's family members, as well as information about the manifestation of a disease or disorder in an individual's family members (i.e., family medical history). Genetic information also includes an individual's request for, or receipt of, genetic services, or the participation in clinical research that includes genetic services by the individual or a family member of the individual, and

the genetic information of a fetus carried by the individual or by a pregnant woman who is a family member of the individual and the genetic information of any embryo legally held by the individual or family member using an assisted reproductive technology. (Equal Employment Opportunity Commission n.d.)

Title I of GINA focuses on genetic nondiscrimination in health insurance and states that health plans may not use genetic information to make eligibility, coverage, underwriting, or premium-setting decisions. Plans cannot ask family members to undergo genetic testing or to provide genetic information. Genetic information obtained intentionally or unintentionally cannot be used for decisions related to plan enrollment. The Medicare supplemental policy and individual health insurance markets are prohibited from imposing pre-existing condition exclusions on the basis of genetic information. Title I also modified the HIPAA Privacy Rule to state that genetic information is health information and prohibits the use and disclosure of genetic information by covered health plans for underwriting purposes (AHIMA 2013a; HHS 2009). There are two exceptions to Title I, which state:

- Health insurers may request genetic information in the case that coverage of a particular claim would only be appropriate if there is a known genetic risk.
- When working in collaboration with external research entities health insurers may request (but not require) in writing that an individual undergo a genetic test. The individual may do so voluntarily, but refusal to participate will have no negative effect on his or her premium or enrollment status. The collected genetic information may be used for research purposes only, and not for underwriting decisions. (NHGRI 2009)

Title II of GINA is the responsibility of the Equal Employment Opportunity Commission (EEOC), which issued final regulations on November 9, 2010, with an effective date of January 10, 2011 (29 CFR Part 1635). Title II "prohibits the use of genetic information in making employment decisions, restricts employers and other entities covered by Title II (employment agencies, labor organizations and joint labor-management training and apprenticeship programs—referred to as "covered entities") from requesting, requiring or purchasing genetic information, and strictly limits the disclosure of genetic information" (EEOC n.d.). GINA specifically addresses the confidentiality of genetic information by stating that

It is also unlawful for a covered entity to disclose genetic information about applicants, employees or members. Covered entities must keep genetic information confidential and in a separate medical file. (Genetic information may be kept in the same file as other medical information in compliance with the Americans with Disabilities Act.) There are limited exceptions to this non-disclosure rule, such as exceptions that provide for the disclosure of relevant genetic information to government officials investigating compliance with Title II of GINA and for disclosures made pursuant to a court order. (EEOC n.d.)

Many states have enacted statutory or regulatory provisions that safeguard genetic information and prohibit discrimination in employment and insurance benefits based on genetic information and mandatory genetic testing for employment and insurance purposes. However, the degree of protection provided by states varies. Some state provisions are less protective than GINA, and some more protective. All entities that are subject to GINA must, at a minimum, comply with applicable GINA requirements as well as more protective state laws. The **National Conference of State Legislatures (NCSL)** maintains information surrounding genetic privacy, employment, and health insurance state anti-discrimination laws. The NCSL website provides current state genetic laws including what protections are offered for genetic information and penalties for privacy violations. The site also outlines consent requirements for performance of genetic tests, accessing genetic information, the retention and disclosure of genetic information, and the personal property rights for genetic information and DNA samples (National Conference of State Legislatures 2008).

In support of protecting genetic information, the Presidential Commission for the Study of Bioethical Issues (PCSBI) issued a report in 2012 that recommended "strong baseline protections for whole genome sequence data to protect individual privacy and data security while also leaving ample room for data sharing opportunities that propel scientific and medical progress" (PCSBI 2012). The commission encouraged the use of informed consent procedures for the sharing of genomic information across state lines and that state and federal governments should have consistent individual privacy protections in place (PCSBI 2012). Subsequently in 2016, President Obama allocated $215 million for the Precision Medicine Initiative to speed patient-centered biomedical discoveries including tools and treatment.

> Through collaborative public and private efforts, the Precision Medicine Initiative will leverage advances in genomics, emerging methods for managing and analyzing large data sets while protecting privacy, and health information technology to accelerate biomedical discoveries. The Initiative will also engage a million or more Americans to volunteer to contribute their health data to improve health outcomes, fuel the development of new treatments, and catalyze a new era of data-based and more precise medical treatment (The White House 2015).

A major objective of the Initiative is commitment to privacy protections that includes addressing legal and technical issues related to privacy and security of data exchange in the context of precision of medicine (The White House 2015). For precision medicine to work, patients must take an active part in their care and sharing of their personal health information. Patient consent for sharing is key, as well as policies and procedures that allow for patient access, use and disclosure of their precision medicine information.

Unfortunately, in the area of direct-to-consumer genetic testing, concerns have arisen that consumers have little protection from unproven or invalid tests which may lead to unnecessary or harmful conclusions regarding consumer health. Although at-home genetic testing has encouraged awareness of genetic diseases, there is no regulatory oversight of the companies offering such tests. Thus, consumers may not be aware of the potential for their genetic information to be used or disclosed in an unauthorized manner by the testing company or aware of the quality of tests performed (National Library of Medicine 2017a). To address concerns, the federal government, and several human genetics organizations have provided "consumer awareness" information regarding direct-to-consumer genetic testing (see figure 15.2) (National Library of Medicine 2017b).

Adoption Information

Adoption is a legal status in which the parental rights and responsibilities of one set of parents are legally terminated and a new parental relationship is established by law (Jones 2017). Parties to an adoption are the adopted individual (adoptee), the biological (natural, birth) parents, and the adoptive parent(s). The rights of each must be considered in light of access to health information. Adoption records include public and nonpublic documents such as the original sealed birth certificate, court documents relating to the adoption process, and records of the adoption agency and/or attorneys involved in the adoption (Adoption.com n.d.). Most state laws deem these records to be confidential and allow their release only with a court order. While health records may not be included in the definition of adoption records, they are nonetheless crucial because of the identifying information and health information they contain.

Figure 15.2 Consumer information on direct-to-consumer genetic tests

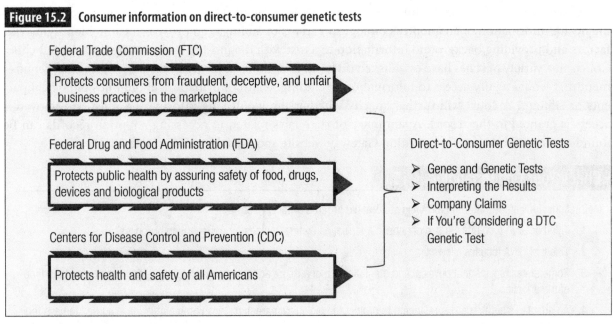

Source: Federal Trade Commission 2014.

Adoption presents a unique challenge to those charged with protecting health information. Previously shrouded in secrecy, many adoptions are now open so that the parties involved know one another's identities. Even in closed adoptions, more emphasis is being placed on blood relatives eventually identifying one another due to health considerations, personal desire, or mere curiosity.

Release of Information to Adopted Persons

A right of access exists for an adoptee's own health records, including the birth record, with all information that identifies the biological parents redacted (removed). Until the adoptee reaches the age of majority, this right of access belongs to the adoptive parents. (When the biological parents' parental rights are terminated, their right of access to the adoptee's health record is also terminated.) Once the adoptee reaches the age of majority, the right of access belongs to the adult adoptee. Policies for the collection and maintenance of adoption information vary from state to state; however, all states have provisions in statutes that allow access to nonidentifying information by an adoptive parent or guardian of an adoptee who is still a minor and then to the adoptee once they reach the age of majority (HHS n.d.a). Some state statutes provide that information regarding the adoptee's physical and mental health be given to the adoptive parents at the time of adoption.

The identity of the biological parents remains confidential unless a registry (often called a mutual consent registry) has been established either by the adoption agency or by state statute that allows adoptees and biological parents to agree to have their identities disclosed (Hughes 2000). For example, the State of Ohio maintains the Ohio Adoption Registry, which was established by the Ohio General Assembly to provide a confidential and voluntary way for adopted Ohioans and their biological families to find one another. The registry resides in the Ohio Department of Health, Office of Vital Statistics (Ohio Department of Health 2015). Unless mandated by court order, health records are not the usual mechanism for parties to an adoption to identify and locate one another. However, requests of this nature may occur, which requires that the healthcare provider have a process in place for preserving the privacy of both parties of concern.

As described above, genetic information has become much more detailed and powerful. Access to the health information of an adoptee's biological parents or siblings can prove critical in identifying risk factors and providing background information to assist with diagnosing and treating the adopted child. Courts in a variety of states have established different thresholds as to what meets a "good cause" requirement that would justify access to information, including health information, about one's biological parents or siblings. A court will further specify whether the identifying information must be removed if access is granted to the record. A summary of state laws related to accessing adoption records can be found at the Child Welfare Information Gateway website sponsored by HHS (HHS 2016a).

Check Your Understanding 15.3

Instructions: Indicate whether the following statements are true or false (T or F).

1. Title I of GINA prohibits the use of genetic information by health plans for underwriting purposes.

2. Title II of GINA focuses allows employers to use genetic information to make employment decisions.

3. Some states provide that physical and mental health of a minor adoptee be given to the adoptive parents at the time of the adoption.

4. An adoptee's birth record is restricted to protect the biological parent(s) unless both parties have agreed to have their identities disclosed in a mutual consent registry.

5. Only the adult adoptee can decide if he or she may access the health information of his or her biological parents for health risk purposes.

Special Access, Request, and Disclosure Situations

Requests for health information vary in terms of what is requested and who is requesting the information. Such requests may be external or internal to an organization and may or may not require patient authorization. Although the general rule for the access, use, or disclosure of patient information is to first obtain the individual's authorization as noted above, there are many exceptions that are based on legal requirements, the best interests of the patient or other parties, or both. The HIPAA Privacy Rule exceptions to the authorization requirement were outlined in chapter 10. Individuals responsible for responding to requests must be trained to deal with each request in accordance with federal and state laws and organizational policy and procedure. This section discusses a variety of situations related to the access, request, and disclosure of health information that have not been discussed elsewhere in this book.

Disclosure of Active Records of Currently Hospitalized or Ambulatory Care Patients

At times, a currently hospitalized patient (**inpatient**) or a patient currently being seen in a clinic setting (**outpatient**) or their personal representative may wish to access, inspect, obtain a copy of, or disclose PHI from the patient's record. The term **active record** is often used to denote the health records of individuals who are currently hospitalized inpatients or outpatients. The Privacy Rule grants individuals the right to access, copy, amend, and disclose their PHI in 45 CFR 164.524 and 45 CFR 164.526, which also states exception to these rights. Individual rights to PHI with exceptions are discussed in detail in chapter 10. If an active inpatient or outpatient wishes to access, copy, amend, or disclose his or her PHI, then the healthcare provider should follow the same policies and procedures in place for patients not currently hospitalized or being treated as an outpatient. More and more healthcare providers are offering patient portals that enable patients to view and copy their personal health records, request test and lab results, request prescription refills and view additional specific information shared by their provider. Procedures should take into consideration what the patient may already have access to and what they wish to still access.

If no exceptions to accessing the information exists, a convenient time and place must be identified where the patient can inspect his or her PHI and obtain copies if requested. If such a request is made, an authorization to release health information must be signed by the patient or his or her personal representative. Because the record is active, the patient should be advised that additional information will be added to the record as the patient continues to receive care while hospitalized or treated as an outpatient. It is suggested that a patient who wishes to access or view his or her record while an inpatient or under current treatment should be provided with the assistance of a physician or other healthcare provider to help the patient in reviewing and understanding the record.

If the patient wishes to have copies of the record sent to another individual, the facility should follow its normal release of information procedure for complying with the request. The date a request was made or received; who made the request; the date the request was honored, and if not honored, why not; what was disclosed; and to whom should be recorded in a log for request-monitoring purposes, and as part of the provider's documentation process for adhering to the HIPAA accounting of disclosures requirements discussed in chapter 10 and in more detail later.

Deceased Patients

HIPAA states that an individual has the same privacy rights in death as they did in life but leaves it up to the states in terms of who qualifies as the deceased person's legal or personal representative for access, use, and disclosure purposes. HITECH modifications to HIPAA provides for flexibility in the disclosure of a decedent's PHI by

1. Removing the PHI status from health records 50 years following the patient's death, and
2. Permitting covered entities (healthcare providers) to disclose decedent records to family members and others involved in the patient's care or payment of care unless doing so would be inconsistent with any known preference of the patient (Hofman 2013).

Although the PHI status has been removed 50 years following a patient's death, it does not mean a healthcare provider must keep a decedent's PHI for 50 years. The Privacy Rule does not address record retention requirements, thus, state retention laws or the providers own record retention procedures should be followed. Upon death, the legal executor or administrator of the estate or the patient's designated personal representative has the right to access the deceased's PHI or records. In the absence of an executor or representative, state law may determine who has access rights. Some states rely on the UHCDA as a guide in identifying a next-of-kin priority such as a spouse, adult child, parent, siblings, or significant other. Other states require that the individual becomes the deceased's official personal representative through appointment by a probate court or court order (Dimick 2013). In some states an individual may authorize for disclosure of his or her PHI, which is valid for two years after the death of the individual, and in other states an authorization is not valid after the individual's death. Thus, state law should be consulted to determine how long after death an authorization remains effective.

The final rule leaves the responsibility up to the CE to have "reasonable assurance" that the person requesting the record has a legitimate right to access it. To avoid conflict, best practices suggest that healthcare providers require requesters to show proof of their relationship to the decedent or present court-authorized documentation showing authority to access the deceased individual's PHI (Dimick 2013).

Disclosure of Information to Medical Examiner or Coroner

Upon death, an **autopsy** may be required to determine the patient's cause of death. The reasons for determining the cause of death are numerous; they include verifying that the death was related to a criminal act, substantiating the cause of death for payment benefits, sudden unexplained or unattended death, accidents, suicide, public health hazards, research, and family history. The Privacy Rule allows the release of PHI without authorization to a medical examiner or coroner for identifying a deceased person, determining cause of death, and other authorized purposes (45 CFR 164.512(g)(1)). State laws define which deaths are reportable to medical examiners and coroners and under what circumstances these public officials may require or decline to perform an autopsy. Authorization by the family or executor of the estate to conduct an autopsy that is deemed a medical examiner or coroner's case is not required.

If the death of the individual is not a medical examiner or coroner's case, the surviving spouse, adult child, parent, adult sibling, grandparent, legal guardian, and/or next of kin of the deceased may request, and subsequently authorize, for an autopsy to be performed. The healthcare organization requires that an authorization form be completed and retained in the health record for evidentiary purposes. A request of this nature is usually made when the cause of death is not known and family member of the deceased feel an autopsy would help resolve concerns regarding the deceased cause of death.

Open Records, Public Records, or Freedom of Information Laws

Open records laws, sometimes called **public records laws**, **sunshine laws**, or freedom of information laws, exist at the federal level and in all 50 states and the District of Columbia. The **Freedom of Information Act** (FOIA) of 1967, amended in 1996 (5 USC 552) to include electronic information, codifies what information is subject to public disclosure, including whether the information is in paper or electronic form. The FOIA specifically provides for public disclosure upon request of many types of information in the possession of federal agencies, except those files that would constitute a clear, unwarranted invasion of personal privacy (5 USC 552(b)(6)). This exemption is used to deny any FOIA requests that include PHI, as previously discussed in chapter 10.

All 50 states and the District of Columbia have public record laws that provide public disclosure upon request of any information from any public body in a state except as otherwise exempted by state regulations. Each state defines its exemptions or exclusions, which often include the withholding of identifiable personal and health information. For example, some exemptions to the Ohio Public Records Law (OH Rev. Code 149.011), as reported in the Reporters Committee for Freedom of the Press *Open Government Guide* (2011), include

> Any record, except births, deaths, and the fact of admission or discharge from a hospital, that pertains to the medical history, diagnosis, prognosis, or medical condition of a patient that is generated and maintained in the process of medical treatment is exempt (Ohio Rev. Code 149.43(A)(1)(a)). Also, records of hospital quality assurance committees and hospital boards or committees reviewing professional qualifications of present or prospective members of the hospital medical staff are exempt from mandatory disclosure (Ohio Rev. Code 2305.251, 2305.25; *State ex rel. Fostoria Daily Review Co. v. Fostoria Hosp. Ass'n*, 44 Ohio St. 3d 111, 541 N.E.2d 587 (1989)). Records containing a trauma center's description of its ability to respond to disasters, mass casualties, and bioterrorism are not public records (Ohio Rev. Code 149.43(A)(1)(x), 3701.072).

There are many other exemptions to the laws, which include issues related to adoption, abortion, law enforcement, and more. What is important is for the healthcare provider to understand that while the intent of the open records laws is to keep society informed of government activities at the federal, state, and local levels, there is a responsibility for agencies that collect and maintain personally identifiable health information to protect the privacy rights of those they serve. These federal and state agencies include government-supported hospitals such as Veterans Affairs hospitals, state-funded or state-supported university medical centers, county and local hospitals and clinics, public health agencies, public health oversight agencies, and public health departments.

Employee Health or Occupational Safety and Health Records

An **occupational health record** may also be known as an employee health record, occupational medical record, or occupational safety and health record. Whichever term is used, it refers to a record kept on an employee that contains information on the health status of the employee. The information may include personal and occupational health histories, medical and drug test results, examinations, physical abilities, immunizations, screenings required by law, biohazardous exposure, occupational illness, and physical limitations (AHIMA 2013c). The employee health record should be kept separately from the employment record of the employee due to the nature of information contained in the record. Employer and occupational healthcare provider access and disclosure of employee health information is dictated by federal and state agency regulations and laws.

Employers are entitled to information regarding an employee's health or medical fitness for work. but not to non-work-related personal health information except as permitted by law. For example, according to the federal **Americans with Disabilities Act (ADA)** (28 CFR Part 35, 36), information regarding an employee medical evaluation is confidential. However, an employer may access information related to fitness for duties, work restrictions, and accommodations. Title II of GINA also offers protection to employees as previously discussed (29 CFR Part 1635). In some situations, federal and state agencies, such as the Occupational Safety and Health Administration (OSHA), ADA, and the Medical Leave Act as a matter of regulation require employers to disclose employee health information to the agency without employee authorization. (AHIMA 2013c).

A sensitive topic related to occupational health records relates to employee drug testing. Employer or workplace drug testing started in the 1980s when the federal government enacted drug-free work programs for federal employees, which have since also been adopted by many state and non-government related employers. Drug testing programs serve as a preventative and deterrent method of supporting a safe, drug-free work environment. Programs of this nature are usually required for pre-employment, pre-promotion, annual physicals, post-accident follow-up, treatment follow-up, or reasonable suspicion purposes. Random drug testing may also occur during employment. Employers may contract with companies to conduct the testing or may require employees to independently undergo drug testing with results submitted back to the employer. Employers must adhere to federal, state and local requirements related to drug testing programs.

SAMHSA (2015) provides resources for establishing a drug-free workplace, such as the "Drug-free Workplace Toolkit." The toolkit suggests that all policies that require testing must be written and communicated to employees in advance. An employer must designate a medical review officer (usually a physician) as the individual who will receive drug test results and report results to appropriate management officials. Drug test results are confidential, but positive results can be cause for termination. Both the results and the subsequent action taken are confidential. In all situations, employees have the right to access the results of drug testing as well as their employee health record under applicable state laws and federal OSHA regulations (29 CFR 1910.20), which ensure that an employee (or designated representative) is given access to his or her health and exposure records within 15 days of a request. Other state regulations may be stricter and preempt the OSHA rule.

Employees should be advised in advance regarding what health records are maintained on them. They should also be notified of any release of such records. Occupational health providers who are CEs must abide by HIPAA rules and obtain patient authorization (or make reasonable efforts to do so) before disclosing health information from an employee health record. Specific authorization may be required for the disclosure of health information relating to HIV or AIDS, substance abuse, and mental health, if more strictly defined by state law. Additionally, many state laws protect the confidentiality of information obtained through employee assistance programs, which provide assessment, intervention, referral for appropriate diagnosis and treatment, and follow-up services to employees whose job performance is impaired by personal concerns such as health, family, financial, alcohol, drug, legal, emotional, or other stressors.

Antiterrorism Initiatives

The federal government enacted two laws in its effort to thwart terrorism and terrorist attacks in the United States, both of which provide access to PHI under certain circumstances. The **Patriot Act** of 2001 was enacted to deter and punish terrorist acts in the United States and around the world and to enhance law enforcement investigations. The goal of the **Homeland Security Act** of 2002 is to prevent terrorist attacks in the United States while reducing vulnerability to terrorism, minimizing its damages, and assisting in recovery from attacks in the United States. Both acts give government authorities the right to access information needed to investigate and deter terrorism (AHIMA 2010).

The Patriot Act allows the director of the Federal Bureau of Investigation or a designee to apply for a production order through the court system to produce tangible items such as documents and records. It also provides sanctions for any unauthorized disclosures of the information obtained by others not involved in the investigation. A healthcare provider who in good faith provided information requested under order would not be held liable for releasing the information (AHIMA Homeland Security Work Group 2010). In contrast, the Homeland Security Act gives the secretary of Homeland Security authority to access information that would include PHI without the authorization of the patient or personal representative (AHIMA Homeland Security Work Group 2010). This act, however, specifically states that PHI is protected from unauthorized disclosure and should be used for the purpose for which it was obtained and that the redisclosure should be restricted to only those involved in the case (AHIMA Homeland Security Work Group 2010).

In essence, the federal government is permitted access to any and all information it deems necessary to protect the country. The healthcare provider should provide the PHI to the requesting authority without delay if appropriate identification of the official is obtained and verified. This should include making a copy of the requester's identification and noting the office location where the information will be taken and the branch of government requesting the information (AHIMA Homeland Security Work Group 2010).

In addition to the above antiterrorism regulation, public health authorities are granted authority through local, state, and federal laws to engage in **syndromic surveillance**. This type of surveillance refers to the "systematic gathering and analysis of health data to rapidly detect clusters of symptoms and health complaints that might indicate an infectious-disease outbreak or other public health threat" (Drociuk et al. 2004). These laws provide public health officials with necessary information to help detect bioterrorism threats and sudden outbreaks of diseases such as West Nile virus, severe acute respiratory syndrome (SARS), and virulent strains of influenza. In support of surveillance, the CDC's National Syndromic Surveillance Program (NSSP) has implemented a "cloud-based BioSense Platform that provides public health departments with a secure integrated electronic health information system with standardized analytic tools and processes ... to rapidly collect, evaluate, share, and store syndromic surveillance data" (CDC 2016). The BioSense Platform also supports the HITECH Meaningful Use program supported by the Centers for Medicare and Medicaid Services (CMS). NSSP has also incorporated the Electronic Surveillance System for the Early Notification of Community Based Epidemics (ESSENCE) into the BioSense Platform. ESSENCE was originally developed to alert health authorities of infectious disease outbreaks, including possible bioterrorism attacks (Coletta n.d.).

Whereas certain uses of the syndromic surveillance data are nonidentifiable, the majority of systems often require medical providers to disclose identifiable health information to state or federal public health agencies. The HIPAA Privacy Rule allows disclosure of health information without patient authorization for public interest and benefits such as public health and safety, it does not compel disclosure. However, most states have regulations that do compel disclosure, with confidentiality controls in place as well. To ensure information is protected, healthcare organizations should implement policies and procedures for disclosing patient information as a result of antiterrorism legislation and other public health syndromic surveillance activity.

Consumer Reporting Agencies

A consumer reporting agency is a company that regularly assembles or evaluates consumer information for the purpose of producing reports. The information collected may be credit information or, in the case of the Medical Information Bureau (MIB), health histories and related issues. Companies that collect credit information are called credit bureaus. Equifax, Experian, and TransUnion are three of the more prominent companies that collect and report on consumer credit (Avery et al. 2003). Insurance companies exchange confidential information with the MIB on individuals who apply for life, health, disability, long-term care, or critical illness insurance. This nationwide specialty consumer reporting agency specializes in fraud detection data, risk management, and actuarial analytics for the insurance industry. Its purpose is to alert a member company when a potential client who has applied for insurance either knowingly or unknowingly omits information from his or her insurance application (MIB 2011). To provide consumers protection against misuse of their health information, the **Fair and Accurate Credit Transactions Act** of 2003 (FACTA) was enacted.

FACTA amended the Fair Credit Reporting Act (FCRA) (15 USC 1681), related to obtaining and using medical (health) information in connection with credit eligibility determination (Privacy Rights Clearinghouse 2011). The rule prohibits a creditor from obtaining and using medical information to decide a consumer's credit eligibility. However, a creditor can obtain and use financial information related to medical debts, expenses, or income (16 CFR 604(g)(2)). A consumer (a patient) must authorize for a consumer reporting agency to share medical information with employers for employment or insurance purposes. Consumer reporting agencies may not report the name, address, or telephone number of any medical information furnisher (such as a healthcare provider) unless the information is coded so as not to identify or infer the provider of care or the individual's medical condition. This restriction does not apply to insurance companies selling only property and casualty insurance (16 CFR 605(a)(6)).

Duty to Warn

As previously discussed in the section on behavioral health information, state laws may permit or even compel psychologists and psychiatrists to use their discretion to warn intended victims of potential harm without the patient's authorization. Such exceptions to state laws that traditionally consider patient–psychologist and patient–physician communications to be privileged serve the public interest by protecting individuals and are compliant with the HIPAA Privacy Rule. Healthcare providers have a duty to exercise reasonable care by warning a patient's intended victim, and the duty to warn supersedes the duty of confidentiality.

Laboratory Test Results

CMS regulates all laboratory testing performed in the U.S. except for research, through the federal **Clinical Laboratory Improvement Amendments** (CLIA) of 1988 (42 CFR 493.3(a)(2)). CLIA was enacted to ensure the accuracy and reliability of all laboratory testing. It permits clinical laboratories to release test results to the individuals responsible for ordering the test and the laboratory that initiated the request. Laboratories can electronically exchange test data but must ensure that an EHR format configures the lab results in the correct format and that lab results are sent to the correct provider (Wiedemann 2011). In 2014, CLIA was amended to remove certain regulatory barriers and HIPAA exceptions for CLIA-certified laboratories and CLIA-exempt laboratories. The amended rule gives patients, patient's designees or personal representative the broad access rights to see or obtain a copy of their PHI, including an electronic copy. Patients may direct the lab that performed the test to send copies of their PHI as requested. Laboratories not subject to HIPAA are not obligated to provide access or send copies but are permitted to do so (McLendon 2014). The rule does not preempt stricter state privacy laws, however it will preempt state laws that provide more narrow access rights. HIPAA gives the laboratory 30 days to release results once a request has been made and additional time under certain circumstances which the lab must explain to the patient in writing. The rule also requires the laboratory to have processes in place to verify the authenticity of the request and to not impose unreasonable verification measures on the patient (45 CFR 164.524).

Payment Requests from Insurance Companies and Government Agencies

Insurance companies commonly request patient information. In accordance with the HIPAA Privacy Rule, requests for payment purposes, including utilization review and medical necessity review, do not require authorization if the information is for the payment of a specific episode of care (45 CFR 164.506). However, other insurance company information requests (for example, for life insurance determinations) require patient authorization. An insurance company acting on behalf of the healthcare organization (for example, obtaining information in a lawsuit in which the insurance company represents the defendant healthcare organization or provider) does not require an authorization. In such a case, the insurance company would function as a business associate. Medicare and Medicaid and agencies working on their behalf, such as Quality Improvement Organizations and fiscal intermediaries, do not require the patient's authorization if the information is required for payment. If the information is required for enrollment, however, patient authorization is required.

The purpose of the request must be determined to comply with HIPAA regulations and accounting of disclosures including additional accounting requirements as defined in the HITECH provisions. Requirements under HITECH will be discussed later in this chapter, in the section Accounting of Disclosures and Tracking Releases.

Medical Emergencies

In **medical emergency** situations, the obligation is to treat the patient and provide whatever information is necessary. This usually entails disclosing patient information without authorization. If such a disclosure occurs, it is prudent to document the content and nature of the disclosure (for example, telephone conversation or electronic transmission) in the health record. Although the HIPAA Privacy Rule does not require authorization for disclosures made for treatment reasons, providers may elect to enforce policies that do require authorization.

An additional consideration associated with medical emergencies is the log or run sheet generated by emergency medical personnel as a result of their response to calls for assistance. The run sheet may contain information such as patient-identifying information, cause for service, condition of individual attended, and where the individual was taken for medical services. This information may be used for reimbursement purposes. Because these documents may be subject to a state's public records laws, state law should be consulted in conjunction with the HIPAA Privacy Rule to ensure proper disclosure.

Public Figures or Celebrities

News media personnel (and others) may have an interest in obtaining information about a public figure or celebrity who is being treated or about individuals involved in events that have cast them in the public eye. The media is not exempt from restrictions imposed by the Privacy Rule facility directory requirement. A healthcare organization may wish to exercise even greater restraint than that mandated by the directory requirement with respect to the media in order to ensure patient confidentiality for noted public figures and celebrities. For example, it is recommended that no information be provided about the location of a patient who is the subject of media inquiry. Special care should be taken to ensure that patients who are the subjects of media inquiry give authorization for any information to be disclosed or for photographs and interviews (Ohio Hospital Association 2005).

A healthcare organization may consider implementing policies and procedures for assigning an alias to patients who are public figures or celebrities and placing their health records in a separate secure area. If information is stored electronically, a process that restricts access on a need-to-know basis should be considered. Media representatives who appear at the organization should always be escorted and restricted from patient care areas. The healthcare organization should appoint a designated spokesperson to address media questions, ensure that staff training occurs regarding the privacy rights of public figures and celebrities, and have staff sign nondisclosure statements (Amatayakul 2003). While individuals who have willingly placed themselves in the public eye have a reduced expectation of privacy, it is nonetheless the obligation of the healthcare provider to take additional precautions to protect the privacy of these individuals and their health information.

Social Security Administration and State Disability Determination Services

Federal and state governments offer rehabilitation and disability services to help people suffering from physical or mental disabilities that affect their ability to work or return to work in a timely manner. These services are administered through the **Social Security Administration** (SSA) and state **disability determination services**. The SSA regulations require that state disability determination services responsible for providing medical evidence must determine whether a resident of a state is or is not disabled under the Social Security disability law. When an individual files a disability application with the SSA, it is transmitted to the state agency that will make the medical decision regarding the claim. The agency sends letters to every medical provider the claimant has listed on their application. The claimant is asked to voluntarily authorize the sending of all medical, school, and other records and information related to his or her case to the SSA and the state agency authorized to process the case by signing disclosure form SSA-827. The SSA has revised the form to comply with the HIPAA Privacy Rule on authorization for use and disclosure of health information.

The SSA processes millions of health records for disability claimants each year. To defray costs and expedite the review process, the SSA and state disability determination services implemented the **Electronic Records Express** (ERE) initiative, which offers providers secure electronic options for submitting records related to disability claims. When a request for records concerning a disability claim is received, the provider may choose to submit the information electronically via the SSA's secure website or fax the information to the state agency handling the disability determination services. The records sent are automatically associated with the applicant's unique disability claim folder (SSA n.d.).

In addition, the SSA has entered into an agreement with several MedVirginia HIEs to process patient disability claims. This has enabled the SSA to reduce the amount of time spent preparing, receiving, and processing patient health records or disability claims (Feldman et al. 2013)). Key to the processing of this information is the patient authorization for access and disclosure of PHI. From a practice perspective, the Healthcare Information and Management Systems Society (HIMSS) offers a document that provides direction on sending records efficiently and securely to the SSA's disability claims system (HIMSS 2007). A link to the document is provided in the references section.

Health Information Handlers: Payment Integrity Review Contractors, Health Information Exchanges

A **health information handler** (HIH) is any organization that handles information on behalf of a provider. For example, most healthcare organizations and providers use an HIH to submit their claims for reimbursement purposes (CMS 2016b). Some examples of HIHs are release of information vendors, HIEs, and EHR vendors. Some HIHs are considered covered entities, business associates, or business associate subcontractors that have agreements with providers to access, use, or disclose PHI. However, HIHs that provide payment oversight for federal government programs such as the Medicare Fee-for-Service program are not required to provide authorization for disclosure of PHI since they fall under the HIPAA exception that allows access and disclosure without authorization for purposes of treatment, payment, and operations (45 CFR 164.501).

Given the massive amount of information and claims handled through the Medicare Fee-for-Service program, CMS has contracted with HIH payment integrity review contractors such as Recovery Audit Contractors (RACs), Medicare Administrative Contractors (MACs), and Zone Program Integrity Contractors (ZPICs) to measure, prevent, identify, and correct incorrect payments and identify fraudulent claims activity (CMS 2016b). These contractors have access to patient information that is submitted to them by healthcare organizations and providers who receive letters requesting that certain medical documentation be released to the review contractors. The healthcare organization may disclose information via paper, disk, or fax. In 2010, CMS implemented a program that enables providers to respond to review contractors and other related HIHs online as well as via paper, disk, or fax through its Electronic Submission of Medical Documentation System (esMD) (CMS 2016a). Phase 2 of the pilot will enable review contractors to send their requests for medical documentation electronically, thus eliminating the paper request. Entities that function as HIEs that have a contract, grant, or cooperative agreement with a federal agency may also participate in the esMD by submitting medical documentation electronically through a gateway service.

Instructions: Indicate whether the following statements are true or false (T or F).

1. In absence of a legal executor or administrator of an estate, states may follow the UHCDA to allow access to the health records of a deceased patient.

2. The Freedom of Information Act, along with state open records laws including public records or sunshine laws, enables federal or state entities to protect personal health information from public access.

3. An employer is entitled to information about an employee's health or medical work fitness for work and non-work related health information.

4. HIPAA does not allow the disclosure of personal health information on a patient who has contacted a disease that is monitored in by public health officials without the patient's authorization.

5. CLIA prohibits a patient from accessing lab results directly for the laboratory conducting the test.

Managing the Release of Information Process

Managing the release of information (ROI) process should be part of an organization or providers information governance program. It is essential to ensuring that a healthcare organization or provider is providing the appropriate safeguards necessary for protecting the privacy, confidentiality, and security of PHI. Complicating the process is whether the information is in paper, electronic, or hybrid form. Whether ROI is handled internally by employed staff or externally by HIHs (which are also business associates) such as copy service vendors or HIEs, it can be costly in terms of time to process requests and address problems resulting from an inadequate management process. Policies and procedures should be in place that support the management practices for access, use, and disclosure of information including responding to subpoenas or court orders.

Quality control practices should address the tracking and monitoring of requests from receipt through final disposition; priority and efficiency of processing requests; and managing productivity, turnaround times, and backlogs (AHIMA 2012, 2013b). Tracking and monitoring requests should include documenting the date on which a request was made or received, who made the request, the date on which the request was honored (and if not honored, why not), what was disclosed, and to whom. Information of this nature may also be encompassed in the process for adhering to the HIPAA accounting of disclosures requirements discussed in chapter 11 and in more detail later. There are many issues to consider when managing an ROI process some of which are discussed below and can be found in additional resources (AHIMA 2012, 2013b; Dunn and Burton 2015)

Definition of LHR and DRS

In managing the ROI process, it is important for the healthcare organization or provider to have defined its legal health record (LHR) and designated record set (DRS) as discussed in chapter 9. Remember, the LHR serves as the organization's business record and is the record that is released upon request (AHIMA 2011). The DRS is broader than the LHR because it includes not only the health record, but also records involved in billing and insurance enrollment and coverage and other documents "used, in whole or in part to make decisions about individuals" (45 CFR 164.501). The DRS inherently includes information in any format and may include videotapes, photographs, cassettes, and other reproductions and duplicates. Knowledge of what constitutes the LHR and DRS helps set parameters for what patient information may be disclosed.

Because the health record may contain a variety of documents that are not directly related to patient treatment they are not considered part of the LHR or included in disclosures. Such documents may include correspondence, information about other family members, copies of insurance cards, records from other providers, authorizations for disclosure of information, internal memoranda about the disclosure of information, and correspondence from and records of requesters. Although not subject to disclosure, such documents may be maintained with the patient paper-based record or scanned into the patient's EHR. Only information that is pertinent and needed for patient care and treatment decisions should be physically incorporated into the health record to be released in response to authorizations, subpoenas, and court orders.

Determining Who Will Disclose/Release Information

A determination must be made regarding which departments will disclose/release information when it is requested, since PHI and electronic PHI (ePHI) can be stored in multiple forms and multiple systems. Departments may be responsible for processing a request for the records that are under their control. For example, radiology may be responsible for directly releasing x-rays or the laboratory for releasing lab results in response. Another alternative is that all requests be handled through the health information management (HIM) department. In this situation, HIM personnel would be responsible for gathering all requested documents, such as health records, billing office records, and x-rays, and releasing them to the requester.

Many HIM departments have moved toward a shared services model with commercial copy service vendors that function as HIHs and business associates. This arrangement allows the healthcare organization to perform front-end functions such as logging ROI requests, confirming validity, identifying what information is to be disclosed, and checking the record for completeness. The copy service vendor usually assumes responsibility for back-office processes such as releasing the record to the requester, communicating with customers, maintaining compliance, invoicing and billing, applying fees to specific types of records, handling postage, and dealing with telephone and walk-in inquiries. Under the shared services model, fees are usually shared between the vendor and the HIM department. Turnaround time for complying with the request tends to decrease with this model, as do customer complaints. When information is disclosed through a copy service vendor, policies and procedures must be clear as to the responsibilities of the vendor versus the responsibilities of the HIM department.

Types of Requests for Access, Use, and Disclosure/Release of PHI

Requests for access, use, and disclosure/release of patient information commonly occur via mail, telephone, or physical presence of the requester, either unannounced (a "walk-in") or by a prearranged on-site review. Requests may also be received electronically via fax or e-mail. In addition, a requester may ask that information be faxed or e-mailed to a given location or sent electronically via a given website. Requests are made directly by the patient or personal representative for inspecting and copying the patient's PHI or disclosing the information to a third party. Requests are also commonly made by third parties such as other healthcare entities, insurance companies, attorneys, health oversight agencies (for example, public health agencies, the SSA, state disability determination services, coroners, RACs, and MACs), and other government-related agencies or HIHs (AHIMA 2013b).

Regardless of the type of request made, if the request is from the patient, a formal authorization form is not required per the HIPAA Privacy Rule; however, many healthcare providers (CEs) will ask the patient to complete an authorization form for the patient's own protection or put their request in writing as long as the CE has informed the patient of this requirement. An authorization is not required for several public interest and benefit situations (45 CFR 164.512) but is required if the requester is a third party to the patient, such as an attorney. If the authorization form is required, then it should include the elements of a valid authorization as defined by the HIPAA Privacy Rule (see figure 10.8 in chapter 10) (45 CFR 164.508).

Verification of Requester

Because providers are not always aware of family situations or other relationships, proof of the requester's relationship to the patient must be verified before health information is disclosed, as required by the HIPAA Privacy Rule (45 CFR 164.514(h)(1)). Such verification generally applies to in-person disclosures in which information is not being released to a destination specified and authorized by the patient. For example, contracted reviewers and representatives of insurance companies or other payers should be required to present documentation of their relationship with the company they represent. A patient's personal representative should also be required to present documentation to appropriate personnel to verify that the requester has the legitimate right to access the information. Whoever the requester is, the HIPAA Privacy and Security Rules require the verification of the identity and authority of the person making the request, if not known, before any information is disclosed (45 CFR 164.514(h)(1); 45 CFR 164.312(d)). If the patient is deceased, policy relating to who can legitimately access the record is followed, as discussed previously.

The validity of the authorization should be verified before information is released. Specifically, the following should be done:

- Check to be sure that all applicable parts of the form have been completed.
- Make sure that the information does not appear to be falsified.
- Check the date of the authorization to be certain it has not expired.
- Compare the patient's signature to one in the actual health record to ensure validity.
- Exercise good judgment to ensure that there is no suggestion in the authorization or circumstances surrounding it that the authorization was not given freely, that releasing the information will damage the relationship between the patient and the facility in which he or she sought treatment, or that disclosing the information will be harmful to the patient.

In addition, all responses to requests should be noted in the organization's procedure for managing requests. It is important for those managing ROI functions to understand each type of request and clearly establish policies and procedures to respond to requests in a time frame set forth by organizational policy and federal and state regulations.

Mail Requests

The most typical request to access, use, or disclose patient information is received through the mail. A letter or a form is received that requests health information to be copied and mailed or sent electronically to the requester. The healthcare organization reviews the authorization, determines if it is valid, and either processes the request or asks for additional information. For example, an insurance company may send a paper authorization requesting a copy of a patient's discharge summary and operation report. Similarly, many payment integrity review contractors such as RACs and MACs may send a written letter requesting medical documentation from patient records. The types of requests received via mail are virtually limitless.

Telephone Requests

Requests by phone tend to come from physician offices, insurance companies, or patients. The healthcare employee who receives a telephone request should request the name, address, telephone number, and, if applicable, the company of the caller to identify the requesting party and verify that the party is entitled to receive the information requested. Once the party is identified and verified, the employee should return the call to disclose the information, if appropriate. In emergencies, the employee should request the calling party to furnish additional pertinent information about the patient that might not be generally known but could be verified by the medical history or some other information found within the patient record. A telephone request can be honored without an authorization if it is for purposes of treatment, payment, or healthcare operations such as transferring the patient to another facility for continuity of care purposes. If the healthcare organization uses a voice mail message system, the voice mail message should request callers to leave their name and callback number or to return the call during working office hours. Patient-identifying information should not be left on the voice mail system as it might not be secure.

Electronic Requests and Requests to Electronically Send Information via Fax or Internet (E-Mail or Web Portal)

Requests may be received via fax, e-mail, patient portal or other electronic means. A process of identifying and verifying the requester must occur before the information is disclosed. There may be a request to fax or e-mail patient information to a given location. If requests of this nature are received, security safeguards should be implemented to ensure the validity of the fax numbers and/or e-mail addresses to which information will be sent; to ensure that the receiving fax machine or e-mail is attended when information is sent; to ensure that a cover sheet containing a confidentiality statement (and a telephone number that an unintended recipient can call to report a transmission error) is used; and to ask the recipient to verify receipt of the transmitted documents (Davis et al. 2006). Guidance for handling fax and e-mail requests was discussed in detail in chapter 13. Figure 13.4 and figure 13.5 offer further recommendations for disclosing PHI by fax and e-mail. If patient makes a request using the e-mail capability of a patient portal provided by his or her provider then additional procedures should be in place to ensure e-mails from patient portals are monitored daily and requests complied within an appropriate amount of time. To facilitate this process, a provider may wish to post a release of information authorization and other applicable forms on their website.

Some requesters are now offering providers the option of sending patient information to a secure website. For example, the SSA and state disability determination services, as discussed previously, have implemented the Electronic Records Express program, which enables providers to submit records related to disability claims to a secure website (SSA n.d.). In addition, the CMS eHeatlh initiative enables providers, review contractors, and HIH to electronically submit requested medical documentation (PHI) through its esMD as previously mentioned (CMS 2016a).

Walk-In Requests

Most unannounced walk-in requests are from patients who wish to inspect or obtain copies of their records; however, third parties may also present themselves unannounced. Ask the individual requesting records for a valid picture identification to verify that the individual is who they say they are. Once the request is determined to be valid, if possible, the requested information should be provided.

Space must be provided for individuals to wait and to review the information requested. Personnel should be present at all times during an on-site review to assist the requester with the record, to assure the record is not altered or documents removed or destroyed, and to answer questions where appropriate. Because of the resources involved with walk-in requests, advance notice by requesters should be encouraged and a scheduled appointment process implemented, such as the one discussed in the next section.

On-Site Record Review Requests

On-site record reviews differ from walk-in requests in that an on-site review is prearranged for a specific day and time when patient information will be made available to the requester. The organization must follow the Privacy Rule time frames when responding to requests, so the setting of appointments must adhere to these time frames. The requesters of on-site reviews are usually attorneys, insurance companies, Quality Improvement Organization representatives, or researchers. Prior to the on-site review, a request should be received and the type of information requested should be specified. If the requester and the authorization for use and disclosure of the information are determined to be legitimate, a time and place for the review is established along with the information requested. As discussed with walk-ins, personnel should be present at all times during on-site reviews to assist the requester with the record, to assure the record is not altered or documents removed or destroyed (if a paper health record) or deleted (if in a EHR system), and to answer questions where appropriate.

Determining If Disclosure Is Appropriate

Once it has been determined that a request is compliant with HIPAA and state regulations, an organization must determine whether the information can be disclosed. State and federal laws should be consulted to ensure no conflicts exist between the two. In addition, records related to adopted children, mental health, substance abuse, HIV/AIDS, potential lawsuits, genetic testing, or minors receiving treatment not requiring parental consent warrant special protections when disclosure or access has been requested.

If there is no conflict, the next step is to determine what content is requested. Dunn (2010) states that requests are often written for "any and all records," which can be problematic to address since there may be multiple records stored in a variety of ways and in a variety of places. Requests for any and all records should be compared to the HIPAA minimum necessary requirement (exceptions are provided in chapter 10). If the request does not meet the requirement, it should be sent back to the sender for clarification (Dunn 2010). Copying documents in a health record or from multiple sites can be costly; thus, verification of the requester's needs should be sought before the request is honored if there is any question or concern regarding what the requester is asking for.

If the request is appropriate and patient information is disclosed, the signed authorization form should be retained with a notation of the specific information disclosed, the reason for disclosure, the date of disclosure, and the signature of the employee who disclosed the information. The actual authorization form does not become part of the LHR or the DRS and should not automatically be disclosed when information from the patient's record is disclosed in the future. For convenience, however, the authorization form may be maintained with the patient record, as noted above.

Subpoena or Court Order

There are times when a health record is required for litigation such as malpractice cases, car accidents, criminal cases, and divorce proceedings. The health record is produced for discovery and litigation purposes through the use of subpoenas and court orders. As discussed in chapter 4, a **subpoena** is a legal tool used to compel one's appearance at a certain time and place to testify (*subpoena ad testificandum*) or produce documents or other tangible items (*subpoena duces tecum*—"bring with") either during the discovery process or at trial. A subpoena can be issued by a state or federal court, a grand jury, a lawyer representing a party in a civil or criminal lawsuit, or a government agency. A **court order** is a document issued by a judge that compels certain action, such as testimony or the production of documents such as health records.

A healthcare provider or organization must have policies and procedures in place that enable it to respond as directed by the subpoena or court order. The process for responding will vary based on state and federal regulations, including HIPAA requirements. Legal counsel should be notified immediately if the provider is party to the litigation. The subpoena or court order may ask for the original health record; however, whenever possible the court should be contacted to request that a copy be placed into evidence rather than the original record. Whether a copy of the record can be provided rather than the original is determined by state or federal regulation. For example, in Ohio a certified copy of the health record can be offered into evidence without the custodian appearance in court if attorneys for both parties stipulate that the records can be offered as evidence (OH Rev. Code 2317.422). If the original record must be submitted, then a process for return of the record must be in place. Whether the record is in paper or electronic form, the facility should have policies and procedures in place for disclosing PHI for discovery (e-discovery) and litigation purposes.

ROI Reimbursement and Fee Structure

The release of health information is a function of doing business, and thus has a cost associated with it. The HIPAA Privacy Rule permits reasonable, cost-based charges for labor, postage, and supplies when fulfilling a patient or personal representative of the patient's request for PHI. If the patient request an electronic copy of his or her PHI that is maintained electronically the charge may not exceed the flat fee of $6.50. Also, HIPAA prohibits a CE to pass along the cost of using an ROI service to the patient (HHS n.d.b). Providers should determine cost-based fees for their operations, taking into consideration state laws on ROI costs and other state and federal programs such as the SSA Electronic Records Express initiative, CMS's esMD system, and meaningful use incentive programs (Dunn 2010). Factors that should be considered in determining the cost of ROI including costs associated with e-discovery are outlined in figures 15.3 and 15.4.

Figure 15.3   Costs factored into ROI costs

- Systems and hardware (such as additional workstations) to accommodate the ROI function
- Applications such as ROI tracking systems
- Peripherals such as copiers, printers, and fax machines
- Forms such as ROI authorization forms and fax cover sheets
- Routine supplies including staples, pens, paper, envelopes, toner, DVDs for scanned documents, and other media
- Postage and labor for handling
- Fees for off-site storage and retrieval
- Overhead such as utilities, space, furnishings, maintenance fees for machines, housekeeping, human resources, and payroll

Source: Dunn 2010.

Figure 15.4 Steps in assessing costs for e-discovery

1. **Identify all places that could store patient information**, both patient-identifiable and non-identifiable. These include data stored in electronic form in equipment (e.g., echocardiogram, EKG, fetal monitoring equipment) and information transmission systems (e-mail, primarily). Electronically stored information was probably catalogued during the facility's efforts to define its designated record set.

2. **Determine how patient-specific data can be extracted** from these other locations. In the case of cancer registry or core measures reporting, these databases often have report generation functions that allow patient-specific data to be printed or exported to an electronic file. However, data in quality assurance or performance improvement and infection control databases may be more difficult to extract

3. **Determine the time and other resources required to extract data** from these files and how long data are stored in them. You will need assistance from your IT department to capture data stored electronically in both equipment and transmission vehicles. Many organizations have established retention techniques that pool or store e-mail and other digital data for a period of time to protect against spoliation.

4. **Inventory this information** to address disclosure costs. An example of an inventory is given in Table 12.1.

5. **Document inventorying effort**. Completely document the initial and ongoing efforts to maintain a current inventory, including the time involved, memoranda used, educational efforts, et cetera. This will help demonstrate that the organization has performed its due diligence in relation to the Federal Rules of Civil Procedure, which applies primarily to data maintained in an electronic format. Outlining files maintained electronically will be important in appealing unreasonable demands in front of the judge.

6. **Apply labor and supply factors**. In the example above, assume that the plaintiff's attorney requires all information from any electronic system and wants it on a CD. The labor cost would be multiplied by 0.5 hours (0.25 for each of the two electronic systems). Supplies include the CD, the current cost of which is easily determined. The time to save the files to a CD would be minimal; however, if multiple documents must be saved, it may be worth inventorying the approximate time to write a document to a CD and then applying that factor to the number of documents requested.

Source: Dunn 2007.

Most states have enacted statutes that control the amount of reimbursement that a healthcare facility or provider can charge. Copy cost and fee schedules vary by state, with some identifying an initial flat fee followed by a per-page fee that usually decreases as the number of pages goes up. For a state-by-state reference guide to health record copying charges, see the following websites at www.lamblawoffice.com (Lamb 2016) or Medicopy.net. Figure 15.5 provides an example of the Ohio Revised Code 3701.741 statue related to ROI copying charges.

If a fee is assessed for a request, the fee schedule must be consulted and an invoice prepared. The fee schedule should be regularly reviewed for compliance with the HIPAA Privacy Rule and applicable state laws. A system should be developed to determine situations in which fees are not assessed, to determine when prepayment is required, and to implement collection procedures for delinquent payments following record disclosure. If a copy service company is used to handle the tasks of responding to requests for information, the company directly bills requesters (patients, attorneys, insurance company representatives, disability determination services, and others) for copying the information. A sales tax may be assessed when information is sent to states where sales tax applies.

Overall, requests for information, whether received by paper or electronically, should be responded to in the same manner as received. While HIPAA's authorization requirements and organizational policy must continue to be followed, documents authorizing the disclosure of information may be retained electronically, along with annotations about the disclosure such as the date information was disclosed and to whom. It is important for providers responsible for releasing information to enter disclosures into a central tracking system. Care should be given to ensure that the process is consistent throughout the

Figure 15.5	State of Ohio law on medical record copying charges

For requests made by *patients or their representatives*, hospitals may charge:
- No record search fee is allowed
- $3.07 per page for the first 10 pages
- $0.64 per page for pages 11–50
- $0.24 per page for pages 51 or higher
- With respect to data recorded other than on paper, $2.10 per page (MRI, x-ray, CAT scan, etc)
- Actual cost of any related postage incurred by the healthcare provider or medical record company

For requests made by *someone other than the patient or patient's representative*:
- Initial search fee of $18.91
- $1.24 per page for the first 10 pages
- $0.64 per page for pages 11–50
- $0.26 per page for pages 51 or higher
- With respect to data recorded other than on paper, $2.10 per page (MRI, x-ray, CAT scan, etc)
- Actual cost of any related postage incurred by the healthcare provider or medical record company

Source: OH Rev. Code 3701.741.

organization, since more than one functional area may disclose patient information. One consideration is to have accounting of disclosures and requests for accounting handled by the HIM department.

Accounting of Disclosures and Tracking Releases

The Privacy Rule requires the tracking and accounting of disclosures of PHI. The accounting requirement currently includes all disclosures made in writing, electronically, by telephone, and/or orally, except for those defined by the Rule as discussed in chapter 11.

A manual or electronic tracking system to account for requesters and recipients of patient information should be in place, along with policies and procedures in support of the process. Most health record copying services also use ROI tracking systems, which are shown in figure 15.6.

Right to Request Restrictions

As described in chapter 11, the Privacy Rule gives patients the right to request that CEs restrict uses and disclosures of their PHI for carrying out TPO (45 CFR 164.522(a)). Covered entities were not required to agree to these requests in the past, although they must abide by requests they agree to. However, HITECH now enables an individual to restrict an organization's ability to disclose information to health plans for payment or operations purposes if the service provided was paid for completely out of the individual's pocket.

Refusal to Disclose Information

In certain circumstances, it may be necessary to refuse to disclose patient information or require additional information or documentation before information is disclosed to the requester. When such situations occur, it is important to have process in place seek assistance from legal counsel if necessary or from

Figure 15.6   Processing ROI request forms received

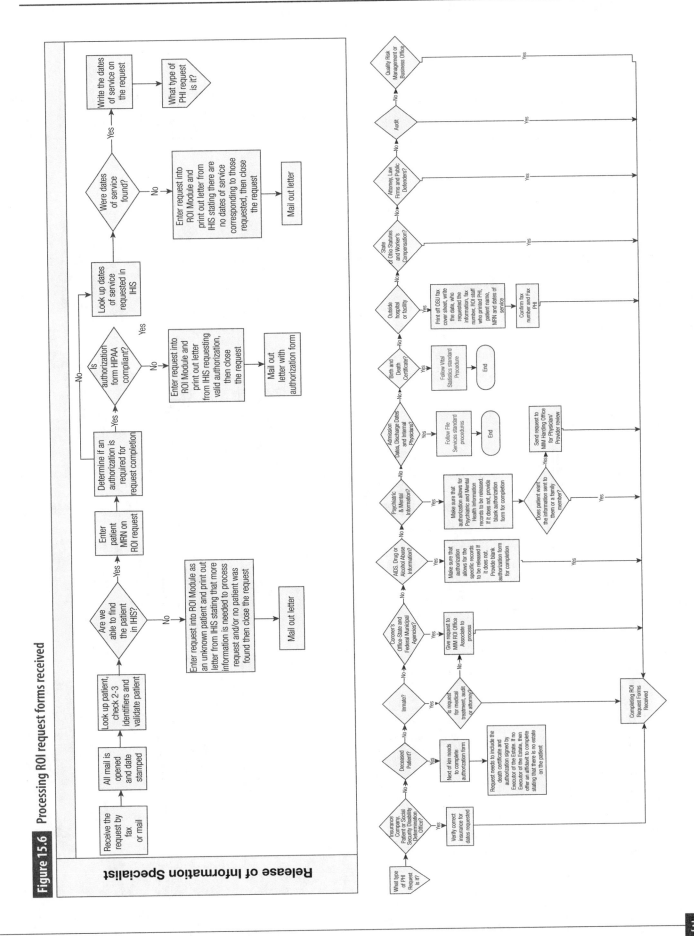

Completing ROI Request Forms Received

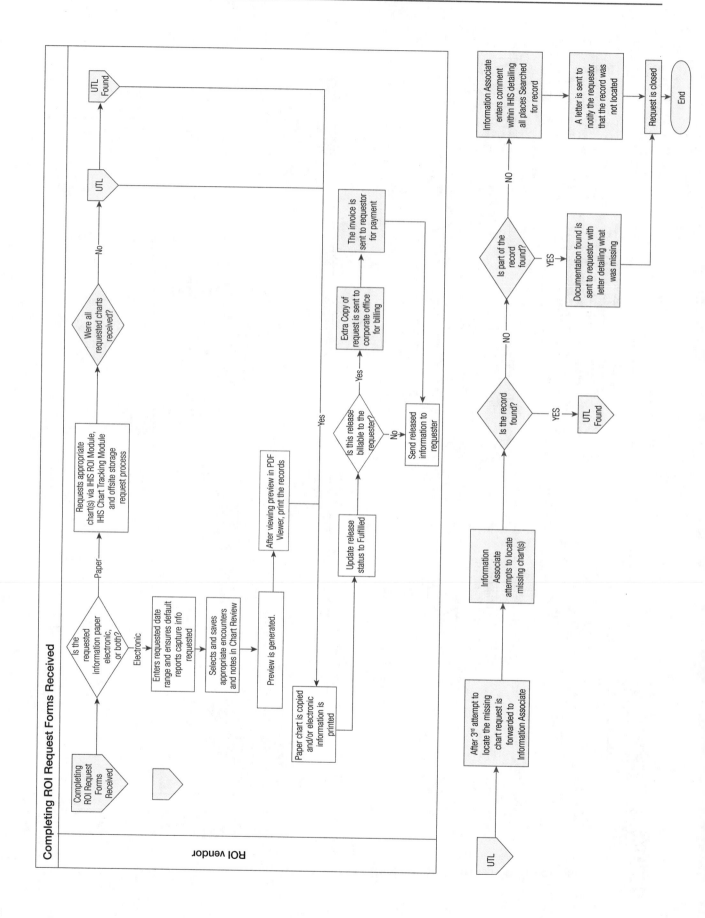

the provider's medical identity theft committee for example. Reasons for refusing to disclose information or requiring additional information are as follows:

- The identity of the person presenting the authorization is in question or the authorization appears to have been completed without the patient's knowledge or after the patient signed the form.
- There is reason to doubt that the person requesting the information is the person named in the authorization.
- The person who signed the authorization is not of legal age.
- There is a question as to the competency of the person who signed the authorization.
- There is a question as to the legal guardian of a minor or incompetent patient or there is documentation of abuse noted in the record.
- The patient has stated that the authorization should not be honored or has revoked the authorization, or the healthcare organization knows that the authorization has been revoked.
- Expiration date or event has passed.
- There is any question as to the authenticity of the patient's signature after comparison of the patient's signature on the authorization with the signature in the medical record.
- There is a question about the patient's ability to understand the authorization.
- There is false information in the form or the form is incomplete.
- There is a question about whether the patient signed the authorization under duress. (Reynolds and Bowman 2016)

Whenever possible and appropriate, requesters should be assisted in completing proper authorizations so that requests can be honored in a timely manner.

Check Your Understanding 15.5

Instructions: Indicate whether the following statements are true or false (T or F).

1. Documents not considered part of the LHR—for example, correspondence, incident reports, and information about other family members—should be released as part of the LHR.
2. Proof of a requester's relationship to a patient must be verified before health information is released to the requester.
3. Regardless of the type of request made, if the request is from the patient, a formal authorization form is required per the HIPAA Privacy Rule.
4. Health organizations and providers may charge a reasonable fee as set by state law for copying health records in response to a request for patient information.
5. HIPAA requires that for the purpose of accounting of disclosures, only PHI that has been released electronically or in writing must be accounted for.

Scenario 15

A 21-year-old man presents himself to the release of information specialist at Metro Medical Center with a request to access his birth records. The young man stated he was adopted and has recently experienced some health complications that his physician suspects are linked to a possible genetic disorder. If he can confirm whether a genetic disorder exists through his mother, the physician will

Scenario 15 (Continued)

be able to establish a more positive and less expensive and invasive treatment protocol for the man. The adoptive parents were able to provide the name of the hospital where he was born and the name of his mother. The young man is requesting access to his birth record, including the medical history of his birth mother who had originally indicated during the adoption process that she wished to remain anonymous. He has submitted his name to the State's Adoption Registry in hopes his biological mother will contact him through the registry. Consider the following:

1. Does the young man have a right to his birth record or his biological mother's medical history? If so, what issues need to be considered before the adoptee is provided with this information?

2. Since genetic information is requested, are there special circumstances to consider before such information is released?

References

Adoption.com. n.d.. Adoption records. https://adoption.com/wiki/Adoption_Records.

AHIMA. 2009. LTC Health information practice & documentation guidelines. http://www.ahima.org.

AHIMA. 2010. Homeland Security Act, Patriot Act, Freedom of Information Act, and HIM. http://www.ahima.org.

AHIMA. 2011. Fundamentals of the legal health record and designated record set. *Journal of AHIMA* 82(2):44–49.

AHIMA. 2012. Practice brief: Management practices for release of information. *Journal of AHIMA* 83(2).

AHIMA. 2013a (January 25). Analysis of modifications to the HIPAA Privacy, Security, Enforcement, and Breach Notification Rules under the HITECH and Genetic Information Nondiscrimination Act: Other modifications to the HIPAA Rules. Chicago: AHIMA.

AHIMA. 2013b. Release of Information Toolkit. A Practical Guide for the Access, Use and Disclosure of Protected Health Information. Chicago: AHIMA. http://www.ahima.org.

AHIMA. 2013c. (April). The privacy and security of occupational health records. *Journal of AHIMA* 84(4):52-56.

AHIMA e-HIM Work Group on Security of Personal Health Information. 2008. Ensuring security of high-risk information in EHRs. *Journal of AHIMA* 79(9):67–71.

AHIMA Homeland Security Work Group. 2010. Practice brief: Homeland security and HIM. *Journal of AHIMA* 75(6):56A–56D.

Amatayakul, M. 2003. Practical advice for effective policies and procedures. *Journal of AHIMA* 74(4):16A–16D.

Asmonga, D. 2008. Getting to know GINA: An overview of the Genetic Information Nondiscrimination Act. *Journal of AHIMA* 79(7):18, 20, 22.

Avery, R., P. Calem, G. Canner, and R. Bostic. 2003. An overview of consumer data and credit reporting. *Federal Reserve Bulletin*, February:48–73. http://www.federalreserve.gov.

Barrett, C., A. Beidler, N. Davis, and B. Glondys. 2016. Using aliases to protect patient privacy in healthcare. *Journal of AHIMA*. 87(11):36–39.

Carpenter, J. 1999. Practice brief: Managing health information relating to infection with human immunodeficiency virus. Web extra. Chicago: AHIMA.

Centers for Disease Control and Prevention. 2006 (September). Revised recommendations for HIV testing of adults, adolescents, and pregnant women in health care settings. *Morbidity and Mortality Weekly Report* 55(RR14):1–17.

Centers for Disease Control and Prevention. 2016. Division of Health Informatics and Surveillance. National Syndromic Surveillance Program Overview. https://www.cdc.gov/nssp.

Centers for Medicare and Medicaid Services. 2016a. Electronic submission of medical documentation overview. https://www.cms.gov.

Centers for Medicare and Medicaid Services. 2016b. Which HIHS offer esMD gateway services to providers? What is a health information handler? https://www.cms.gov.

Coletta, M. n.d. CDC NSSP ESSENCE. In-Person Training Workshop. http://www.cdc.gov/nssp/documents/essence-training-presentation-phi-conference.pdf.

Davis, N., et al. 2006. Practice brief: Facsimile transmission of health information. Web extra. Chicago: AHIMA.

Department of Health and Human Services. n.d.a. Child welfare information gateway. State statutes search. https://www.childwelfare.gov/.

Department of Health and Human Services. n.d.b. Individuals' right under HIPAA to access their health information 45 CFR 164.524. http://www.health.gov.

Department of Health and Human Services. n.d.c. Office of National Coordinator. Advancing privacy and security in health information exchange. http://www.healthit.gov.

Department of Health and Human Services. 2006. HIPAA frequently asked questions for professionals. Answer ID; 209. https://www.hhs.gov/hipaa/for-professionals/faq.

Department of Health and Human Services. 2009. Office for Human Research Protections. Guidance on the Genetic Information Nondiscrimination Act: Implications for investigators and institutional review boards. http://www.hhs.gov/ohrp/policy/gina.html.

Department of Health and Human Services. 2011. HIPAA Privacy Rule accounting of disclosures under the Health Information Technology for Economic and Clinical Health Act. 45 CFR Part 164. *Federal Register* 76 (104): 31426–31449.

Department of Health and Human Services. 2013. Modifications to the HIPAA Privacy, Security, Enforcement, and Breach Notification Rules under the Health Information Technology for Economic and Clinical Health Act and the Genetic Information Nondiscrimination Act: Other Modifications to the HIPAA Rules; Final Rule. 45 CFR Parts 160 and 164. *Federal Register* 78(17):5566-5702.

Department of Health and Human Services Office of National Coordinator. 2015. Connecting Health and Care for the Nation. A Shared Nationwide Interoperability Roadmap. Final Version 1.0. http://www.healthit.gov.

Department of Health and Human Services. 2016a. Child welfare information gateway. Access to adoption records: Summary of state laws. http://www.childwelfare.gov.

Department of Health and Human Services. 2016b. Confidentiality of substance use disorder patient records: proposed rule. *Federal Register*. 81(26):6988–7024.

Department of Health and Human Services. 2016c. HIPAA Privacy Rule and the National Instant Criminal Background Check System (NICS). https://www.hhs.gov/hipaa/for-professionals/special-topics/NICS/index.html.

Dimick, C. 2013. Accessing deceased patient records—FAQs (2013 update). AHIMA blog post. April 1. http://journal.ahima.org/2013/04/01/.

Drociuk, D., J. Gibson, and J. Hodge. 2004. Health information privacy and syndromic surveillance systems. *Morbidity and Mortality Weekly Report* 53(Suppl.):221–225.

Dunn, R. 2007. Calculating the costs of e-discovery. *Journal of AHIMA* 78(10): 64–65, 72.

Dunn, R. 2010. Release of information: Costs remain high in a hybrid, highly regulated environment. *Journal of AHIMA* 81(11):34–37.

Dunn, R. and B. Burton. 2015. The Practical Guide to Release of Information: ROI in a HITECH World, 2nd ed. Marblehead, MA: HCPro.

Equal Employment Opportunity Commission. n.d. Genetic information discrimination. http://www.eeoc.gov.

Federal Trade Commission. 2014. Direct-to-consumer genetic tests. https://www.consumer.ftc.gov/articles/0166-direct-consumer-genetic-tests

Feldman, S., T. Horan, and D. Drew. 2013. Understanding the value proposition of health information exchange: the case of uncompensated care cost recovery. *Health Systems* 2(2):134–146.

Fuller, B., and K. Hudson. 2006. Genetic information. Chapter 18 in *Ethical Challenges in the Management of Health Information*, 2nd ed. Edited by Harman, L. Sudbury, MA: Jones and Bartlett.

Healthcare Information and Management Systems Society. 2007. Sending records efficiently and securely to the Social Security Administration's disability claims system. http://www.himss.org/.

HealthInfoLaw.org. 2015a. Fast facts: Who owns medical records?

HealthInfoLaw.org. 2015b. States with laws relating to medical records collection, retention, and access.

Hofman, J. 2013. Privacy after death. *Journal of AHIMA* 84(4):32–35.

Hughes, G. 2000. The ins and outs of adoption information provision. *In Confidence* 8(1):6–7.

Johns, M. 2015. *Enterprise Health Information Management and Data Governance.* Chicago: AHIMA.

Jones, M. 2017. Adoption information. In *Ethical Challenges in the Management of Health Information*, 3nd ed. Edited by Harman, L. and F. Cornelius. Sudbury, MA: Jones and Bartlett.

Lamb, T. 2016. Medical records copying charges. http://www.lamblawoffice.com.

Law Center to Prevent Gun Violence. 2016. Mental health reporting. http://smartgunlaws.org/gun-laws/policy-areas/background-checks/mental-health-reporting/.

McLendon, K. 2014. Law changes patient access to clinical lab reports. *Journal of AHIMA.* 85(10):60–62.

Medical Information Bureau. 2011. Consumer guide. http://www.mib.com.

National Conference of State Legislatures. 2008. Genetic privacy laws. http://www.ncsl.org.

National Human Genome Research Institute. 2009. Title I of the Genetic Information Nondiscrimination Act of 2008 (GINA). http://www.genome.gov.

National Library of Medicine. 2017a. What is direct-to-consumer genetic testing? https://ghr.nlm.nih.gov/primer/testing/directtoconsumer.

National Library of Medicine. 2017b. Help me understand genetics: Genetic testing. https://ghr.nlm.nih.gov/.

Ohio Department of Health. 2015. Office of Vital Statistics Adoption information. http://www.odh.ohio.gov.

Ohio Hospital Association. 2005. Media guide for Ohio hospitals. http://www.ohanet.org.

Presidential Commission for the Study of Bioethical Issues (PCSBI). 2012. Privacy and Progress in Whole Genome Sequencing. https://bioethicsarchive.georgetown.edu/pcsbi/node/764.html

Privacy Rights Clearinghouse. 2011. Fact sheet 6a: Facts on FACTA, the Fair and Accurate Credit Transaction Act. http://www.privacyrights.org.

Randolph, S., and L. Rinehart-Thompson. 2006. Drug, alcohol, sexual and behavioral information. Chapter 20 in *Ethical Challenges in the Management of Health Information*, 2nd ed. Edited by Harman, L. Sudbury, MA: Jones and Bartlett.

Reporters Committee for Freedom of the Press. 2011. *Open Government Guide.* Access to public records and meetings in OHIO. 6th ed. Washington, DC: RCFP. http://www.rcfp.org.

Research Triangle Institute (RTI). 2009. Privacy and security solutions for interoperable health exchange: Report on state medical record access laws. Chicago: RTI International.

Reynolds, R. and E. Bowman (eds). 2016. *Tennessee Health Information Management Association Handbook.* THIMA Legislative Committee. Nashville, TN: THIMA. http://www.thima.org/resources/legal/.

Rinehart-Thompson, L. and S. Randolph. 2017. Substance Abuse, Behavioral Health and Sexual Information. In *Ethical Challenges in the Management of Health Information*, 3nd ed. Edited by Harman, L and F. Cornelius. Sudbury, MA: Jones and Bartlett.

Roach, W., R. Hoban, B. Broccolo, A. Roth, and T. Blanchard. 2006. *Medical Records and the Law*, 4th ed. Sudbury, MA: Jones and Bartlett.

Schlossberger, E., and L. Hecker. 1996. HIV and family therapists' duty to warn: A legal and ethical analysis. *Journal of Marital and Family Therapy* 22(1):27–40.

Sharp, M. and C. Madlock-Brown. 2016. Data Management. In *Health Information Management: Concepts, Principles, and Practice*, 5th ed. Edited by Ouchs, P. and A. Watters. Chicago: AHIMA.

Social Security Administration (SSA). n.d. Electronic record express. https://www.ssa.gov/ere/.

Substance Abuse and Mental Health Services Administration. 2004. The confidentiality of alcohol and drug abuse patient records regulation and the HIPAA Privacy Rule: Implications for alcohol and substance abuse programs. http://www.samhsa.gov.

Substance Abuse and Mental Health Services Administration. 2010. Frequently asked questions: Applying the substance abuse confidentiality regulations to health information exchange (HIE). http://www.samhsa.gov.

Substance Abuse and Mental Health Services Administration. 2011. Applying the Substance Abuse Confidentiality Regulations 42 CFR Part 2. http://www.samhsa.gov.

Substance Abuse and Mental Health Services Administration. 2015. Drug-free Workplace Toolkit. http://www.samhsa.gov.

The White House. 2015 (January 15). Office of the Press Secretary. Fact Sheet: President Obama's Precision Medicine Initiative. https://www.whitehouse.gov.

Thomson Reuters. 2016. FindLaw State medical records laws. FindLaw. http://statelaws.findlaw.com/health-care-laws/medical-records.html.

Uniform Law Commission. 2016. Health-Care Decisions Act summary. Chicago: National Conference of Commissioners on Uniform State Laws. http://uniformlaws.org.

Wiedemann, L. 2011. Correcting lab results in an EHR. *Journal of AHIMA* 81(5):38–39.

Cases, Statutes, and Regulations Cited

Tarasoff v. the Regents of the University of California, 17 CA 3d 425, 551 P.2d 334, 131 CA Rptr. 14 (1976).

16 CFR 604(g)(2): Fair Credit Reporting Act. 2006.

16 CFR 605(a)(6): Fair Credit Reporting Act. 2006.

28 CFR Part 35, 36: Americans with Disabilities Act (ADA). 1990.

29 CFR 1910.20: Access to employee exposure and medical records. 2003.

29 CFR Part 1635: Genetic Information Nondiscrimination Act. 2008.

42 CFR 2.11 Part 2: Definitions. 1987.

42 CFR 2.14(c)(2): Minor patients. 1987.

42 CFR 493.3(a)(2): Clinical Laboratory Improvements Act. 1988.

45 CFR 160.103: Definitions. 2006.

45 CFR 164.310(a)(1): Facility access controls. 2006.

45 CFR 164.312(d): Device and medic controls. 2006.

45 CFR 164.501: Definitions. 2006.

45 CFR 164.502(b): Minimum necessary. 2006.

45 CFR 164.506: Uses and disclosures to carry out treatment, payment, or health care operations. 2006.

45 CFR 164.508: Uses and disclosures for which authorization is required. 2006.

45 CFR 164.510(a): Use and disclosure for facility directories. 2006.

45 CFR 164.512: Uses and disclosures for which an authorization or opportunity to agree or object is not required. 2006.

45 CFR 164.512(g)(1): Uses and disclosures about decedents. 2006.

45 CFR 164.514(h)(1): Verification requirements. 2006.

45 CFR 164.520(b)(1)(v)(C): Notice of privacy practices for protected health information. 2002.

45 CFR 164.522(a): Rights to request privacy protection for protected health information. 2006.

45 CFR 164.524: Access of individuals to protected health information. 2006.

45 CFR 164.524(c)(4): Fees. 2006.

45 CFR 164.526: Amendment of protected health information. 2006.

45 CFR 164.528(c)(2): Provisions of the accounting. 2006.

5 USC 552: Freedom of Information Act. Amended 1996.

5 USC 552(b)(6): Exemption: Personal and medical files. 2004.

15 USC 1681: Fair Credit Reporting Act. 2004.

OH Rev. Code 149.011: Ohio public records law. 2004.

OH Rev. Code 2317.422: Authentication of nursing, rest, community alternative home and adult care facilities records. 2010.

OH Rev. Code 3701.24.3, 3701.243: Disclosure of HIV test results or diagnosis. 2000.

OH Rev. Code 3701.741: Fees for providing copies of medical records. 2011.

TN Code Ann. 33-8-202: Outpatient mental health treatment. 2002.

TN Code Ann. 36-6-103: Rights of noncustodial parents. 1987, 1989.

TN Code Ann. 68-10-115: Immunity from liability for informing person of potential HIV infection. 1993.

Fair and Accurate Credit Transaction Act of 2003. Public Law 108-159.

Genetic Information Nondiscrimination Act of 2008. Public Law 110-233.

Homeland Security Act of 2002. Public Law 107-296.

Patriot Act of 2001. Public Law 107-06.

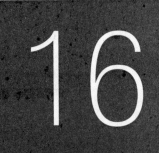

Required Reporting and Mandatory Disclosure Laws

Melanie S. Brodnik, PhD, RHIA, FAHIMA

Learning Objectives

- Describe the four elements of the HIPAA Privacy Rule that relate to required reporting laws
- Identify the HIPAA exceptions that allow the release of health information without patient authorization
- Discuss the common state reporting requirements related to abuse and neglect of children, the elderly, and the disabled
- Describe state responsibility for reporting vital statistics including births, deaths, fetal deaths and induced termination of pregnancy, and reportable deaths
- Contrast requirements for the reporting of communicable diseases to public health entities
- Discuss federal and volunteer reporting requirements that do not require patient authorization
- Compare various clinical, disease, and outcome-based registries and how patient privacy is protected
- Discuss how an entity may be protected when disclosing patient information not required by law to public health authorities

Key Terms

- Birth certificate
- Birth defects registry
- Cancer registry
- Communicable disease
- Coroner
- Death certificate
- Diabetes registry
- Fetal death
- Healthcare Integrity and Protection Data Bank (HIPDB)

- Health Care Quality Improvement Act
- Histocompatibility
- Immunization registry
- Implant registry
- Medical device
- Medical device reporting
- Medical examiner
- MedWatch
- National Practitioner Data Bank (NPDB)

- Notifiable disease
- Organ Procurement and Transplantation Network (OPTN)
- Organ Procurement Organization
- Prescription drug monitoring program
- Qualified clinical data registry
- Registry

- Safety Information and Adverse Event Reporting Program
- Transplant registry
- Trauma registry
- Traumatic injury
- Unusual event
- Vital record
- Workers' compensation

To protect the health and safety of a community, state and federal reporting laws require certain healthcare organizations and providers to report specific information, including protected health information (PHI), to government and quasigovernment agencies. The Health Insurance Portability and Accountability Act (HIPAA) identifies 12 exceptions to the Privacy Rule that permit the use or disclosure of PHI without patient authorization, as discussed in chapter 10 and 11. In general, the mandatory disclosure laws address issues related to disease prevention and control, and community health and safety. These laws require the disclosure of PHI without patient authorization and offer protection from civil liability to those who disclose the information as a matter of law. The reporting laws usually stipulate that the information collected is not considered public information and that patient privacy and confidential information are also protected. The laws vary from state to state, most of which fall under the auspices of state public health departments, while federal reporting laws fall under various departments at the federal level. This chapter addresses common reporting requirements mandated by state laws, such as abuse and neglect of children, the elderly, and the disabled; communicable diseases; suspicious or unattended deaths; vital statistics; and registries. It also addresses some of the common federal mandatory and volunteer reporting systems related to Medicare and Medicaid programs, quality measures and oversight, medical devices, registries, and national health statistics.

HIPAA and Required Reporting

Four elements of the HIPAA Privacy Rule as discussed in chapter 10 and 11 should be considered when addressing required reporting and mandatory disclosure laws related to PHI:

Disclosure without patient authorization or agreement - Under the HIPAA Privacy Rule no PHI is to be used or disclosed without patient authorization or agreement unless the Privacy Rule provides an exception to the authorization requirement. There are 12 exceptions to the rule that relate to public interest and benefit activities that serve society and national priority purposes (see figure 16.1). Most states have statutory requirements that parallel the Privacy Rule exceptions, and other federal reporting requirements that call for PHI without patient authorization.

Preemption - When federal and state laws conflict, the federal law must be followed unless the state law is more stringent on the matter, in which case it may preempt federal law. HIPAA allows for state law to prevail if the laws, include state procedures for the reporting of disease or injury, child abuse, birth, or death, or for the conduct of public health surveillance, investigation, or intervention (45 CFR 160.203). State reporting requirements that collect and store PHI can, therefore, be followed as exceptions to the doctrine of preemption.

Notice of Privacy Practices - Although an individual has a right to adequate notice of the uses and disclosures of his or her PHI (45 CFR 164.520) information reported under state and federal laws or statutes without patient authorization should be included in the Notice of Privacy Practices. An example of wording from a Notice of Privacy Practices is provided in appendix 10.A.

Accounting of disclosures - The Privacy Rule requires that required reporting by law or regulation must be included in an accounting of disclosures. Disclosures should be recorded in a central tracking

Figure 16.1   Public interest and benefit exceptions permitting use or disclosure of PHI without patient authorization

1. Required by law (45 CFR 164.512(a))
2. Public health activities (45 CFR 164.512(b))
3. Victims of abuse, neglect, domestic violence (45 CFR 164.512(c))
4. Health oversight activities (45 CFR 164.512(d))
5. Judicial and administrative proceedings (45 CFR 164.512(e))
6. Law enforcement purposes (45 CFR 164.512(f))
7. Decedents (45 CFR 164.512(g))
8. Cadaveric organ, eye, or tissue donation (45 CFR 164.512(h))
9. Research (45 CFR 164.512(i))
10. Prevent or lessen serious threat to health or safety (45 CFR 164.512(j))
11. Specialized government functions (45 CFR 164.512(k))
12. Workers' compensation (45 CFR 164.512(l))

Item to be Reported	Responsible Hospital Department
Births, fetal deaths	Labor and Delivery
Deaths	Morgue/Bereavement Department
Child or elder abuse	Social Services
Notifiable diseases	Infectious Disease
Statewide cancer registry	Cancer Registry
Trauma	Trauma Registry
Medical examiners cases	Risk Management

Table 16.1 Reporting of disclosures by responsible department

system that enables areas responsible for disclosing information under mandatory reporting laws to record disclosures. A healthcare organization or provider should make a list of these departments and the types of required disclosures made by each department so that when a patient requests an accounting of disclosures, the list can be referenced for items to be included in the accounting. See table 16.1 for an example of such a list.

Common State Reporting Requirements

All states have laws, codes, statutes, or regulations that require the reporting of certain diseases or events. Reported data provide information on the incidence and prevalence of diseases, possible high-risk populations, survival statistics, and trends over time. Data may be collected using a variety of methods including interviews, physical examination of individuals, and review of health records.

Abuse and Neglect of Children

Reporting abuse and neglect of children is routinely required by state laws and is reportable to local or county law enforcement or county children's services boards in the county where the incident occurred. According to the federal Child Abuse Prevention and Treatment Act of 1996 (CAPTA) (42 USC 5101 et seq.), as amended by the CAPTA Reauthorization Act of 2010 (42 USC 5101§3), child abuse and neglect are

> … at minimum, any recent act or failure to act on the part of a parent or caretaker which results in death, serious physical or emotional harm, sexual abuse or exploitation; or an act or failure to act which presents an imminent risk of serious harm.

CAPTA further defines sexual abuse as

> The employment, use, persuasion, inducement, enticement, or coercion of any child to engage in, or assist any other person to engage in, any sexually explicit conduct or simulation of such conduct for the purpose of producing a visual depiction of such conduct; or

> The rape, and in cases of caretaker or interfamilial relationships, statutory rape, molestation, prostitution, or other form of sexual exploitation of children, or incest with children (42 USCA 5106(g)(4)).

Each state has its own child abuse and neglect civil or criminal statutes based on the federal law. State child protective services are mainly responsible for the safety and overall well-being of children. In general, five types of abuse are recognized by state law: neglect, physical abuse, sexual abuse, parental substance abuse, and emotional abuse. The state statutes tend to define a child for reporting purposes as any person under the age of 18 years or any physically or mentally handicapped person up to the age of 21 years. Many state statutes define the persons who can be reported as perpetrators of abuse or neglect. These individuals usually have some relationship or responsibility for the child such as parents, guardians, foster parents, relatives, or other caregivers (Child Welfare Information Gateway 2014).

State laws identify who must report child abuse and neglect, the time frame for reporting, and the kind of information reported. The most commonly cited individuals required to report include healthcare practitioners, police officers, educators, human service workers, and others who are aware of the abuse or neglect of a child. These individuals are afforded protection from civil or criminal liability through state statutes for reporting abuse and neglect made in good faith (Pozgar 2016). In addition, most states have incorporated waivers into their rules that preempt state physician-patient privilege and Federal Alcohol and Drug Abuse Act restrictions on disclosure of patient information if the person whose information is being requested is under prosecution for abuse (Roach et al. 2006).

Most states require that known or suspected abuse and neglect must be verbally reported immediately with written reports to follow in a prescribed time frame. The information typically required in these reports includes:

- Name of child and parents, or other custodial person
- Address of child and parents, or other custodial person
- Age of child
- Nature and extent of current or previous known or suspected injuries, abuse, or neglect
- Any other information that would be useful in establishing cause of injuries, abuse, or neglect (Pozgar 2016)

The health records of the abused or neglected child may be subject to disclosure without authorization. Such state laws do not conflict with the HIPAA Privacy Rule because such disclosures are permissible without authorization, either under the public interest and benefit exceptions of "required by law," "public health activities," or "disclosures about victims of abuse, neglect, or domestic violence," or as provided by the preemption exception. If a state law permits, but does not require, disclosure of this information, steps must be taken to ensure that the individual agrees to the disclosure or the healthcare organization believes disclosure is necessary to prevent serious harm to the individual or others. If the individual is not capable of agreeing, it must be confirmed by a public authority authorized to receive the information that the information will not be used against the individual and that delay in disclosing the information will likely have an adverse effect (45 CFR 164.512(c)).

Abuse and Neglect of the Elderly and Disabled

The Older Americans Act of 1965 (OAA) funded critical services for older or elderly individuals, 60 years of age and older (42 USC 3002). In April 2016, Congress passed legislation to reauthorize the act, now known as the Older Americans Act Reauthorization Act of 2016 (Pub. L. 114-144). The reauthorized act promotes practices for responding to elder abuse, neglect, and exploitation in long-term care facilities and for states to submit information on elder abuse. The term "disability" is defined in the law as meaning:

. . . a disability attributable to mental or physical impairment, or a combination of mental and physical impairments, that results in substantial functional limitations in one or more of the following areas of major life activity:

1. Self-care
2. Receptive and expressive language
3. Learning
4. Mobility
5. Self-direction
6. Capacity for independent living
7. Economic self-sufficiency
8. Cognitive functioning
9. Emotional adjustment (42 USC 3002)

Abuse of the elderly and disabled includes physical, emotional or psychological, and sexual abuse; financial or material exploitation; neglect; self-neglect and abandonment (Stiegel 2015). State laws vary on the definitions of elderly and disabled as well as the definitions of abuse, neglect, and exploitation. Some states have laws that address abuse, neglect, and exploitation separately as well as criminal laws that specifically define and outline penalties for elder abuse. There may be separate laws covering abuse in the home setting (domestic abuse) versus abuse in an institutional setting such as a nursing home. These laws are commonly grouped under the term adult protective services (APS) which function to provide safety and well-being for the elderly and adults with special needs (Stiegel 2015).

At the federal level, Section 1150B of the Social Security Act as part of the Patient Protection and Affordable Care Act of 2010 (ACA) requires specific individuals in Medicare and Medicaid funded long-term care facilities to report any reasonable suspicion of a crime committed against a resident of a facility. Reporting of a suspicious crime must be made to the law enforcement agency of jurisdiction and the state survey agency (CMS 2012). The facilities that must comply with this requirement include

- Nursing facilities
- Skilled nursing facilities
- Hospices that provide services in long-term care facilities
- Intermediate care facilities for the mentally retarded (CMS 2012).

State laws also vary regarding the required reporting of abuse of the elderly and disabled. The laws often mandate who must report suspected abuse and whether failure to report the abuse is a crime. Alabama law, for example, requires physicians, practitioners of the healing arts, and caregivers to report physical abuse, neglect, exploitation, sexual abuse, or emotional abuse (AL Code 38-9-8). Florida law, on the other hand, requires any person to report abuse, neglect, or exploitation of vulnerable persons (FL Stat. Ann. 415.101 et seq.).

Such state laws do not conflict with HIPAA because under either the public interest and benefit exceptions of "required by law" or "regarding victims of abuse, neglect, domestic violence," or as provided by the preemption exception, such disclosures are permissible without authorization. If a state law permits, but does not require, disclosure of this information, steps must be taken to ensure that the individual agrees to the disclosure or the healthcare organization or provider believes disclosure is necessary to prevent serious harm to the individual or others. If the individual is not capable of agreeing, it must be confirmed by a public authority authorized to receive the information that the information will not be used against the individual and that delay in disclosing the information will likely have an adverse effect (45 CFR 164.512(c))

Check Your Understanding 16.1

Instructions: Indicate whether the following statements are true or false (T or F).

1. Healthcare providers must report their suspicion of child abuse.

2. Individuals who report neglect or abuse of children are protected from civil liability as long as they are reporting concern in good faith.

3. Information reported without patient authorization under federal laws should be included in the Notice of Privacy Practices.

4. State required reporting laws are an exception to the doctrine of preemption.

5. Abuse of the elderly is limited to physical neglect of an elder person.

Vital Records

Vital records are those concerned with births, deaths, marriages, divorces, abortions, and fetal deaths. In the United States, the National Center for Health Statistics (NCHS) of the Department of Health and Human Services (HHS) is responsible for working with state vital statistics laws and regulations for the reporting of vital statistics. At the federal level, the Model State Vital Statistics Act and Regulations provide uniform guidance to states related to the definitions, registration practices, disclosure procedures, and other processes that comprise states' vital statistics functions (NCHS 1992). The information is used to generate statistics such as birth and death rates as well as to identify trends in areas such as causes of death and types of birth defects. The NCHS creates standard certificates of live birth and death that contain the minimum data required for the certificates to serve as models for the states. Each state can then modify the standard forms to meet their specific data collection needs.

Vital record information from the states is shared with the NCHS. Using this information, the states and the federal government provide statistics on the vital events within their jurisdiction. The information required commonly includes demographic information as well as medical information. Cases are sometimes reported without PHI; however, most of the time PHI is included in the data since there must be a way to connect the certificate with the actual case, if required. State laws requiring the reporting of vital statistics do not conflict with the HIPAA Privacy Rule because, under the public interest and benefit exception of "public health activities" or as provided by the preemption exception, such disclosures are permissible without authorization.

Birth Certificates

A **birth certificate** must be filed for every live birth regardless of where it occurred. Information needed to complete the birth certificate may be obtained from the mother or father, mother and child attending physician, and hospital or physician records. If the birth occurred within a hospital, it is generally the hospital's responsibility to file the birth certificate with the health department's office of vital statistics. The birth certificate form has two parts. The first part includes identifying information about the parents and the child. In the second part, there is information about the mother's pregnancy and any birth defects in the newborn. The second part serves a statistical purpose only and is not a part of the official birth certificate. Regarding paternity, most state laws delineate how a father may be acknowledged on the birth certificate if the father is not married to the mother at the time of the birth. State law also defines what surname for the child is entered on the certificate.

Death Certificates

When someone dies, state law requires that a **death certificate** be completed. The funeral director or other person responsible for internment or cremation of remains generally has responsibility for filing the death certificate within a prescribed time frame as defined by state law. The death certificate includes identifying information about the deceased as well as information about the cause of death. The physician must provide the cause of death and sign the death certificate within a certain amount of time as defined by state law. The original death certificate must be filed with the local health department's department of vital statistics in the county where the death occurred.

Communicable Diseases

A **communicable disease** is one that can be transmitted from an infected person, animal, or inanimate reservoir to a susceptible person or host by either direct or indirect contact. States require the reporting of "notifiable" communicable diseases through state laws for the purpose of tracking outbreaks and preventing the spread of the disease. State health departments or agencies serve as the state entities responsible for administering communicable disease reporting requirements. State laws define what diseases are reportable, by whom, and how they should be reported. Lists of diseases vary from state to state and may include certain quarantine diseases such as cholera, plague, Ebola, and yellow fever as required by the World Health Organization.

Notifiable diseases may be classified according to their potential for endemic or epidemic spread and danger to public health. How a disease is reported will depend on its classification. The more dangerous or problematic the disease, the more quickly it must be reported. Twenty-four hours is the usual reporting time for a confirmed case or for a suspected case once it is known. However, in certain cases dealing with

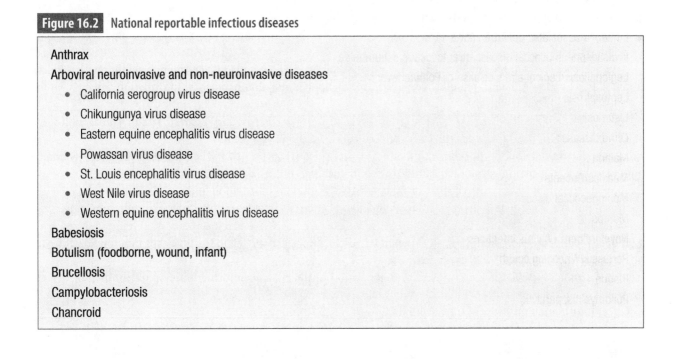

Figure 16.2 National reportable infectious diseases

Anthrax

Arboviral neuroinvasive and non-neuroinvasive diseases
- California serogroup virus disease
- Chikungunya virus disease
- Eastern equine encephalitis virus disease
- Powassan virus disease
- St. Louis encephalitis virus disease
- West Nile virus disease
- Western equine encephalitis virus disease

Babesiosis

Botulism (foodborne, wound, infant)

Brucellosis

Campylobacteriosis

Chancroid

Figure 16.2 National reportable infectious diseases (Continued)

Chlamydia trachomatis infection

Cholera

Coccidiodomyscosis/Valley fever

Congenital syphilis

Cryptosporidiosis

Cyclosporiasis

Dengue virus infections

Diphtheria

Ebola viruses (various types)

Ehrlichiosis/Anaplasmosis

- *Anaplasma phagocytophilum infection*
- *Ehrlichia chaffeenis infection*
- *Ehrlichia ewingii infection*
- Undetermined

Giardiasis

Gonorrhea

Haemophilus influenzae, invasive disease

Hansen disease (leprosy)

Hantavirus infection, non-hantavirus pulmonary syndrome

Hantavirus pulmonary syndrome

Hemolytic uremic syndrome, post-diarrheal

Hepatitis (A, B, C acute and chronic)

HIV infection*

- HIV infection, adult/adolescent (age ≥ 13 years)
- HIV infection, child (age ≥ 18 months and < 13 years)
- HIV infection, pediatric (age < 18 months)

Influenza-associated pediatric mortality

Invasive pneumococcal disease/streptococcus pneumoniae

Legionellosis/Legionnaire's disease or Pontiac fever

Leptospirosis

Listeriosis

Lyme disease

Malaria

Measles/Rubeola

Meningococcal disease

Mumps

Novel influenza A virus infections

Pertussis/Whooping cough

Plague

Poliomyelitis, paralytic

Figure 16.2 National reportable infectious diseases (Continued)

Poliovirus infection, nonparalytic

Psittacosis

Q Fever (acute, chronic, rabies)

Rabies, animal

Rabies, human

Rubella/German measles

Rubella, congenital syndrome

Salmonellosis

Severe Acute Respiratory Syndrome–associated Coronavirus (SARS-CoV) disease

Shiga toxin-producing *Escherichia coli* (STEC)

Shigellosis

Smallpox

Spotted Fever Rickettsiosis

Streptococcal toxic-shock syndrome

Streptococcus pneumoniae, invasive disease

Syphilis (primary, secondary, latent, neuro, stillborn, congenital)

Tetanus/*C. tetani*

Toxic-shock syndrome (other than Streptococcal)

Trichinellosis (Trichinosis)

Tuberculosis

Tularemia

Typhoid fever

Vancomycin-intermediate *Staphylococcus aureus* (VISA)

Vancomycin-resistant *Staphylococcus aureus* (VRSA)

Varicella/chickenpox

Varicella (deaths only)

Vibriosis

Viral Hemorrhagic Fevers, due to:

- Yellow fever
- Zika virus disease, congenital infection

Source: CDC 2016a.

*AIDS has been reclassified as HIV stage III.

newborns, such as inflammation of the eyes, the reporting time may be six hours. Figure 16.2 lists the nationally notifiable infectious diseases as specified by the Centers for Disease Control and Prevention (CDC 2016a).

Laws require that diseases be reported in writing, verbally, or through other rapid means of communication. Laws also identify what specific information must be reported, such as the patient's name, age, gender, and address; details of the illness; and other pertinent information. In some cases, such as sexually transmitted diseases like syphilis, HIV, and AIDS or diseases such as hepatitis or tuberculosis, information is required pertaining to contacts the infected person under investigation has had with other individuals to limit further spread of the disease. Responsibility for notifying individuals who have had contact with the infected person is defined by state law.

State laws define who must report communicable diseases. In most cases, the reporting individual is the attending physician or a person (or delegated representative) in charge of a hospital, emergency room, clinic, diagnostic laboratory, or other entity providing care or treatment and having knowledge of the case. State laws may also grant the appropriate state health director or representative the right to access and copy the patient's health record without the patient's authorization. Most state laws include regulations that, despite required reporting, keep information confidential and indicate that it will not be released or made public upon subpoena, court order, discovery, search warrant, or otherwise except in special situations as further defined by state law (TN Code Ann. 68-10-113). In addition, some state laws specify that the public health authorities must be provided access to records of patients with notifiable diseases during the investigation of the disease. Under such laws, patient authorization is not required for such access (OH Admin. Code 3701-3-08).

State laws requiring the reporting of communicable diseases do not conflict with HIPAA because, under the public interest and benefit exception of "public health activities" or as provided by the preemption exception, such disclosures are permissible without authorization. The HIPAA Privacy Rule, under the public health activities exception, further permits a covered entity (CE) to disclose PHI to persons who may have been exposed to a communicable disease or may be at risk of contracting or spreading a disease or condition, provided that the CE is authorized by law to make such notification as part of a public health intervention (45 CFR 164.512 (b)).

Induced Termination of Pregnancy (Abortion)

Most state laws require the healthcare organization where an induced termination of pregnancy was performed to file a report on the termination of pregnancy. If the induced termination of pregnancy did not occur in a healthcare facility such as a clinic or hospital, then the attending physician who administered care to the patient after the induced termination is responsible for filing a report. Usually, information identifying the individual patient or physician is not required in the reporting of induced abortions. Information that is typically reported pertains to the patient's date of birth, race, marital status, and county and state of residence; the type of procedure performed; and resulting complications, if any. In some states, physicians and facilities are required to report injuries or death to a mother due to an induced abortion.

Birth Defects

Birth defect information may be obtained from birth certificates filed with the state. Such information is used to determine trends in birth defects and to look for ways to prevent them. State laws requiring the reporting of birth defects do not conflict with HIPAA because, under the public interest and benefit exception of "public health activities" or as provided by the preemption exception, such disclosures are permissible without authorization.

Reportable Deaths

State laws have developed requirements for certain deaths—such as accidental, homicidal, suicidal, sudden, and those suspicious in nature—to be reported, usually to the medical examiner or coroner.

In addition, deaths resulting from abortion or induced termination of pregnancy are reportable. A **medical examiner** is typically a physician with pathology training given the responsibility by a government, such as a county or state, for investigating suspicious deaths. A **coroner** is typically an appointed or elected official, who may or may not be a physician, with the responsibility for investigating suspicious deaths.

Physicians, squad members, or law enforcement members acting in their duties are required to notify the medical examiner or coroner of any death that may fit one of the categories mentioned above. Healthcare entities such as hospitals must have clearly defined policies and procedures for reporting such deaths, especially since individuals may be brought to the emergency room dead on arrival (DOA) or may expire shortly thereafter from what might be any of the types of death noted above.

Suspicious deaths are of particular interest to state law enforcement. For example, Mississippi defines a suspicious death as a "'**death affecting the public interest**' [which] means any death of a human being where the circumstances are sudden, unexpected, violent, suspicious or unattended" (MS Code 41-61-53). These deaths affect the public interest because they may be indicative of a crime or they may identify a cause of death that needs to be remedied, such as a death from carbon monoxide poisoning due to a faulty furnace. The information commonly reportable to the coroner or medical examiner includes

- Name and address of the deceased
- Age of the deceased, if known
- Marital status of the deceased
- Ethnicity of the deceased
- Time of accident or onset of cause of death
- Place, mode, and manner of injury
- Place of death
- Time of death
- Location of body
- Other pertinent data
- Name of person reporting the case, including date and time
- Name of physician who pronounced person dead

Medical examiners and coroners have the right to receive medical information needed to investigate the case without authorization and may have subpoena powers to collect such information. State laws requiring the reporting of suspicious deaths do not conflict with HIPAA because such disclosures are permissible without authorization, either under the public interest and benefit exceptions of "public health activities," "disclosures for law enforcement purposes," or "about decedents," or as provided by the preemption exception.

Wounds: Knife, Gunshot, Burns

Like suspicious deaths, wounds such as knife wounds, gunshot wounds, and burns are commonly indicative of crimes and must be reported to legal authorities. State laws requiring the reporting of knife and gunshot wounds as well as burns do not conflict with HIPAA because such disclosures are permissible without authorization, either under the public interest and benefit exceptions of "public health activities," "disclosures for law enforcement purposes," or (if applicable) "about decedents," or as provided by the preemption exception.

Fetal Deaths

Fetal deaths must also be reported. A **fetal death** refers to the death of a fetus of a particular weight or gestation, frequently 500 grams or more or 22 or more completed weeks of gestation, though the weight and week gestation may vary from state to state. The definition of a fetal death is generally as found in the Vermont statute:

> … the complete expulsion or extraction from the mother of a product of conception; the death is indicated by the fact that after such separation, the fetus does not breathe or show any other evidence of life such as beating of the heart, pulsation of the umbilical cord, or definite movement of voluntary muscles. (VT Stat. 18-6-107 5221)

In most states, the remains of a fetal death cannot be interred until a certificate of fetal death is completed. Depending on state law, the responsibility for completing the fetal death certificate may lie with the designated person in the institution where the fetal death occurred, the funeral director or other person responsible for internment or cremation of remains, or, if the fetal death occurred outside an institution, the physician in attendance at or immediately after the delivery. If no one was in attendance and the dead fetus is brought to the hospital, the hospital should notify the medical examiner, who will file the fetal death certificate. The information requested in a fetal death certificate includes information about the parents as well as information about the pregnancy and the fetus.

Unusual Events and Other State Reporting Requirements

States sometimes require the reporting of certain **unusual or adverse events** for other public health prevention and control programs. Examples include adverse medical events such as medication errors, transfusion reactions, falls resulting in fractures, wrong patient or wrong site surgical procedures, and operative complications. Such laws have resulted from recent concerns about patient safety and may apply to any type of healthcare facility. At least 26 states and the District of Columbia have implemented systems for the mandatory reporting of adverse medical events resulting in patient deaths or serious harm (Hanlon et al. 2015).

Most states have implemented **prescription drug monitoring programs** (PDMPs) in an effort to identify inappropriate and illegal activities involving controlled prescription drugs. States define which controlled drugs they wish to monitor and require pharmacies to report on the dispensing of these drugs. The information collected, at minimum, includes the physician name, Drug Enforcement Administration (DEA) registration number, the individual the drug was dispensed to, and the name of the drug. The information is submitted to a state data bank, which is used to monitor the dispensing of drugs. The information collected may be shared with healthcare providers or law enforcement agencies as defined by state law.

The Nuclear Regulatory Commission (NRC) has oversight responsibility for the medical use of ionizing radiation. The NRC has entered into licensing agreements with the majority of states to oversee the possession and use of radiation byproduct, source, and special nuclear material by the medical community. A listing of state radiation regulations and legislation is posted on the NRC website (NRC n.d.). Medical centers must report information on their use of radioactive materials and any misadministration of the material. If a medical event occurs, it must be reported to the state agency and the NRC (10 CFR 35.3045). The event notification information is public record and is posted daily on the commission's website (NRC 2016). Identifiable PHI is eliminated from the reports, but location and reporting individuals are not.

Other state agencies such as Medicaid and maternal and child health programs that provide state assistance to individuals who qualify for services have access to PHI by virtue of state regulation. The type and amount of PHI collected and maintained depends on the program.

In all situations discussed previously, the reporting of PHI is permissible without authorization since they fall under the public interest and benefit exception of "required by law" or "to prevent or lessen a serious threat to health or safety."

Workers' Compensation for Occupational Illness, Injury, and Death

All states have enacted **workers' compensation** legislation to ensure that employees who are injured on the job or become ill as a result of a job are provided with some means of support while recovering from their illness or injury. The laws also provide benefits to the surviving spouse and dependents if the worker dies as a result of work-related illness or injury while working (Cornell University Law School 2010). Employers must have workers' compensation insurance or group insurance or be self-insured.

When an employee becomes ill or injured as a result of a work-related situation, the employee or employee representative may file a workers' compensation claim as defined by the state. In doing so, the employee usually signs an authorization to release his or her medical information to the workers' compensation entity. See figure 16.3 for Ohio's Bureau of Workers' Compensation Authorization for Release of Medical Information form. State workers' compensation laws require employers to collect and maintain information on the employee's illness, injury, or death, which may include medical information requested from healthcare facilities in which the individual received care. The information may be disclosed to other entities in the state or to the federal government for reporting purposes without the patient's or family's authorization. The information is used to determine if the individual or family should receive compensation for the injury, illness, or death. The information collected usually includes the following:

- Injured worker's name
- Social Security number, address, home and work phone
- Date of birth
- Gender
- Date of injury, disease, or death
- Occupation or job title
- Description of accident
- Type of injury or disease and parts of body affected
- Place of accident or exposure on employer premises
- Date hired
- Date employer notified of injury, illness, or death

Regarding workers' compensation for federal employees, the federal government offers federal employees a compensation program similar to state programs. The federal government's program is administered through the Office of Workers' Compensation Programs of the US Department of Labor. The federal workers' compensation program falls under the same HIPAA Privacy Rule provision as that of the state workers' compensation programs.

State laws requiring employers and healthcare providers to report occupational illnesses, injuries, and deaths for the purpose of establishing workers' compensation do not conflict with HIPAA under the public interest and benefit exception of workers' compensation. The employer or healthcare provider is permitted to disclose PHI as necessary to comply with a state's compensation laws (45 CFR 164.512(a); 45

Figure 16.3 Workers' compensation authorization to release medical information

Ohio

Bureau of Worker's Compensation

Authorization to Release Medical Information

Instructions

You can obtain this form online at www.bwc.ohio.gov

- Please print or type.
- List the provider(s) you are authorizing to release medical records in the space indicated on this form.
- Please sign and date the form, and send it to the customer service office where your claim is located or to your self-insured employer.

Injured worker name (first, M.I., last)			Date of injury	Claim number
Address	City		State	Nine-digit ZIP code
Employer name		Employer MCO or QHP		

I, the above-named injured worker, understand I am allowing the Opportunities for Ohioans with Disabilities and the providers (persons or facilities) named here (_____
_____) that attend or examine me to release the following medical, psychological and/or psychiatric information (excluding psychotherapy notes) that are related causally or historically to physical or mental injuries relevant to my workers' compensation claim:

- Pathology slides and immunohistochemical staining results, if applicable;
- Hospital admission history and physical; emergency room reports; hospital discharge summaries; physician office notes; physical therapist, occupational therapist or athletic trainer assessments and progress notes; consultation reports; lab results; medical reports; surgical reports; diagnostic reports; procedure reports; nursing home and skilled nursing facilities documentation; home nursing progress notes; or other listed below.

_____.

I understand I am authorizing the release of this information to the following: the Ohio Bureau of Workers' Compensation (BWC), the Industrial Commission of Ohio, the above-named employer, the employer's managed care organization or qualified health plan and any authorized representatives.

I understand this information is being released to the above-referenced persons and/or entities for use in administering my workers' compensation claim.

This authorization to release medical, psychological and/or psychiatric information shall remain in effect for as long as my workers' compensation claim remains open under Ohio law. I understand I have the right to revoke this authorization at any time. However, I must submit my revocation in writing and file it with BWC or my self-insured employer. My decision to revoke this authorization will be effective, except in the case that any provider referenced above already has relied on my authorization and released information.

I understand the provider(s) referenced above may not make my completing and signing this authorization a condition of my treatment.

I understand the parties I am authorizing the release of information to are exempted from the federal privacy requirements of the Health Insurance Portability and Accountability Act of 1996 as they administer workers' compensation programs. Information disclosed pursuant to this authorization may be redisclosed by them and may no longer be protected by the federal privacy requirements. I understand such redisclosures may include but are not limited to the following:

- A copy of the medical information the employer receives may be forwarded to BWC by the employer;
- A copy of the medical information will be available to me or my physician of record upon request to BWC or to the employer.

Injured worker (or guardian or personal representative) signature	Date

If signed by the injured worker's guardian or personal representative, provide a description of the guardian or personal representative's authority to sign on behalf of the injured worker _____
_____.

BWC-1224 (Rev. 9/24/2013)
C-101

Source: Ohio Bureau of Workers' Compensation 2013.

CFR 164.502(b)(2)(iv)). The patient or family does not have the right to restrict the healthcare provider from this disclosure if the disclosure is required by state compensation laws. If a healthcare organization is asked for information related to a worker's previous condition not related to the claim for compensation, the organization must seek the worker's authorization before disclosing the information (45 CFR 164.508).

WorkersCompensation.com provides a workers' compensation guide to compensation law, information, and resources by state (WorkersCompensation.com 2016).

Check Your Understanding   16.2

Instructions: Indicate whether the following statements are true or false (T or F).

1. States can modify birth and death certificate information as long as certificates contain the minimum data required by the NCHS.

2. The responsibility for notifying individuals who have had contact with an individual with an infected communicable disease is the person who has the disease.

3. In the case of a suspicious death, a medical examiner or coroner has the right to receive medical information without authorization.

4. The National Regulatory Commission (NRC) posts daily medical events related to radiation on their website which includes PHI in addition to the location and reporting person.

5. The patient or family does not have the right to restrict a healthcare provider from disclosing PHI if the disclosure is required by state worker's compensation laws.

National Reporting Requirements

In addition to state laws requiring reporting of conditions and circumstances, there are federal mandatory reporting requirements, along with volunteer reporting systems hosted by agencies such as the CDC.

Reporting of Serious Occurrences or Deaths Related to Restraint or Seclusion

Federal regulations require reporting to appropriate authorities any deaths or serious occurrences related to patients who have been restrained or placed in seclusion. In addition, most states have implemented regulations similar to, or in tandem with, federal regulations. The Conditions of Participation (CoP) regarding patient rights applies to all Medicare- and Medicaid-participating healthcare entities such as hospitals (short-term acute care, critical access, psychiatric, children's), and rehabilitation, long-term care, and alcohol and drug facilities. The CoP contains six standards requiring facilities to notify patients of their rights in regard to their care and addressing privacy and safety, confidentiality of health records, and freedom from seclusion and restraints used in behavior management unless clinically necessary. There are specific documentation requirements for orders to be written, time limitations, and notes regarding ongoing observation and monitoring and continuing assessments of the need for restraints.

In December 2006, the CoP Patient Rights final rule (42 CFR 482.13(g)) for hospitals was published and specified that a hospital accredited by the Joint Commission or the American Osteopathic Association is deemed to meet all Medicare requirements and thus must report the following information:

- Each death that occurs while a patient is in restraint or seclusion.
- Each death that occurs within 24 hours after the patient has been removed from restraint or seclusion.

- Each death known to the hospital that occurs within one week after restraint or seclusion where it is reasonable to assume that use of restraint or placement in seclusion contributed directly or indirectly to a patient's death. "Reasonable to assume" in this context includes, but is not limited to, deaths related to restrictions of movement for prolonged periods of time, chest compression, restriction of breathing, or asphyxiation (42 CFR 482.13(g)).

The hospital must report the death to the Centers for Medicare and Medicaid Services (CMS) Regional Office by telephone, facsimile or electronically as determined by CMS no later than the close of business the next CMS business day following knowledge of the patient's death. Hospital staff must document in the patient's health record the date and time the death was reported. The facility must also record the death in an internal log or other system within seven days of the death. The entry must document the patient's name, date of birth, date of death, name of attending physician or other licensed practitioner responsible for the patient's care, medical record number, and primary diagnosis. This information must be made available in either written or electronic form to the CMS upon request (42 CFR 482.13(g)). In all of the previously mentioned situations, the death would also be reported to a state agency as determined by state law.

The Children's Health Act of 2000, signed into law on October 17, 2000, establishes national standards that restrict the use of restraints and seclusion in all psychiatric facilities that receive federal funds and in "non-medical community-based facilities for children and youth." In those settings, the use of restraints and seclusion is restricted to emergency safety situations. In the case of a minor, the parent or legal guardian must be notified no later than 24 hours after the occurrence (42 CFR 483.374). The information must include the patient's name, a description of the occurrence, and contact information for the facility.

These requirements do not conflict with the HIPAA Privacy Rule because such reporting meets the public interest and benefit exception of either "required by law" or "to prevent or lessen a serious threat to health or safety," and patient authorization is not required.

National Reporting of Quality Measures

Medicare, in collaboration with the Joint Commission and other private organizations, has developed several quality measures for hospitals, physician's offices, nursing homes, and other provider entities for the purpose of improving the quality and safety of patient care. The PHI collected is used for retrospective analysis and real-time reporting that enables healthcare organizations to comprehensively evaluate and manage quality improvement efforts. Some of the reporting activities are mandatory and some are voluntary (see table 16.2). Data may be submitted to federally supported Quality Improvement Organizations (QIOs) and Clinical Data Abstraction Centers (CDACs), the CDC, or other reporting organizations. Chapter 17 provides additional information on CMS quality reporting programs.

The CMS has several mandatory quality reporting initiatives in place that require hospitals and other healthcare organizations to report data. In all cases the confidentiality of patient information is maintained. The reported data are shared through websites that enable comparison among all doctors, hospitals, and other healthcare organizations. Recent regulations, such as Section 3004 of the 2010 Affordable Care Act, establish mandatory quality reporting requirements for long-term care hospitals, inpatient rehabilitation facilities, and hospice programs, which went into effect in 2014. Previous legislation has already made reporting mandatory for hospitals. A Medicare provider that fails to comply with the data reporting requirements is subject to a 2 percent reduction of reimbursement. Healthcare organizations

Table 16.2 Examples of national quality reporting initiatives

Initiative	Who	Purpose
Hospital Consumer Assessment of Healthcare Providers and Systems (HCAHPS)	Hospitals	Samples discharged patients on their experience in hospital related to communication, cleanliness of facility, pain management, discharge information, overall satisfaction with hospital
Hospital Quality Alliance (HQA)	Hospitals	Reporting on 22 clinical process and two 30-day mortality (outcome) measures on: • Acute myocardial infarction (AMI) • Heart failure (HF) • Pneumonia (PN) • Surgical Care Improvement Project (SCIP)
National Healthcare Safety Network (NHSN)	Hospitals, dialysis centers, ambulatory surgical centers, long-term care facilities	Surveillance system that collects data on healthcare-associated infections, adherence to clinical practices known to prevent healthcare-associated infections, incidence or prevalence of multidrug-resistant organisms within their organizations, trends and coverage of healthcare personnel safety and vaccination, and adverse events related to the transfusion of blood and blood products
Nursing Home Improvement Feedback Tool (NHIFT)	Nursing homes	Free, computer-based, process-of-care data collection tool that assists nursing homes in collecting data and viewing process measure scores for four clinical topics: depression, pain, physical restraints, and pressure ulcers
Physician Quality Reporting Initiative (PQRI)	Physician practices	Voluntary reporting of specified quality measures, which will earn participating physician a payment bonus, subject to a cap

Source: CMS 2011.

must provide copies of health records to Recovery Audit Contractors (RACs), Medicare Administrative Contractors (MACs), and Medicaid Integrity Contractors (MICs), whose responsibilities include but are not limited to measuring, preventing, identifying, and correcting incorrect payments under the Tax Relief and Health Care Act of 2006 and other federal healthcare reform legislations (Premier Advisor Live 2011).

In all of the programs just mentioned, the reporting of data is permissible under the Privacy Rule as "required by law," "for the purpose of research," or "to prevent or lessen a serious threat to health or safety."

National Practitioner Data Bank

As with any profession, there are times when certain individuals either intentionally or unintentionally engage in behavior that results in an adverse action occurring, such as malpractice, negligence, or fraud and abuse of insurance claims, to name a few. To address such problems, Congress passed the Health Care Quality Improvement Act (Public Law 99-660) in 1986 to encourage peer oversight of incompetent or unethical healthcare providers by protecting healthcare peer review bodies from liability damages when investigating problem practitioners. Title IV of the Act created the National Practitioner Data Bank (NPDB) to collect and release information related to the competence and conduct of physicians, dentists and other healthcare practitioners. The NPDB became operational in 1990 (42 USC 11133(a)(1)).

In 1996, HIPAA legislation established the **Healthcare Integrity and Protection Data Bank (HIPDB)** under Section 1128E of the Social Security Act to collect adverse actions against healthcare providers, suppliers, or practitioners involved in fraud and abuse activities and to maintain a database of these findings. The data collection program did not include settlements in which no findings of liability were made. Healthcare organizations wishing to hire or work with practitioners or suppliers would as part of their due diligence request information from both databases. (42 USC 1301, 1128E).

In 2010, the ACA authorized HHS to merge the HIPDB with the NPDB to eliminate duplication and "improve the quality of healthcare and encourage state licensing boards, hospitals and other healthcare entities, and professional societies to identify and discipline those who engage in unprofessional behavior and to restrict the ability of incompetent physicians, dentists, and other healthcare practitioners to move from State to State without disclosure or discovery of previous medical malpractice payment and adverse action history" (HHS 2015).

In 2013, the **NPDB** formally become the information clearinghouse that receives reportable adverse action information on healthcare providers, practitioners, or suppliers from federal and state government agencies, hospitals, health plans, malpractice payers, and others, and discloses the information to those who have access rights to the information. See tables 16.3 and 16.4 for a listing of who is required to report,

Table 16.3 National data bank reporting requirements for Title IV

Law	Who Reports?	What is Reported?	Who is Reported?	Who May Query
Title IV	Medical malpractice payers	Medical malpractice payments resulting from a written claim or judgment	Practitioners	Hospitals (required by law)
	State medical and dental boards	Certain adverse licensure actions related to professional competence or conduct	Physician and dentists	Other health care entities with formal peer review
	Hospitals	Certain adverse clinical privileges actions related to professional competence or conduct	Physician and dentists	Professional societies with formal peer review
	Other healthcare entities with formal peer review		Other practitioners (optional)	State medical and dental boards and other State licensing boards
	Professional societies with formal peer review	Certain adverse professional society membership actions related to professional competence or conduct	Physician and dentists	
			Other practitioners (optional)	Plaintiff's attorney/ pro se plaintiff (limited circumstances)
	DEA	DEA controlled-substance registration actions*	Physician and dentists	Health care practitioners (self-query)
	OIG	Exclusions from participation in Medicare, Medicaid, and other Federal health care programs*	Practitioners	Researchers (de-identified statistical data only)

*This information is reported to the NPDB under Title IV based on a memorandum of understanding.
Source: HHS 2015 NPDB Guidebook C-7.

Table 16.4 National data bank reporting requirements for Sections 1921 and 1128E

Law	Who Reports?	What is Reported?	Who is Reported?	Who May Query
Section 1921	Peer review organizations	Negative actions or findings by peer review organizations	Practitioners	Hospitals and other health care entities*
	Private accreditation organizations	Negative actions or findings by private accreditation organizations	Entities, providers, and suppliers	
	State licensing and certification authorities	State licensing and certification actions	Practitioners, entities, providers, and suppliers	Professional societies with formal peer review*
	State law enforcement agencies***	Exclusions from a State health care program	Practitioners, providers, and suppliers	Quality improvement organizations*
	State Medicaid fraud control units	Health care-related civil judgments in State court		State licensing and certification authorities
	State agencies administering or supervising administration of State healthcare programs***	Health care-related State criminal convictions		Agencies administering Federal health care programs, including private entities administering such programs under contract
		Other adjudicated actions or decisions		Federal licensing and certification agencies
	State prosecutors			Health plans
Section 1128E	Federal agencies	Federal licensing and certification actions**	Practitioners, providers, and suppliers	State law enforcement agencies***
	Federal prosecutors	Exclusions from a Federal health care program**		State Medicaid fraud control units***
	Health plans	Health care-related Federal or State criminal convictions**		State agencies administering or supervising the administration of State health care programs***
		Health care-related civil judgments in Federal or State court		Federal law enforcement officials and agencies
		Other adjudicated actions or decisions		Practitioners, entities, providers, and suppliers (self-query)
				Researchers (de-identified, statistical data only)

*These entities have access to most of the information reported under Section 1921 and Section 1128E.

**Reported by Federal agencies only.

***NPDB regulations define "state law or fraud enforcement agency" as including but not limited to these entities.

Source: HHS 2015 NPDB Guidebook C-8.

what information is reported, who is reported, and who may query by laws. For example, a hospital must report to the NPDB adverse actions against a physician on staff (such as suspension of privileges) lasting more than 30 days, medical malpractice payments, and settlement reports. When evaluating a provider's application for privileges, the facility must query the NPDB. Data bank information provides additional details regarding an applicant but does not supersede the normal investigation practices. Hospitals must query the NPDBs about staff members every two years. It's important to note that practitioners may also provide input to the database in their defense if deemed necessary.

Information reported to the data banks is considered confidential and is not disclosed except as specified by regulation. For example, a practitioner or physician access the information reported on them and entities engaged in professional review activity. The receipt, access, use, and disclosure of information from the data banks do not conflict with the HIPAA Privacy Rule because they meet the public interest and benefit "required by law" exception.

Medical Device Reporting

The Food and Drug Administration (FDA) is the federal oversight body "responsible for protecting the public by assuring the safety, efficacy and security of human and veterinary drugs, biological products, medical devices, our nation's food supply, cosmetics, and products that emit radiation" (FDA 2015d). The Center for Devices and Radiological Health (CDRH) is the unit within the FDA that oversees "access to safe, effective, and high quality medical devices and safe radiation-emitting products" (FDA 2015a).

A **medical device** is defined as an instrument, apparatus, or other article that is used to prevent, diagnose, mitigate, or treat a disease or to affect the structure or function of the body, with the exception of drugs. Examples of medical devices are x-ray machines, sutures, defibrillators, vascular grafts, syringes, surgical lasers, heating pads, bone screws, gauze pads, patient restraints, wheelchairs, infusion pumps, and hospital beds. A serious injury or illness as a result of a medical device is identified as one that:

- Is life-threatening
- Results in permanent impairment of a body function or permanent damage to a body structure
- Necessitates medical or surgical intervention to preclude permanent impairment of a body function or permanent damage to a body structure (21 USC 360i(b))

The FDA requires **medical device reporting** of deaths and severe complications thought to be due to a device to be reported to the FDA and the manufacturer. To facilitate reporting, the FDA categorizes medical devices into one of three classes, with Class I representing devices that are considered to be low-risk and exempt from pre-market review by the FDA. Class II devices are considered to have moderate to well-understood risks and are usually subject to premarket review. Class III devices may pose the greatest risk, thus, are subject to premarket approval and other regulatory controls. With the increased use of health information technology (HIT) and digital health devices, such as wearable devices, mobile medical devices, telemedicine, medical device data systems, and wireless devices, the FDA has issued guidance to manufacturers, distributors and other entities regarding regulatory authority related to selected mobile applications (FDA 2015e). Figure 16.4 provides examples of mobile applications that are also subject to the class ratings and that the FDA will regulate, those it may regulate, and those it will not regulate.

To date, the FDA does not regulate electronic health record systems (EHRs) although a number of data integrity failures have been reported (ECRI 2013). Instead, the FDA has worked collaboratively with the Office of the National Coordinator for Health IT (ONC) and the Federal Communications Commission (FCC) to supports a risk-based regulatory framework that promotes innovation while

Figure 16.4	Examples of mobile medical applications and FDA responsibility

FDA regulates mobile apps that:

- Use a sensor, lead or electrode such as electrocardiograph, electronic stethoscope, accelerometer, nystagmograph, audiometer, tremor transducer, EEG.
- Connect to an existing device type to control its operation or function such as infusion pump, implantable neuromuscular stimulator, blood pressure cuff, calibrate hearing aids.
- Display, transfer, store, or convert patient-specific medical device data such as medical device data system, bedside, cardiac, perinatal monitors, PACS.

FDA may exercise enforcement discretion on mobile apps that:

- Help patients maintain behavioral coping skills.
- Provide periodic educational information, reminders, motivational guidance
- Use GPS location information to alert asthmatics of environmental conditions
- Allow a user to, collect, log, track, and trend data, such as blood glucose, blood pressure, heart rate, weight or other data from a device to share with a heath care provider, or upload to an online (cloud) database, personal or electronic health record.
- Meet the definition of MDDS and connect to a nursing central station and display medical device data to a physician's mobile platform for review.

FDA does not regulate mobile apps that:

- Provide access to electronic copies such as medical dictionaries, abbreviations, e-books, audio books.
- Are used as educational tools for medical training such as interactive videos, flash cards, simulated games or scenario, surgical training videos.
- Are intended for general patient education and facilitate patient access to commonly used reference information.
- Automate general office operations in healthcare setting such as billing codes, insurance claims, and patient satisfaction surveys.
- Are generic aids or purpose products, such as magnifying glass, allow patients to interact through email, video communication or web-based link.

Source: FDA et al. 2015e.

protecting patient safety, and avoiding unnecessary or duplicative regulation (FDA et al. 2014). While the FDA, ONC, and FCC work together on patient safety issues, users of HIT and EHRs are encouraged to voluntarily report problems with EHRs. Reporting of these problems may include PHI without patient authorization.

Prior to 1990, FDA required reporting focused on adverse consequences related to FDA-regulated drugs, biologics, dietary supplements, and cosmetics. The Safe Medical Devices Act of 1990 (SMDA) (21 USC 360i(b)) and the subsequent Medical Device Amendments of 1992 expanded required reporting by user facilities and manufacturers to report to the FDA deaths and serious injuries from medical devices that have or may have caused or contributed to a patient's death or injury. User facilities and manufacturers must also maintain an adverse event file. User facilities include hospitals, ambulatory surgical facilities, nursing homes, outpatient treatment facilities, or outpatient diagnostic facilities (FDA 2016). Mandatory reporting must be done electronically through the FDA's **Safety Information and Adverse Event Reporting Program,** or **MedWatch.** Reporting can be done using the MedWatch online form or an electronic equivalent (FDA 2015c). User facilities and manufacturers have different requirements for when they must report, and to whom which are outlined in table 16.5. Data typically reported includes the following items:

Table 16.5 Summary of medical device reporting requirements

Reporter	Report What?	To Whom	When?
User Facility	Deaths	FDA and manufacturer	Within 10 work days
	Serious injuries*	Manufacturer, FDA only if manufacturer unknown	Within 10 work days
	Semiannual report of death and serious injuries	FDA	January 1 and July 1
Manufacturer	30-day reports of deaths, serious injuries* and malfunctions	FDA	30 days from becoming aware
	Baseline report to identify and provide basic data on each device that is subject of a report	FDA	With 30-day report when device is reported for 1st time
	5-day report on events that require immediate remedial action and other types of events designated by FDA	FDA	Within 5 work days
	Annual certification of compliance with regulation	FDA	When firm submits annual registration

*Serious injury definition no longer necessitates immediate intervention, just medical or surgical intervention
Source: FDA Medical Device Reporting for User Facilities 2016.

- User facility report number
- Name and address of the device manufacturer
- Device brand name and common name
- Product model, catalog, serial, and lot numbers
- Brief description of the event reported to the manufacturer and/or the FDA
- Where the report was submitted (for example, to the FDA, manufacturer, or distributor) (FDA 2015c)

In addition to mandatory reporting requirements, the FDA encourages health professionals and consumers to voluntarily report adverse events, observed or suspected to be related to products, technologies or EHR systems as noted above. Voluntary reporting is also done through MedWatch. Voluntary reporting of problems or events may include PHI without patient authorization.

The HIPAA Privacy Rule specifically allows medical device reporting (45 CFR 164.512(b)) without patient authorization as follows:

1. To collect or report adverse events (or similar activities with respect to food or dietary supplements), product defects or problems (including problems with the use or labeling of a product), or biological product deviations

2. To track FDA-regulated products

3. To enable product recalls, repairs, replacements, or lookback (including locating and notifying individuals who have received products that have been recalled or withdrawn or are the subject of lookback)

4. To conduct post-marketing surveillance

Under the Freedom of Information and Privacy Acts, however, prior to any public disclosure, the FDA is required to delete any personal, medical, and similar information that would constitute a clear unwarranted invasion of personal privacy, in addition to trade secrets and confidential commercial or financial information related to the manufacturer or identifying information of the reporter of the event.

Organ Procurement Reporting

In 1984, the National Organ Transplant Act established the **Organ Procurement and Transplantation Network (OPTN)** to facilitate patient and donor organ matching opportunities. The law established nonprofit organ procurement organizations who all must be members of the OPTN (Organdonor.gov n.d.). Currently there are 58 OPOs in the U.S. who are responsible for the evaluation and procurement of donor organs for organ transplantation. Each state has one to five OPOs that hospital work with in regard to organ donation and procurement. The Federal Conditions of Participation for Hospitals requires that a hospital must have an agreement with an OPO and a protocol in place to notify the organization that a specified organ donor has died in the hospital or for whom death is imminent (42 CFR 482.45). Hospitals must also work with the OPO to conduct annual death record reviews (42 CFR 482.45). A hospital is not violating patient confidentiality by contacting the OPO and providing information about an individual who has died or whose death is imminent if the patient has identified him or herself as an organ donor either through prior advance directive documentation or while hospitalized with permission granted by the patient or the patients next of kin. Although the statute and regulations are not explicit in establishing that such notification does not violate patient confidentiality, it is implicit in the law. There is no requirement in the statute or regulations that the family be informed about the hospital's notification of the OPO before the OPO can be contacted. (Reynolds and Bowman 2016). Further, this federal law does not conflict with HIPAA because, under the public interest and benefit exception of "for cadaveric organ, eye or tissue donation," such disclosures are permissible without authorization.

Occupational Fatalities, Injuries, and Illnesses

The Federal Occupational Safety and Health Act (29 CFR 1904.0) of 1970 established the Occupational and Health Administration (OSHA) under the auspices of the Department of Labor. The regulation requires employers to report work-related fatalities, injuries, and illnesses to OSHA. According to the regulation, such events must be reported if they result in (29 CFR 1904.7(a)):

> … death, days away from work, restricted work or transfer to another job, medical treatment beyond first aid, or loss of consciousness. You must also consider a case to meet the general recording criteria if it involves a significant injury or illness diagnosed by a physician or other licensed healthcare professional, even if it does not result in death, days away from work, restricted work or job transfer, medical treatment beyond first aid, or loss of consciousness.

Federal law requiring the reporting of occupational fatalities, injuries, and illnesses does not conflict with HIPAA because, under the public interest and benefit exception of "public health activities" or as provided by the preemption exception, such disclosures are permissible without authorization. Healthcare facilities may be required to release medical information relevant to the fatality, injury, or illness to appropriate authorities. Chapter 20 addresses OSHA requirements and employee workplace safety in more detail.

Check Your Understanding   16.3

Instructions: Indicate whether the following statements are true or false (T or F).

1. A hospital must report to the CMS Regional Office the death of a patient within 24 hours after the patient has been removed from restraint.

2. The reporting of quality measures that includes PHI is mandatory by federal law.

3. When a physician applies for staff privileges a hospital must query the NPDB only if the physician requests that the hospital does so.

4. The FDA does not regulate electronic health records but it does regulate a number of health IT applications that may pose a risk to the health or safety of a patient.

5. When an employee is injured at work, he must authorize disclosure of his PHI before it can be reported to OSHA.

Clinical, Disease and Outcome-Based Registries

The term **registry** refers to a program that collects and stores data, and the records that are created through this process. Registries are designed and used for a broad range of purposes in public health and medicine, from evaluating patient care to monitoring defective devices; examples include

- Assessing natural history, including estimating magnitude of a problem; determining underlying incidence or prevalence rate; examining trends of disease over time; conducting surveillance; assessing service delivery and identifying groups of high risk; documenting types of patients served by a healthcare provider; and describing and estimating survival
- Determining clinical effectiveness, cost-effectiveness, or comparative effectiveness of a test or treatment, including evaluating the acceptability of drugs, devices, or procedures for reimbursement
- Measuring or monitoring safety and harm of specific products and treatments, including conducting comparative evaluation of safety and effectiveness
- Measuring or improving quality of care, including conducting programs to measure and/or improve the practice of medicine and/or public health (Gliklich and Dreyer 2014, 10–11)

The National Committee on Vital and Health Statistics states that a registry is an organized system for the collection, storage, retrieval, analysis, and dissemination of information on individuals who have a particular disease or condition or prior exposure to a substance or circumstance that may cause an adverse health effect (Gliklich and Dreyer 2014). Registries are usually secondary data sources and are maintained for a variety of purposes by a variety of entities. Federal and state regulation may require registries for collecting extensive information on particular diseases used for setting health policy, disease prevention and control, reporting of quality measures, research, and other reporting purposes. Registries are maintained by healthcare providers, professional organizations, researchers, disease specific agencies, consortiums or vendors independently of what may be required by federal or state regulation. The types of registries vary, as does the information collected by the registries.

Common among registries however, are the requirements that the patient data submitted to the registry be maintained in a confidential manner and that the identity of the patient be protected from disclosure. For the most part, registries are maintained by HIPAA-covered entities (or their business associates) and are subject to the HIPAA Privacy Rule. Healthcare organizations releasing the data do so under the HIPAA Privacy Rule's public interest and benefit exception of "public health activities."

Registries maintained by healthcare organizations and providers typically use data from patient health records under the healthcare operations provision, so individual patient authorization is not required for the data to be included in the registry. If the registry is maintained by a private organization for research purposes; however, the registry is subject to the research requirements of the Privacy Rule (Gliklich and Dreyer 2014). Some common types of registries are described next.

Federal Registry for Implantable Cardiac Defibrillators (ICDs)

In January 2005, Medicare expanded its coverage of implantable cardiac defibrillators (ICDs) to eligible Medicare beneficiaries. As a requirement for covering the cost of ICDs, hospitals are required to submit data to the Medicare ICD registry. On April 1, 2006, Medicare contracted with the American College of Cardiologists (ACC) National Cardiovascular Data Registry (NCDR) to assume responsibility for the ICD registry. Every hospital that seeks reimbursement for ICDs must participate in the registry (CMS 2015). This requirement does not conflict with the HIPAA Privacy Rule because it meets the public interest and benefit exception of required by law, for the research, or prevent or lessen a serious threat to health or safety (see figure 16.1). In addition to the ICD registry, the NCDR coordinates seven other hospitals and two outpatient non-government-mandated national clinical data registries related to carotid artery stenting and endarterectomy procedures, cardiac catherizations, and quality improvement products (NCDR n.d.). The PHI collected in these registries also does not conflict with the HIPAA Privacy Rule because the information meets the exception related to "the purpose of research".

Cancer Registries

State-based **cancer registries** are data systems that collect, manage, and analyze data about cancer cases and cancer deaths. In each state, medical facilities (including hospitals, physician's offices, therapeutic radiation facilities, freestanding surgical centers, and pathology laboratories) are required to report data to a central cancer registry as defined by state law. The data reported to a central statewide registry or incidence surveillance program are in turn reported to the CDC. In 1992, the Cancer Registries Act established the National Program of Cancer Registries (NPCR), which is administered by the CDC. State cancer surveillance programs, assisted by the NPCR, collect data on the occurrence of cancer, type, extent, location, and type of initial treatment, which are then used to determine trends, allocate resources, and advance research (CDC 2016b). For example, according to Ohio law (ORC 3701.262)

> … each physician, dentist, hospital or person providing diagnostic or treatment services to patients with cancer shall report each case of cancer to the Ohio Cancer Incidence Surveillance System (OCISS) at the Ohio Department of Health (ODH). … A reportable case is defined as: any primary malignant neoplasm with the exception of basal and squamous cell carcinoma of the skin and carcinoma in-situ of the cervix diagnosed and/or treated in any person in Ohio on or after Jan. 1, 1992, as well as cases of benign and borderline intracranial and nervous system (CNS) tumors diagnosed on or after Jan. 1, 2004. (Ohio Department of Health 2016)

Confidentiality of the data reported by healthcare facilities to state registries is protected as defined by state law. In addition, the NPCR requires that all registries that submit data to the program have a security policy in place.

Trauma Registries

Trauma registries maintain databases on patients with severe traumatic injuries. A **traumatic injury** is a wound or other injury caused by an external physical force such as an automobile accident, a shooting, a stabbing, or a fall. Information collected by the trauma registry may be used for performance improvement and research in trauma care. Trauma registries may be facility-based or may include data for a region or state.

The information collected by trauma registries may include patient demographics, injury location, injury date and time, cause of injury, safety equipment used, prehospital assessment/treatment, emergency department or admission assessment/treatment, hospital assessment/treatment, disposition and diagnosis (including injury severity scores), and patient outcome. The entities usually required to report trauma are healthcare facilities of all types, other state agencies as required by state regulation, and medical examiners or coroners. Not every patient who is injured qualifies for inclusion in a trauma registry, so state regulations must be reviewed to determine what constitutes a trauma patient. For example, the New York State Trauma Registry defines a trauma patient as having at least one injury that falls within the ICD-10 diagnosis code range of 800–959.9, that includes burns, hypothermia, smoke inhalation, hanging, drowning, abuse, and DOAs (dead on arrival) (New York State Department of Health 2016). Tennessee has a registry specific to traumatic brain and spinal cord injuries as well as a general trauma registry (TN Code Ann. 68-55-101; TN Code Ann. 68-11-259). Ultimately, the information from a trauma registry might be used to assess the need for a state public health law, such as a motorcycle helmet law, or for other public safety concerns.

Immunization Registries

Immunization registries have been implemented in many states to collect and maintain vaccination records on children and in some cases adults in an effort to promote disease prevention and control. These registries are different in that while they require the reporting of PHI, they also allow access to this information by the individual or his or her representative whose data is recorded in the registry. The reasons some state immunization registries have moved in this direction can be summed up as outlined by the Georgia Immunization Registry:

- Assure that all persons in Georgia receive appropriate, timely immunizations to lead healthy, disease-free lives
  - Assist providers and public health officials in reminding individuals when they or their children need or are past due for vaccination(s)
  - Assist public health officials in assessing and improving community immunization status
- Assure access to up-to-date immunization records of Georgians
  - Assist providers in evaluating the immunization status of their patients
  - Avoid duplicate immunizations
- Meet the needs of Georgia's Immunization Registry mandate
- Provide a Registry that is cost-effective, user friendly, and efficient (Georgia Department of Public Health 2012)

The party responsible for reporting immunizations is the healthcare entity (or its designee) that administers a vaccine licensed by the FDA (e.g., physicians, public health departments or agencies, hospitals, and clinics). Registries usually collect patient identification information, immunization received, date administered, by whom, and where. The registry records and tracks this information, which is then made available to healthcare providers, parents, and legal guardians. Access to the information through the Internet or in some other format is usually delineated by state regulation or guidelines. The state of Wisconsin's immunization program offers a public immunization record access hyperlink that gives people the ability to look up their immunization record in the Wisconsin Immunization Registry (Wisconsin Department of Health Services 2016.).

Birth Defects Registries

Birth defects registries collect information on newborns with birth defects. Usually maintained by the state, these registries serve a variety of purposes. They provide information on the incidence of birth defects to study causes and prevention of birth defects, to monitor trends in birth defects, to improve medical care for children with birth defects, and to target interventions for preventable birth defects, such as folic acid to prevent neural tube defects. Information for birth defects registries may come from reporting by healthcare facilities and providers as well as from birth, fetal death, and death certificates. For example, the Florida Birth Defects Registry (FBDR) passive case ascertainment methodology involves the linkage of multiple secondary "source" datasets including Florida Division of Public Health Statistics and Performance Management birth records, the Agency for Health Care Administration (AHCA) hospital inpatient and ambulatory discharge databases, Regional Perinatal Intensive Care Centers (RPICC) data, Children's Medical Services (CMS) case management records, and CMS Early Steps data (FBDR n.d.).

The type of data collected in birth defects registries includes demographic information; birth weight; status at birth, including live-born, stillborn, or aborted; autopsies; cytogenetics results; whether the infant was a single or multiple birth; mother's use of alcohol, tobacco, or illicit drugs; father's use of drugs and alcohol; and family history of birth defects.

Diabetes Registries

Since diabetes is such a serious public health problem, many states have passed legislation in support of diabetes programs including the establishment of **diabetes registries**. These registries have been developed to follow diabetic patients for assistance in managing diabetes care as well as for research. Patients whose diabetes is not kept under good control frequently have numerous complications. The diabetes registry can track whether a patient has been seen by a physician to prevent complications. Diabetes registries are typically kept in ambulatory care settings, since this is where most diabetic care is provided.

On a global level, the Diabetes Collaborative Registry (DCR) is a "cross-specialty clinical registry designed to track and improve the quality of diabetes and metabolic care across the primary care and specialty care continuum" (DCR n.d.). The registry is led by the American College of Cardiology in partnership with the American Diabetes Association, the American College of Physicians, the American Association of Clinical Endocrinologists and the Joslin Diabetes Center. The registry collects data from primary care physicians, endocrinologists, cardiologists and other providers of diabetic care (DCR n.d.).

Implant Registries

An implant is a material or substance inserted into the body, such as breast implants, heart valves, and pacemakers. **Implant registries** have been developed for tracking the performance of implants, including complications, deaths, and defects resulting from implants, as well as implant longevity. Implants are considered Class III medical devices and thus are regulated by the FDA. The safety of implants has been questioned recently in several highly publicized cases. For example, there have been questions about the safety of silicone breast implants, metal on metal hip implants, and temporomandibular joint implants (FDA 2015b). In such cases, it is often difficult to ensure that all patients with the implants have been notified of the safety questions. Some implant registries were developed in response to these types of situations. Implant registries help healthcare providers in complying with the legal requirement for reporting of medical device adverse events. Demographic data on patients receiving implants are included in the registry as well as the other data items mentioned above to facilitate reporting.

Transplant Registries

Transplant registries serve a variety of purposes. Some organ transplant registries maintain databases of patients in need of organs so when an organ becomes available there is a way to allocate the organ to the patient with the highest priority. In other cases, the purpose of the registry is to provide a database of potential donors for transplants using live donors, such as bone marrow transplants. Posttransplant information also is kept on organ recipients and donors.

Because transplant registries are used to try to match donor organs with recipients, they are often national or even international in scope. Examples of national registries include the United Network for Organ Sharing (UNOS) and the registry of the National Marrow Donor Program (NMDP).

Data collected in the transplant registry may also be used for research, policy analysis, and quality control. The type of information collected varies according to the type of registry. Pretransplant data about the recipient include demographic data, patient's diagnosis, patient's status codes regarding medical urgency, patient's functional status, whether the patient is on life support, previous transplantations, and **histocompatibility** (compatibility of donor and recipient tissues). For donor registries, information on donors varies according to whether or not the donor is living. For organs harvested from patients who have died, information is collected on the cause and circumstances of the death, organ procurement and consent process, medications the donor was taking, and other donor history. For a living donor, information collected includes the relationship of the donor to the recipient (if any), clinical information, information on organ recovery, and histocompatibility.

Qualified Clinical Data Registries

A **qualified clinical data registry** (QCDR) is an entity that collects clinical data and submits it to CMS on behalf of physicians or physician group practices who are voluntarily participating in the federally sponsored Physician Quality Reporting System (PQRS). The QCDR "is a CMS-approved entity that collects medical and /or clinical data for the purposes of patient and disease tracking to foster improvement in the quality of care provided to patients" (CMS 2016a). Entities that have qualified as a clinical data registry are subject to the HIPAA Privacy Rule. If independent physicians and physician group practices participate in PQRS, they may avoid Medicare Part B Physician Fee Schedule negative payment adjustments. A QCDR may also collect and submit quality measures from the following entities:

- Clinical & Group Consumer Assessment of Healthcare Providers and Systems (CAHPS)
- National Quality Forum (NQF) endorsed measures
- Measures used by boards or specialty societies (like those mentioned above)
- Measures used by regional quality collaborations (CMS 2016b)

Disclosures to Public Health Authorities Not Required by Law

Covered entities may disclose PHI to public health entities even if law does not specifically require the disclosure, if the disclosure is for the purpose of:

> . . . preventing or controlling disease, injury, or disability, including, but not limited to, the reporting of disease, injury, vital events such as birth or death, and the conduct of public health surveillance, public health investigations, and public health interventions; or, at the direction of a public health authority, to an official of a foreign government agency that is acting in collaboration with a public health authority. (45 CFR 164.512(b))

For example, information about an individual with a disease might be disclosed in order to determine the cause of the disease and prevent it from spreading (CDC 2003). In such cases, it is necessary for the facility to verify the identity of the person requesting the information if the request is made in person, or to determine the authority for the request using methods such as requiring a statement on official letterhead from the public health entity (CDC 2003). Another example may occur if several individuals over a week's time arrive at the emergency department complaining of an illness that they seem to have picked up at a local bar in town. The hospital will report the finding to the public health department providing the patient PHI in order for the health department to interview the patients involved to determine what commonality they may have all been exposed thus, resulting in illness.

Check Your Understanding 16.4

Instructions: Indicate whether the following statements are true or false (T or F).

1. Statewide cancer registries are frequently required to report data to the NCHS.
2. Depending on state law, an individual may access his or her PHI housed in an immunization registry.
3. Because implants are classified as Class III medical devices, they are not regulated by the FDA, and PHI would not be found in an implant registry.
4. Transplant registries may include data about organ donors as well as organ recipients.
5. A covered entity cannot disclose a patient's PHI to a public health entity even if it is to prevent the spread of a disease unless the patient authorizes the disclosure.

Scenario 16

On Thursday, a 75-year-old patient at Wesley Glen Senior Living Facility became agitated and physically abusive to himself and others, so was placed in wrist and ankle restraints. An hour later, staff found the patient unconscious and called the EMT squad for assistance. The patient was taken to the medical center emergency department (ED), where he awoke and once again became physically abusive. The physician ordered the patient to be restrained to protect the patient and others while the physician examined the patient. Upon examining the patient, the physician noted that the patient had multiple bruises on his back, buttocks, and thighs. In addition, the patient had a cardiac defibrillator implanted during his last inpatient visit. The hospital had received a medical device alert notice regarding the implant device, and was notifying patients with the device to contact their physician for follow-up. The patient was sedated and the restraints removed. However, 15 hours later, the patient expired. The hospital reported the death to the medical examiner and coroner office. Consider the following:

Scenario 16 (Continued)

1. Why is the hospital required to report this patient's death to the medical examiner or coroner? Do medical examiners or coroners have the right to receive patient information needed to investigate a case?

2. What additional required reporting must be done by Wesley Glen and the hospital about the patient's death?

3. Who is responsible for notifying the hospital that a medical device in use may cause harm to patients? If the patient's death was attributed to the cardiac implant defibrillator, what is the hospital's responsibility for reporting the death to the FDA? How is the death reported?

References

Centers for Disease Control and Prevention. 2003. HIPAA Privacy Rule and public health: Guidance from CDC and the US Department of Health and Human Services. http://www.cdc.gov.

Centers for Disease Control and Prevention. 2016a. Nationally notifiable infectious diseases, United States 2016. http://www.cdc.gov.

Centers for Disease Control and Prevention. 2016b. National Program of Cancer Registries. http://www.cdc.gov/cancer/npcr/about.htm.

Centers for Medicare and Medicaid Services. 2011. Quality Initiatives: General information. http://www.cms.gov.

Centers for Medicare and Medicaid Services. 2012. Memorandum reporting reasonable suspicion of a crime in a long-term-care facility (LTC): Section 1150B of the Social Security Act. http://www.cms.gov.

Centers for Medicare and Medicaid Services. 2015. ICD registry. http://www.cms.hhs.gov.

Centers for Medicare and Medicaid Services. 2016a. Qualified clinical data registry reporting. https://www.cms.gov/Medicare/Quality-Initiatives-Patient-Assessment-Instruments/PQRS/Qualified-Clinical-Data-Registry-Reporting.html.

Centers for Medicare and Medicaid Services. 2016b. Physician Quality Reporting System (PQRS): qualified clinical data registry participation made simple. https://www.cms.gov/Medicare/Quality-Initiatives-Patient-Assessment-Instruments/PQRS/Downloads/2016PQRS_QCDR_MadeSimple.pdf.

Child Welfare Information Gateway. 2014. Definitions of child abuse and neglect. Washington, DC: US Department of Health and Human Services, Children's Bureau. http://www.childwelfare.gov.

Cornell University Law School. 2010. Workers' compensation: An overview. http://www.law.cornell.edu/.

Department of Health and Human Services Health Resources and Services Administration. 2015. NPDB Guidebook. https://www.npdb.hrsa.gov/.

Diabetes Collaborative Registry. n.d. Diabetes Collaborative Registry Transforming the future of diabetes care. https://www.ncdr.com/WebNCDR/Diabetes/publicpage.

ECRI Institute. 2013. Top 10 health technology hazards for 2014. *Guidance Article*. November. 354–380.

Florida Birth Defects Registry. n.d. Birth defects surveillance in Florida. http://www.fbdr.org/Data_Research/research_data.html.

Food and Drug Administration, Federal Trade Commission, and Office of the National Coordinator for Health Information Technology. 2014. FDASIA health IT report proposed strategy and recommendations for a risk-based framework. http://www.fda.gov/downloads/AboutFDA/CentersOffices/OfficeofMedicalProductsandTobacco/CDRH/CDRHReports/UCM391521.pdf.

Food and Drug Administration. 2015a. Center for Devices and Radiological Health. http://www.fda.gov.

Food and Drug Administration. 2015b. Implants and prosthetics. http://www.fda.gov/MedicalDevices/ProductsandMedicalProcedures/ImplantsandProsthetics/default.htm.

Food and Drug Administration. 2015c. Mandatory reporting requirements: Manufacturers, importers and devise users facilities. http://www.fda.gov.

Food and Drug Administration. 2015d. What we do. http://www.fda.gov.

Food and Drug Administration Center for Devices and Radiological Health, Center for Biologics Evaluation and Research. 2015e. Mobile medical applications: Guidance for industry and Food and Drug Administration staff. http://www.fda.gov/downloads/MedicalDevices/DeviceRegulationandGuidance/GuidanceDocuments/UCM263366.pdf#page=23.

Food and Drug Administration. 2016. Medical device reporting for user facilities. http://www.fda.gov/downloads/MedicalDevices/DeviceRegulationandGuidance/GuidanceDocuments/UCM095266.pdf.

Georgia Department of Public Health. 2012. Keeping Georgians healthy. Georgia Registry of Immunization Transactions Services (GRITS). https://dph.georgia.gov/sites/dph.georgia.gov/files/Immunizations/Publications-GRITS-brochure.pdf.

Gliklich, R. and N. Dreyer, eds. 2014. *Registries for Evaluating Patient Outcomes: A User's Guide*, 3rd ed. Rockville, MD: Agency for Healthcare Research and Quality.

National Cardiovascular Data Registry. n.d. About NCDR. http://www.ncdr.com.

National Center for Health Statistics. 1992. Model State Vital Statistics Act and Regulations. http://www.cdc.gov.

New York State Department of Health. 2016. New York State Trauma Registry. Data dictionary. http://www.health.ny.gov/professionals/ems/state_trauma/docs/trauma_data_dictionary_v9_01-2016.pdf.

Nuclear Regulatory Commission. 2016. Event notification reports. http://www.nrc.gov.

Nuclear Regulatory Commission. n.d. State regulations and legislation. http://www.nrc.gov.

Organdonor.gov. n.d. Find your organ procurement organization. https://organdonor.gov/awareness/organizations/local-opo.html.

Ohio Bureau of Workers' Compensation. 2013. Authorization to release medical information. BWC-1224 (Rev. 9/24/2013). http://www.ohiobwc.com.

Ohio Department of Health. 2016. Specialized registry: Cancer case report. https://www.ohiopublichealthreporting.info/Enrollment/MeaningfulUse/CancerReporting.

Pozgar, G. 2016. *Legal Aspects of Health Care Administration*, 12th ed. Sudbury, MA: Jones and Bartlett.

Premier Advisor Live. 2011. Compliance with revenue audits: RACS, MACS, MICS and ZPICs. http://www.premierinc.com/advisorlive/Presentations/rac011211.pdf.

Reynolds, R. and E. Bowman (eds). 2016. *Tennessee Health Information Management Association Handbook*. THIMA Legislative Committee. Nashville, TN: THIMA. http://www.thima.org/resources/legal/.

Roach, W., R. Hoban, B. Broccolo, A. Roth, and T. Blanchard. 2006. *Medical Records and the Law*, 4th ed. Sudbury, MA: Jones and Bartlett.

Hanlon, C., K. Sheedy, T. Kniffin, and J. Rosenthal. 2015. 2014 guide to state adverse event reporting systems. National Academy for State Health Policy. http://www.nashp.org/sites/default/files/2014_Guide_to_State_Adverse_Event_Reporting_Systems.pdf.

Stiegel, L. 2015. Template for state-specific adaption of legal issues related to elder abuse. A Desk guide for law enforcement. American Bar Association Commission on Law and Aging. http://www.americanbar.org.

Wisconsin Department of Health Services. 2016. Wisconsin Immunization Registry. http://www.dhs.wisconsin.gov.

WorkersCompensation.com. 2016. Workers' compensation: The workers' comp service center. http://www.workerscompensation.com.

Cases, Statutes, and Regulations Cited

10 CFR 35.3045: Report and notification of a medical event. 2003.

29 CFR 1904.0: Purpose. 2001.

29 CFR 1904.7(a): Recording and reporting occupational injuries and illness; Recordkeeping forms and recording criteria, basic requirements. 2001.

42 CFR 482.13(g): Standard: Death reporting requirements. 2012.

42 CFR 482.45: Organ, tissue, and eye. 1998.

42 CFR 483.374: Facility reporting. 2001.

45 CFR 160.203: General rules and exceptions. 2002.

45 CFR 164.502(b)(2)(iv): Uses and disclosures of protected health information. 2002.

45 CFR 164.508: Uses and disclosures for which an authorization is required. 2002.

45 CFR 164.512(a): Uses and disclosures required by law. 2002.

45 CFR 164.512(b): Uses and disclosures for public health activity. 2002.

45 CFR 164.512(c): Abuse, neglect, and domestic violence. 2002.

45 CFR 164.512(d): Health oversight activities.

45 CFR 164.512(e): Judicial and administrative proceedings.

45 CFR 164.512(f): Law enforcement purposes.

45 CFR 164.512(g): Decedents.

45 CFR 164.512(h): Cadaveric organ, eye, or tissue donation.

45 CFR 164.512(i): Research purposes.

45 CFR 164.512(j): Avert a serious threat to health or safety.

45 CFR 164.512(k): Specialized government functions.

45 CFR 164.512(l): Workers' compensation.

45 CFR 164.520: Notice of privacy practices for protected health information. 2002.

21 USC 360i(b): Records and reports on devices; general rule.

42 USC 1301, 1128E: Health Care and Abuse Data Collection Program.

42 USC 11133(a)(1): Reporting of certain professional review actions by healthcare entities. 1986.

42 USC 3002: The Older Americans Act. 2006.

42 USC 5101 et seq.: Child Abuse Prevention and Treatment Act. 1996

42 USC 5101§3: CAPTA Reauthorization Act. 2010.

42 USCA 5106g(4): CAPTA Reauthorization Act. 2010.

AL Code 38-9-8: Reports by physicians of physical, sexual, or emotional abuse, neglect or exploitation. 2000.

FL Stat. Ann. 415.101 et seq.: Adult Protective Services Act. 2004.

MS Code 41-61-53: Reporting cases of disease. 1986.

OH Admin. Code 3701-3-08: Release of patient's records. 2009.

ORC 3701.262: Cancer incidence surveillance system rules. 2013.

S.192 Older Americans Reauthorization Act of 2016. Public Law 114-144.

TN Code Ann. 68-10-113: Sexually transmitted diseases, confidentiality of information. 1992.

TN Code Ann. 68-11-259: Establishing a trauma registry, compliance, confidentiality. 2005.

TN Code Ann. 68-55-101: Head and spinal cord injury information system, chapter definitions. 2015.

VT Stat. 18-6-107 5221: Fetal deaths. 1973.

Resources

Child Welfare Information Gateway. State statutes search, https://www.childwelfare.gov/survey/.

National Center on Elder Abuse. Administration on Aging. State Resources. Department of Health and Human Services. http://www.ncea.aoa.gov/Stop_Abuse/Get_Help/State/index.aspx.

National Institutes of Health. List of registries. https://www.nih.gov/health-information/nih-clinical-research -trials-you/list-registries.

New York County District Attorney Office. 2013 Nationwide Survey of Mandatory Reporting Requirements for Elderly and/or Vulnerable Persons. http://www.napsa-now.org/wp-content/uploads/2014/11/Mandatory -Reporting-Chart-Updated-FINAL.pdf.

Risk Management, Quality Improvement, and Patient Safety

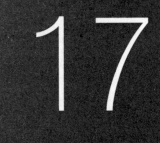

Chapter

17

Melanie S Brodnik, PhD, RHIA, FAHIMA and
Rebecca B. Reynolds, EdD, MHA, RHIA, CHPS, FAHIMA

Learning Objectives

- Distinguish between quality, quality improvement, risk management, and patient safety
- Contrast the typical steps one would find in a risk management program. and discuss the tools used in support of risk management activities
- Summarize the federal regulations and government initiatives in support of quality and patient safety
- Differentiate between the voluntary quality and patient safety reporting programs

Key Terms

- Adverse patient occurrences (APOs)
- Agency for Healthcare Research and Quality (AHRQ)
- Beneficiary and Family Centered-Quality Improvement Organizations (BFCC-QIOs)
- Captain of the ship
- Center for Quality Improvement and Patient Safety (CQuiPS)
- Charitable immunity
- Claims management program
- Darling case
- Enterprise risk management

- Health Care Quality Improvement Act of 1986
- Healthcare Research and Quality Act of 1999
- Healthgrades
- Health Plan Report Card
- Incidents
- Leapfrog Group
- National Committee for Quality Assurance (NCQA)
- National Patient Safety Goals
- National Quality Strategy
- Near misses (or close calls)
- Occurrence screening
- Patient Protection and Affordable Care Act

- Patient safety
- Patient Safety and Quality Improvement Act of 2005
- Patient Safety Organization (PSO)
- Patient safety work product
- Peer Review Organizations (PROs)
- Professional Standards Review Organizations (PSROs)
- Quality
- QualityCheck.org
- Quality improvement
- Quality Improvement Organizations (QIOs)

- Quality Innovation Network-Quality Improvement Organization (QIN-QIOs)
- Report cards
- Risk analysis
- Risk and opportunity identification
- Risk control techniques
- Risk evaluation
- Risk financing
- Risk management
- Risk treatment
- Root cause analysis
- Sentinel events
- Unsafe conditions

No matter whom is asked—patients, providers, administrators, employers, scientists, or policymakers—everyone shares an interest in healthcare quality. However, depending on the individual, quality can mean different things to different people. From a patient's perspective, quality can mean, "Did I get better after I went to the doctor?" whereas a provider might ask, "Did the patient get the right intervention at the right time?" An administrator may want to know, "Has our facility met all the required quality standards for accreditation?" while an employer may wonder, "Have I provided my employees with health plans that will provide preventive care and reduce sick days?" A scientist may want to know, "How does this new technology produce better results than the existing technology and is it safe?" while a policymaker might ask, "How do we make sure patients are protected from harm or death as a result of the care they receive? Whichever way healthcare quality is perceived it basically means, "doing the right thing, at the right time, in the right way, for the right person - and having the right results" (AHRQ n.d.c). Healthcare quality affects lives, and directly and indirectly impacts healthcare costs.

Overall, the cost of medical errors, and liability insurance used by organizations to protect against financial loss related to medical errors and other types of negligence increased significantly during the 1980s through the 1990s. By 2002, one-third of hospitals experienced an increase of 100 percent or more in liability insurance premiums and over one-fourth of hospitals reported a reduction or complete discontinuation of a service as a result of increasing liability premiums (*Journal of Healthcare Risk Management* 2007). Since 2002, efforts to address the malpractice crisis as discussed in chapter 6 along with an increased focus on quality improvement, patient safety and risk management efforts have resulted in a decline of approximately 4.5 percent per year of adverse effects among hospitalized patients (Kronick et al. 2016). In addition, there has been a savings of $12 billion in Medicare spending as result of these efforts (HHS 2015). Much has been done over the last 40 years to advance quality healthcare while reducing the cost associated with delivering care, however, more still needs to be done.

At the heart of advancing positive patient outcomes and reducing the costs associated with poor quality care are the interrelated concepts of risk management, quality improvement, and patient safety. This chapter will discuss the evolution of these concepts, including the legal and regulatory implications that support safe, efficient, quality patient care.

Differences between Quality, Risk Management, Quality Improvement, and Patient Safety

Before addressing risk management and quality improvement, it is important to understand the meaning of healthcare **quality**. In short, "quality healthcare means doing the right thing, at the right time, in the right way, for the right person—and having the best possible results" (AHRQ n.d.c). **Quality improvement** refers to the overall processes a facility has in place to make sure healthcare is safe, effective, patient-centered, timely, efficient, and equitable. Quality improvement is sometimes referred to as quality management. In comparison, healthcare **risk management** refers to the processes in place to identify, evaluate, and control risk to minimize potential for patient harm (AHIMA 2014). Risks may be operational, financial, human, strategic, legal/regulatory or technological (ASHRM 2014b). Although quality improvement and risk management programs may have different roles their goal is the same: **patient safety**. Both strive to make patient care "continually safer by reducing harm and preventable mortality" (IHI 2016).

From a clinical standpoint, there is an inter-relationship between quality improvement and risk management that stems from similarities in their underlying processes. By implementing effective quality improvement processes, an organization increases its chances of improved clinical outcomes and decreases its chances of unexpected financial loss associated with poor outcomes. Additionally, by implementing effective risk management processes, an organization reduces its chances of financial loss from unplanned or unexpected events and promotes good clinical outcomes.

Quality improvement and risk management programs have evolved concurrently over the past 40 years. An effective quality and risk management program is focused on improving the quality and safety of patient care. It incorporates the identification, analysis, evaluation, and elimination or reduction of possible risks to the institution's patients, visitors, and employees. The quality improvement or management department may have responsibility for the risk management program or the in-house legal department may handle risk management. In larger organizations, these functions may operate as separate departments.

Departments such as health information management (HIM) may assist with quality or risk program efforts by performing, for example, occurrence screening. This entails analyzing records for evidence of unplanned or unexpected events. HIM departments may also assist various quality or risk management committees with follow-up activities.

Check Your Understanding 17.1

Instructions: Indicate whether the following statements are true or false (T or F).

1. Occurrence screening refers to analyzing records for evidence of unplanned or unexpected events.
2. Patient safety is the ultimate goal of quality improvement and risk management activities.
3. Risks are always isolated and remain confined to one area.

Risk Management

According to the American Society for Healthcare Risk Management, risk management is defined as

A systematic and scientific approach...to identify, evaluate, reduce or eliminate the possibility of an unfavorable deviation from expectation and thus, to prevent the loss of financial assets, resulting from injury to patients, visitors, employees, independent medical staff, or from damage, theft or loss of property belonging to the healthcare entity or persons mentioned. (ASHRM 2003)

The risk of financial liability can be found in many situations: a nurse may administer the incorrect dose of a medication, a hospital visitor may slip and fall on a freshly mopped surface, or a natural disaster may destroy patient records. If an organization is ordered to pay damages in a negligence case or fines in an agency enforcement action, it has incurred this kind of financial liability. In other words, its financial liability has arisen from unplanned, accidental events.

To protect from such events, ASRHM suggests implementing an **enterprise risk management (ERM)** approach, which is a structured process that focuses on identifying and eliminating the financial impact and volatility of a portfolio of risks rather than on risk avoidance alone (ASHRM 2014a). ERM is important in healthcare because risks are not isolated and risks in one area can easily and often impact other departments and the organization overall (ASHRM 2014a). ERM varies from traditional risk management by looking at the probability that adverse events will occur and what the liability might be.

For example, a large integrated healthcare systems enterprise risk management program manages risk through its compliance committee and HIPAA program. A risk tool is used to score risk items. The tool takes into consideration inherent risks, likelihood of risk, and controls to determine residual risk. Through reporting and environmental assessments presented to the compliance committee, potential events are identified that may affect the medical center and determine residual risks. The committee votes to either accept the risk or take action to address the risk. A similar risk assessment process is followed for all the information systems used to address HIPAA security. Scores are determined based on risk, which the Privacy and Security Officer and Committee, along with the HIPAA Steering Committee determine to accept the risk or implement action to address the risk. In the past, healthcare providers such as hospitals were not concerned with financial loss as a result of legal protection, such as the doctrine of charitable immunity, discussed below.

Background

Historically, as charitable institutions, early hospitals were shielded from liability for negligence by the doctrine of **charitable immunity** as discussed in chapter 6. The rationale for charitable immunity was grounded in the belief that donors would not make contributions to hospitals if they thought their donation would be used to litigate claims, combined with concern that a few lawsuits could bankrupt a hospital. Hospitals were also protected by early "**captain of the ship**" case law holding physicians solely responsible for all aspects of the patient's care, including care provided by hospital staff. The role of the hospital was simply to provide a place for the physician to conduct his treatment—any negligence associated with that treatment was the responsibility of the physician.

Over the years, the doctrine of charitable immunity was eliminated by state legislatures and case law, and the door to hospital liability was opened. The 1965 **Darling case**—*Darling v. Charleston Community Memorial Hospital*—is often credited as the landmark case for extending liability for negligence to hospitals. In that case, the plaintiff's broken leg had to be amputated after the hospital failed to notice that it had become gangrenous underneath the cast. In reviewing the case, the Illinois Supreme Court recognized that hospitals had evolved beyond simply furnishing facilities for treatment. Specifically, the court acknowledged that hospitals "regularly employ on a salary basis a large staff of physicians, nurses and interns, as well as administrative and manual workers, and they charge patients for medical care and treatment, collecting for such services, if necessary, by legal action." The court also noted, "The Standards for Hospital Accreditation, the state licensing regulations and the defendant's bylaws demonstrate that the medical profession and other responsible authorities regard it as both desirable and feasible that a hospital assume certain responsibilities for the care of the patient." The court ultimately determined that it was reasonable to conclude that the hospital itself was negligent when it failed to have adequate nursing staff capable of recognizing the progressive gangrenous condition of the plaintiff's leg and when it failed to require consultation of the plaintiff's condition by members of the hospital's surgical staff with expertise in the plaintiff's condition. After the *Darling* case and other "pro-plaintiff" changes in the law, the frequency and severity of malpractice claims increased dramatically in the early 1970s, as discussed in chapter 6 (Danzon 1982). At the same time, many major malpractice insurers left the insurance market and insurance rates for physicians and hospitals significantly increased. Some physicians and hospitals found it difficult, if not impossible, to obtain malpractice insurance (Mello et al. 2003). The resulting financial pressure led hospitals to explore the need to develop and implement risk management programs in order to control their risk of financial loss (ASHRM 2005).

By 1980, ASHRM (2005) provided a national voice for risk managers and guidance for organizing risk management programs, identifying risk, and gaining provider involvement in risk management programs, and continues to do so today. By the mid-1980s, lawsuits against hospitals for corporate negligence were increasing. As a result, state legislatures began passing laws requiring hospitals to implement risk management programs. During the late 1980s, the Joint Commission established its first standards for the loss control and prevention components of risk management programs (*Journal of Healthcare Risk Management* 1992).

Since the early years, the field of risk management has continued to evolve with the changing healthcare environment. Today, risk management programs are closely aligned or integrated with patient safety and quality activities. Risk management functions may now assume a more enterprise-wide approach to protecting the financial assets and reputation of an organization while preventing harm to patients, employees and others (ECRI 2014).

Organization and Operation of Risk Management

Although standards for patient quality are found in both federal and state law and accreditation standards, risk management programs are most commonly governed by state law. State law defines the minimum scope and components of a risk management program, as well as any applicable certification standards for risk management professionals. Most of these laws identify risk in terms of incidents of actual harm or reasonable likelihood of harm to a patient resulting from substandard care, medical errors, or impaired providers. States generally require risk management programs to include a system for the investigation and analysis of the frequency and causes of incidents, measures to minimize the occurrence of incidents and their resulting injuries, and a formalized reporting system for reporting incidents to a designated individual (for example, risk manager, chief of staff, or chief administrator) (KS Stat. Ann. 65-4922).

Many healthcare facilities have risk management programs that encompass more than the baseline patient-safety aspects required by state law and include areas such as billing compliance, privacy compliance, and workplace safety. Regardless of its scope, any enterprise risk management program must be integrated throughout the organization and have support from top executives.

Steps

The steps of risk management can vary depending on the type of risk being addressed. For example, the specific steps taken to monitor, investigate, and prevent medication errors will be different than those steps taken to monitor, investigate, and prevent patient falls. However, from a broader perspective, an integrated enterprise-wide risk management program should consist of at least four key components (see figure 17.1).

Risk Identification

Risk identification refers to a systematic means of identifying potential risks. The process should include a review of adverse events, committee reports, root cause analysis, patient satisfaction surveys and various other tools. These risks should be compiled on a risk list that is maintained to capture potential risks to the organization. After the risk list is developed, the next step is to categorize the risks into domains.

Figure 17.1 The integrated enterprise-wide risk management program

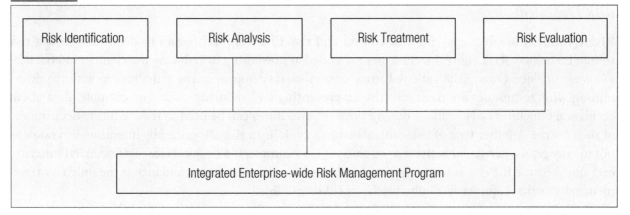

Source: Adapted from ASHRM 2014a.

ASHRM identifies eight domain areas which include operational, clinical or patient safety, strategic, financial, human capital, legal/regulatory, technology and hazard (ASHRM 2014a, b). Next, risk drivers for each domain should be identified. The focus should be on identification of risks that are likely to occur with an understanding that it is not likely that all risks can be predicted. There will be some risks that may have a low probability of occurrence but a catastrophic impact.

An additional method for identifying risk is **occurrence screening**, defined in the Joint Commission Sentinel Event Glossary of Terms as

> A system for concurrent or retrospective identification of **adverse patient occurrences** (APOs) through medical chart-based review according to objective screening criteria. Examples of criteria include admission for adverse results of outpatient management, readmission for complications, incomplete management of problems on previous hospitalization, or unplanned removal, injury, or repair of an organ or structure during surgery. (Joint Commission 2016a)

In addition to the Joint Commission standards, ASHRM also suggests that organizations define categories of preventable harm and establish common definitions for variations in care. These include pre-patient events, safety events and serious safety events (SSE). A SSE can occur in any healthcare setting as a "deviation from generally-accepted practice or process that reaches the patient and causes severe harm or death" (ASHRM 2012). ASHRM offers a two-part white paper on SSEs called "Getting to Zero" which is designed to eliminate harm from delivery of care and provide guidance in designing harm classification systems and scales (ASHRM 2012, 2014c).

Risk Analysis

Risk analysis involves the process of identifying which risks should be proactively addressed and which risks are lower in priority. ASHRM recommends that each level of safety event be expanded and the level of harm from death to almost happened, be defined as well as a suggested follow-up analysis for each category and level of harm be developed (ASHRM 2014a). ASHRM also recommends that follow-up analysis include root cause analysis, common cause analysis, error detection analysis, and culpability/accountability review. The white paper contains a guide for organizations to develop a risk analysis.

Risk Treatment

Risk treatment involves applying risk control and risk financing techniques to determine how a risk should be treated. **Risk control techniques** are aimed at preventing or reducing the chances or effects of a loss occurrence. Often, data gathered from internal quality improvement activities can assist in determining what techniques are most effective in preventing and reducing risks. For example, data about accidental punctures or lacerations during surgical procedures can be used to reduce future occurrences of such events. Another type of risk control involves avoiding a risk altogether by intentionally choosing not to engage in a particular activity or operation. For example, if a hospital closes its neonatal intensive care unit because the risk is too high, risk avoidance has occurred. Risk avoidance is the only risk treatment activity that completely eliminates the possibility of loss.

Risk financing refers to the methods used to pay for the costs associated with claims and other expenses. The most common form of risk financing is the purchase of liability insurance. Simply stated, liability insurance is a contract requiring the insurer to pay for certain losses sustained by the insured in exchange for a premium. In today's market, it can be difficult for individuals and organizations to use liability insurance to finance risk because insurance may be completely unavailable or too expensive.

Risk Evaluation

Risk evaluation involves evaluating each piece of the process in order to determine whether objectives are being met. For example, in evaluating the risk identification step, the following questions should be asked: Have exposures been missed in the identification activity? If so, why? What adjustments are necessary to improve this phase? Is useful data being gathered? Are exposures being updated with other current data input? (ASHRM 2014a)

In evaluating risk analysis, the following questions are suggested: Does the analysis capture important quantitative data and consider important qualitative issues? Is the analysis being used to make decisions on risk treatment? With respect to the evaluation of risk treatment, suggested questions are: Are risk control and financing methods used for each exposure type? Are exposures actually evaluated to determine which treatment methods are appropriate? What are the current insurance market conditions concerning the availability and cost of insurance coverage?

Tools Supporting Risk Management

Any time an adverse event occurs at a facility, the potential exists for financial loss as well as damage to the facility's reputation. Risk management programs may use a variety of tools, such as risk assessment tools. For example, when designed and implemented effectively, a **claims management program** can help prevent or reduce financial loss in the occurrence of an adverse event. Claims management generally requires knowledge about a facility's insurance policies, a system to identify potential loss quickly, and the ability to accurately estimate potential liability.

Incident Reports

An incident report is an important tool that assists risk managers with identifying and responding to adverse events and other patient safety events or occurrences that are inconsistent with the standard of care (figure 17.2). As discussed in chapter 5, incident reporting serves to:

- Describe the unexpected occurrence or incident
- Provide the foundation for an investigation of the occurrence or incident
- Provide information necessary for taking remedial or corrective action
- Provide data useful for identifying risks of future similar occurrences (Dunn 2003, 49)

Incident reports may serve as key evidence in litigation proceedings. As a risk management tool, it is important that employees understand when to fill out incident reports and what information should be included in those reports (figure 17.3). Event reporting should be part of a facility's culture that also includes policies identifying which patient safety events or errors should be reported and to whom as well as the steps required to complete incident reporting. Generally, incidents should be documented by the individual(s) who witnessed the event or who were involved in the occurrence as soon as reasonably possible after an event (Dunn 2003). Documentation of incidents should be objective and concise and only present the facts of a situation. Helpful questions to ask include "the five Ws":

1. What? Describe what happened in detail.

2. When? Give the date and time of the incident.

3. Where? Describe the incident's location.

4. Who? Tell who did what to whom and who witnessed the incident.

5. Why? Did equipment fail? Did someone fail to perform a certain test? (Dunn 2003)

Figure 17.2 Incident reporting process

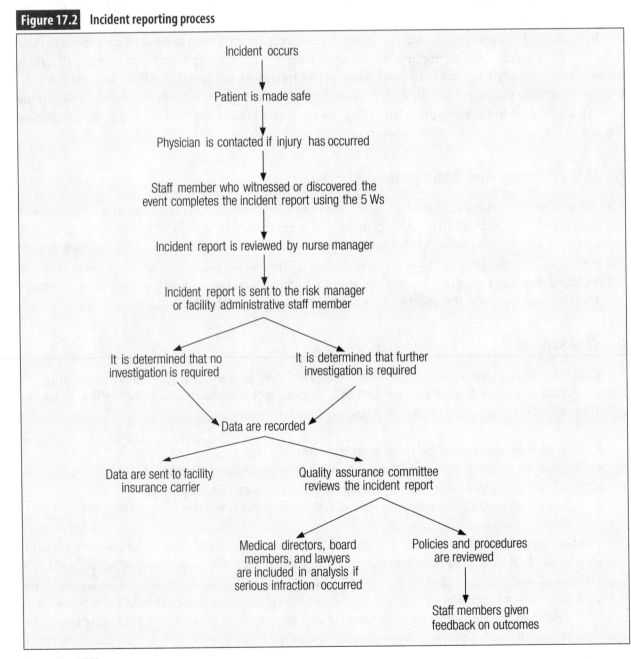

Source: Dunn 2003.

Figure 17.3	Data to be included in incident reports

Patient data	• Monitors in use
• Age	• Patient diagnosis and condition
• Medical record number	• Physician's examination data, if appropriate, and signature with date
• Patient name	• Physiological consequences
Event data	• Reason for hospitalization, if appropriate
• Bed rail status	• Signature of person completing report with date
• Condition of individuals involved	• Manager of department
• Date and time of event	• Person completing report
• Description of occurrence by observer	• Physician
• Equipment in use	• Witnesses
• Exact location of event	• Follow-up data
• Identification of causative and contributing factors (for example, staffing patterns, experience level of staff members, fatigue, complexity of patient management)	• Classification section for retrieval, trend analysis, and future outcomes and recommendations for prevention
• Medical and nursing personnel present	• Section for evaluation and follow-up of patient harm

Source: Dunn 2003.

Some organizations choose to restrict incident reporting to the first four questions, and to leave the "why" question to the subsequent investigation of the incident. This often occurs in states where incident reports are not well protected from discovery. However, in some states they are protected by regulation. This usually occurs when regulations also require reporting of incidents or adverse events (see figure 17.4). Since incident reports are considered privileged communication, they are not part of or filed in the patient's record but kept separately in a private location usually managed by risk management.

Health Records and Risk Management

The health record plays a key role in risk management and quality improvement efforts in that information in the record may be used to determine whether there has been a deviation from the standard of care, the extent of a party's injuries, and what may have caused those injuries. The record becomes a tool of proof of care. After an adverse event, the record should be sequestered in a secure place and its access monitored in order to prevent any tampering with the record contents. In the case of electronic records, user rights to edit a record may need to be suspended. Such a process may help alleviate the risk that documentation in the patient records was altered, stolen, clarified or tampered with in any way. Alterations or clarifications of health records can cast a shadow of fault over a facility and should be prevented.

No matter how high the quality of care actually provided, poor health record documentation practices can give the appearance of poor quality care. The integrity of documentation is extremely important and, in many provider organizations, is supported through clinical documentation improvement (CDI) activities. Thus, it is critical for all staff (including providers, risk managers, and HIM and informatics professionals) to recognize good and poor documentation practices and understand what constitutes the organizations legal health record as discussed in chapter 9.

Figure 17.4 Tennessee health data reporting act of 2002 (unusual events reporting)

Tennessee Health Data Reporting Act of 2002 (Unusual Events Reporting) requires that the affected patient and the patient's family, as appropriate, be notified of if an incident has occurred (TN Code Ann. 68-11-211). The law requires hospitals and other healthcare facilities to report unusual events within seven days to the Department of Health and provide a correction notice report. Tennessee law defines an unusual event as, "An unusual event is an unexpected occurrence or accident resulting in death, life-threatening or serious injury to a patient that is not related to a natural course of the patient's illness or underlying condition. An unusual event also includes an incident resulting in the abuse of a patient." The law also provides protection for reporting events. According to the law, the information received in event reports and corrective action plans is considered confidential and is not subject to subpoenas or discovery or admissible in any civil or administrative proceeding other than disciplinary proceedings by the Department of Health or regulatory board (TN Code Ann 68-11-211).

Source: TN Code Ann 68-11-211.

Peer Review and National Practitioner Data Bank

Two other tools used by risk management programs relate to peer review records and the National Practitioner Data Bank (NPDB). The **Health Care Quality Improvement Act of 1986,** as it relates to peer review records discussed in chapter 16, ensures that a facility has sufficient information to evaluate and monitor the professional qualifications and practice of healthcare providers. Facilities must report adverse actions (such as suspensions of privileges) lasting more than 30 days, medical malpractice payments, and settlement reports to the NPDB. As discussed in chapter 19, when evaluating a provider's application for staff privileges, the facility must query the data bank, and every two years thereafter to ensure no problems have arisen with the provider's performance that may jeopardize quality of care and patient safety.

Check Your Understanding   17.2

Instructions: Indicate whether the following statements are true or false (T or F).

1. Hospitals were exonerated from liability as a result of the Darling vs. Charleston landmark case.
2. Risk management programs are most commonly governed by state law.
3. A risk and opportunity identification process is very useful since it can predict all risks an organization may be exposed to.
4. A claims management program can help prevent financial loss if an adverse event occurs.
5. An incident report should be completed by an individual who was involved or witnessed the event.
6. Hospitals may choose to contact the NPDB when reviewing an individual's credential for staff privileges.

The Joint Commission - Quality and Patient Safety

The Joint Commission (formally the Joint Commission on Accreditation of Hospitals) was founded in 1951 to accredit hospitals that met minimum health and safety standards. Today it offers a variety of accreditation and certification programs designed to continuously improve the safety and quality of care provided to the public. Currently, the Joint Commission evaluates and accredits or certifies more than 21 thousand healthcare organizations and programs in the United States, covering the following service areas:

- ambulatory health care
- behavioral health care

- critical access hospital
- disease-specific care
- home care
- hospital
- laboratory services
- nursing care center
- office-based surgery (The Joint Commission 2016a)

The Joint Commission accreditation standards are designed to address an organization's level of performance in specific functional areas, such as patient safety, patient treatment, and infection control (Joint Commission 2016a). In 1979, the Joint Commission quality assurance standard required select hospital departments to conduct at least four medical record audits a year. Data from these audits were used to validate the quality of care patients received, and to correct problems if found. Subsequently, in 1984, the Commission strengthened the quality functions in hospitals with its Quality and Monitoring Standard.

An important aspect of the Joint Commission's focus on quality was its policy on sentinel events. The policy was originally adopted in 1996 and updated in 2014 to help hospitals and other healthcare organizations, to learn from their adverse events and improve patient safety. Adverse events were identified as **sentinel events** and defined as

> a patient safety event that reaches a patient and result in any of the following: death, permanent harm or sever temporary harm and intervention required to sustain life. Such events are called "sentinel" because they signal the need for immediate investigation and response (Joint Commission 2016c).

It is important to note that sentinel events and medical errors are not the same thing. Not all sentinel events occur because of a medical error and not all medical errors result in sentinel events (Joint Commission 2013). The Joint Commission website contains a sentinel events glossary of terms that should be referenced to avoid confusion and potential miscommunication about these terms.

The goals of the Joint Commission policy are to have a positive impact in improving patient care by focusing the attention of an organization such as a hospital that has experienced a sentinel event on understanding the causes that underlie the event and on making changes in the organization's systems and processes to reduce the probability of such an event in the future as well as to increase the general knowledge about sentinel events, their causes, and strategies for prevention.

The Joint Commission organizes sentinel events into reviewable and non-reviewable categories. Reviewable events include the following:

- The event has resulted in an unanticipated death or major permanent loss of function, not related to the natural course of the patient's illness or underlying condition
- The event was one of the following (even if the outcome was not death or major permanent loss of function unrelated to the patient's illness or underlying condition):
  - Suicide of any patient receiving care, treatment, and services in a staffed around-the-clock care setting or within 72 hours of discharge, including from the hospital's emergency department (ED)
  - Abduction of any patient receiving care, treatment, and services

- Any elopement (that is, unauthorized departure) of a patient from a staffed around the-clock care setting (including the ED), leading to death, permanent harm, or severe temporary harm to the patient
- Hemolytic transfusion reaction involving administration of blood or blood products having major blood group incompatibilities (ABO, Rh, other blood groups)
- Rape, assault (leading to death, permanent harm, or severe temporary harm), or homicide of a staff member, licensed independent practitioner, visitor, or vendor while on site at the hospital
- Invasive procedure, including surgery, on the wrong patient, at the wrong site, or that is the wrong (unintended) procedure
- Unintended retention of a foreign object in a patient after an invasive procedure, including surgery
- Severe neonatal hyperbilirubinemia (bilirubin >30 milligrams/deciliter)
- Prolonged fluoroscopy with cumulative dose >1,500 rads to a single field or any delivery of radiotherapy to the wrong body region or >25 percent above the planned radiotherapy dose
- Fire, flame, or unanticipated smoke, heat, or flashes occurring during an episode of patient care
- Unanticipated death of a full-term infant
- Discharge of an infant to the wrong family
- Any intrapartum (related to the birth process) maternal death
- Severe maternal morbidity (Joint Commission 2013)

The Joint Commission categorizes "near misses" and other specific events as non-reviewable but an organization may still evaluate such events as part of its performance improvement activities.

The Joint Commission accreditation standards require that a healthcare organization has an organization-wide, integrated patient safety program as part of the organizations performance improvement activities. The program must relate to the management of sentinel events. Each organization must develop its own definition of a sentinel event for purposes of establishing procedures for identifying, reporting, and managing these events. While the organization's overall definition of *sentinel event* must be consistent with that of the Joint Commission, it can tailor specific terms such as *unexpected*, *serious*, and *the risk thereof* to its own needs (Joint Commission 2013).

Second, organizations are expected to identify and respond appropriately to all sentinel events. This involves conducting a comprehensive systematic analysis, developing an action plan, implementing improvements, and monitoring the effectiveness of those improvements. Organizations are encouraged to use the process of **root cause analysis** (RCA) to investigate sentinel events (Joint Commission 2016e). This process refers to a structured method of identifying the physical, human or organizational causes of an event, how the causes contributed to the event, and developing a process to prevent reoccurrence of the event (NPSF 2016).

Accredited organizations are not required, but are highly encouraged to, self-report sentinel events to The Joint Commission. The deidentified data collected is added to the Joint Commission's Sentinel Event Database. The database is used to provide information on the type and frequency of sentinel events, and root causes along with lessons learned. Information from that database is shared through the Commission's patient safety newsletter, *Sentinel Event Alert* (Joint Commission Perspective 2014). The Joint Commission regularly reports sentinel event statistics on a quarterly basis. For example, in the first two quarters of 2016, 439 sentinel events were reported with unintended retained foreign bodies and falls representing the most frequently reported events (AHRQ 2016).

The Joint Commission Safety Goals

Each year, the Joint Commission publishes **National Patient Safety Goals** designed to improve patient safety in specific healthcare areas identified as problematic. These goals and corresponding requirements for meeting those goals are primarily based on informal recommendations made in the *Sentinel Event Alert* and information from the Joint Commission's sentinel event database. Specific goals and requirements are developed by the Sentinel Event Advisory Group. As part of the accreditation process, organizations are evaluated for their compliance with specific requirements related to patient safety goals applicable to their setting (Joint Commission 2016c). The National Patient Safety Goals for various organizations can be found on the Joint Commission website. The 2016 National Patient Safety Goals for hospitals includes many requirements that support proper documentation, including the following:

- Use at least two patient identifiers (neither to be the patient's room number) whenever administering medications or blood products, taking blood samples and other specimens for clinical testing, or providing any other treatments or procedures
- Prior to the start of any invasive procedure, conduct a final verification process (such as a "time out") to confirm the correct patient, procedure, and site using active—not passive—communication techniques
- Improve the effectiveness of communication among caregivers. For verbal or telephone orders or for telephonic reporting of critical test results, verify the complete order or test result by having the person receiving the order or test result "read-back" the complete order or test result
- Standardize a list of abbreviations, acronyms, and symbols that are not to be used throughout the organization
- Measure, assess and, if appropriate, take action to improve the timeliness of reporting, and the timeliness of receipt by the responsible licensed caregiver, of critical test results and values (Joint Commission 2016c)

Check Your Understanding 17.3

Instructions: Indicate whether the following statements are true or false (T or F).

1. A non-reviewable sentinel event would be the suicide of a patient with 72 hours of discharge from a facility.
2. A root cause analysis process includes developing a process to prevent reoccurrence of the event.
3. Joint Commission–accredited organizations are expected to have an organization wide, integrated patient safety program.
4. Organizations are encouraged to self-report sentinel events to the Joint Commissions Sentinel Event Database.
5. The Joint Commission Patient Safety Goals include many requirements that support the significance of proper clinical documentation.

Quality Improvement and Patient Safety

Efforts to address quality improvement in healthcare were originally driven by The Joint Commission in the early 1960s, with its subsequent focus on patient safety in the last 20 years. The federal government's focus on quality and patient safety began in 1965 when the government became a major player in the financing of healthcare services for the elderly, disabled, and poor. Passage of Public Law 89-97,

Title XVIII Medicare and Title XIX Medicaid of the Social Security Act (42 USC 1395; 1396) in 1965 set forth minimum health and safety standards for hospital participating in Medicare. If a hospital met Joint Commission standards then they were deemed to have met the Conditions of Participation required by Medicare.

In 1972, Congress amended the Social Security Act to establish **Professional Standards Review Organizations (PSROs)** to ensure that hospital services for Medicare and Medicaid patients were medically necessary and appropriate (Sprague 2002). PSROs conducted utilization reviews to justify hospital admissions and to lower patient lengths of stay as one method of reducing healthcare costs for the government. This process often involved policing providers and punishing those deemed not in compliance with applicable standards of care. Under the PSRO system, physicians were allowed to review cases involving their own colleagues and competitors. PSROs also supported the Joint Commission's requirement for hospitals to conduct performance audits which the PSROs called medical quality reviews. In 1979, the Joint Commission implemented a quality assurance standard which eventually resulted in the establishment of quality departments in US hospitals and shortly thereafter, risk management departments (Joint Commission 2015).

In 1982, under the Medicare Utilization and Quality Care Program, Congress replaced PSROs with 54 **Peer Review Organizations (PROs)**. Under the Centers for Medicare and Medicaid (CMS), the PROs statement of work (SOW) required the PROs to continue to conduct utilization review of hospital services and review of medical necessity of care. Peer review activities were revised, and reviewing physicians were restricted from reviewing local colleagues or competitors to prevent conflicts of interest (Sprague 2002). From its inception until 2001 the PROs SOWs have focused on a collaborative relationship with providers to create cooperative programs for improving healthcare.

By the mid 1980s, most hospitals had established formal quality improvement and risk management departments to fulfill Joint Commission standards, adhere to federal government quality requirements and address rising malpractice issues. As mentioned earlier in 1986, Congress passed the Health Care Quality Act which offers individuals legal immunity for participating in peer review activities. The Act also established standards and requirements for peer review processes and established the **National Practitioner Data Bank (NPDB)** as discussed previously in this chapter and in chapter 16.

While much had been accomplished to address quality and risk concerns throughout the 1980s and 90s, it wasn't until the 1999 Health and Medicine Division of the National Academies of Sciences, Engineering, and Medicine (formerly Institute of Medicine or IOM) sentinel report, *To Err is Human: Building a Safer Health Systems*, that patient safety took center stage. The report stated that there were many preventable errors causing patients deaths and that the industry should do more to prevent such errors. The report called for better analysis of errors and near misses and the need to build safety into processes of care as a way to reduce errors (IOM 1999). Subsequently, in 2001, the IOM released a second report, *Crossing the Quality Chasm: A new Health System for the 21st Century*, which identified the need for healthcare to be safe, patient-centered, efficient, effective, equitable, and timely (IOM 2001). The report emphasized that reducing risk and ensuring safety requires processes in place that will help prevent and mitigate errors. Also, information on an organization's performance on safety and patient satisfaction should be transparent and made available to consumers, employers and government (IOM 2001). The reports recognized the importance of using health information technology to promote patient safety and prevent harm.

These two reports essentially laid the groundwork for the subsequent enactment of numerous federal, state and public-private initiatives to improve patient safety and quality care while reducing healthcare costs.

Government Focus on Patient Safety

To address the challenges identified in the IOM study Congress passed the **Healthcare Research and Quality Act of 1999** which created the federal **Agency for Healthcare Research and Quality (AHRQ)**. AHRQ's purpose was and still is to build private–public partnerships to conduct and support research to

- identify the causes of preventable healthcare errors and patient injury in healthcare delivery;
- develop, demonstrate, and evaluate strategies for reducing errors and improving patient safety; and
- disseminate such effective strategies throughout the healthcare industry (AHRQ 2012).

The **Center for Quality Improvement and Patient Safety (CQuiPS)** was established within AHRQ to oversee a number of quality and patient safety programs including the yearly publication of the National Healthcare Quality and Disparities Report Program. These reports share trends in patient safety, and data on quality and access to healthcare on a yearly basis (AHRQ 2012).

In 2001, the Department of Health and Human Services (HHS) and CMS launched a number of quality and patient safety initiatives such as renaming PROs, **Quality Improvement Organizations (QIOs)**, to better reflect the government's overall mission to work with healthcare providers to improve quality of healthcare (Sprague 2002). The QIOs' assumed responsibilities for providing specific consultation and quality improvement resources to a wide range of providers, including hospitals, physician practices, managed care organizations, and others (CMS 2016).

Many of the quality and patient safety efforts required the reporting and sharing of healthcare data as means of providing accountability and transparency of healthcare quality to the public. The Office of the National Coordinator for Health Information Technology (ONC) was created in 2004 to coordinate nationwide efforts to advance the use of health information technology (health IT) and electronic exchange of health information as one means of supporting quality and patient safety efforts (ONC 2016). Over the years, the ONC has addressed privacy and security concerns related to the electronic sharing of primary and secondary data for quality, patient safety and risk management. Under HIPAA and HITECH as discussed in chapters 10, 11, and 15, a covered entity (CE) can disclose protected health information (PHI) to another CE or CE's business associate (BA) for treatment and health care operations (ONC OCR 2016). Health care operations may include the following:

- Conducting quality assessment and improvement activities
- Conducting patient safety activities as defined in applicable regulations
- Conducting population-based activities relating to improving health or reducing healthcare cost
- Evaluating performance of healthcare providers and/or plans
- Supporting fraud and abuse detection and compliance programs (ONC OCR 2016)

Recognizing the importance of sharing data, in 2005, the **Patient Safety and Quality Improvement Act** (Pub. L. 109-41) was passed with an effective date of 2009. The goal of the **Patient Safety Rule** (42 CFR 3.102(b)(1)(i)) was to improve patient safety by encouraging clinicians and hospitals to voluntarily report their confidential quality and patient safety data on events that adversely affected patients. The rule gave AHRQ oversight responsibility for the creation and monitoring of **Patient Safety Organizations (PSOs)** which are public and private data organizations that collect, analyze, and aggregate patient safety data at the local, regional, and national levels. To facilitate data reporting of adverse events, AHRQ recommended two common formats: generic ones that apply to all patient safety events and event-specific ones that relate to certain high frequency event types. AHRQ further suggested that reportable patient safety events such as medication errors or hospital acquired infections include the following:

- **Incidents:** patient safety events that reached the patient, whether or not there was harm involved
- **Near misses (or close calls):** patient safety events that did not reach the patient
- **Unsafe conditions:** circumstances that increase the probability of a patient safety event occurring (AHRQ n.d.b)

Currently there are over 80 certified PSOs that collect, compile, analyze, and maintain confidential medical error information that is voluntarily reported by healthcare providers (AHRQ n.d.a). To encourage reporting and sharing of data, the Patient Safety Rule provides for confidential and privilege protections for hospitals and clinicians voluntarily reporting adverse events that affect patients. To protect information from discovery it must be identified as a **patient safety work product** which includes any data, reports, records or written or oral material developed by the provider or the PSO for patient safety purposes. The Office for Civil Rights (OCR) has responsibility for enforcing the confidentiality provisions of the Patient Safety Rule as it relates to PSOs (AHRQ n.d.a.). In addition, many states have enacted statutes that require providers to report data to the state related to adverse-events, monitoring, and investigation of patient safety problems as well.

In 2009, HITECH provided investment in the information systems infrastructure of hospitals, physician practices and clinics and strengthened aspects of the HIPAA Privacy Rule which enabled the sharing of PHI with other CEs or BAs. It created opportunities for QIOs to assist eligible providers in becoming meaningful users of HIT and EHRs, and to meet the requirements for submitting electronic clinical quality measures (eCQM) to required reporting programs as part of quality and patient safety efforts (CMS 2016).

In 2010, the **Patient Protection and Affordable Care Act (ACA)** was passed as a way to increase access to high-quality, affordable healthcare for all Americans (CMS 2016). The ACA implemented quality initiatives targeted to "avoid costly mistakes and readmissions, keep patients healthy, reward quality instead of quantity, and create a health information technology infrastructure that enables new payment and delivery models to work" (Sebelius 2013). A number of pay-for-performance programs have been implemented which reduces provider payments if required quality and patient safety measures are not met.

The ACA mandated that HHS establish a **National Quality Strategy (NQS)** to guide quality efforts. The Strategy was developed through a collaborative process that included hundreds of stakeholders and was published in 2011 (HHS 2011a). The strategy's three aims and six priorities (see figure 17.5) have guided HHS, CMS, and AHRQ program development related to improving the delivery of healthcare services, patient outcomes, and overall population health (AHRQ 2016).

As part of the NQS in 2014, CMS restructured the QIOs to enable innovation, foster learning organizations, eliminate disparities, and strengthen the health information infrastructure and data systems (CMS 2016). In the QIOs 11th SOW, the QIOs were reconfigured into two types: **Beneficiary and Family Centered-Quality Improvement Organizations (BFCC-QIOs)** and **Quality Innovation Network-Quality Improvement Organizations (QIN-QIOs).** The BFCC-QIOs perform the quality of care (medical case) reviews and medical necessity reviews. Two organizations have been identified who cover all 50 states and three territories to address Medicare beneficiaries' quality of care concerns and hear appeals from providers, patients and others. Fourteen QIN-QIOs have been identified who work with providers, stakeholders, and Medicare beneficiaries to improve patient safety, reduce harm, engage patients and families, and improve clinical care at the local and regional levels. The QIN-QIOs support advanced quality improvement and data analytical methods to accomplish four major goals:

Figure 17.5 HHS national quality strategy aims and priorities

AIMS

- Better Care: Improve the overall quality, by making health care more patient-centered, reliable, accessible, and safe.
- Healthy People/Healthy Communities: Improve the health of the U.S. population by supporting proven interventions to address behavioral, social and, environmental determinants of health in addition to delivering higher-quality care.
- Affordable Care: Reduce the cost of quality health care for individuals, families, employers, and government.

PRIORITIES

- Making care safer by reducing harm caused in the delivery of care.
- Ensuring that each person and family are engaged as partners in their care.
- Promoting effective communication and coordination of care.
- Promoting the most effective prevention and treatment practices for the leading causes of mortality, starting with cardiovascular disease.
- Working with communities to promote wide use of best practices to enable healthy living.
- Making quality care more affordable for individuals, families, employers, and governments by developing and spreading new health care delivery models.

Source: HHS 2011b

- Promote effective prevention and treatment of chronic disease by promoting safe care that is patient and family-centered, reliable and accessible
- Make care safer and reduce harm caused in the delivery of care
- Promote effective communication and coordination of care
- Make care more affordable (CMS 2016)

In 2016, CMS published its Quality Strategy fashioned after the NQS. Its Strategy focused on ways CMS pays providers to incentivize quality instead of quantity, ways to cut down on inefficiencies and over use of healthcare services, better use and access to data and health information technology for decision making, and innovative ways to communicate with providers and consumers to make care more person-centered (CMS 2016). CMS is using its Strategy to help align its initiatives to ensure high quality healthcare for everyone.

An important caveat to quality, risk management and patient efforts is the work ONC has been doing to ensure the use of health IT and EHRs are safe in and of themselves. There is no argument that health IT systems have improved patient safety. However, with the increased use of medical technology and health IT including EHRs concern for the safe use of the technology itself has risen. The literature has reported that adverse events have occurred as a result of malfunctioning and/or problems with application software. The ONC in collaboration with federal partners and other public-private stakeholders are working to "improve the safety and safe use of health IT as well as the use of health IT to improve patient safety" according to a number of available resources found on the ONC website (ONC n.d).

Reporting of Quality and Patient Safety Measures

Both government and private entities monitor healthcare quality and patient safety initiatives through required or voluntary reporting of quality measures. Data reported is shared through comparison sites or what some term as **report cards**. These sites are designed to empower consumers with more access to information on patient safety and quality measures. Table 16.2 in chapter 16 lists several of the required government reporting programs that have evolved over the last 20 years. In addition to these initiatives, there are several voluntary programs supported by groups that at times may be politically active and advocate for laws that support greater patient safety and quality improvement. Several of these voluntary programs are discussed below.

Healthgrades

Healthgrades is an independent organization online resource that provides profiles and ratings on numerous hospitals and physicians in the United States (Healthgrades 2016a). It obtains information from government and commercially available sources on provider organizations and physicians. Each year, Healthgrades publishes its list of America's 100 Best Hospitals, urging consumers to "do their homework when selecting hospitals…since not all hospitals perform equally" (Healthgrades 2016a). In addition, Healthgrades offers yearly awards that focus on patient experience and patient safety. The Outstanding Patient Experience Award is based on an evaluation of 14 patient experience measures from data collected from the Hospital Consumer Assessment of Healthcare Providers and Systems (HCAHPS) survey of hospital patients. The Award evaluates data from the occurrence of observed incidents and expected performance for select patient safety indicators as defined by AHRQ. In 2016, Healthgrades awarded 466 hospitals with the Patient Safety Award, indicating that "patient safety is strongly associated with high quality care" (Healthgrades 2016b). Healthgrades protects the information on its website by using an identify-verification system used by health information exchanges and through security procedures that watch for abnormalities in the data.

The Joint Commission

The Joint Commission publishes hospital core performance measurement data on its website at **QualityCheck.org** (Joint Commission 2016d). Consumers can search for an organization, check on its performance based on the Joint Commission performance measures, and determine the organization's accreditation status.

The Leapfrog Group

The **Leapfrog Group** is a nonprofit voluntary organization that was founded in 2000 by large employers and other purchasers to promote transparency, value, and excellence in healthcare. The group is comprised of private and public-sector companies and purchasers representing more than 34 million Americans and more than $62 billion in healthcare expenditures. Its goals are to reduce preventable medical mistakes and improve the quality and affordability of health care (Leapfrog Group n.d.c). To achieve these goals the Leapfrog Group supports the following programs:

- **Leapfrog Hospital Survey:** This yearly survey "collects, analyzes and disseminates hospital data which is used by employers, health plans, vendors, and others to design benefits plans, recognize high performing hospitals, and steer employees and members toward facilities most capable of offering safe, quality care" (Leapfrog Group n.d.b). Survey results are made available through Leapfrog's "Compare Hospital" website.
- **Hospital Safety Score:** Leapfrogs Blue Ribbon Panel assigns an A, B, C, D or F grade to more than 2,500 hospitals based on their ability to prevent harm. The score is based on national, publicly

reported measures of patient safety data (Leapfrog Group n.d.a). Safety scores are made available through the "Hospital Safety Score" website.

- **Leapfrog Value-Based Purchasing (VBP) Platform:** Leapfrog applies its VBP Platform methodology to hospitals' survey results and gives each facility an overall value score. The value score enables the plan to rank the hospitals and set benchmarks for financial awards or incentives, such as allocating the highest rewards to hospitals scoring in the top decile. All participating hospitals receive a report detailing their Survey performance and results twice per year (Leapfrog n.d.d).

National Committee for Quality Assurance (NCQA)

The **National Committee for Quality Assurance (NCQA)** is another voluntary private non-profit organization that develops quality standards and performance measures for a broad range of health care entities. It provides information on hundreds of health plans on its **Health Plan Report Card** website (NCQA n.d.a). Every year, NCQA publishes *The State of Health Care Quality Report*, which focuses on key quality issues in the United States. The report provides data on "performance trends over time, tracks variation in care and recommends quality improvements" (NCQA n.d.b).

Organization and Operation of Quality and Patient Safety Management

The challenge for hospitals, physician practices, nursing homes, and other providers is to assure their organization meets the regulatory and accrediting body requirements for sound quality improvement, risk management and patient safety programs. Quality, patient safety, and risk management departments must have policies, procedures, and processes in place to address these requirements and to ensure they are working in tandem with QIN-QIOs and other quality, patient safety entities. With the growing use of EHRs and the legitimate sharing of data internal and external to an organization greater emphasis is placed on using data for decision making related to cost, access, quality and patient safety activities. Health information management and informatics professionals are key contributors in the development of processes to ensure the integrity of the data used in reporting quality and patient safety measures and the systems necessary to assure the privacy and security of the data that is collected and shared.

Check Your Understanding | 17.4

Instructions: Indicate whether the following statements are true or false (T or F).

1. Healthcare providers voluntarily report confidential quality and patient safety data on events that adversely affect patients to Patient Safety Organizations.
2. Providers who engage in peer review activities relate to patient safety and quality of healthcare have legal immunity for their involvement.
3. Safety work products related to adverse event data that are shared with PSOs does are always discoverable in a litigation situation.
4. HHS and CMS quality strategies are guided by 3 aims: better care, healthy people/healthy communities, and affordable care.
5. Healthgrades represents one of many required programs for reporting of quality and patient safety measures.

Scenario 17

Al Harman was a patient in Ross Community Hospital for a ruptured appendix, which resulted in an appendectomy and 4 weeks of intensive antibiotic therapy. The severity of Mr. Harman's condition was exacerbated by his obesity and the length of time from his first symptom and when he sought care. During his stay, he complained to the charge nurse that he was not receiving an adequate dose of antibiotics which was the cause of his infection and the length of his stay in the hospital. The charge nurse followed the hospital's risk management procedure, objectively documented the patient's complaint in the patient's record, and completed an incident report.

1. If a lawsuit is subsequently brought against the hospital, what role does the patient's record play in this situation?

2. Decide whether the incident report would or would not be subject to discovery by Mr. Harman's attorney.

3. Judge whether this incident represents a sentinel event as defined by The Joint Commission.

References

Agency for Healthcare Research and Quality. 2012. Advancing Patient Safety - A Decade of Evidence, Design, and Implementation. http://www.ahrq.gov/professionals/quality-patient-safety/patient-safety-resources/resources/advancing-patient-safety/index.html.

Agency for Healthcare Research and Quality. 2016. 2015 National Healthcare Quality and Disparities Report and 5th Anniversary Update on the National Quality Strategy. http://www.ahrq.gov/research/findings/nhqrdr/nhqdr15/index.html.

Agency for Healthcare Research and Quality PSNET. 2016. Sentinel Event Statistics 1995–2016. https://psnet.ahrq.gov/resources/resource/4007/sentinel-event-statistics-1995-2016

Agency for Healthcare Research and Quality. n.d.a. Patient Safety Organization (PSO) Program. https://www.pso.ahrq.gov/faq#whatrolewillocrhave

Agency for Healthcare Research and Quality. n.d.b. Patient Safety Organization (PSO) Program Common Formats. https://www.pso.ahrq.gov/common

Agency for Healthcare Research and Quality. n.d.c. Your guide to choosing quality health care: A quick look at quality. http://www.ahrq.gov.

American Health Information Management Association *Pocket Glossary of Health Information Management and Technology* 4th ed. 2014.

American Society for Healthcare Risk Management. 2000. Risk management program development tool kit, sample excerpt.

American Society for Healthcare Risk Management. 2003. Barton Certificate in Healthcare Risk Management program glossary.

American Society for Healthcare Risk Management. 2005. Celebrating 25 years, 1980–2005: A brief history of ASHRM. http://www.ashr.org.

American Society for Healthcare Risk Management. 2012. Serious Safety Events: Getting to Zero. White Paper Ed. No. 1. http://www.ashrm.org/pubs/files/white_papers/SSE%20White%20Pape_10-5-12_FINAL.pdf.

American Society for Healthcare Risk Management. 2014a. Enterprise risk management: A framework for success. http://www.ashrm.org/pubs/files/white_papers/ERM-White-Paper-8-29-14-FINAL.pdf.

American Society for Healthcare Risk Management. 2014b. Healthcare risk management: The path forward. http://www.ashrm.org/pubs/white_papers.dhtml#erm.

American Society for Healthcare Risk Management. 2014c. Serious Safety Events: Getting to Zero. White Paper Ed. No. 2. http://www.ashrm.org/pubs/files/white_papers/SSE-2_getting_to_zero-9-30-14.pdf

Centers for Medicare and Medicaid Services. 2016. Quality Improvement Organizations. https://www.cms.gov.

Cox, C.H. 2002 (June). Notice of loss requirements—Risk primer. *Risk & Insurance* 13(7):12.

Danzon, P.M. 1982. *The Frequency and Severity of Malpractice Claims*. Santa Monica, CA: Rand. http://www.rand.org.

Department of Health and Humans Services. 2011a. National Quality Strategy will promote better health, quality care for Americans. http://www.hhs.gov.

Department of Health and Human Services. 2011b. Report to Congress: National Strategy for Quality Improvement in Health Care. http://www.healthcare.gov.

Department of Health and Human Services. 2015. Better, smarter, healthier: In historic announcement, HHS sets clear goals and timeline for shifting Medicare reimbursements from volume to value. http://www.hhs.gov/news.

Dunn, D. 2003 (June). Incident reports: Their purpose and scope. *AORN Journal* 78(1):46, 49–61, 65–66, 67–70.

ECRI Institute. 2014 (November). Patient safety, risk and quality. *Healthcare Risk Control*. https://www.ecri.org/components/HRC/Pages/RiskQual4.aspx.

Healthgrades. 2016a. Healthgrades announces America's Best Hospitals for 2016. http://www.healthgrades.com.

Healthgrades. 2016b. Healthgrades releases its 2016 Outstanding Patient Experience Award and 2016 Patient Safety Excellence Award recipients. https://www.healthgrades.com.

Institute for Healthcare Improvement. 2016. Patient safety. http://www.ihi.org.

Institute of Medicine. 1999. *To Err Is Human*. Washington, DC: National Academies Press.

Institute of Medicine. 2001. *Crossing the Quality Chasm: A New Health System for the 21st Century*. Washington, DC: National Academies Press.

Joint Commission. 2013. Sentinel event (SE). http://www.jointcommission.org/assets/1/6/CAMH_2012_Update2_24_SE.pdf.

Joint Commission. 2015. The Joint Commission: Over a century of quality and safety. https://www.jointcommission.org/assets/1/6/TJC_history_timeline_through_2015.pdf.

Joint Commission. 2016a. Facts about patient safety. https://www.jointcommission.org/facts_about_patient_safety/

Joint Commission. 2016b. Most commonly reviewed sentinel event types. https://www.jointcommission.org/assets/1/18/Event_type_2Q_2016.pdf.

Joint Commission. 2016c. National Patient Safety Goals. https://www.jointcommission.org/standards_information/npsgs.aspx.

Joint Commission. 2016d. Quality Check. https://www.qualitycheck.org/

Joint Commission. 2016e. Sentinel Event Policy and Procedures. http://www.jointcommission.org.

Joint Commission Perspectives. 2014. Why organizations self report sentinel events to the Joint Commission. 34(9): 11–12. https://www.jointcommission.org/assets/1/18/Why_Organizations_Self_Report_Sentinel_Events_to_The_Joint_Commission.pdf.

Journal of Healthcare Risk Management. 2007 (January 1). Cost of adverse events borne by provider. Academic OneFile. http://www.gale.cengage.com.

Kronick, R., S. Arnold, and J. Brady. 2016. Improving safety for hospitalized patients much progress but many challenges remain. *JAMA* 316(5):489–490.

The Leapfrog Group. n.d.a. Hospital Safety Score. http://www.leapfroggroup.org/data-users/hospital-safety-score.

The Leapfrog Group. n.d.b. Leapfrog Hospital Survey. http://www.leapfroggroup.org/data-users/leapfrog-hospital-survey.

The Leapfrog Group. n.d.c. Raising the bar for safer healthcare. http://www.leapfroggroup.org/about

The Leapfrog Group. n.d.d. Leapfrog Value-Based Purchasing Platform. http://www.leapfroggroup.org/data-users/leapfrog-value-based-purchasing-platform.

Mello, M.M., D.M. Studdert, and T.A. Brennan. 2003. The new medical malpractice crisis. *New England Journal of Medicine* 348(23):2281–2284.

National Committee for Quality Assurance. n.d.a. About NCQA. http://www.ncqa.org.

National Committee for Quality Assurance. n.d.b. The State of Health Care Quality Report. http://www.ncqa.org /report-cards/health-plans/state-of-health-care-quality.

National Patient Safety Foundation. 2016. RCA2. Improving root cause analyses and actions to prevent harm. https://c.ymcdn.com/sites/npsf.site-ym.com/resource/resmgr/PDF/RCA2_v2-online-pub_010816.pdf.

Office of the National Coordinator for Health Information Technology. 2016. About ONC. https://www.healthit .gov/newsroom/about-onc.

Office of the National Coordinator for Health Information Technology. n.d. ONC Health IT Safety Program – Progress on Health IT Patient Safety Action and Surveillance Plan. https://www.healthit.gov/sites/default/files /ONC_HIT_SafetyProgramReport_9-9-14_.pdf.

Office of the National Coordinator for Health Information Technology and Office for Civil Rights. 2016. Permitted uses and disclosures: Exchange for health care operations. https://www.healthit.gov/sites/default/files /exchange_health_care_ops.pdf.

Sebelius, K. 2013(March 20). The Affordable Care Act at three: Paying for quality saves health care dollars. Health Affairs Blog. http://healthaffairs.org/blog/2013/03/20/the-affordable-care-act-at-three-paying-for-quality -saves-health-care-dollars/.

Sprague, L. 2002. Contracting for quality: Medicare's Quality Improvement Organizations. *NHPF Issue Brief* 774.

Cases, Statutes, and Regulations Cited

Darling v. Charleston Community Memorial Hospital, 33 IL 2d 326, 211 N.E.2d 253, 14 A.L.R.3d 860. 1965.

42 CFR 3.102(b)(1)(i): Process and requirements for initial and continued listing of patient safety organizations (PSOs). 2005.

KS Stat. Ann. 65-4922: Kansas Risk Management Statute, healthcare providers.

Pub. L. 106-129: Healthcare Research and Quality Act of 1999.

Pub. L. 109-41: Patient Safety and Quality Improvement Act of 2005.

Pub. L. 107-204: Sarbanes-Oxley Act of 2002.

Pub. L. 111-148 (Sec. 10326): Patient Protection and Affordable Care Act of 2010.

TN Code Ann. 68-11-211: Health Data Reporting Act: Unusual Events Reporting. 2002.

Corporate Compliance

Sue Bowman, MJ, RHIA, CCS, FAHIMA

Learning Objectives

- Differentiate among the concepts of fraud, waste, and abuse
- Describe common types of healthcare fraud and abuse
- Identify the major federal laws governing healthcare fraud and abuse
- Describe federal government initiatives to enforce healthcare fraud and abuse laws and also prevent fraud from occurring
- Explain fraud prevention strategies, including the fundamental elements of a corporate compliance program, the risks of non-compliance, and effective strategies for risk mitigation

Key Terms

- Abuse
- Accountable Care Organization (ACO)
- Advisory opinion
- Civil Monetary Penalties (CMP) Law
- Compliance officer
- Corporate code of conduct
- Corporate compliance
- Corporate compliance program
- Corporate integrity agreement (CIA)
- Deficit Reduction Act of 2005

- False Claims Act (FCA)
- Federal Anti-Kickback Statute (AKS)
- Federal Physician Self-Referral Statute
- Fraud
- Fraud Enforcement and Recovery Act (FERA)
- Health Care Fraud Prevention and Enforcement Action Team (HEAT)
- Health Insurance Portability and Accountability Act
- Improper payment

- Knowing standard
- Medicaid Integrity Contractor
- National Benefit Integrity Medicare Drug Integrity Contractor
- Patient Protection and Affordable Care Act (ACA)
- Provider Self-Disclosure Protocol
- Qui tam relator
- Recovery Audit Contractor
- Referral
- Remuneration
- Safe harbor

- Sherman Antitrust Act
- Stark Law
- Supplemental Medical Review Contractor
- Unbundling
- Upcoding
- Waste
- Whistleblower
- Zone Program Integrity Contractor

Introduction

In an era of increased regulatory oversight, expanded enforcement efforts, and heightened expectations for corporate accountability, corporate compliance has become an important aspect of organizational culture and operations. **Corporate compliance** refers to adherence to the laws and regulations passed by official regulating bodies as well as general principles of ethical conduct (Society of Corporate Compliance and Ethics n.d.). In order to establish effective internal controls to promote adherence to federal and state laws, regulations, and other applicable requirements, organizations have established corporate compliance programs. Implementation of an effective corporate compliance program significantly reduces the risk of unlawful or improper conduct, criminal and civil liability, and the risk of a government audit, and also promotes an ethical organizational culture.

Corporate compliance in the context of healthcare means meeting the statutory and regulatory requirements set out for particular activities in the provision of healthcare (AHLA n.d.b). Given the highly complex and regulated nature of the healthcare industry, and as the federal government's enforcement efforts and penalties evolve, staying abreast of compliance requirements continues to be a challenge for healthcare organizations, particularly the personnel responsible for the management and integrity of healthcare information. The Government Accountability Office (GAO) has designated Medicare a high-risk program, in part because the program's size and complexity make it vulnerable to fraud, waste, and abuse (GAO 2014). The federal government has engaged in aggressive efforts to combat fraud and abuse. Since 1996, Congress has taken a number of steps to increase Medicare program integrity funding and oversight, including (GAO 2014):

- Creation of the Medicare Integrity Program and establishment of dedicated funding for activities targeted toward fraud, waste, and abuse in federal healthcare programs (Health Insurance Portability and Accountability Act of 1996)
- Requiring the Centers for Medicare and Medicaid Services (CMS) to implement a national Recovery Audit Program (Tax Relief and Health Care Act of 2006)
- Provision of additional funding for program integrity activities and requiring CMS to extend the Medicare Recovery Audit Program to Medicare Parts C and D (Patient Protection and Affordable Care Act of 2010)
- Making compliance programs a condition of enrollment in federal healthcare programs and requiring CMS to develop core elements for such programs (Patient Protection and Affordable Care Act of 2010)
- Requiring the use of predictive analytics to identify and prevent fraud in Medicare Fee-for-Service programs (Small Business Jobs Act of 2010).

The Department of Health and Human Services (HHS) has indicated that eliminating fraud, waste and abuse is a top priority (DOJ 2015b). HHS and the Department of Justice (DOJ) announced in 2015 that more than $27.8 billion has been returned to the Medicare Trust Fund over the life of the Health Care Fraud and Abuse Control (HCFAC) Program, which was established as part of the Health Insurance Portability and Accountability Act of 1996 (HIPAA). This program has returned $7.70 for each dollar invested in cases involving healthcare fraud in federal programs (DOJ 2015b). As a result of the government's fraud initiatives, the development of formal corporate compliance programs has become a core function in healthcare organizations.

In this chapter, healthcare fraud and abuse are defined and common types of fraud and abuse are identified; key federal fraud statutes federal enforcement initiatives are described; and fraud prevention strategies, particularly development of a corporate compliance program, are discussed. While this chapter will focus on federal laws and enforcement, it is important to keep in mind that states also have insurance fraud laws and penalties and have also required health insurers to meet certain standards of fraud detection. The chapter concludes with a detailed discussion of the role of corporate compliance programs and the standards, policies, and procedures that healthcare organizations should have in place to assure they are in compliance with government-funded healthcare programs.

What are Fraud and Abuse?

Fraud in healthcare is defined independently by a number of legal authorities, but all definitions share common elements:

- A false representation of fact
- A failure to disclose a fact that is material (relevant) to a healthcare transaction
- Damage to another party that reasonably relies on the misrepresentation or failure to disclose

The National Health Care Anti-Fraud Association (NHCAA) (n.d.) defines healthcare fraud as an intentional deception or misrepresentation that the individual or entity makes knowing that the misrepresentation could result in some unauthorized benefit to the individual, the entity, or some other party.

The Centers for Medicare and Medicaid Services (CMS) have defined fraud as an "intentional deception or misrepresentation that an individual knows, or should know, to be false, or does not believe to be true, and makes, knowing the deception could result in some unauthorized benefit to himself or some other person(s)" (CMS 2006).

It's important to keep in mind that all improper payments do not constitute fraud. The majority of improper payments are due to unintentional errors. An **improper payment** has been defined by the federal government as any payment that should not have been made or that was made in an incorrect amount (including overpayments and underpayments) under statutory, contractual, administrative, or other legally applicable requirements (31 USC 3321). There are a number of causes of improper payments, including billing for services with insufficient or lack of clinical documentation, incorrect coding, or providing services that do not meet payment policy requirements. Many improper payments to providers and suppliers relate to claims for which the information in the patient's health record did not support the services billed (Agrawal et al. 2013).

While they are not necessarily fraud, improper payments of any type cause significant financial impact. For consumers, improper payments can mean higher premiums and out-of-pocket expenses, as well as potentially reduced benefits. For employers, improper payments increase both the cost of providing insurance benefits and the overall cost of doing business (Agrawal et al. 2013). Patients also can potentially be harmed through the compromising of their health records, by the inclusion of erroneous medical information in the case of medical identity theft, which can result in inappropriate care.

Anyone who has received an overpayment from a federal healthcare program is legally obligated to report and return the overpayment within 60 days after the date on which the overpayment was identified or the date any corresponding cost report is due, if applicable, whichever date is later. In February 2016, CMS published a final rule describing providers' and suppliers' obligation to report and return overpayments and the process by which they should do so. Failure to return an overpayment within the required timeframe may result in liability under the False Claims Act, Civil Monetary Penalties Law, or exclusion from federal healthcare programs which are discussed in more detail below (CMS 2016).

Healthcare **abuse** refers to provider, supplier, and practitioner practices that are inconsistent with accepted sound fiscal, business, or medical practices, which directly or indirectly may result in

- Unnecessary costs to the healthcare program
- Improper payment
- Services that fail to meet professionally recognized standards of care or are medically unnecessary
- Services that directly or indirectly result in adverse patient outcomes or delays in appropriate diagnosis or treatment (CMS 2011)

According to CMS, the primary difference between fraud and abuse is intention. Abuse occurs when healthcare providers or suppliers perform actions that directly or indirectly result in unnecessary costs to any healthcare benefit program (CMS 2014b). Although there is no specific legal definition, **waste** generally refers to overutilization or inappropriate utilization of services and misuse of resources. It is not considered a criminal or intentional act (National Association of Medicaid Directors 2012).

Common Types of Healthcare Fraud and Abuse

Healthcare fraud is a significant national problem, affecting federal, state, and private health insurance programs. Fraud not only drives up healthcare costs, but also reduces the funds available for legitimate healthcare services and endangers the long-term solvency of federal healthcare programs (Agrawal et al. 2013). Only a small percentage of the estimated four billion healthcare claims submitted each year are fraudulent. Taken in total, however, the resulting cost is high, and the scope of activity is wide.

Although the actual cost of healthcare fraud is unknown, the NHCAA estimates that the financial losses due to healthcare fraud are in the tens of billions of dollars each year. In 2012, the Institute of Medicine (IOM) estimated that the U.S. healthcare system loses about $765 billion a year to waste. Of that $765 billion, about $210 billion is attributable to unnecessary services, $190 billion to excess administrative costs, $130 billion to inefficiently delivered services, $105 billion to excessive prices, $75 billion to fraud, and $55 billion to missed prevention opportunities (IOM 2012).

Healthcare organizations should assess their risk areas to identify vulnerabilities to unlawful or improper conduct. According to the NHCAA, the most common types of healthcare fraud include

- Billing for services that were never rendered (either by using actual patient information to fabricate entire claims or by padding claims with charges for services or procedures that were not provided or performed)
- Billing for more expensive services or procedures than were actually provided or performed, also known as **upcoding**, which often includes falsifying the patient's diagnosis so that it supports the fraudulent service or procedure
- Performing medically unnecessary services in order to increase revenue
- Misrepresenting noncovered services as covered services
- Falsifying a patient's diagnosis to justify tests or treatments that aren't medically necessary
- **Unbundling** (billing individual components of a complete procedure or service separately)
- Billing patients more than the co-pay amount for services that were prepaid or paid in full by the benefit plan under the terms of a managed care contract
- Accepting kickbacks for patient referrals
- Waiving patient co-pays or deductibles and overbilling the health plan (NHCAA n.d.)

Common types of Medicare and Medicaid fraud and abuse include

- Incorrect reporting of diagnoses or procedures to maximize payments (such as upcoding)
- Billing for services not furnished and/or supplies not provided
- Billing for unnecessary services or items
- Billing deliberately for duplicate payment for the same services or supplies, billing both Medicare and the beneficiary for the same service, or billing both Medicare and another insurer in an attempt to get paid twice
- Altering claim forms, electronic claim records, clinical documentation, etc., to obtain a higher payment amount than justified

- Soliciting, offering, or receiving a kickback, bribe, or rebate (for example, compensation in exchange for patient referrals)
- "Unbundling" charges
- Billing non-covered or non-payable items or services as covered or payable items or services
- Medical identity theft (misuse of a person's medical identity to wrongfully obtain healthcare goods, services, or funds) (CMS 2011, 2015d)

The most frequent type of Medicare fraud arises from a false statement or misrepresentation made, or caused to be made, that is material to entitlement or payment under the Medicare program (CMS 2015a).

Physician Self-Referral

Physician self-referral, or the practice of a physician referring a patient to a medical facility in which he has a financial interest, is a significant fraud risk area. This type of arrangement is viewed as involving an inherent conflict of interest, as the physician stands to financially benefit from the referral. It may also encourage over-utilization of healthcare services, thereby driving up healthcare costs.

As fee-for-service reimbursement models shift to value-based models, physician compensation agreements are shifting to reflect a focus on value as well. Healthcare organizations are still obligated to ensure new compensation models comply with all federal laws, including prohibitions against self-referral and payment for referrals, unless the arrangement is protected by an exception, safe harbor, or waiver. Regardless of whether physician compensation models include quality metrics, potential liability under the Federal Physician Self-Referral Statute (Stark Law) will be a potential issue if the value or volume of referrals is a factor in compensation arrangements. Later in this chapter, the Stark Law and waivers of certain fraud and abuse laws for new payment and service delivery models will be discussed.

Electronic Health Records

Electronic health record (EHR) vendors have introduced a variety of tools to facilitate the coding process and clinical documentation capture that can potentially lead to fraud and abuse, including documentation that reflects services that were never rendered, a higher complexity of services than actually provided, or medical conditions that don't exist. Examples of these features include copying and pasting text (either within or between different patient records), creation of default notes, single-click template notes, "make me an author," evaluation and management (E/M) code optimization alerts, and drop-down boxes containing only the highest-paying diagnosis or procedure options (Simborg 2011). Templates can drive both unnecessary and inaccurate information, which can lead to overpayments and false claims allegations, as well as raising questions regarding the validity of the record if template documentation is contradicted by other information in the record.

Benefits of EHR tools should be weighed against the potential for creating inaccurate or fraudulent documentation. Policies and procedures should be established for the proper use of these tools to ensure compliance with governmental, regulatory, and industry standards, with consideration being given to disabling some of them or limiting their use when they are deemed high-risk for fraud and abuse vulnerabilities. Organizations should also establish requirements for participation in education in the proper use of EHR tools and ongoing monitoring to ensure their use is in compliance with organizational policies and procedures.

Check Your Understanding 18.1

Instructions: Indicate whether the following statements are true or false (T or F).

1. If an overpayment is not returned to Medicare within 30 days, it becomes a violation of the False Claims Act.
2. The primary difference between fraud and abuse is intention.
3. Billing for services never rendered is one of the most common types of healthcare fraud.
4. Paying physicians for referrals is a practice encouraged by Medicare.
5. Some electronic health record features increase fraud and abuse risks.

Key Federal Fraud Statutes

Health information management and informatics professionals should be aware of the major statutes, rules, and regulations related to compliance. Because they change quickly, it is imperative to monitor them regularly to ensure that an organization or provider is following the most current version of the laws. Federal and state statutes, rules, and regulations must be understood since a claim of ignorance will not excuse the organization or provider from penalties. Federal statues impacting compliance, fraud, and abuse are discussed below.

False Claims Act

The **False Claims Act** of 1986 (FCA) (31 USC 3729, 18 USC 287) is the government's primary litigation tool for combating fraud. It provides that anyone who "knowingly" submits, or causes the submission of, false claims to the federal government is liable for civil and/or criminal penalties. This includes not only those with actual knowledge of the false claim, but also those who act in deliberate ignorance of the truth or falsity of the information and those who act in reckless disregard of the truth or falsity of the information. No specific intent to defraud the government is required. Examples of FCA violations include upcoding, billing for unnecessary services, billing for services or items not rendered, and billing for services performed by an excluded provider. Providers who fail to return Medicare or Medicaid over-payments can face liability under the FCA.

Violations of the FCA may result in damages up to three times the amount of the erroneous payment plus penalties up to $11,000 for each false claim submitted. In addition to bringing about civil penalties, submitting false claims is a criminal offense. An organization can be fined either $500,000 or twice the false claim amount, whichever is greater, and an individual can be fined either $250,000 or twice the false claim amount, whichever is the larger sum, and can be imprisoned for up to five years. The burden of proof is higher in criminal prosecutions than in civil cases. In a civil FCA action, the standard is a "preponderance of the evidence," whereas in a criminal FCA case, the government must prove beyond a reasonable doubt that the defendant knew the claim was false. FCA violations can also lead to exclusion from federal healthcare programs.

Civil legal actions under the FCA may be brought not only by the government, but also by private individuals (**whistleblowers**), such as competitors or an employee of the organization, on behalf of the government. These individuals, known as *qui tam* **relators**, are entitled to a percentage of the recovery when the legal action is successful. If the government believes the claim lacks merit and declines to intervene, the *qui tam* relator may elect to prosecute the action without the government, in which case his percentage of the recovery in successful legal actions is higher. The FCA provides protection to *qui tam* relators who are discharged, demoted, suspended, threatened, harassed, or in any other way discriminated against in the terms or conditions of their employment as a result of their furtherance of an action under the FCA. Remedies include reinstatement with seniority comparable to what the qui tam relator would have had if not for the discrimination, two times the amount of any back pay, interest on any back pay, and compensation for any special damages sustained as a result of the discrimination, including litigation costs and reasonable attorney's fees.

What Constitutes a False Claim?

To establish liability under the FCA, the government or whistleblower must establish that the claim was false or fraudulent. Since the FCA does not specifically define what constitutes a false claim, the standard has been developed through case law. There are two general types of healthcare claims that the government considers false: 1. furnishing inaccurate or misleading information to the government to obtain payment or approval of a claim, such as upcoding or submitting claims for services not rendered; and 2. omission of information from a claim or implicitly certifying compliance with rules, without actually complying with the rules.

The Knowing Standard

Falsity alone is not enough to impose FCA liability. The **knowing standard** refers to the fact that the provider must have knowingly submitted the false claim. The FCA defines "knowing" and "knowingly" to mean that a person

- Has actual knowledge of the information,
- Acts in deliberate ignorance of the truth or falsity of the information, or
- Acts in reckless disregard of the truth or falsity of the information.

No proof of specific intent to defraud is required. Therefore, submission of claims in a sloppy, unsupervised fashion without due care regarding the accuracy of the claim can constitute reckless disregard and create an FCA violation.

Interpreting the law is sometimes difficult for providers. When a provider acts in accordance with one interpretation of the law, even if the government has another interpretation, the FCA action should not succeed. If a provider's actions are based on the advice of legal counsel, it may also be difficult to prove intent to violate the FCA. However, as a practical matter, many providers settle such cases rather than proceeding to trial to defend the action, which makes the FCA a powerful government enforcement tool.

Fraud Enforcement and Recovery Act

The **Fraud Enforcement and Recovery Act of 2009 (FERA)** (Pub. L. 111-21) amended the FCA. It expanded the potential for liability under the FCA and also expanded the government's investigative powers. FERA eliminated the requirement that a person must present a false claim to a US government officer or employee or a member of the US armed services in order to be liable under the FCA. With the passage of this legislation, the FCA penalties apply to "any person who knowingly presents, or causes to be presented, a false or fraudulent claim for payment or approval," regardless of to whom the claim was made. The statutory definition of a "claim" has been expanded to include claims submitted "to a contractor, grantee, or other recipient, if the money or property is to be spent or used on the Government's behalf, or to advance a Government program or interest" (31 USC 3729). This revision substantially broadens the types of payments that fall within the scope of the FCA, such as claims submitted to Medicare and Medicaid managed care plans and other federally funded healthcare payers. These amendments to the FCA are intended to ensure that those who submit false or fraudulent claims or make false statements related to a claim—to any contractor, subcontractor, or entity to which payment is made by the government—are liable to the same extent that they would be if they made such claims or provided such information to the government itself.

Further, FERA established that FCA penalties apply to "any person who knowingly makes, uses, or causes to be made or used, a false record or statement material to a false or fraudulent claim." A violation of the FCA also occurs when any person "knowingly makes, uses, or causes to be made or used, a false record or statement material to an obligation to pay or transmit money or property to the Government, or knowingly conceals or knowingly and improperly avoids or decreases an obligation to pay or transmit money or property to the Government" (31 USC 3729).

"Material" is defined as "having a natural tendency to influence, or be capable of influencing, the payment or receipt of money or property" (31 USC 3729). These revisions allow the government and whistleblowers to pursue violations of regulatory statutes with penalty provisions as FCA cases and to pursue false documents that are "material to an obligation to pay or to transmit money ... to the Government," regardless of whether a false claim has been submitted (Pub. L. 111-21). For example, a physician who creates backdated health records to support a claim already submitted could be liable under this provision. Also, since the definition of "obligation" expressly includes retention of overpayments, FERA makes it clear that providers have an affirmative duty to notify the applicable entity and repay the overpayment.

FERA also expanded anti-retaliation protections for whistleblowers by allowing nonemployees, including contractors and agents, to sue for retaliation. In addition, FERA expanded the US Attorney General's authority to issue civil investigative demands and broadened the government's authority to share documents obtained through subpoena with *qui tam* relators and other parties.

Federal Anti-Kickback Statute

The **Federal Anti-Kickback Statute (AKS)** (42 USC 1320a–7b) prohibits knowingly and willfully offering, paying, soliciting, or receiving remuneration, directly or indirectly, in order to induce business for which payment may be made under any federal healthcare program. The only exceptions are voluntary safe harbors, which protect certain payment and business practices that might otherwise result in prosecution for an AKS violation (42 CFR 1001.952). Remuneration covered by the AKS includes, but is not limited to, kickbacks, bribes, and rebates. **Remuneration** is defined broadly to include the transfer of anything of value, directly or indirectly, overtly or covertly, in cash or in kind. Prohibited conduct includes not only remuneration intended to induce referrals, but also remuneration intended to induce the purchasing, leasing, ordering, or arranging for any good, facility, service, or item paid for by a federal healthcare program.

Violators may be subject to criminal or civil penalties. Criminal penalties include fines up to $25,000 per violation and a maximum of a 5-year prison term per violation. Possible civil/administrative penalties include FCA liability, civil monetary penalties, and program exclusion. Civil penalties can include up to $50,000 per violation plus three times the amount of the kickback (HHS OIG n.d.e).

Safe Harbors

Safe harbor regulations protect certain payment and business practices that could potentially implicate the AKS from criminal and civil prosecution. To be protected by a safe harbor, an arrangement must fit squarely in the safe harbor and satisfy all of its requirements (HHS OIG n.d.a, n.d.f). Some of these safe harbors are similar to, or the same as, exceptions under the Stark Law. The Office of Inspector General (OIG) has created a number of regulatory safe harbors covering such arrangements as

- Space and equipment rentals
- Personal services and management contracts
- Sale of practice
- Bona fide employment arrangements
- Group purchasing organizations
- Coinsurance and deductible waivers
- Increased coverage, reduced cost-sharing amounts, or reduced premium amounts offered by health plans
- Price reductions offered to health plans
- Practitioner recruitment
- Investments in group practices
- Referral arrangements for specialty services
- Electronic prescribing items and services
- Electronic health records items and services (42 CFR 1001.952)

A common theme that runs through these safe harbors is the intent to protect certain arrangements in which commercially reasonable items or services are exchanged for fair market value compensation. The statute does not define the term "fair market value" but makes it clear that fair market values cannot vary based on referrals or the additional value that one party would attribute to property as a result of its proximity or convenience to sources of Medicare or Medicaid business or referrals.

Safe Harbor for Electronic Health Records Items and Services

The safe harbor for "electronic health records items and services," which is also an exception under the Stark Law, is of particular interest to health information management and informatics professionals. This safe harbor is intended to protect beneficial arrangements that would eliminate perceived barriers to the adoption of EHRs without creating undue risk that the arrangements might be used to induce or reward the generation of federal healthcare program business (HHS OIG 2006, 2013a). The EHRs safe harbor protects certain arrangements involving the provision of interoperable EHR software or information technology and training services. To fit within the safe harbor, certain EHR donation regulations must be met (42 CFR 1001.952(y)) (see Figure 18.1).

In 2015, the OIG issued an alert to remind the public about how information blocking may affect safe harbor protection under the AKS. Per the OIG, the third EHR safe harbor conditions are directly relevant to the issue of information blocking. As stated in figure 18.1, the donor (or any person on the donor's behalf) must not take any action to limit or restrict the use, compatibility, or interoperability of the items or services with other electronic prescribing or [EHR] systems (including, but not limited to, health information technology applications, products, or services). Donations of items or services that have limited or restricted interoperability due to action taken by the donor or by any person on the donor's behalf (which could include the recipient acting on the donor's behalf) would fail to meet this condition. Failure to meet this condition would mean that the safe harbor would not apply and the arrangement would be subject to case-by-case review under the AKS.

Figure 18.1 Electronic health records safe harbor under the Anti-Kickback statute

- The items and services are provided to an individual or entity engaged in the delivery of health care by an individual or entity, other than a laboratory company, that provides services covered by a Federal health care program and submits claims or requests for payment, either directly or through reassignment, to the Federal health care program, or a health plan
- The software is interoperable at the time it is provided to the recipient (software is deemed to be interoperable if, on the date it is provided to the recipient, it has been certified by a certifying body authorized by the National Coordinator for Health Information Technology to an edition of the electronic health record certification criteria identified in the then-applicable version of 45 CFR part 170)
- The donor (or any person on the donor's behalf) does not take any action to limit or restrict the use, compatibility, or interoperability of the items or services with other electronic prescribing or electronic health records systems (including, but not limited to, health information technology applications, products, or services)
- Neither the beneficiary nor the recipient's practice (or any affiliated individual or entity) makes the receipt of items or services, or the amount or nature of the items or services, a condition of doing business with the donor
- Neither the eligibility of a beneficiary for the items or services, nor the amount or nature of the items or services, is determined in a manner that directly takes into account the volume or value of referrals or other business generated between the parties
- The arrangement is set forth in a written agreement
- The donor does not have actual knowledge of, and does not act in reckless disregard or deliberate ignorance of, the fact that the beneficiary possesses or has obtained items or services equivalent to those provided by the donor
- For items or services that are of the type that can be used for any patient without regard to payer status, the donor does not restrict, or take any action to limit, the recipient's right or ability to use the items or services for any patient
- The items and services do not include staffing of the recipient's office and are not used primarily to conduct personal business or business unrelated to the recipient's clinical practice or clinical operations
- Before receipt of the items and services, the beneficiary pays 15 percent of the donor's cost for the items and services. The donor (or any affiliated individual or entity) does not finance the recipient's payment or loan funds to be used by the beneficiary to pay for the items and services
- The donor does not shift the costs of the items or services to any Federal health care program.

Source: HHS OIG 2006, 2013a
Note: This safe harbor is scheduled to sunset on December 31, 2021.

OIG has indicated that such donations would be suspect under the law as they would appear to be motivated, at least in part, by a purpose of securing federal healthcare program business (HHS OIG 2013a).

Civil Monetary Penalties Law

In order to combat an increase in healthcare fraud and abuse, Congress enacted the **Civil Monetary Penalties (CMP) law** under section 1128A of the Social Security Act (42 USC 1320a–7a) in 1981. As one of several administrative remedies, the CMP law authorized the Secretary and Inspector General of HHS to impose CMPs, assessments, and program exclusions on individuals and entities whose wrongdoing caused injury to HHS programs or their beneficiaries. The CMP law authorizes penalties of up to $50,000 per violation and assessments of up to three times the amount claimed for each item or service, or up to three times the amount of remuneration offered, paid, solicited, or received. Violations that may result in imposition of civil monetary penalties include

- Presenting a claim that an individual or entity knows or should know is for an item or service not provided as claimed or that is false and fraudulent

- Presenting a claim that an individual or entity knows or should know is for an item or service for which Medicare will not pay
- Violating the Anti-Kickback Statute

The Federal Civil Penalties Inflation Adjustment Improvements Act of 2015, part of the Bipartisan Budget Act (Pub. L. 114-74), required federal agencies to update the level of their civil monetary penalties to account for inflation, with automatic annual adjustments thereafter.

Federal Physician Self-Referral Statute (Stark Law)

The **Federal Physician Self-Referral Statute** (42 USC 1395nn), also known as the **Stark Law**, prohibits physicians from referring Medicare or Medicaid patients for certain designated health services to an entity in which the physician or a member of his immediate family has an ownership or investment interest, or with which he or she has a compensation arrangement, unless an exception applies. The entity is prohibited from presenting or causing to be presented claims to Medicare (or billing another individual, entity, or third party payer) for those referred services. The Stark Law is a strict liability statute, meaning that proof of specific intent to violate the law is not required. Penalties include repayment of claims, fines, and potential exclusion from participation in federal healthcare programs.

Referral means, for Medicare Part B services, "the request by a physician for the item or service" and, for all other Medicare and Medicaid services, "the request or establishment of a plan of care by a physician which includes the provision of the designated health service" (42 USC 1395(h)(5)(A)) (see figure 18.2 for a list of designated health services). Under the Stark Law, certain referral relationships are deemed not to constitute a referral if the services are furnished by (or under the supervision of) a specialist pursuant to a consultation. Specifically, the Stark Law excludes from the term "referral":

- A request by a pathologist for clinical diagnostic laboratory tests and pathological examination services
- A request by a radiologist for diagnostic radiology services
- A request by a radiation oncologist for radiation therapy, if such services are furnished by or under the supervision of the pathologist, radiologist, or radiation oncologist

Figure 18.2 Designated health services under the Stark Law

1. Clinical laboratory services.
2. Physical therapy services.
3. Occupational therapy services.
4. Outpatient speech-language pathology services.
5. Radiology services, including magnetic resonance imaging, computerized axial tomography scans, and ultrasound services.
6. Radiation therapy services and supplies.
7. Durable medical equipment and supplies.
8. Parenteral and enteral nutrients, equipment, and supplies.
9. Prosthetics, orthotics, and prosthetic devices and supplies.
10. Home health services.
11. Outpatient prescription drugs.
12. Inpatient and outpatient hospital services.

Source: 42 USC 1395nn.

Figure 18.3	Stark Law exceptions to the referral prohibition

- Academic medical centers
- Assistance to compensate a nonphysician practitioner
- Bona fide employment relationships
- Certain arrangements with hospitals
- Community-wide health information systems
- Compliance training
- Dialysis-related drugs
- Electronic health records items and services
- Electronic prescribing items and services
- Eyeglasses and contact lenses following cataract surgery
- Fair market value compensation
- Implants furnished by an Ambulatory Surgical Center
- Indirect compensation arrangements
- In-office ancillary services

- Intra-family rural referrals
- Isolated financial transactions
- Medical staff incidental benefits
- Nonmonetary compensation within certain limits
- Personal service arrangements
- Physician recruitment
- Physician services
- Preventive screening tests, immunizations, and vaccines
- Rental of equipment
- Rental of office space
- Retention payments in underserved areas
- Risk-sharing arrangements
- Services furnished by an organization (or its contractors or subcontractors) to enrollees in certain prepaid health plans
- Timeshare arrangements

Source: 42 CFR 411.355, 411.357.

Penalties for violating the Stark Law include denial of payment, refunds of amounts collected in violation of the statute, a civil monetary penalty of up to $15,000 for each bill or claim a person knew or should have known was for a service for which payment may not be made, three times the amount of the improper payment the designated health service entity received from the Medicare program, and a civil monetary penalty of up to $100,000 for each arrangement or scheme that the physician or entity knew or should have known had a principal purpose of ensuring referrals that, if directly made, were in violation of the Stark Law.

The Stark Law does, however, provide a number of specific exceptions to the referral prohibition and gives the Secretary of HHS the authority to create regulatory exceptions for financial relationships that do not pose a risk of program or patient abuse. Refer to figure 18.3 for the types of services (subject to specified conditions) included in these exceptions.

Changes to Stark Regulations in 2016 Medicare Physician Fee Schedule Final Rule

The calendar year 2016 Medicare Physician Fee Schedule Final Rule made modifications in Stark Law regulatory provisions, including the addition of two new exceptions to the self-referral prohibition and providing several regulatory clarifications intended to reduce perceived or actual violations without increasing the risk of abuse of federal programs (Taft 2015; CMS 2015e). The first new exception permits payment by hospitals, Federally Qualified Health Centers, and Rural Health Clinics to physicians for the purpose of recruiting and compensating non-physician practitioners under certain conditions. This exception was added due to the recognition that the supply of primary care physicians will be inadequate to meet the demand for primary care services and also the growing role for non-physician practitioners in evolving care delivery models. The second new exception allows time-share arrangements for the use of office space, equipment, personnel, items, supplies, and other services. This exception provides flexibility for a hospital or physician practice to ask a specialist from another community to provide services in space owned by the hospital or practice on a limited or as-needed basis. Neither of these new exceptions can involve arrangements that are conditioned on patient referrals (CMS 2015e).

The 2016 final rule clarified that a split-billing arrangement does not create a financial relationship pursuant to the physician self-referral statute when both the hospital and physician bill independently for their services. Per CMS, a physician's use of hospital space to provide services to the hospital's patients is not itself "remuneration," and therefore does not create a financial relationship between the hospital and the physician, if both the hospital and the physician independently bill for their respective services (CMS 2015e).

CMS also provided clarification that for the purpose of complying with the signature requirement, only physicians who stand in the shoes of their physician organization are parties to an arrangement. However, for Stark Law purposes other than the signature requirement, all physicians in a physician organization, including employees and independent contractors, are considered to be parties to the arrangement. Thus, compensation arrangements between a physician practice and a hospital are considered direct compensation arrangements between the hospital and each physician who provides care through the practice, regardless of whether the physician is an owner of the physician practice organization, an employee, or an independent contractor. Therefore, for example, compensation paid to a physician organization cannot take into account the referrals of *any* physician in the physician organization (Taft 2015).

Check Your Understanding 18.2

Instructions: Indicate whether the following statements are true or false (T or F).

1. For a provider to be liable under the False Claims Act, there must be proof of a specific intent to defraud.
2. To fit within the Anti-Kickback Statute safe harbor for "electronic health records items and services," the software must be interoperable.
3. The Stark Law is another name for the Anti-Kickback Statute.
4. The Stark Law is the government's primary litigation tool for combating fraud.
5. Risk-sharing arrangements are a Stark Law exception to the referral prohibition.

Sherman Antitrust Act

The **Sherman Antitrust Act** (15 USC 1–7), passed in 1890, is one of several antitrust laws, including the Clayton Act of 1914. They collectively make it illegal to restrain trade through contracts or conspiracies, and they prohibit price fixing and mergers that lessen competition. There are civil and criminal sanctions. The Federal Trade Commission (FTC) and the Department of Justice enforce these laws. Their respective websites contain information about healthcare issues. Healthcare mergers and joint ventures among providers for the purchase of equipment are examples of arrangements that must be carefully reviewed to ensure that competition is not hindered and that consumers are not harmed. Credentialing and peer review processes also may be scrutinized to ensure that privileges are not denied or restricted to limit competition. Physicians and hospitals cannot set different prices for services for one group of consumers, such as members of a particular health plan.

Health Insurance Portability and Accountability Act

The **Health Insurance Portability and Accountability Act of 1996 (HIPAA)** established a criminal federal offense of "healthcare fraud." This statutory provision prohibits knowingly and willfully executing a scheme or artifice to defraud any healthcare benefit program or to obtain, by means of false or fraudulent pretenses, representations, or promises, any of the money or property owned by, or under the custody or control of, any healthcare benefit program, in connection with the delivery of or payment for healthcare benefits, items, or services (18 USC 1347). A person need not have actual knowledge of this section or specific intent to commit a violation. Penalties may include fines, imprisonment, or both.

HIPAA also significantly expanded the OIG's sanction authorities. It extended the application and scope of the current civil monetary penalty and exclusion authorities beyond programs funded by HHS to all federal healthcare programs (such as Tricare, Veterans Affairs, and the Public Health Service). HIPAA also significantly revised and strengthened the OIG's CMP authorities pertaining to violations under Medicare and state healthcare programs. The maximum penalty amount per false claim was increased from $2,000 to $10,000, and the amount of authorized assessments was raised from double to triple the amount claimed. HIPAA allowed CMPs to be assessed for incorrect coding, medically unnecessary services, and persons offering remuneration to induce a beneficiary to order from a particular provider or supplier receiving Medicare or state healthcare funds. A new CMP was established for the false certification of eligibility for Medicare-covered home health services (HHS OIG 2000a).

Deficit Reduction Act

The **Deficit Reduction Act of 2005 (DRA)** (42 USC 1396a(a)(68)) is particularly significant to compliance because it began the process of transforming compliance programs from voluntary to mandatory. This act contains the Employee Education about False Claims Recovery provision, which requires any entity that annually receives or makes at least $5 million in Medicaid payments to establish written policies for all employees of the entity (including management) and for any contractor or agent of the entity. This written policy must provide detailed information about the FCA, administrative remedies for false claims and statements, any state laws pertaining to civil or criminal penalties for false claims and statements, and whistleblower protections under such laws, with respect to the role of such laws in preventing and detecting fraud, waste, and abuse in federal healthcare programs. The entity's written policies must include detailed provisions regarding the entity's policies and procedures for detecting and preventing fraud, waste, and abuse. The entity's employee handbook must include a specific discussion of the federal and state laws pertaining to false claims and statements, the rights of employees to be protected as whistleblowers, and the entity's policies and procedures for detecting and preventing fraud, waste, and abuse.

Compliance with the DRA provisions became effective January 1, 2007. Failure to comply may result in the affected entity being ineligible to receive Medicaid payments. Also, any affected entity that knowingly violates these requirements may be penalized for submitting false claims under the FCA.

Patient Protection and Affordable Care Act

The **Patient Protection and Affordable Care Act of 2010** (Pub. L. 111–148) (generally referred to as ACA) expanded the federal government's ability to combat fraud and abuse, including:

- Increased funding for enforcement efforts
- Expansion of the Recovery Audit Program to include Medicare Parts C and D and Medicaid
- Limitations on the FCA's public disclosure standard for whistleblower suits by
  - Narrowing the definition of what constitutes "publicly disclosed information" so that a whistleblower suit cannot be barred unless substantially the same allegations or transactions

were publicly disclosed in a federal criminal, civil, or administrative hearing in which the Government or its agent is a party, in a congressional, GAO, or other federal report, hearing, audit, or investigation, or from the news media, and

- o Broadening the definition of the original source exception to the public disclosure bar to include any individual who has knowledge that is independent of and materially adds to the publicly disclosed allegations or transactions, and who voluntarily provided the information to the government before filing suit.
- Amended the statutory exception for in-office ancillary services in the Stark Law by requiring physicians to inform patients in writing that they may obtain Designated Health Services from other entity outside the physician's group practice
- Requiring Medicare and Medicaid overpayments to be reported and returned within 60 days of the date on which the overpayment was identified, or the date a corresponding cost report is due (if applicable), whichever is later
- Added penalties for:
  - o Failing to report or return a known overpayment
  - o Failing to give the OIG timely access for audits, investigations, evaluations, and such
  - o False statements material to a false or fraudulent claim for payment for an item or service furnished under a federal healthcare program
- Required states to terminate individuals or entities from their state Medicaid programs if they have been terminated from Medicare or another state's Medicaid program
- Required Medicaid programs to exclude an individual or entity that owns, controls, or manages another entity that has failed to repay overpayments, been suspended, terminated, or excluded from Medicaid participation, or is affiliated with any such entity

The ACA required development and implementation of a corporate compliance program as a condition of enrollment in Medicare, Medicaid, and/or the Children's Health Insurance Program (CHIP), thus essentially making compliance programs mandatory rather than voluntary. Additionally, the ACA required the HHS Secretary, in cooperation with the HHS Inspector General, to establish a voluntary, Medicare self-referral disclosure protocol that sets forth a process for providers and suppliers to self-disclose actual or potential violations of the Stark Law (HHS OIG 1998b). Under authority granted by this provision, the Secretary may reduce the amount owed for violations of the physician self-referral statute if the provider or supplier self-disclosed the violation. The Provider Self-Disclosure Protocol is discussed in further detail later in this chapter.

Waivers of Fraud and Abuse Laws

The ACA promulgates the testing of innovative payment and service delivery models for patients covered by federal healthcare programs in order to reduce costs, and improve the coordination, quality, and efficiency of healthcare services. Congress authorized the Secretary to waive certain fraud and abuse laws as may be necessary to carry out the testing of these new models. Payment and service delivery models developed by the Center for Medicare and Medicaid Innovation for which fraud and abuse waivers have been issued include Bundled Payment for Care Improvement Models, Comprehensive End-Stage Renal Disease Care Model, and the Comprehensive Care for Joint Replacement Model. CMS noted that Individuals or entities seeking waiver protection should keep in mind that a waiver will apply to their arrangement(s) only if they are eligible to use the waiver and all conditions of the waiver are met (CMS 2015b).

The ACA also required the establishment of a Medicare shared savings program to promote accountability for a Medicare patient population and coordinate items and services under Medicare Parts A and B and encourage investment in infrastructure and redesigned care processes for high quality and efficient service delivery. Under this program, **Accountable Care Organizations (ACOs)**, or groups of providers and suppliers meeting certain criteria that work together to manage and coordinate care for Medicare fee-for-service beneficiaries, that meet certain quality performance standards can share in any savings they achieve for the Medicare program.

The shared savings program focuses on coordinating care between and among providers, including those that are potential referral sources for one another. This coordination potentially implicates fraud and abuse laws that address financial arrangements between sources of federal healthcare program referrals and those seeking such referrals. The ACA authorized the waiver of fraud and abuse laws as necessary to carry out the shared savings program. Per an October 2015 Final Rule, waivers of the application of the Stark Law, AKS, and the Civil Monetary Penalties Law provision relating to beneficiary inducements were instituted for certain ACO arrangements. CMS and OIG noted that a waiver of a fraud and abuse law is not needed for an arrangement that does not implicate the specific fraud and abuse law, or implicates the law, but either fits within an existing exception or safe harbor, as applicable, or does not otherwise violate the law (CMS and HHS OIG 2015).

Exclusion Statute

The OIG has the authority to exclude individuals and entities from federally funded healthcare programs pursuant to sections 1128 and 1156 of the Social Security Act. They are required to exclude providers and suppliers convicted of

- Medicare fraud
- Patient abuse or neglect
- Felony convictions related to fraud, theft, embezzlement, breach of fiduciary responsibility, or other financial misconduct in connection with the delivery of a healthcare item or service
- Felony convictions for unlawful manufacture, distribution, prescription, or dispensing of controlled substances
- The OIG also has the discretion to impose exclusions for other reasons. Exclusion from participation in a federal healthcare program means that, for a designated period, Medicare, Medicaid, and other federal healthcare programs will not pay for any items or services furnished, ordered, or prescribed by the excluded individual or entity. At the end of an exclusion period, an excluded provider must affirmatively seek reinstatement (reinstatement is not automatic) (42 USC 1320a–7).

The OIG's List of Excluded Individuals/Entities (OIG Exclusion List) provides information to the healthcare industry, patients and the public regarding individuals and entities currently excluded from participation in Medicare, Medicaid and all other federal healthcare programs. Civil monetary penalties may be imposed against healthcare providers and entities that employ or enter into contracts with excluded individuals or entities, and no payment will be provided for any items or services furnished, ordered, or prescribed by an excluded individual or entity. Therefore, it is important for healthcare organizations to routinely check the OIG Exclusion List to ensure that potential and current employees or contractors and physicians and other practitioners who order items and services that the provider renders are not excluded.

State Healthcare Fraud Laws

Many states also have enacted laws that address healthcare fraud and abuse. These state laws apply to all payers, not just federal healthcare programs. Some states have enacted laws that prohibit self-referral, which is the referral of patients for healthcare services by a physician or other healthcare professional to healthcare facilities in which that healthcare professional has an investment or other financial interest. Some state laws are similar to the Stark Law, while other states only require the referring physician or other healthcare professional to disclose their financial interests in a healthcare facility prior to the referral.

Many states have enacted laws that prohibit certain financial arrangements between healthcare practitioners that constitute illegal remuneration in return for the referral of patients, such as kickbacks or bribes. States also may have laws prohibiting fee-splitting among healthcare professionals and others in return for patient referrals. Private insurers also have taken measures to control healthcare fraud and may work with state or federal agencies to report or detect healthcare fraud.

Interaction among the Laws

The interaction among the laws can be convoluted. For example, neither the AKS nor the Stark Law contains a private right of action allowing a private plaintiff to file a lawsuit. Nevertheless, the government and *qui tam* plaintiffs have successfully argued that violations of the AKS and Stark Law can serve as the basis for a claim under the FCA. According to this theory, a claim to the government is rendered "false" for the purposes of the FCA if the medical services or items were furnished in violation of the AKS or Stark Law, even though the services or items provided were themselves appropriate and proper. Despite vigorous opposition by the healthcare industry and defense attorneys, a number of courts have accepted these theories. It is important that competent legal counsel be consulted on these matters as the laws, regulations, and case law change frequently.

Check Your Understanding 18.3

Instructions: Indicate whether the following statements are true or false (T or F).

1. Mergers of healthcare organizations are subject to the Sherman Antitrust Act.

2. The Deficit Reduction Act extended the application and scope of the current civil monetary penalty and exclusion authorities beyond programs funded by HHS to all federal healthcare programs.

3. The Patient Protection and Affordable Care Act added penalties for failing to report or return a known overpayment.

4. Waivers of the Stark Law, False Claims Act, and the Civil Monetary Penalties Law provision relating to beneficiary inducements apply to certain ACO arrangements.

5. When a provider is excluded from federal healthcare programs, services he orders for a beneficiary of one of these programs will be paid as long as the service is furnished by a non-excluded provider.

Federal Enforcement of Fraud and Abuse Laws and Regulations

The federal government has made major strides in combating healthcare fraud, through enforcement of applicable laws and a number of other actions. For example, in fiscal year 2014, the federal government's healthcare fraud enforcement efforts recovered more than $3 billion in taxpayer dollars. A total of 734 defendants were convicted of healthcare fraud-related crimes (CMS 2015c). The federal government is using a two-pronged strategy to combat fraud and abuse. Under new authorities granted by the ACA, programs have been implemented that move away from the "pay and chase" approach (namely, post-payment recovery of funds lost due to fraudulent claims) toward the use of powerful anti-fraud tools aimed at preventing healthcare fraud and abuse before it occurs (DOJ 2015b). Several examples of federal government settlements involving fraud allegations are listed in figure 18.4. These settlements

---

Figure 18.4 | **Example of recent federal government fraud settlements**

1. Thirty-five people pled guilty to their roles in a long-running and elaborate bribery scheme, which involved the acceptance of bribes in exchange for laboratory test referrals (DOJ 2015a).

2. The former owner and chief executive officer, the chief operating officer, and the chief financial officer of the now-closed Sacred Heart Hospital were convicted by a jury after a nearly two-month trial of collectively paying hundreds of thousands of dollars in illegal kickbacks in exchange for the referral of hospital patients who were insured by Medicare and Medicaid (DOJ 2015c).

3. Sixteen hospitals agreed to collectively pay $15.69 million to resolve False Claims Act allegations that they sought and received Medicare reimbursement for medically unnecessary psychotherapy services (DOJ 2015d).

4. A national Medicare fraud takedown resulted in charges against 243 individuals for their alleged participation in Medicare fraud schemes involving approximately $712 million in false billings. The defendants were charged with various healthcare fraud-related crimes, including conspiracy to commit healthcare fraud, violations of the anti-kickback statutes, money laundering and aggravated identity theft. The charges were based on a variety of alleged fraud schemes involving various medical treatments and services, including home healthcare, psychotherapy, physical and occupational therapy, durable medical equipment (DME), and pharmacy fraud (DOJ 2015e).

5. Adventist Health System agreed to pay $115 million to settle allegations that it violated the False Claims Act by maintaining improper compensation arrangements with referring physicians and by miscoding claims. Adventist allegedly submitted false claims to the Medicare and Medicaid programs for services rendered to patients referred by employed physicians who received bonuses based on a formula that improperly took into account the value of the physicians' referrals to Adventist hospitals. Adventist also allegedly submitted bills to Medicare for its employed physicians' professional services containing certain improper coding modifiers, and thereby obtained greater reimbursement for these services than entitled (DOJ 2015g).

6. Court issued a $237 million judgment against a South Carolina hospital for illegally billing the Medicare program for services referred by physicians with whom the hospital had improper financial relationships. The hospital entered into contracts with a number of specialist physicians that required the physicians to refer their outpatient procedures to the hospital and, in exchange, paid them compensation that far exceeded fair market value and included part of the money the hospital received from Medicare for the referred procedures (DOJ 2015h).

7. Nearly 500 hospitals paid more than $250 million to resolve False Claims Act allegations related to implantation of cardiac devices in Medicare patients in violation of a Medicare coverage policy (DOJ 2015i).

8. Thirty-two hospitals located throughout 15 states paid more than $28 million to settle allegations that they submitted false claims to Medicare for minimally-invasive kyphoplasty procedures. The hospitals allegedly often billed Medicare for kyphoplasty procedures on a more costly inpatient basis, rather than an outpatient basis, in order to increase their Medicare billings (DOJ 2015j).

9. The former owner and operator of three medical clinics was sentenced to 78 months in prison for his role in a scheme that submitted more than $4.5 million in fraudulent claims to Medicare. He and his co-conspirators paid illegal cash kickbacks to patient recruiters who brought Medicare beneficiaries to the clinics. They also billed Medicare for lab tests and other services that were not medically necessary or were not actually provided to the Medicare beneficiaries, which they supported with false documentation they created (DOJ 2016a).

10. Miami physician plead guilty for $20 million Medicare healthcare fraud scheme. In exchange for kickbacks and bribes, he and his co-conspirators wrote prescriptions for home healthcare and other services for Medicare beneficiaries that were not medically necessary or not provided and falsified patient records to make it appear as if the beneficiaries qualified for these services (DOJ 2016b).

---

were made possible as a result of federally mandated fraud and abuse programs, some of which are discussed next.

Health Care Fraud and Abuse Control Program

As mentioned at the beginning of the chapter, HIPAA established a comprehensive program to combat fraud committed against all health plans, both public and private. The legislation required the establishment of the national Health Care Fraud and Abuse Control (HCFAC) program, under the joint direction of the Attorney General and the Secretary of HHS acting through the Department's Inspector General (CMS 2015f). The HCFAC program is designed to coordinate federal, state, and local law enforcement activities with respect to healthcare fraud and abuse.

Healthcare Fraud Prevention Partnership (HFPP)

The Healthcare Fraud Prevention Partnership (HFPP) is a voluntary public-private partnership between the federal government, state officials, law enforcement, private health insurance plans and associations, and healthcare anti-fraud associations. The goal of this partnership is to foster a proactive approach to detect and prevent healthcare fraud through data and information sharing. In addition to exchanging information between the public and private sectors, the HFPP leverages various analytic tools against multiple data sets (CMS n.d.a).

Healthcare Fraud Prevention and Enforcement Action Team (HEAT)

The **Health Care Fraud Prevention and Enforcement Action Team (HEAT)** is a joint HHS and DOJ initiative to combat Medicare and Medicaid fraud. This team is using real-time data analysis to investigate healthcare fraud cases, rather than a prolonged subpoena and account analyses, resulting in much shorter periods of time between fraud identification, arrest and prosecution (HHS and DOJ, n.d.).

The mission of HEAT is

- To marshal significant resources across government to prevent waste, fraud, and abuse in the Medicare and Medicaid programs and crack down on the fraud perpetrators who are abusing the system and costing us all billions of dollars.
- To reduce skyrocketing healthcare costs and improve the quality of care by ridding the system of perpetrators who are preying on Medicare and Medicaid beneficiaries.
- To highlight best practices by providers and public sector employees who are dedicated to ending waste, fraud, and abuse in Medicare.
- To build upon existing partnerships between DOJ and HHS, such as our Medicare Fraud Strike Force Teams, to reduce fraud and recover taxpayer dollars. (DOJ n.d.)

The joint HHS/DOJ Medicare Fraud Strike Force is a multi-agency team of federal, state, and local investigators designed to fight Medicare fraud. Strike Force teams are located in healthcare fraud "hot spot" geographic locations and use advanced data analysis techniques to identify possible fraud. Since 2007, Strike Force teams have charged more than 2,300 defendants with defrauding Medicare of more than $7 billion and convicted approximately 1,800 defendants of felony healthcare fraud offenses (HHS and DOJ n.d.). In 2015, HEAT coordinated the largest-ever national healthcare fraud takedown involving $712 million in fraudulent billing (DOJ 2015e).

Centers for Medicare and Medicaid Services (CMS)

CMS, through its Center for Program Integrity, is responsible for, either directly or through oversight, a number of anti-fraud initiatives, such as tracking medical identity theft, using predictive modeling to identify suspect claims before payment, and suspending payments during the investigation of a credible allegation of fraud (CMS 2015c). Its efforts have been aimed at fraud prevention rather than the "pay and chase" approach. (namely, postpayment recovery of funds lost due to fraudulent claims) (GAO 2013). Since the concept of "program integrity" spans the entire spectrum of improper payments, from fraud to abuse, errors, and waste in the healthcare system, the goal of the CPI goes beyond fraud prevention and detection to ensuring that correct payments are made to legitimate providers for covered, appropriate, and reasonable services for eligible beneficiaries.

Similar to the technology used by credit card companies, CMS' Fraud Prevention System (FPS) applies advanced analytics to the Medicare Fee-for-Service claims. The FPS identifies aberrant and suspicious billing patterns, which trigger actions that can be quickly taken to prevent payment of fraudulent claims. Providers with aberrant billing patterns can be more readily identified and investigations prioritized (DOJ 2015b, GAO 2013).

Comprehensive Error Rate Testing (CERT) Program

CMS implemented the Comprehensive Error Rate Testing (CERT) program to measure improper payments in the Medicare Fee-for-Service program. A sample of Medicare claims is reviewed by an independent medical review contractor to determine if they were paid properly under Medicare coverage, coding, and billing rules. If these criteria are not met or the provider fails to submit medical records to support the claim billed, the claim is counted as either a total or partial improper payment and the improper payment may be recouped (for overpayments) or reimbursed (for underpayments). The annual Medicare fee-for-service improper payment rate is then calculated, which is published in the HHS Agency Financial Report. For example, the fiscal year (FY) 2015 improper payment rate was 12.1 percent, representing $43.3 billion in improper payments. Error categories identified in CERT reports include no documentation, insufficient documentation, lack of medical necessity, incorrect coding, and other. The improper payment rate is not a fraud rate, but rather a measurement of payments that did not comply with Medicare requirements. The CERT program cannot identify fraudulent claims. The CMS improper payment estimates are widely thought to understate the true size of the fraud, waste, and abuse problem (Energy and Commerce Committee 2013).

CMS Contractors

Two types of CMS contractors, Medicare Administrative Contractors and program integrity contractors, play a role in ensuring proper Medicare and Medicaid payments or preventing, detecting, and investigating possible fraud and abuse in federal healthcare programs. Program integrity contractors are further divided into five subtypes.

Medicare Administrative Contractors (MACs)

Since the inception of Medicare, private health insurers have processed medical claims for Medicare beneficiaries. These entities were originally known as Part A Fiscal Intermediaries and Part B Carriers. The Medicare Prescription Drug Improvement and Modernization Act of 2003 required CMS to replace Fiscal Intermediaries and Carriers with MACs. MACs are private health plans that have been awarded a geographic jurisdiction to process Medicare Parts A and B medical claims or Durable Medical Equipment claims for Medicare Fee-for-Service beneficiaries.

Medicare uses prepayment review to deny claims that should not be paid and postpayment review to recover payment from improperly paid claims. As claims make their way through Medicare's electronic claims processing systems, they are subject to prepayment edits. For automated edits, if a claim does not meet the edit criteria, it is automatically denied. Claims that fail manual prepayment edits are flagged for human review. The GAO recommended that increased use of prepayment edits would help prevent improper Medicare payments (GAO 2014).

Program Integrity Contractors

CMS Program Integrity Contractors are a nationally coordinated Medicare/Medicaid program integrity team of contractors. They are listed next in order of relevance or interest to the HIM and informatics community:

- Zone Program Integrity Contractors (ZPICs)
- Recovery Audit Contractors (RACs)
- Medicaid Integrity Contractors (MICs)
- National Benefit Integrity (NBI) Medicare Drug Integrity Contractor (MEDIC)
- Supplemental Medical Review Contractor (SMRC)

Zone Program Integrity Contractors (ZPICs) In 1999, CMS began transferring the responsibility for detecting and deterring fraud and abuse in Medicare Parts A and B from Fiscal Intermediary and Carrier fraud units to Program Safeguard Contractors (PSCs). The Program Safeguard Contractors were responsible for identifying and investigating potential fraud in specific parts of Medicare (such as Part A) in particular states or regions. In 2008, CMS began replacing PSCs with ZPICs, reducing the total number of contractors and granting additional responsibilities to ZPICs to investigate potential fraud across the Medicare Fee-for-Service programs (HHS OIG 2007; GAO 2013).

The primary goal of Zone Program Integrity Contractors (ZPICs) is to investigate instances of suspected fraud, waste, and abuse in Medicare Parts A and B programs. ZPIC responsibilities include

- Investigating fraud leads, including referrals from CMS' Fraud Prevention System
- Performing data analysis to identify cases of suspected fraud, waste, and abuse
- Making referrals to law enforcement for potential prosecution
- Providing support for ongoing investigations
- Identifying improper payments to be recovered

The seven Zone Program Integrity Contractor zones align with Medicare Administrative Contractor jurisdictions.

Recovery Audit Contractors (RACs) Medicare Recovery Audit Contractors (RACs) carry out the mission of the Medicare Fee-for-Service Recovery Audit Program, which is to identify and correct Medicare improper payments through the efficient detection and collection of overpayments made on claims of healthcare services provided to Medicare beneficiaries, and the identification of underpayments to providers so that CMS can implement actions that will prevent future improper payments (CMS n.d.c). The ACA required states to establish Medicaid RAC programs for the purpose of identifying underpayments and overpayments and recouping overpayments.

There are two types of Medicare RAC review. In an automated review, a claim determination is made at the system level with a human review of the medical record. Automated review may only be used when making Medicare coverage and coding determinations if there is certainty that the service is not covered or is incorrectly coded and there is a written Medicare policy, Medicare article, or Medicare-sanctioned coding guideline (such as a CPT statement or *Coding Clinic* statement). Automated review may be used when the Recovery Auditor makes other determinations (such as a duplicate claim) where there is certainty that an overpayment or underpayment exists. Overpayment determinations resulting from an automated review are communicated to the provider. In a complex review, a claim determination is made using human review of medical records or other documentation. Complex medical review is used in situations where there is a high probability (but not certainty) that the service is not covered or where no Medicare policy, Medicare article, or Medicare-sanctioned coding guideline exists. Whenever performing complex coverage or coding reviews, the RAC is required to ensure that coverage and medical necessity determinations are made by RNs or therapists and that coding determinations are made by certified coders. The results of every complex review, regardless of whether an improper payment was identified, are communicated to the provider. Providers have the right to appeal overpayments and underpayments determined during the RAC review process (CMS n.d.d).

RAC audits have had a significant impact on healthcare providers, especially health information management functions. RAC audits are very complex, and the appeal process is complicated and requires extensive technical expertise. Provider organizations have established systems and processes for managing and tracking RAC record requests, responses, and deadlines and for handling appeals. Internal audits of RAC focus areas have also become an essential function in order to reduce the risk of a RAC audit.

Medicaid Integrity Contractors (MICs) There are three types of Medicaid Integrity Contractors (MICs): review, audit and education. The MICs support state Medicaid program integrity efforts; conduct post-payment audits; and identify overpayments and refer them to states for collection. The objective of MICs is to ensure that paid claims are

- For services provided and properly documented
- For services billed properly, using correct and appropriate procedure codes
- For covered services
- Paid according to federal and state laws, regulations, and policies (CMS 2011)

National Benefit Integrity (NBI) Medicare Drug Integrity Contractor (MEDIC) The NBI MEDIC investigates fraud, waste, and abuse in the Medicare Parts C and D programs.

Supplemental Medical Review Contractor (SMRC) The SMRC is charged with performing, and or providing support for, a variety of tasks aimed at lowering improper payment rates and increasing efficiencies of the medical review functions of the Medicare and Medicaid programs.

Department of Justice

The prosecution and prevention of healthcare fraud is an important priority for the US Department of Justice (DOJ). As noted earlier in this chapter, the DOJ plays a critical role in HEAT. United States Attorneys' Offices play a major role in healthcare fraud enforcement by bringing criminal and affirmative civil cases to recover funds wrongfully taken from the Medicare Trust Funds and other taxpayer funded healthcare systems as a result of fraud, waste, and abuse. Civil and criminal healthcare fraud referrals are often made to United States Attorneys' Offices through other law enforcement agencies. The other principal source of referrals of civil cases for United States Attorneys' Offices is through the filing of *qui tam* complaints. Civil and criminal Assistant United States Attorneys litigate a wide variety of healthcare fraud matters, including false billings by physicians and other providers of medical services, overcharges by hospitals, Medicaid fraud, and kickbacks to induce referrals of Medicare or Medicaid patients, fraud by pharmaceutical and medical device companies, home health and hospice fraud, and failure of care allegations against nursing home owners (HHS OIG 2016).

The Fraud Section of the DOJ Criminal Division initiates and coordinates complex healthcare fraud prosecutions and supports the United States Attorneys' Offices with legal and investigative guidance and training and trial attorneys to prosecute healthcare fraud cases. The DOJ Civil Division's Commercial Litigation Branch (Fraud Section) investigates complex healthcare fraud allegations and files suit under the FCA to recover money on behalf of defrauded federal healthcare programs. The Fraud Section works closely with the United States Attorneys' Offices and often team with the Consumer Protection Branch, OIG, state Medicaid Fraud Control Units and other law enforcement agencies to pursue allegations of healthcare fraud (HHS OIG 2016).

In 2015, the DOJ announced policy changes designed to step up efforts to hold individuals, rather than just the corporate entity, accountable for corporate wrongdoing, in both civil and criminal matters. In a memorandum from the Deputy Attorney General (known as the "Yates Memo"), federal prosecutors were advised that criminal and civil corporate investigations should focus on individuals from the inception of the investigation. Absent extraordinary circumstances or approved departmental policy, the DOJ will not release culpable individuals from civil or criminal liability when resolving a matter with a corporation (DOJ 2015f).

Department of Health and Human Services Office of Inspector General

The HHS OIG is responsible for protecting the integrity of HHS programs and operations and the well-being of beneficiaries by detecting and preventing fraud, waste, and abuse; identifying opportunities to improve program economy, efficiency, and effectiveness; and holding accountable those who do not meet program requirements or who violate federal healthcare laws. Their mission encompasses more than 100 programs administered by HHS at agencies including CMS, Administration for Children and Families, Centers for Disease Control and Prevention, Food and Drug Administration, Indian Health Services, and National Institutes of Health.

The OIG carries out its mission to protect the integrity of HHS programs and the health and welfare of the people served by those programs through a nationwide network of audits, investigations, and evaluations, as well as outreach, compliance, and educational activities.

OIG Work Plan

The annual OIG Work Plan summarizes new and ongoing reviews and activities the OIG plans to pursue with respect to HHS programs and operations during the current fiscal year and beyond. To develop its work plan, the OIG assesses relative risks in HHS programs and operations to identify those areas most in need of attention and, accordingly, to set priorities for resource allocation. The factors the OIG considers when evaluating potential projects to undertake include

- Mandatory requirements for OIG reviews, as set forth in laws, regulations, or other directives
- Requests made or concerns raised by Congress, HHS management, or the Office of Management and Budget
- Top management and performance challenges facing HHS

- Work performed by other oversight organizations, such as the GAO
- Management's actions to implement OIG recommendations from previous reviews; and
- Potential for positive impact

For example, one project identified in the Fiscal Year 2017 OIG Work Plan is a "Review of CMS Action on CERT Data." As part of this review, the OIG planned to determine if CMS took action on its previous recommendation to use CERT data to target error-prone providers and reduce payment errors. They also intended to analyze CERT data to identify errors and potential patterns where further interventions could reduce payment errors (FY 2017 OIG Work Plan).

Corporate Integrity Agreements

A **corporate integrity agreement (CIA)** is an enforcement tool used by the HHS OIG to improve the quality of healthcare and to promote compliance with healthcare regulations (AHLA n.d.a). It is essentially a compliance program imposed by the government, with substantial government oversight and outside expert involvement in the organization's compliance activities. The OIG negotiates CIAs with healthcare providers and other entities as part of the settlement of federal healthcare program investigations arising under a variety of civil false claims statutes. Providers or entities agree to the obligations, and in exchange, OIG agrees not to seek their exclusion from participation in Medicare, Medicaid, or other federal healthcare programs. A material breach of the terms of a CIA may result in the provider's exclusion from participation in federal healthcare programs.

CIAs have many common elements, but each one addresses the specific facts at issue and often attempts to accommodate and recognize many of the elements of preexisting voluntary compliance programs. A comprehensive CIA typically lasts five years and includes requirements to

- Hire a compliance officer or appoint a compliance committee
- Develop written standards and policies
- Implement a comprehensive employee training program
- Retain an independent review organization to conduct annual reviews
- Establish a confidential disclosure program
- Restrict employment of ineligible persons
- Report overpayments, reportable events, and ongoing investigations/legal proceedings
- Provide an implementation report and annual reports to OIG on the status of the entity's compliance activities (HHS OIG n.d.c)

Fraud Alerts and Advisory Opinions

The OIG uses fraud alerts as a vehicle to identify fraudulent and abusive practices within the healthcare industry. For example, a fraud alert issued by the OIG in 2014 addressed compensation paid by laboratories to referring physicians for blood specimen collection, processing, and packaging, and for submitting patient data to a registry or database. Specifically, it described two specific trends OIG had identified involving transfers of value from laboratories to physicians that they believe presented a substantial risk of fraud and abuse under the AKS (HHS OIG 2014).

OIG also issues **advisory opinions** about the application of OIG's fraud and abuse authorities to the requesting party's existing or proposed business arrangement. While these advisory opinions are made available to the public through this OIG website, advisory opinions are binding and may legally be relied upon only by the requestor. One purpose of the advisory opinion process is to provide meaningful advice on the application of the anti-kickback statute and other OIG sanction statutes in specific factual situations.

Advisory opinions may address what constitutes prohibited remuneration, whether an arrangement fits an exception or safe harbor, what constitutes inducement to reduce or limit services, and whether the activity described would constitute grounds for the imposition of sanctions. Advisory opinions have been issued on a variety of topics including percentage compensation arrangements, joint ventures, beneficiary inducement, discounts, and waivers of deductibles and copayments. There have also been numerous informal letters issued by the OIG relating to subjects such as discounts and the provision of free items or services. Most of these and other federal government documents related to healthcare fraud and abuse are included on the OIG's website (HHS OIG n.d.d).

Provider Self-Disclosure Protocol

As part of a legal and ethical duty to deal with federal healthcare programs with integrity, healthcare organizations have an obligation to take measures to detect and prevent fraudulent and abusive practices, including the implementation of specific procedures and mechanisms to investigate and resolve instances of potential fraud involving federal healthcare programs. The **Provider Self-Disclosure Protocol** is a mechanism for providers to voluntarily disclose self-discovered evidence of potential fraud to the OIG. This protocol gives providers the opportunity to avoid the costs and disruptions associated with a federal investigation and civil or administrative litigation. It is intended to facilitate the resolution of only matters that, in the provider's reasonable assessment, are potential violations of federal criminal, civil, or administrative laws. The Provider Self-Disclosure Protocol provides guidance on how to investigate the improper conduct, quantify damages, and report this conduct to the OIG to resolve the provider's liability under the OIG's civil monetary penalty authorities. Good faith disclosure of potential fraud is reviewed as one indication of a robust and effective compliance program (HHS OIG 1998b, 2013b).

Matters involving only overpayments or errors that do not suggest that violations of law have occurred should be brought directly to the attention of the entity that processes the relevant claims and issues payment, such as a Medicare Administrative Contractor (HHS OIG 1998b, 2013b).

Check Your Understanding 18.4

Instructions: Indicate whether the following statements are true or false (T or F).

1. The federal government's primary approach to combating healthcare fraud is "pay and chase."

2. The Health Care Fraud Prevention and Enforcement Action Team (HEAT) uses real-time data analysis to investigate healthcare fraud cases.

3. The Medicare Fee-for-Service improper payment rate calculated through the Comprehensive Error Rate Testing (CERT) program is widely regarded to be an accurate reflection of the true size of the fraud, waste, and abuse problem.

4. The Government Accountability Office recommended that increased use of prepayment edits would help prevent improper Medicare payments.

5. All billing errors that result in overpayments by a federal healthcare program should be reported to the government through the Provider Self-Disclosure Protocol.

Fraud Prevention Strategies

Steps providers can take to prevent fraud and abuse include

- Becoming familiar with the laws and regulations governing healthcare
- Being aware of the organization's fraud and abuse risk areas
- Screening potential and existing employees and contractors for current exclusions, or grounds for exclusion, from federal healthcare programs
- Properly managing financial relationships
- Implementing a corporate compliance program

Corporate Compliance Programs

As stated earlier, corporate compliance is adherence to the laws and regulations passed by official regulating bodies as well as general principles of ethical conduct (Society of Corporate Compliance and Ethics, n.d.). A **corporate compliance program** is an internal set of policies, processes, and procedures that an organization implements to help it act ethically and lawfully (GAO 2014). Organizational compliance efforts are designed to establish a culture within a hospital that promotes prevention, detection, and resolution of instances of conduct that do not conform to federal and state law, and federal, state, and private payer healthcare program requirements, as well as the hospital's ethical and business policies. In practice, the compliance program should effectively articulate and demonstrate the organization's commitment to the compliance process. While implementing a compliance program may not completely eliminate fraud and abuse, a sincere effort to comply with applicable statutes and regulations as well as government and private payer healthcare program requirements helps a provider fulfill its legal duty to ensure that it is not submitting false or improper claims and significantly reduces the risk of unlawful or improper conduct.

According to the OIG, the benefits of implementing a compliance program may include

- The formulation of effective internal controls to ensure compliance with statutes, regulations, and rules
- A concrete demonstration to employees and the community at large of the organization's commitment to responsible corporate conduct
- The ability to obtain an accurate assessment of employee and contractor behavior
- An increased likelihood of identifying and preventing unlawful and unethical behavior
- The ability to quickly react to employees' operational compliance concerns and effectively target resources to address those concerns
- An improvement in the quality, efficiency, and consistency of providing services
- A mechanism to encourage employees to report potential problems and allow for appropriate internal inquiry and corrective action
- A centralized source for distributing information on healthcare statutes, regulations and other program directives
- A mechanism to improve internal communications
- Procedures that allow prompt and thorough investigation of alleged misconduct
- Through early detection and reporting, minimizing loss to the Government from false claims, and thereby reducing the organization's exposure to civil damages and penalties, criminal sanctions, and administrative remedies (HHS OIG 2000b)

While implementation of a corporate compliance program in most healthcare organizations is voluntary, the ACA contains a provision requiring providers and suppliers to establish a compliance program as a condition of enrollment in federal healthcare programs. This legislation also requires the Secretary of HHS to establish core elements for compliance programs within a particular industry or sector, and gave HHS the discretion to determine the timeline for establishing these core elements and the required implementation date. At press time, HHS has only issued core elements and a timeline for mandatory compliance programs in Medicare Advantage Plans and Medicare Prescription Drug Plans, not for other types of providers or suppliers. The ACA mandated the implementation of a compliance program in nursing facilities by March 2013 and set forth required elements for this program.

The OIG will consider the existence of an effective compliance program that pre-dated a federal investigation when addressing the appropriateness or severity of administrative penalties. In addition to mitigating fines and penalties, corporate compliance programs help organizations identify problems and improve performance. The adoption of a compliance program may help an organization avoid the imposition of a corporate integrity agreement (CIA), which was described earlier in this chapter. The OIG generally requires a CIA as a condition of settling a fraud and abuse investigation, but if a healthcare organization can demonstrate that it has an "effective" compliance program in place, the OIG may not require the execution of a CIA. If a CIA is required, it may not be as intrusive and may allow the organization to perform its own compliance functions, such as auditing, rather than requiring a more expensive third-party auditor, referred to as an independent review organization.

The Federal Sentencing Guidelines outline seven steps as the hallmark of an effective program to prevent and detect violations of law (USSC 2015) (see figure 18.5). These seven steps were the basis for the OIG's recommendations regarding the fundamental elements of an effective compliance program.

Figure 18.5   Seven steps for an effective compliance program

1. Establish standards and procedures to prevent and detect criminal conduct.

2. Assign responsibility to oversee compliance with the standards and procedures to specific individual(s) within high-level personnel of the organization.

3. Use reasonable efforts not to include within the substantial authority personnel of the organization any individual whom the organization knew, or should have known through the exercise of due diligence, has engaged in illegal activities or other conduct inconsistent with an effective compliance and ethics program.

4. Communicate periodically and in a practical manner its standards and procedures, and other aspects of the compliance and ethics program, to members of the governing authority, high-level personnel, substantial authority personnel, the organization's employees, and, as appropriate, the organization's agents, by conducting effective training programs and otherwise disseminating information appropriate to such individuals' respective roles and responsibilities.

5. Take reasonable steps to ensure that the organization's compliance and ethics program is followed, including monitoring and auditing to detect criminal conduct; to evaluate periodically the effectiveness of the organization's compliance and ethics program; and to have and publicize a system, which may include mechanisms that allow for anonymity or confidentiality, whereby the organization's employees and agents may report or seek guidance regarding potential or actual criminal conduct without fear of retaliation.

6. Promote and enforce the compliance program consistently throughout the organization through appropriate incentives to perform in accordance with the compliance and ethics program; and appropriate disciplinary measures for engaging in criminal conduct and for failing to take reasonable steps to prevent or detect criminal conduct.

7. After criminal conduct is detected, take reasonable steps to respond appropriately to the criminal conduct and to prevent further similar criminal conduct, including making any necessary modifications to the organization's compliance program.

Source: US Sentencing Commission 2015.

Both the Federal Sentencing Guidelines and compliance guidance issued by the OIG emphasize that a compliance program must be tailored to meet the specific needs of the organization, taking into account the size of the organization, the likelihood that certain offenses may occur because of the nature of the business, and the prior history of the organization. The OIG guidance provides specific recommendations for the structure and components of an effective compliance program.

The OIG has issued specific compliance guidance for the following entities (HHS OIG 1998a, 2005):

- Hospitals
- Clinical laboratories
- Home health agencies
- Third-party medical billing companies
- Durable medical equipment providers
- Hospices
- Medicare+Choice organizations
- Nursing facilities
- Ambulance suppliers
- Individual and small group physician practices
- Pharmaceutical manufacturers
- Recipients of US Public Health Service (PHS) research awards
- Part D plan sponsors (included in the Medicare Prescription Drug, Improvement and Modernization Act of 2003)

According to the OIG, these are the fundamental elements of an effective compliance program:

- Implementing written policies, procedures, and standards of conduct
- Designating a compliance officer and compliance committee
- Conducting effective training and education
- Developing effective lines of communication
- Conducting internal monitoring and auditing
- Enforcing standards through well-publicized disciplinary guidelines
- Responding promptly to detected offenses and undertaking corrective action

The core elements established by HHS for mandatory compliance programs in Medicare Advantage Plans and Medicare Prescription Drug Plans are consistent with the above elements contained in OIG guidance for effective compliance programs. The ACA added an eighth element for the mandatory compliance program for nursing facilities, requiring periodic reassessment of the compliance program to identify changes necessary to reflect changes within the organization and its facilities.

Elements of a Corporate Compliance Program

An effective corporate compliance program is one of the most effective tools to minimize a healthcare organization's fraud and abuse exposure. The adoption and implementation of compliance programs significantly advance the prevention of fraud, abuse, and waste while at the same time furthering the fundamental mission of all hospitals, which is to provide quality care to patients. Any entity engaged in submitting claims to Medicare cannot afford to be without a compliance program in these times of shrinking Medicare reimbursement and ever-increasing regulatory requirements that impact healthcare providers, particularly physicians.

A successful compliance program addresses the public and private sectors' mutual goals of reducing fraud and abuse, enhancing healthcare providers' operations, improving the quality of healthcare services, and reducing the overall cost of healthcare services (HHS OIG 1998a, 2005). Additional benefits include

- Demonstration of an organization's commitment to honest and responsible corporate conduct
- Increased likelihood of preventing, identifying, and correcting unlawful and unethical behavior at an early stage
- Encouragement of employees to report potential problems to allow for appropriate internal inquiry and corrective action
- Through early detection and reporting, minimization of any financial loss to government and taxpayers, as well as any corresponding financial loss to the hospital

A sincere effort by healthcare providers to comply with federal and state laws and regulations through an effective compliance program is a mitigating factor in reducing a provider's liability. It is not enough to have a compliance program—the organization must be able to demonstrate that its program is effective. To demonstrate that its compliance program is effective, every healthcare organization must include an evaluation and measurement of effectiveness as a component of its program (Bowman 2007).

Adopting and implementing an effective compliance program requires a substantial commitment of time, energy and resources by senior management and the hospital's governing body. An effective compliance program and plan should include the elements explained as follows.

Standards of Conduct

The compliance plan should include the organization's standards of conduct, often referred to as a **corporate code of conduct**. The standards of conduct express the organization's commitment to ethical behavior. The code should be the organization's constitution, detailing the fundamental principles, values, and framework for action within the organization. The code of conduct helps to define the organization's culture. It must include a clearly delineated commitment to compliance by the hospital's senior management and its divisions. Standards of conduct should state the organization's mission, goals, and ethical requirements of compliance and reflect a carefully crafted, clear expression of expectations for all governing body members, officers, managers, employees, physicians, and, where appropriate, contractors and other agents. Standards should be distributed to, and comprehensible by, all employees (HHS OIG 1998a).

Designation of a Compliance Officer

In order for a corporate compliance program to be effective, there must be appropriate oversight. OIG compliance guidance calls for someone to be responsible for the overall administration of the compliance activities in an organization. This oversight responsibility may be the individual's sole duty or added to other management responsibilities, depending upon the size and resources of the hospital and the complexity of the task. For multi-facility organizations, the OIG encourages coordination with each facility owned by the corporation or foundation through the use of a headquarters **compliance officer**, communicating with parallel positions in each facility, or regional office, as appropriate (HHS OIG 1998a). A compliance officer must have the appropriate authority and power to carry out the duties of the position in relationship to the laws and regulations governing compliance. The OIG recommends that a compliance committee be established to advise the compliance officer and assist in the implementation of the compliance program (HHS OIG 1998a, 2000b).

Policies and Procedures

The compliance plan must include policies and procedures that define the process for compliance and claims submission in the organization, including policies for identifying and reporting overpayments. The policies and procedures should be concise and easy to read and understand. These documents become a teaching tool for staff education and training. Policies and procedures should be reviewed and revised accordingly as part of the annual review of the compliance program. All staff members should have a current copy of the compliance plan containing the current policies and procedures.

Compliance in healthcare requires monitoring of activities that are highly vulnerable to fraud or other violations. Policies and procedures should include a risk assessment plan. Some regulatory risk areas are common to all healthcare providers. Areas of particular interest include referral relationships and arrangements, billing practices, privacy breaches, and adverse medical events. Risks may be identified through internal sources, such as employee reports to an internal compliance hotline or internal audits, OIG-issued documents such as its annual work plan, consultants, competitors, or news media (HHS et al. 2015). Specific examples of potential risks include

- Coding and billing issues (for example, upcoding, unbundling, duplicate billing)
- Documentation of reasonable and necessary services
- Consistent reporting of all compliance activities, including any potential instances of violation of Medicare laws and regulations (such as the Stark Laws)
- Accuracy of claims submission; payments to limit or reduce services
- Compliance with the Emergency Medical Treatment and Active Labor Act (EMTALA; see chapter 14)
- HIPAA Privacy and Security Rules and transaction standards
- Compliance with the Medicare Two-Midnight Rule (Under the two-midnight rule, an inpatient admission is generally appropriate for Medicare Part A payment if the physician [or other qualified practitioner] admits the patient as an inpatient based upon the expectation that the patient will need hospital care that crosses at least two midnights, with certain limited exceptions)

Risk assessment plans should take recent industry trends into account, including the increasing emphasis on quality, industry consolidation, and changes in insurance coverage and reimbursement. New reimbursement models (for example, value-based purchasing, bundling of services for a single payment, and global payments for maintaining the health of individual patients or entire patient populations) lead to new incentives and compliance risks. New payment models have incentivized consolidation among healthcare providers and more employment and contractual relationships, such as those between hospitals and physicians (HHS et al. 2015).

Education and Training

Education and training are essential elements of a compliance plan and should occur as part of a new employee's orientation to the organization and as an ongoing continuing education activity for staff. Compliance orientation should be provided to all new staff members, including physicians. The training should focus on compliance policies and procedures, with each staff member receiving a copy of the organizational compliance plan. Topics covered in the training should include corporate ethics, federal and state statutes and regulations, and payer policies. For staff involved in coding and billing, educational topics should include proper coding, and billing practices, proper documentation to support claims, and payer requirements. Staff and physicians should understand their role in the compliance program and how to report compliance concerns, in an anonymous manner if they so choose. Compliance education and training must be as detailed and as frequent as required by the size of the organization and the frequency of changes in laws and regulations.

Attendance records should be kept, along with detailed records of new hire compliance orientation and training as well as records of ongoing education and training of staff. The modalities used for education and training may include in-service sessions, teleconferences, reading material, and videoconferencing, to name a few.

Open Lines of Communication

Open lines of communication are an important element of compliance activity. Key to this element of a compliance program is a mechanism for staff members to report compliance violations or suspected violations. The OIG encourages the use of hotlines, e-mails, newsletters, suggestion boxes, and other forms of information exchange to maintain open lines of communication (HHS OIG 1998a, 2000b). Every healthcare provider should develop a procedure for reporting violations and ensure that all staff members understand how to report compliance concerns.

It is important that the procedure for reporting allow staff members to report anonymously if they choose to do so. This may be accomplished by a dedicated phone line to the compliance officer, a report form that can either be placed in a specified secure location (similar to a suggestion box) accessible only to the compliance officer, anonymous reporting via the organization's intranet, or a hotline operated by a third party to ensure anonymity.

In smaller organizations, an open-door policy is encouraged. Ideally, a staff member would have no fear of reporting a compliance concern. Built into the compliance plan should be a clear statement of disciplinary action taken against anyone in authority who punishes or causes any measure of retribution to a staff person who reports a compliance concern in good faith. Similarly, all staff members should be made aware that it is their responsibility to report compliance concerns and that they could face disciplinary action if they were aware of a compliance violation and did not report it.

Open communication means that everyone in the organization is mutually committed to maintaining compliance with the appropriate laws and regulations and ultimately committed to doing the right thing.

Auditing and Monitoring

An ongoing evaluation process is critical to a successful compliance program. The compliance program should be flexible enough to accommodate responding to current areas of priority with Medicare and other payers. The auditing and monitoring activities should be pertinent, focused, and ongoing while recognizing that it is not possible to monitor everything that is done all the time. High-priority targets for auditing and monitoring activities include identified high-risk areas (such as OIG focus areas published in the annual OIG Work Plan), problem-prone activities (such as patterns of coding errors or claims denials), and high-dollar and high-volume services. Monitoring techniques may include sampling protocols that permit the compliance officer to identify and review variations from an established baseline.

Significant variations from the baseline should trigger a reasonable inquiry to determine the cause of the deviation. Compliance reports created by ongoing monitoring processes, including reports of suspected noncompliance, should be maintained by the compliance officer and shared with the hospital's senior management and the compliance committee.

Audits should also be conducted to assess compliance with the Health Insurance Portability and Accountability Act (HIPAA), the Health Information Technology for Economic and Clinical Health Act (HITECH), and associated regulatory requirements, in order to ensure that privacy and security of personal health information are appropriately safeguarded.

Offense Detection and Corrective Action Initiatives

Responding to detected offenses and engaging in corrective action initiatives are core principles in determining whether the compliance program is effective or not. Effective action must be taken when problems are identified, and future monitoring must be done to ensure the problems stay solved.

Upon reports or reasonable indications of suspected noncompliance, it is important that the chief compliance officer or other management officials initiate prompt steps to investigate the conduct in question to determine whether a material violation of applicable law or the requirements of the compliance program has occurred, and if so, take steps to correct the problem. As appropriate, such steps may include an immediate referral to criminal and/or civil law enforcement authorities, a corrective action plan, a report to the Government, and the submission of any overpayments, if applicable. The outcome of the investigation may be any one of the following: no problem was found; a problem was found but is believed to be isolated and not likely to occur again; or a problem was found and needs corrective action—for example, not a violation of a law but an aberrant billing practice by one provider. If a problem is verified, then the corrective action plan should be appropriate to the seriousness of the offense. The following are sample actions that could be taken on confirmed compliance violations or errors:

- In-service education or retraining
- Fine or penalty
- Discipline
- Termination

Where potential fraud is not involved, the OIG recommends that the organization use normal repayment channels to return overpayments as they are discovered. However, even if the organization's billing department is effectively using the overpayment detection and return process, the OIG believes that the organization needs to alert the compliance officer to those overpayments that may reveal trends or patterns indicative of a systemic problem (HHS OIG 1998a, 2000b). For potential criminal violations, the entity, in collaboration with legal counsel, should self-disclose the violation to the appropriate government or law enforcement agency. As mentioned before, all actions conducted during the investigation of compliance issues and actions taken should be carefully documented and maintained in the files of the compliance officer.

Enforcing Disciplinary Standards through Well-Publicized Guidelines

An effective compliance program should include disciplinary policies that set out the consequences of violating the organization's standards of conduct, policies, and procedures. Enforcement and disciplinary provisions are necessary to add credibility and integrity to a compliance program. As with failure to investigate compliance violations and develop corrective action plans, if appropriate discipline is withheld, the compliance program is rendered ineffective and is not taken seriously by the staff.

Disciplinary action may be appropriate where a responsible employee's failure to detect a violation is attributable to his or her negligence or reckless conduct. Each situation must be considered on a case-by-case basis to determine the appropriate response (HHS OIG 2000b). Disciplinary actions should be appropriate to the compliance violation and, in some cases, they should reflect whether the violation is part of a pattern of behavior or a first offense. The range of disciplinary standards for improper conduct should be published and disseminated and employees should be educated regarding these standards. The consequences of noncompliance should be consistently applied and enforced (HHS OIG 1998a, 2000b). Discipline should be fair and consistent. Following is an example of inconsistent discipline:

A large hospital employs five coders in the HIM Department. In the spring of the year, one of the coders is found to be upcoding all pneumonia cases in order to maximize the DRG and reimbursement. She is terminated. The next year, a new coder is found to be coding all urinary tract infections as septicemia in order to maximize reimbursement. This employee is suspended for two weeks without pay and brought back to full employment.

Where appropriate, peer review should be part of the investigative process for physicians under disciplinary review. Obviously, in the case of a criminal offense, discipline would ultimately be determined by the court system.

Disciplinary actions might include, but are not limited to, the following:

- Oral (or verbal) warnings
- Written reprimands or warnings
- Probation
- Demotion
- Temporary suspension
- Termination
- Restitution of damages
- Referral for criminal prosecution

Check Your Understanding 18.5

Instructions: Indicate whether the following statements are true or false (T or F).

1. A corporate compliance program is an internal set of policies, processes, and procedures that an organization implements to help it act ethically and lawfully.
2. An effective compliance program is a mitigating factor in reducing a provider's liability under fraud and abuse laws.
3. The seven fundamental elements of an effective compliance program recommended by the OIG are based on HHS regulatory standards.
4. Oversight of the compliance program is primarily the responsibility of the organization's general counsel.
5. Detection of compliance violations is an important part of an effective compliance program.

Scenario 18.1

A registration employee in the cardiac catheterization laboratory noticed that one physician was providing the identical diagnosis as the reason for the procedure for all of his patients presenting for services in this department. None of the other physicians reported the exact same diagnosis for all of their patients. The physician in question also has a much higher number of referrals to the cardiac catheterization lab than other physicians. This employee does not have access to patients' health records, so she cannot check to see if the diagnosis is supported by documentation in the patients' medical records.

1. What should the employee do?
2. What steps should the employee's supervisor take?
3. What course(s) of action on the part of the facility might be appropriate to resolve this matter?
4. What potential federal statute(s) or law(s) may be at issue here?

Scenario 18.2

A hospital compliance auditor noticed during a routine audit that an unusually high number of pressure ulcers submitted on claims over the last six months were coded as stage 3 or 4. A deeper analysis of the medical records revealed that an upgrade in the computer-assisted coding software had resulted in a glitch whereby the system was automatically assigning the codes for either a stage 3 or 4 pressure ulcer regardless of the stage identified in the clinical documentation. While the coders were supposed to review auto-assigned codes, they had missed the errors in the pressure ulcer codes. Since a stage 3 or 4 pressure ulcer is a major complication/comorbidity in the Medicare MS-DRG system, the coding error had led to inappropriate higher-paying MS-DRGs in some cases.

1. What should the auditor do?
2. What should be the next step to confirm whether incorrect codes were submitted and resulted in overpayment?
3. If overpayments did occur, should the hospital just keep quiet about it and assume that other errors likely resulted in underpayments, so the overpayments and underpayments would probably balance each other out? If not, what actions should be taken?
4. Failure to report overpayments may result in liability under what federal statue(s) and/or law(s)?

References

Agrawal, S., B. Tarzy, L. Hunt, J. Taitsman, and P. Budetti. 2013 (August). Expanding physician education in health care fraud and program integrity. *Academic Medicine* 88(8):1081–1087.

American Health Lawyers Association. n.d.a. Corporate Integrity Agreements (CIAs). https://www.healthlawyers.org/hlresources/Health%20Law%20Wiki/Corporate%20Integrity%20Agreements%20(CIAs).aspx.

American Health Lawyers Association. n.d.b. Corporate compliance. https://www.healthlawyers.org/hlresources/Health%20Law%20Wiki/Corporate%20Compliance.aspx.

Bowman, S. 2007. *Health Information Management Compliance: Guidelines for Preventing Fraud and Abuse.* Chicago: AHIMA.

Centers for Medicare and Medicaid Services. 2006. Glossary. https://www.cms.gov/.

Centers for Medicare and Medicaid Services. 2011. Medicaid program integrity manual. https://www.cms.gov/Regulations-and-Guidance/Guidance/Manuals/Downloads/mpi115c17.pdf.

Centers for Medicare and Medicaid Services. 2014a. Medicare fraud and abuse: Prevention, detection, and reporting. https://www.cms.gov/Outreach-and-Education/Medicare-Learning-Network-MLN/MLNProducts/downloads/Fraud_and_Abuse.pdf.

Centers for Medicare and Medicaid Services. 2014b. National Training Program, Module 10. Medicare and Medicaid fraud and abuse prevention. https://www.cms.gov/Outreach-and-Education/Training/CMSNationalTrainingProgram/Downloads/2014-Medicare-and-Medicaid-Fraud-and-Abuse-Prevention-Workbook.pdf.

Centers for Medicare and Medicaid Services. 2015a. Common types of health care fraud. https://www.cms.gov/Medicare-Medicaid-Coordination/Fraud-Prevention/Medicaid-Integrity-Education/Downloads/fwa-factsheet.pdf.

Centers for Medicare and Medicaid Services. 2015b. Fraud and abuse waivers. https://www.cms.gov/.

Centers for Medicare and Medicaid Services. 2015c. Fraud, waste, and abuse toolkit. Health Care fraud and program integrity: An overview for providers. https://www.cms.gov/Medicare-Medicaid-Coordination/Fraud-Prevention/Medicaid-Integrity-Education/Downloads/fwa-overview-booklet.pdf.

Centers for Medicare and Medicaid Services. 2015d. Medicare program integrity manual. https://www.cms.gov/Regulations-and-Guidance/Guidance/Manuals/downloads/pim83c04.pdf.

Centers for Medicare and Medicaid Services. 2015e. Medicare program; Revisions to payment policies under the physician fee schedule and other revisions to Part B for CY 2016. *Federal Register* 80 (220):71300–71341.

Centers for Medicare and Medicaid Services. 2015f. The Health Care Fraud and Abuse Control Program Protects Consumers and Taxpayers by Combating Health Care Fraud. https://www.cms.gov/Newsroom/MediaReleaseDatabase/Fact-sheets/2015-Fact-sheets-items/2015-03-19.html.

Centers for Medicare and Medicaid Services. 2016. Medicare Program; Reporting and Returning of Overpayments. *Federal Register* 81(29):7654–7684.

Centers for Medicare and Medicaid Services. n.d.a. Healthcare Fraud Prevention Partnership. https://hfpp.cms.gov/about/.

Centers for Medicare and Medicaid Services. n.d.b. Comprehensive Error Rate Testing (CERT). https://www.cms.gov/Research-Statistics-Data-and-Systems/Monitoring-Programs/Medicare-FFS-Compliance-Programs/CERT/index.html?redirect=/cert.

Centers for Medicare and Medicaid Services. n.d.c. Medicare Fee for Service Recovery Audit Program. https://www.cms.gov/research-statistics-data-and-systems/monitoring-programs/medicare-ffs-compliance-programs/recovery-audit-program/.

Centers for Medicare and Medicaid Services. n.d.d. Statement of Work for the Part A/B Medicare Fee-for-Service Recovery Audit Program – Regions 1–4. https://www.cms.gov/Research-Statistics-Data-and-Systems/Monitoring-Programs/Medicare-FFS-Compliance-Programs/Recovery-Audit-Program/Downloads/New_RAC-SOW-Regions-1-4-clean.pdf.

Centers for Medicare and Medicaid Services and Department of Health and Human Services Office of Inspector General. 2015. Medicare Program; Final Waivers in Connection With the Shared Savings Program. *Federal Register* 80(209):66726–66730.

Department of Health and Human Services and Department of Justice. n.d. Healthcare Fraud Prevention and Enforcement Action Team (HEAT). https://www.stopmedicarefraud.gov/aboutfraud/heattaskforce/.

Department of Health and Human Services Office of Inspector General. 1998a. Compliance program guidance for hospitals. *Federal Register* 63(35):8987–8998. http://oig.hhs.gov.

Department of Health and Human Services Office of Inspector General. 1998b. Publication of the OIG's Provider Self-Disclosure Protocol. *Federal Register* 63 (210): 58399–58403.

Department of Health and Human Services Office of Inspector General. 2000a. Health care program: Fraud and abuse; Revised OIG civil money penalties resulting from Public Law 104-191. *Federal Register* 65(81):24400–24419.

Department of Health and Human Services Office of Inspector General. 2000b. Publication of the OIG Compliance Program Guidance for Nursing Facilities. *Federal Register* 65(52):14289–14305.

Department of Health and Human Services Office of Inspector General. 2005. Supplemental compliance program guidance for hospitals. *Federal Register* 70(19):4858–4856. http://oig.hhs.gov.

Department of Health and Human Services Office of Inspector General. 2006. Medicare and state health care programs: Fraud and abuse; Safe harbors for certain electronic prescribing and electronic health records arrangements under the Anti-Kickback Statute. *Federal Register* 71 (152): 45110–45111. https://www.gpo.gov/fdsys/pkg/FR-2006-08-08/pdf/06-6666.pdf.

Department of Health and Human Services Office of Inspector General. 2007. Medicare's program safeguard contractors: Activities to detect and deter fraud and abuse. http://oig.hhs.gov/oei/reports/oei-03-06-00010.pdf.

Department of Health and Human Services Office of Inspector General. 2013a. Medicare and state health care programs: Fraud and abuse; Electronic health records safe harbor under the Anti-Kickback Statute. *Federal Register* 78(249):79202–79219. https://www.gpo.gov/fdsys/pkg/FR-2013-12-27/pdf/2013-30924.pdf.

Department of Health and Human Services Office of Inspector General. 2013b. Provider Self-Disclosure Protocol. http://oig.hhs.gov/.

Department of Health and Human Services Office of Inspector General. 2014 (June 25). Special Fraud Alert: Laboratory payments to referring physicians. http://oig.hhs.gov.

Department of Health and Human Services Office of Inspector General. 2015 (October 6). OIG policy reminder: Information blocking and the Federal Anti-Kickback Statute. http://oig.hhs.gov/.

Department of Health and Human Services Office of Inspector General. 2016 (February). The Department of Health and Human Services and the Department of Justice Health Care Fraud and Abuse Control Program Annual Report for Fiscal Year 2015. https://oig.hhs.gov/publications/docs/hcfac/FY2015-hcfac.pdf.

Department of Health and Human Services Office of Inspector General. Fiscal Year 2017 HHS OIG Work Plan. https://oig.hhs.gov/reports-and-publications/archives/workplan/2017/HHS%20OIG%20Work%20Plan%202017.pdf.

Department of Health and Human Services Office of Inspector General. n.d.a. A roadmap for new physicians—Avoiding Medicare and Medicaid fraud and abuse laws. http://oig.hhs.gov/.

Department of Health and Human Services Office of Inspector General. n.d.b. Compliance guidance. http://oig.hhs.gov.

Department of Health and Human Services Office of Inspector General. n.d.c. Corporate integrity agreements. http://oig.hhs.gov.

Department of Health and Human Services Office of Inspector General. n.d.d. Fraud Alerts. http://oig,hhs.gov.

Department of Health and Human Services Office of Inspector General. n.d.e. Provider Compliance Training. Comparison of the Anti-Kickback Statute and Stark Law. http://oig.hhs.gov/compliance/provider-compliance-training/files/StarkandAKSChartHandout508.pdf

Department of Health and Human Services Office of Inspector General. n.d.f. Safe harbor regulations. http://oig.hhs.gov.

Department of Health and Human Services Office of Inspector General, Association of Healthcare Internal Auditors, American Health Lawyers Association, and Health Care Compliance Association. 2015. Practical guidance for health care governing boards on compliance oversight. http://oig.hhs.gov/compliance/compliance-guidance/docs/Practical-Guidance-for-Health-Care-Boards-on-Compliance-Oversight.pdf.

Department of Justice. 2015a (February 4). Press release: Doctor admits taking bribes in test-referral scheme with New Jersey clinical lab. https://www.justice.gov/usao-nj/pr/doctor-admits-taking-bribes-test-referral-scheme-new-jersey-clinical-lab-0.

Department of Justice. 2015b (March 19). Press Release: Departments of Justice and Health and Human Services announce over $27.8 billion in returns from joint efforts to combat health care fraud. http://www.justice.gov/opa/pr/departments-justice-and-health-and-human-services-announce-over-278-billion-returns-joint.

Department of Justice. 2015c (March 19). Press release: Owner and executives convicted in Medicare referral kickback conspiracy at closed Sacred Heart Hospital. https://www.justice.gov/usao-ndil/pr/owner-and-executives-convicted-medicare-referral-kickback-conspiracy-closed-sacred.

Department of Justice. 2015d (May 7). Press release: Sixteen hospitals to pay $15.69 million to resolve False Claims Act allegations involving medically unnecessary psychotherapy services. https://www.justice.gov/opa/pr/sixteen-hospitals-pay-1569-million-resolve-false-claims-act-allegations-involving-medically.

Department of Justice. 2015e (June 18). Press release: National Medicare fraud takedown results in charges against 243 individuals for approximately $712 million in false billing. https://www.justice.gov/opa/pr/national-medicare-fraud-takedown-results-charges-against-243-individuals-approximately-712.

Department of Justice. 2015f (September 9). Memorandum on individual accountability for corporate wrongdoing. http://www.justice.gov/.

Department of Justice. 2015g (September 21). Adventist Health System agrees to pay $115 million to settle False Claims Act allegations. https://www.justice.gov/opa/pr/adventist-health-system-agrees-pay-115-million-settle-false-claims-act-allegations.

Department of Justice. 2015h (October 16). Press release: United States resolves $237 million False Claims Act judgment against South Carolina hospital that made illegal payments to referring physicians. https://www.justice.gov/opa/pr/united-states-resolves-237-million-false-claims-act-judgment-against-south-carolina-hospital.

Department of Justice. 2015i (October 30). Press release: Nearly 500 hospitals pay United States more than $250 million to resolve False Claims Act allegations related to implantation of cardiac devices. https://www.justice.gov/opa/pr/nearly-500-hospitals-pay-united-states-more-250-million-resolve-false-claims-act-allegations.

Department of Justice. 2015j (December 18). Press release: 32 hospitals to pay U.S. more than $28 million to resolve False Claims Act allegations related to kyphoplasty billing. https://www.justice.gov/usao-wdny/pr/32-hospitals-pay-us-more-28-million-resolve-false-claims-act-allegations-related.

Department of Justice. 2016a (January 4). Press release: Owner of three Los Angeles clinics sentenced to 78 months in prison for Medicare fraud. https://www.justice.gov/opa/pr/owner-three-los-angeles-clinics-sentenced-78-months-prison-medicare-fraud.

Department of Justice. 2016b (February 9). Press release: Miami physician pleads guilty for role in $20 million health care fraud scheme. https://www.justice.gov/usao-sdfl/pr/miami-physician-pleads-guilty-role-20-million-health-care-fraud-scheme.

Department of Justice. n.d. Health Care Fraud Unit. https://www.justice.gov/criminal-fraud/health-care-fraud-unit.

Energy and Commerce Committee. 2013 (February 25). Memorandum on hearing entitled "Fostering innovation to fight waste, fraud and abuse in health care." http://docs.house.gov/meetings/IF/IF14/20130227/100329/HMTG-113-IF14-20130227-SD001-U1.pdf.

Government Accountability Office. 2013. Medicare program integrity: Contractors reported generating savings, but CMS could improve its oversight. http://www.gao.gov/assets/660/658565.pdf.

Government Accountability Office. 2014. Testimony before Subcommittee on Health, Committee on Ways and Means, House of Representatives. MEDICARE FRAUD: Progress made, but more action needed to address Medicare fraud, waste, and abuse. http://www.gao.gov/assets/670/662845.pdf.

Institute of Medicine. 2012. Best care at lower cost: The path to continuously learning health care in America. http://iom.nationalacademies.org/Reports/2012/Best-Care-at-Lower-Cost-The-Path-to-Continuously-Learning-Health-Care-in-America.aspx.

National Association of Medicaid Directors. 2012. Rethinking Medicaid program integrity: Eliminating duplication and investing in effective, high-value tools. http://medicaiddirectors.org/wp-content/uploads/2015/08/namd_medicaid_pi_position_paper_final_120319.pdf.

National Health Care Anti-Fraud Association. n.d. The problem of health care fraud. http://www.nhcaa.org.

Simborg, D. 2011. There is no neutral position on fraud! *Journal of the American Medical Informatics Association* 18(5):675–677.

Society of Corporate Compliance and Ethics. n.d. https://www.corporatecompliance.org/.

Taft. 2015 (November 12). News and Events. CMS final rule includes revisions to Stark Law. http://www.taftlaw.com/.

US Sentencing Commission. 2015. Federal sentencing guidelines, section 8B2.1: Effective compliance and ethics program. http://www.ussc.gov.

Federal Statutes and Regulations Cited

42 CFR 411.350 et seq.: Financial Relationships Between Physicians and Entities Furnishing Designated Health Services. 2004.

42 CFR 411.355: General exceptions to the referral prohibition related to both ownership/investment and compensation. Amended 2010.

42 CFR 411.357: Exceptions to the referral prohibition related to compensation arrangements. Amended 2016.

42 CFR 1001.952(y). Safe Harbor Anti-Kickback. Exceptions. Amended 2016.

15 USC 1–7: Sherman Antitrust Act. 1890. Amended 1914.

18 USC 287: Criminal False Claims Act. 1986.

18 USC 1347: Criminal Health Care Fraud. Amended 2010.

31 USC 3729–3733: Civil False Claims Act. 1986. Amended 2010.

31 USC 3730(e)(4)(A)(B), 42 USC 1320a–7k(d): Patient Protection and Affordable Care Act. 2010.

31 USC 3321: Improper Payments Information Act of 2002. Amended, 2010, 2012.

42 USC 1320a–7: Exclusion. Amended 2010.

42 USC 1320a–7a: Civil monetary penalties 1128A. Amended 2010.

42 USC 1320a–7b: Federal Anti-Kickback Statute. Amended 2010.

42 USC 1395nn, 42 USC 1396b: Physician Self-Referral Statute (Stark Law). Amended 2010.

42 USC 1396a(a)(68): Deficit Reduction Act. 2006.

Fraud Enforcement and Recovery Act of 2009. Public Law 111-21.

Patient Protection and Affordable Care Act of 2010. Public Law 111-148.

Small Business Jobs Act of 2010. Public Law 111-240.

Bipartisan Budget Act of 2015. Public Law 114-74.

Medical Staff

Rebecca B. Reynolds, EdD, MHA, RHIA, CHPS, FAHIMA, and Melanie S. Brodnik, PhD, RHIA, FAHIMA

Learning Objectives

- Discuss the relationship of a healthcare organization's governing board to its medical staff
- Describe the components of medical staff bylaws as required by the Joint Commission accreditation standards for medical staff
- Identify the various categories of medical staff membership
- Explain the significance of the medical staff credentialing process
- Describe the process of applying for medical staff privileges, including primary source verification, and how privileges are determined
- Discuss the duties and rights of a medical staff and issues related to disciplinary action, suspension of privileges, and due process under the law

Key Terms

- Accreditation Council for Graduate Medical Education (ACGME)
- American Board of Medical Specialties (ABMS)
- *Comprehensive Accreditation Manual for Hospitals*
- Credentialing
- Credentials verification organization (CVO)
- Deemed status
- Due process
- Focused professional practice evaluation
- Locum tenens
- Medical staff
- Medical staff bylaws
- Medical staff executive committee
- National Association of Medical Staff Services (NAMSS)
- National Committee for Quality Assurance (NCQA)
- Ongoing professional practice evaluation
- Primary source verification

The **medical staff** of a healthcare organization is comprised of individuals who have been granted clinical privileges to provide care to patients in the organization. The medical staff includes physicians and other healthcare providers such as nurse practitioners, physician assistants, dentists, optometrists, pharmacists, podiatrists, and psychologists who may be employed by the healthcare organization or who may function as independent contractors. In either situation, the practitioner is governed by medical staff bylaws that are compliant with governing body bylaws, facility polices, laws, and regulations. The medical staff bylaws define the responsibilities and obligations of the practitioner to provide quality patient care. The bylaws are typically voted upon by the medical staff and approved by the healthcare organization's governing board, which must ensure that the medical staff is competent to treat patients. To practice in a healthcare organization, a physician or care provider must apply for and be admitted to the medical staff. The application process includes a credentialing procedure that verifies the background of the care provider and assists in defining the type of appointment granted to the practitioner. The credentialing process requires continuing review of credentials and renewal of staff appointments on a regular basis. This chapter provides a brief review of the governing board responsibilities of an organization and how it delegates power to the medical staff to provide quality patient care. It discusses the components of medical staff bylaws and the application process for granting medical staff privileges. It covers the process of medical staff credentialing and the duties and rights of the medical staff with regard to patient care and documentation requirements. The chapter also discusses issues related to granting or denial of medical staff privileges as well as consequences for not adhering to the bylaws.

Governing Board

The governing board as discussed in chapter 7 has ultimate responsibility for the quality of care and financial well-being of the healthcare organization as described in governing body bylaws. Typical responsibilities of a hospital board include the following:

- Define the mission and purpose of the organization
- Select (hire the chief executive officer [CEO])
- Review and support the CEO
- Ensure adequate organization planning
- Ensure the financial health of the organization (fiduciary duty)
- Ensure the quality of patient care
- Enhance the public image of the organization
- Serve as a court of appeals (for due process of the medical staff)
- Assess the performance of the board of directors (BOD)

The composition of the board for a hospital may include physicians, community leaders, religious leaders, businesspeople, and attorneys. Members of the board are usually appointed, but the structure may allow for elected positions as well. The business model for healthcare organizations particularly hospitals is unique in that the hospital relies on the medical staff to admit and treat patients, which ultimately generates business for the organization. In order for a patient to receive care, a physician or other authorized-care provider, as designated by state licensing law, must order the treatment or service delivered to the patient. Thus, the board delegates power to the organized medical staff to provide patient care and to ensure quality of care for the patients in the facility.

The governing board must ensure that its medical staff members are qualified, competent, and up-to-date on the education and training required to provide appropriate medical care and avoid legal risk. The board hires the healthcare administrator or chief executive officer (CEO), who reports directly to the board and works with the organized medical staff to provide patient care services. The CEO is responsible for the overall management of the healthcare facility while the organized medical staff is responsible for oversight of the quality of patient care and is also directly accountable to the governing board. A sample organizational chart for a healthcare organization is shown in figure 19.1.

To fulfill its responsibilities, the medical staff is governed by bylaws that are voted upon by the medical staff and approved by the governing board of the organization.

Medical Staff Bylaws

The requirement for an organized medical staff is found in state licensure standards, as well as the accreditation standards of many standard-setting organizations. See figure 19.2 for a list of standards organizations that govern medical staff quality. Because the Joint Commission is the dominant accrediting organization in the United States for hospitals and other types of healthcare organizations, it is important to

Figure 19.1 Organization chart

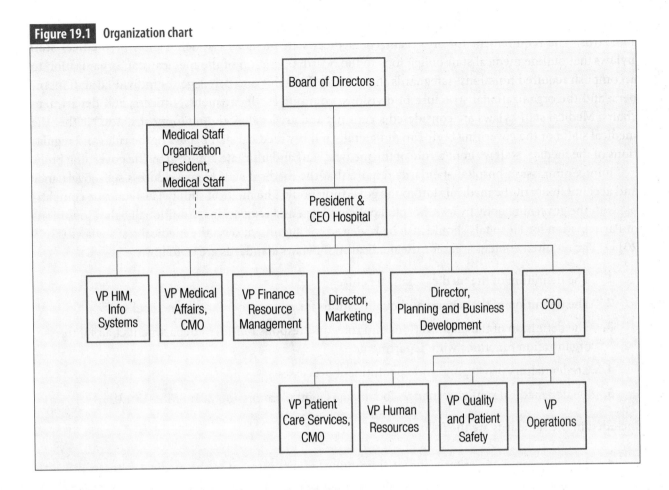

Figure 19.2 Medical staff quality and standards organizations

- Accreditation Association for Ambulatory Health Care
- Accreditation Commission for Healthcare
- Accreditation Council for Graduate Medical Education
- American Association for Ambulatory Surgery Facilities
- American Board of Medical Specialties
- American Medical Association Masterfile request
- American Osteopathic Association/Healthcare Facilities Accreditation Program
- Center for Improvement in Healthcare Quality
- Commission on Accreditation of Rehabilitation Facilities
- Community Health Accreditation Program
- DNV Healthcare
- Federation of State Medical Boards
- The Joint Commission
- National Committee for Quality Assurance
- National Practitioner Data Bank
- National Quality Forum
- URAC/American Accreditation Healthcare Commission

understand the Joint Commission medical staff standards and the liabilities for noncompliance of these standards. The requirement for an organized medical staff includes the delineation of **medical staff bylaws** that outline medical staff obligations to the board; operation of the medical staff organization to accomplish required functions; safeguards that protect the rights and privileges of individual staff members; and the organizational structure of divisions, committees, departments, officers, and department chairs. Medical staff bylaws are considered a contract and are legally binding in most states. Neither the medical staff nor the governing body can unilaterally modify medical staff bylaws or the rules and regulations of the medical staff without a vote of the medical staff and ultimate approval by the governing body.

Joint Commission hospital standards require that the medical staff bylaws address self-governance and accountability of the medical staff to the governing body. The medical staff bylaws must be compatible with the governing body bylaws, hospital policies, laws, and regulations. Additionally, the Conditions of Participation for Hospitals should also be reviewed for alignment with the medical staff bylaws (HHS 2011). The required content areas for the medical staff bylaws standards are as follows:

1. The definition of the medical staff structure
2. The definition of the criteria and qualifications for appointment to the medical staff
3. The definition of the qualifications and roles and responsibilities of department chairs if the organization functions with departments
4. Credentialing, privileging, and appointment processes
5. Related medical staff governance documents (Joint Commission 2016, MS.01.01.01)

Included in the standards are the following:

- The definition of the criteria and qualifications for appointment to the medical staff
- The qualifications and roles and responsibilities of the department chair
- A description of the **medical staff executive committee** including the function, size, composition, and methods for selecting and removing its members and the medical staff officers
- A statement empowering the medical staff executive committee to act for the organized medical staff between meetings of the medical staff
- A description of indications for automatic suspension or summary suspension of a practitioner's medical staff membership and clinical privileges
- A description of when automatic suspension or summary suspension procedures are implemented
- A description of the mechanism to recommend medical staff membership or terminations, suspensions, or reductions in privileges
- A description of the mechanism for a fair hearing and appeal process
- A description of the credentialing and privileging processes
- A description of the process of appointment to membership of the medical staff (Joint Commission 2016, MS.01.01.01)

The standards require that the organized medical staff operate under the direction of the medical staff officers and a committee structure. The medical staff officers typically consist of a president, president-elect, chief of staff, and vice chief of staff, with the president-elect transitioning to president and the vice chief of staff transitioning to the chief of staff position. Depending on the size and organization of the medical staff, there might be an associate chief of staff for each department. In the case of multisite facilities with a common organized medical staff, there might be an associate chief of staff for each department from each facility that shares a common medical staff. This provides greater representation for the medical staff in larger facilities.

Often the president of the medical staff serves as the chair of the medical staff executive committee and presides over meetings of the general medical staff. By virtue of position, the president of the medical staff is typically a member of the hospital board and serves as a spokesperson for the medical staff in its public relations and external professional capacities. Additionally, the leadership of the medical staff consists of a chair of each clinical department and chairs of major medical staff committees. See figure 19.3 for a list of typical medical staff committees. The chair of each clinical department (such as medicine, surgery, pediatrics) is usually an appointed position to minimize the pressures on this individual to enforce rules. The chair typically serves a term greater than one year and tends to be an established, experienced, and respected member of the medical staff.

Medical Staff Executive Committee

The Joint Commission requires that the medical staff executive committee be comprised of elected members of the medical staff who are authorized to act on behalf of the medical staff. Only those physicians who are medical doctors (MD), clinical psychologists, doctors of osteopathy (DO), or oral surgeons and dentists (DDS) approved by the board for medical staff membership may serve as members of the medical staff executive committee and have voting rights. Others may belong to the committee as ex officio members without voting rights. An example of an ex officio member would be the organization CEO. The Joint Commission requires that hospitals who use Joint Commission accreditation for **deemed status** have a medical staff executive committee (Joint Commission 2016, MS.02.01.01). Deemed status enables a healthcare organization that is Joint Commission-accredited to use its accreditation status in lieu of a separate Medicare or Medicaid Conditions of Participation healthcare organization certification process. In small hospitals, the entire medical staff may serve as the executive committee. Regardless of the size of the medical staff, the medical staff executive committee must follow the function and structure as described in the medical staff bylaws for the organization.

Figure 19.3 List of typical medical staff committees

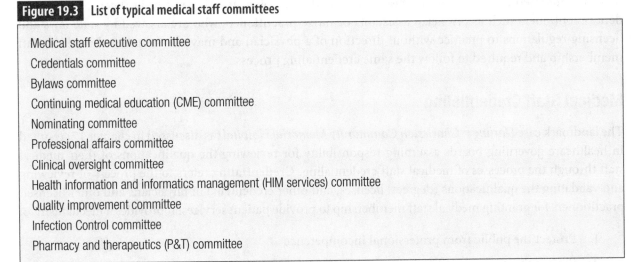

Medical staff executive committee
Credentials committee
Bylaws committee
Continuing medical education (CME) committee
Nominating committee
Professional affairs committee
Clinical oversight committee
Health information and informatics management (HIM services) committee
Quality improvement committee
Infection Control committee
Pharmacy and therapeutics (P&T) committee

Note: These are hospital-wide medical staff committees. Each department typically has a medical staff department committee that conducts the business of the specific department.

Table 19.1	Classification (categories) of medical staff membership
Active (regular)	This category has all the responsibilities of medical staff membership and all the privileges. They can serve as medical staff officers and chair medical staff committees.
Associate	This category has all the responsibilities of medical staff membership and all the privileges. However, they cannot serve as medical staff officers or chair medical staff committees.
Courtesy	This category is reserved for those medical staff who have a primary clinical practice at another facility. It allows for a limited number of hospital admissions without the responsibilities of membership.
Consulting	This category is intended for those medical staff who do not admit patients but who serve as consultants to other members of the medical staff. They typically do not have to attend committee meetings and cannot serve as medical staff officers.
Honorary	This category is intended for those medical staff who practice very little and may not admit patients, but their reputation and previous service to the hospital is such that the hospital wishes to recognize their contribution.
Affiliate	This category is designated for those non-physicians who are allowed to join the staff. There may be restrictions on what role these members have on committees and what, if any, voting privileges they have.

Categories of Medical Staff Membership

The medical staff bylaws describe the classifications or categories of medical staff membership. Table 19.1 details several typical categories. The distinction between categories of members of the medical staff is important since this defines the responsibilities and privileges of each member. Multiple categories of membership provide flexibility and allow for a larger pool of staff to assist with patient care needs. The organized medical staff defines the scope of practice via the privileges that are extended to practitioners.

The medical staff is comprised of those medical staff members who are granted permission or clinical privileges to provide care to patients in the hospital. The medical staff may be comprised of physicians, dentists, optometrists, pharmacists, podiatrists, and psychologists. There may be licensed independent practitioners such as physician assistants or nurse practitioners who are allowed by state laws and licensing regulations to practice without direction of a physician and may also be granted medical staff membership and required to follow the same credentialing process.

Medical Staff Credentialing

The landmark case *Darling v. Charleston Community Memorial Hospital* (as discussed in chapter 17) resulted in healthcare governing boards assuming responsibility for reviewing the qualifications of their medical staff through the processes of medical staff credentialing. **Credentialing** refers to the process of reviewing and validating the qualifications (degrees, licenses, and other credentials) of physicians and other licensed practitioners for granting medical staff membership to provide patient services. It provides a mechanism to:

1. Protect the public from professional incompetence
2. Protect the medical staff from working with incompetent professionals
3. Protect the facility from liability due to providing inadequate care
4. Protect the rights of the medical staff from unfair restrictions on their practice

The **National Association of Medical Staff Services (NAMSS)** recommends 13 criteria for review that should be included in the medical staff bylaws, rules and regulations and other governance documents. The credentialing review should also detect professional incompetence, malevolence, behavioral problems, and other red flags (NAMSS 2014). This review should also include the **Accreditation Council for Graduate Medical Education (ACGME)** Common Program Requirements including patient care and procedural skills, medical knowledge, practice-based learning and improvement, systems-based practice, professionalism, and interpersonal and communication skills (ACGME 2015). A functional credentialing process results in the granting of privileges to practice at a site based on the practitioner's credentials. It protects the self-governance of the professional community and allows a medical staff to regulate its practices within a healthcare organization.

Anyone who applies for medical staff privileges must go through the credentialing process maintained by the healthcare organization where they wish to practice. All healthcare providers are subject to the same credentialing process as defined by the organization's medical staff bylaws and employment criteria. The Joint Commission requires that for facilities using Joint Commission accreditation for deemed status that the surgical services area maintain a current roster of each practitioner's surgical privileges (Joint Commission 2016, MS.06.01.06).

Other non-physician allied health professionals (such as nurse anesthetists, occupational therapists, and physical therapists) who are not considered part of the medical staff may also go through the credentialing process depending on the policy of the healthcare organization. These individuals may be licensed through a state licensing board, and in some cases, professional certifications, before they are allowed to practice in a given discipline. For the most part, these individuals work under the direction and supervision of a physician. However, in some states non-physician healthcare providers such as physical therapists are allowed to offer services without a physician's order. The ability to practice without physician oversight for some disciplines is seen as one way of lowering healthcare costs and addressing physician workforce shortages.

Check Your Understanding 19.1

Instructions: Indicate whether the following statements are true or false (T or F).

1. The medical staff has the ultimate responsibility for the quality and financial well-being of the health organization.

2. Medical staff bylaws are considered a contract and are legally binding in most states.

3. The executive committee of the medical staff does not have to follow the medical staff bylaws.

4. If a practitioner is assigned a medical staff category of "associate," he or she can chair the medical staff executive committee.

5. The classification of medical staff membership impacts a provider's ability to admit patients to a healthcare facility.

Joining the Medical Staff

Healthcare organizations must have rigorous processes in place to ensure that only competent, qualified physicians and other licensed independent practitioners are providing patient care. Hospitals and other healthcare organizations typically have a dedicated medical staff office or individual (medical staff coordinator) responsible for oversight of the credentialing and privileging processes. Joining the medical staff begins with a written application. The application for appointment and reappointment to the medical staff is usually a lengthy and detailed document that attempts to gather information about the medical education, training, and professional experiences of the practitioner. Common categories of information found on an application are listed in figure 19.4.

Primary Source Verification

Once the application is received, the process of verifying all the information begins. The practitioner is responsible for the accuracy, truthfulness, and completeness of the information on any medical staff credentialing or privileging application. Therefore, all practitioners are required to sign an attestation statement attesting to the accuracy, truthfulness, and completeness of the information they have provided on the application. Verification of practitioners' credentials, from the originating sources, is known as **primary source verification**. This means that a facility must obtain a copy of the medical school transcript from the medical school and cannot rely on documents obtained from others. Credentialing standards of the Joint Commission, Medicare Conditions of Participation for Hospitals, and the **National Committee for Quality Assurance (NCQA)** require verification from the primary source of information on the medical staff application. An example would be obtaining an official certified transcript directly from the medical school, the primary source, rather than accepting an unofficial copy from the applicant. In addition, the hospital or healthcare organization must verify that the individual requesting approval is the same individual identified in the credentialing documents by viewing a valid government photo identification card such as a driver's license (Joint Commission 2016, MS.06.01.03).

Methods for conducting primary source verification of credentials may include direct correspondence, telephone verification, secure electronic verification from the original qualification source, and obtaining reports from a **credentials verification organization (CVO)**. A CVO gathers and verifies the background, licensing, schooling, continuing education, and other performance measures of an applicant for a healthcare organization. The hospital or healthcare organization may contract with the CVO to serve as their authorized agent to query or report to the National Practitioner Data Bank (NPDB) as required by law (HHS 2015).

Figure 19.4 Common categories of information on a medical staff application

- Personal information (including residence status)
- Medical education
- Formal medical training
  - Residency
  - Fellowship
- Practice information
- Hospital affiliations
- Fellowship/teaching appointments
- Licensure (active)
- Medical society memberships
- Board certification
- Other certifications
- Peer references
- Professional liability insurance
- Disclosure of conflicts of interest*
- Privileges requested and specialty

*The American Medical Association's policy, "Conflict of Interest Guidelines for Organized Medical Staffs," is available on their website.
Source: AMA 2005.

National Practitioner Data Bank

Chapter 16 discussed the evolution of the NPDB and its reporting requirements as mandated by law. The law also singles out hospitals as the only healthcare entities that are mandated by law to query the NPDB when verifying the background of a healthcare practitioner for medical staff appointment, clinical privileges or professional peer review activity. Hospitals must query the database every two years (biennially) in accordance with medical staff reappointment and clinical privilege re-delineation, or when a practitioner seeks additional or temporary privileges (HHS 2015). When a practitioner is filling in for another, often referred to as **locum tenens**, for any length of time that individual must also go through the hospital's credentialing process, which requires querying the NPDB. Figure 19.5 provides a list of the types of information a hospital may receive based upon its query of the NPDB. Failure to query the NPDB may leave hospital open to litigation if a problem arises with the practitioner's performance in the future (HHS 2015).

Healthcare organizations also have a duty to share information on practitioners upon a legitimate request. In *Kadlec Medical Center v. Lakeview Anesthesia Associates*, the Louisiana Federal Court found that hospitals have a duty to disclose information about their current or former medical staff members to other healthcare providers in order to protect future patients when a physician in this case moves on. This case has a significant impact on primary source verification because it is no longer sufficient to state that a physician once served on the medical staff. Information regarding disciplinary action should include the same information hospitals are required to report to the federal NPDB as discussed in chapter 16. Another example of this is detailed in figure 19.6.

Office of the Inspector General

The medical staff office should also check the Office of the Inspector General (OIG) list of individuals and organizations that have been excluded from participation in Medicare, Medicaid, and all federal healthcare programs. A healthcare organization that knowingly hires an excluded provider may face civil monetary penalties. Some states also publish a list of providers excluded from state programs. This list should also be referenced. In Tennessee there is a list of terminated providers that may be accessed on the Division of Health Care Finance & Administration page (TennCare n.d.).

Figure 19.5 List of types of information accessible to hospitals from NPDB

- Medical malpractice payment information
- Licensure actions by boards of medical examiners
- Licensing and certification actions taken by States
- Federal licensing and certification actions
- Adverse actions taken by health care entities against clinical privileges, including professional review actions taken by professional societies
- Negative actions or findings by peer review organizations or private accreditation entities
- Health care-related criminal convictions
- Health care-related civil judgments
- Exclusions from participating in Federal or State health care programs
- Other health care-related adjudicated actions or decisions

Source: HHS 2015, 61.

Figure 19.6   The case of Dr. Michael Swango

Michael Swango began his medical career as a resident at a large Midwestern teaching hospital in the early 1980s. He was asked to leave the residency program shortly thereafter due to performance problems. Upon leaving he moved from job to job in several states assuming a variety of names, and for a time worked in Zimbabwe. However, wherever Dr. Swango worked a pattern of mysterious deaths occurred. He was eventually convicted of 4 murders he confessed to but was believed to have committed at least 35 murders of patients and friends by lethal injection or poison. Dr. Swango is now serving a life sentence for murder. Had healthcare entities who hired and ultimately fired him been able to access information on the adverse actions taken against him by a variety of employers, the pattern of his behavior may have been caught much earlier, thus saving lives. Unfortunately, this is an extreme example, but nonetheless one that supports the importance of hospitals and other healthcare entities reporting to, and querying the NPDB.

Source: Stewart, J. 1999. *Blind Eye: How the Medical Establishment Let a Doctor Get Away with Murder.* New York: Simon & Schuster.

Review of Credentials Documents

All credentialing documents are presented to the credentialing committee for review and recommendation. The recommendation is then presented to the medical staff executive committee, who recommends approval or disapproval to the board. Ultimately, the board has the responsibility for selecting medical staff members and granting privileges to a practitioner.

Credentialing for Health Plans

Certain types of health insurance plans have specific requirements for providers to be credentialed in order to be eligible to submit claims, receive reimbursement and be listed on provider panels of a health plan. This is similar to a healthcare organization's medical staff credentialing process. Typically a provider has to already be credentialed by a healthcare organization before the provider may apply for credentialing to a health plan. Many health plans use the Council for Affordable Quality Healthcare (CAQH) to coordinate the credentialing process and serve as a CVO (CAQH n.d.).

Determination of Clinical Privileges

The determination or delineation of clinical privileges is the process whereby the medical staff determines what clinical treatment and clinical procedures a practitioner is authorized to perform. The privileging decision is made by comparing the qualifications of the applicant with predetermined criteria deemed necessary to perform the privileges being requested. The processes for medical staff appointment and clinical privileges are typically the same, and a practitioner may apply for them simultaneously. In the 2016 Joint Commission *Comprehensive Accreditation Manual for Hospitals* (CAMH), there are six areas of general competencies developed by the ACGME and the **American Board of Medical Specialties (ABMS)**, which should be incorporated into the comprehensive evaluation of a practitioner's professional practice. These general competencies include patient care, medical/clinical knowledge, practice-based learning and improvement, interpersonal and communication skills, professionalism, and systems-based practice (Joint Commission 2016, MS.06.01.03.)

The 2016 CAMH also includes concepts of **focused professional practice evaluation** and **ongoing professional practice evaluation**. Focused evaluation is defined as a time-limited period during which an organization evaluates and determines a practitioner's professional performance of privileges. It will occur in all requests for new privileges and when there are concerns regarding the provision of safe, high-quality care by a current medical staff member. Ongoing evaluation refers to documenting data on credentialed staff on an ongoing basis rather than at the two-year reappointment process. These two evaluations encourage the medical staff to create continuous evaluations of performance. The Joint Commission also requires continuous queries of the NPDB for compliance (2016). The board is ultimately responsible for ensuring that medical staff members are qualified, and it may be held liable for the negligent acts of its practitioners. Healthcare facilities have a duty to select competent practitioners and to protect patients from the negligent acts of practitioners.

Center for Medicare and Medicaid Services (CMS) and the Joint Commission both have options for credentialing of providers that perform telemedicine services at the facility. The facility can use the same process of credentialing as other providers. The facility may use the information provided by the distant site and then use that to start the process at the facility. If the facility wants to rely on the credentialing process at the distant site then a contract must be in place and there must be a data sharing agreement (Joint Commission 2016; CMS 2011).

Medical Staff Duties and Rights

One of the responsibilities of medical staff membership is the duty or obligation to provide patient care, treatment, and service as needed to patients. Physicians are allowed access to hospital facilities to admit and render treatment to their patients. As a result, the physician must respond to calls from the emergency department regarding patients and provide consultation services, when appropriate, for patients regardless of their payer source. This means that a physician must treat patients with whom he or she does not have an established relationship and who may or may not have the capacity to pay the hospital or the physician. This is a potential area for sanctions if members of the medical staff refuse to take calls or do not provide the appropriate level of care to patients. Facilities that use Joint Commission accreditation for deemed status are required to have a doctor of medicine or osteopathy on duty at all times (Joint Commission 2016, MS.03.01.05).

The frequency of physician or other healthcare provider on-call time is typically established by clinical department rules and may vary based on the categories of the medical staff. For example, a physician classified as an active member of the medical staff may be required to be on call on a regular schedule, whereas a physician classified as courtesy may not be required to take call. The trade-off for these categories is that physicians with greater rights also have greater responsibilities, and vice versa. The physician classified as courtesy may be able to admit only five patients per year while the physician classified as an active member of the medical staff may have an unlimited ability to admit patients.

Additional responsibilities of active members of the medical staff include service on medical staff committees. There may be standing committees such as the credentials committee, performance improvement committee, infection committee, critical care committee, and other functional committees to improve patient care quality and safety. Attendance is required at medical staff meetings, and a member of the medical staff office typically coordinates and records attendance at these meetings. A physician who misses too many meetings, as delineated in the medical staff bylaws, is reported to the department chair along with the chair of the committee. The medical staff bylaws typically include a progressive discipline plan for physicians who either do not attend meetings or do not meet other obligations as specified in the medical staff bylaws.

In teaching facilities members of the medical staff are required to supervise fellows, residents, and interns. The medical staff must define the responsibility of the licensed independent provider who has responsibility for the professional graduate education program. Medical staff rules, policies, procedures, or bylaws must designate participants in professional graduate education programs who may write patient care orders, and what entries require countersignature by the supervising licensed independent practitioner (Joint Commission 2016, MS.04.01.01).

Health Record Integrity and Documentation Requirements

There is generally a medical staff committee responsible for patient record issues, including electronic health records (EHRs). Individual medical staff members must adhere to bylaws related to timely completion of health records as well as documentation guidelines and requirements. This also supports an organization's patient safety and quality efforts and helps to minimize legal risk and vulnerability to lawsuits. Overall, the concern is that failure to document may compromise patient care.

Typical medical staff bylaws provide for timely completion of health records, including legibility requirements (or, alternatively, use of the institution's EHR or health information system to record patient notes); communication and coordination of care with other members of the staff; and completion of reports of history and physical examinations, operative notes, and other required documents based on best practices and facility policies. Failure to comply with any of the provisions of health record documentation may result in progressive discipline up to and including suspension of medical staff membership. Information about incomplete and delinquent records is typically reported by the HIM department during committee meetings. Because of this, it is important to acknowledge the medical staff bylaws, Joint Commission standards, Medicare and Medicaid Conditions of Participation, state statutes, and other facility licensure requirements regarding the documentation requirements and timely completion of health records.

Disciplinary Actions and Suspension

Physicians and other healthcare providers agree to adhere to the bylaws in order to have access to healthcare facility resources including the operating room, emergency department, cardiac catheterization lab, radiology services, and other equipment and personnel that assist the provider in the diagnosis and treatment of patients. Physicians who have patient performance issues and noncompliant documentation practices (for example, incomplete documentation or inappropriate references in the health record to patients and staff in the health record) may face disciplinary action. Physicians may be suspended from admitting patients for failure to complete health records timely.

Hospitals typically have procedures to notify the admissions department, surgical care department, and other key hospital departments when a practitioner's privileges are suspended. Depending on their staff privileges, suspension limits or restricts the ability of healthcare providers to admit patients or schedule time in the operating room. Hospital bylaws should prohibit the practice of partners admitting patients on behalf of the suspended physician. Admission patterns should be reviewed to ensure that suspended physicians are following the suspension regulations set forth in the bylaws. Any adverse action against a practitioner's medical staff membership or clinical privileges is a reportable event to the NPDB. The medical staff services office typically communicates this action to the NPDB.

Due Process and Antitrust Issues

In healthcare employment and medical staff privileges, healthcare facilities must be cognizant of an individuals' right to liberty, property and the ability to make a living as protected by due process and antitrust laws. As discussed in chapter 3, **due process** provides an individual with the right to fair treatment under the law. Thus, due process is required in hiring, disciplining, or other actions that affect a practitioner's medical staff privileges or employment. Government regulations, court decisions and Joint Commission standards compel healthcare facilities to resolve conflicts related to employment and medical staff privileges (for example, termination of employment or adverse credentialing) through internal procedures that exercise due process. Such procedures allow for notice and the opportunity to be heard through a fair hearing in which the individual can voice objections to the organization's proposed actions. Due process should be evident in the facility's policies and procedures and medical staff bylaws.

To protect from antitrust issues as discussed in chapter 7, medical staff bylaws must clearly state the process for granting medical and professional staff membership, and clinical privileges, and the process required for thorough investigation of all applicable qualifications and clinical performance. Care must be exercised not only in drafting the bylaws and associated rules and regulations, but also in adhering to them at all times when considering medical staff applications and requests for privileges. The criteria for granting or denying specific privileges are often left to each clinical department to determine, but they must be fair, not violate the rights of any federally protected class of persons, and not be designed to favor those already on staff or restrain competition by keeping otherwise qualified practitioners off the staff.

Scenario 19

A clinical documentation improvement (CDI) specialist notices that one of the physicians from the cardiac catheter lab is now performing procedures in the operating room. Although this may be appropriate, the CDI specialist has worked in the facility a number of years and is not aware of any advanced training that would qualify this physician to perform procedures in the operating room.

1. What should the CDI specialist do?
2. What course of action should the facility take?
3. What course of action should the medical staff take?
4. What are the potential liabilities for the facility and the medical staff member?

References

Accreditation Council for Graduate Medical Education (ACGME). 2015 (July 1). Common Program Requirements. http://www.acgme.org.

Centers for Medicare and Medicaid. 2011 (July). Center for Medicaid, CHIP, and Survey Certification /Survey and Certification Group. https://www.cms.gov/Medicare/Provider-Enrollment-and-Certification /SurveyCertificationGenInfo/downloads/SCLetter11_32.pdf.

Council for Affordable Quality Healthcare. n.d. CAQH ProView FAQs. http://www.caqh.org.

Department of Health and Human Services. 2011. Conditions of Participation for Hospitals. 42 CFR. Part 482. https://www.gpo.gov/fdsys/granule/CFR-2011-title42-vol5/CFR-2011-title42-vol5-part482/content-detail .html.

Department of Health and Human Services. 2015. *NPDB Guidebook*. Rockville: HHS. http://www.npdb.hrsa.gov /resources/aboutGuidebooks.jsp.

Joint Commission. 2016 (September). *Comprehensive Accreditation Manual for Hospitals (CAMH)*. Oakbrook Terrace, IL: Joint Commission.

National Association of Medical Staff Services (NAMSS). 2014 (February). The ideal credentialing standards: Best practice criteria and protocol for hospitals. http://www.namss.org.

TennCare Division of Health Care Finance and Administration. n.d. Terminated provider list. https://www.tn.gov /tenncare/topic/terminated-provider-list.

Cases, Statutes, and Regulations Cited

Darling v. Charleston Community Memorial Hospital, 33 IL 2d 326, 211 N.E.2d 253, 14 A.L.R.3d 860 (IL Sep 29, 1965).

Kadlec Medical Center v. Lakeview Anesthesia Associates, No. Civ.A. 04-0997 (E.D.La. May 19, 2005).

Workplace Law

Rebecca Reynolds, EdD, MHA, CHPS, RHIA, FAHIMA,
and Melanie S. Brodnik, PhD, RHIA, FAHIMA

Learning Objectives

- Identify the major laws related to discrimination prevention in the work setting
- Explain the components of the Fair Labor Standards Act and related laws in regard to wages, overtime, compensation, and benefits
- Discuss the federal laws that enable union activity in healthcare and their relationship to healthcare workers
- Describe the components of the Occupational Safety and Health Act and how employees are protected by the Act

Key Terms

- Age Discrimination in Employment Act of 1967
- Americans with Disabilities Act of 1990
- Arbitration
- Collective bargaining
- Compensation
- Consolidated Omnibus Budget Reconciliation Act of 1986 (COBRA)
- Employee Retirement Income Security Act of 1974 (ERISA)
- Equal Employment Opportunity Act of 1972 (EEOA)
- Equal Employment Opportunity Commission (EEOC)
- Equal Pay Act of 1963
- Exempt employee
- Fair Labor Standards Act of 1938 (FLSA)
- Genetic Information Nondiscrimination Act of 2008 (GINA)
- Grievance procedure
- Immigration Reform and Control Act of 1986
- Labor-Management Relations Act of 1947
- National Labor Relations Act of 1935 (Wagner Act)
- National Labor Relations Board (NLRB)
- Nonexempt employee
- Pregnancy Discrimination Act of 1973
- Title VII of the Civil Rights Act of 1964
- Uniform Guidelines on Employee Selection Procedures
- Union steward

The healthcare industry operates within the constraints of numerous laws and standards designed to support the delivery and financing of quality healthcare while protecting the rights and responsibilities of healthcare consumers and providers. The delivery of quality healthcare depends on personnel or human resources who "do no harm." Human resources are protected in the workplace by employment laws that function to protect both employee and employer. The goal of workplace law is to strike a balance between employee and employer that protects the employee from personal injury, prejudice, unfair wages, whistleblower discrimination, duress, and unwanted sexual advances while allowing the employer to pursue desired business outcomes (Department of Labor n.d.). Federal employment laws deal with employee-employer issues, whereas federal labor laws often refer to employer-union issues or other labor protections.

Managing department staff requires an understanding of the federal and state laws that govern employment. Most healthcare organizations have a human resources department or someone dedicated to human resources oversight who can assist managers in ensuring that proper labor practices are in place. This chapter provides an overview of common workplace laws. The civil rights of employees are discussed in terms of discrimination related to age, color, national origin, race, religion, and sex. Wage and salary regulations are introduced along with employee occupational and safety laws. The chapter closes with a discussion of fair labor practices and laws related to union activity and collective bargaining.

Discrimination and Related Laws

Discrimination laws focus on issues that protect applicants and employees from discrimination in all aspects of employment. The United States **Equal Employment Opportunity Commission (EEOC)** is responsible for enforcing federal laws that prohibit discriminating against a job applicant or employee on the basis of

- Age
- Disability
- Equal pay/Compensation
- Genetic information
- Harassment
- National origin
- Pregnancy
- Race/Color
- Religion
- Retaliation
- Sex
- Sexual harassment

In addition, the EEOC oversees discrimination or retaliation against an individual who has complained about discrimination, filed a charge of discrimination, or participated in an employment discrimination investigation or lawsuit (EEOC n.d.a). The laws apply to all types of work situations, as listed in figure 20.1. The EEOC enforces laws, works to prevent discrimination, and investigates job discrimination complaints. The **Equal Employment Opportunity Act of 1972 (EEOA)** gives the EEOC authority to sue in federal courts when there is reasonable cause to believe discrimination has occurred. If a complaint cannot be settled, the EEOC can file a federal lawsuit against the employer. EEOC complaints are generally handled through field offices at the state or local agency level.

To assist employers in the hiring process and to help alleviate potential discrimination issues related to hiring, the EEOC (n.d.b) publishes **Uniform Guidelines on Employee Selection Procedures**. The overriding principle is that employee selection must be made on qualifications related to job performance and prohibits discrimination in employment practices on the basis of race, color, religion, sex, or national origin (Society for Human Resources Management 1978).

An overview of discrimination statutes and regulations follows.

Civil Rights Act and Related Acts

Title VII of the Civil Rights Act, passed in 1964, and as amended by the EEOA, prohibits discrimination based on age, race, color, national origin, sex, religion, disability, political beliefs, and marital or familial status. The EEOC was created and implemented as part of the Civil Rights Act for the purpose of enforc-

Figure 20.1 Aspects of employment affected by discrimination laws

- Hiring and firing
- Compensation, assignment, or classification of employees
- Transfer, promotion, layoff, or recall
- Job advertisements
- Recruitment
- Testing
- Use of company facilities
- Training and apprenticeship programs
- Fringe benefits
- Pay, retirement plans, and disability leave
- Other terms and conditions of employment
- Discriminatory practices under these laws also include
- Harassment on the basis of race, color, religion, sex, national origin, disability, or age
- Retaliation against an individual for filing a charge of discrimination, participating in an investigation, or opposing discriminatory practices
- Employment decisions based on stereotypes or assumptions about the abilities, traits, or performance of individuals of a certain sex, race, age, religion, or ethnic group or individuals with disabilities
- Denying employment opportunities to a person because of marriage to, or association with, an individual of a particular race, religion, or national origin or an individual with a disability. Title VII also prohibits discrimination because of participation in schools or places of worship associated with a particular racial, ethnic, or religious group

Source: EEOC 2009.

ing laws against discrimination as discussed above. The Civil Rights Act prohibits not only *intentional discrimination* but also *practices* that have the effect of discriminating against individuals because of their race, color, national origin, religion, or sex. In 1991, the Civil Rights Act was expanded to authorize compensatory and punitive damages in cases of intentional discrimination (EEOC n.d.a).

Many healthcare organizations have diversity awareness programs as well as cultural competency programs to raise awareness about diversity and the need for cultural sensitivity. Many organizations have programs that correspond to national diversity holidays. The Joint Commission cultural competency standards relate to the need to effectively communicate with each patient and family. The Joint Commission has published roadmaps on advancing effective communication, cultural competency and family centered care along with a focus on lesbian, gay, bisexual, and transgender community (Joint Commission n.d.).

Age Discrimination

Age discrimination involves treating an applicant or employee less favorably because of age. The **Age Discrimination in Employment Act of 1967** (29 USC 621-34) protects individuals 40 years and older; however, some states have laws that protect younger workers. Age discrimination applies to any aspect or terms of employment (hiring, promotion, discharge, pay, fringe benefits, job training, classification, or referral). It also includes harassing someone (verbally or in writing) because of his or her age or condoning a hostile or offensive work environment (EEOC n.d.c).

Table 20.1 Workplace auxiliary aids for people with hearing and sight disabilities

Sign language interpreter	Assistive listening devices
• Assistive listening devices	• Strobe lighting for emergency notifications and alerts
• Augmentative communication devices	• Telephone headset
• Communication access real-time translation (CART)	• Video relay service
	• Work area adjustments

Source: EEOC n.d.d.

Disability Discrimination

Disability discrimination occurs when an employer treats someone with a disability unfavorably because of the disability. The **Americans with Disabilities Act of 1990** (ADA) and the ADA Amendments Act of 2008 (ADAAA) (42 USC 12101 et seq.) protects individuals with disabilities, which are broadly defined to include physical conditions, psychological conditions, contagious diseases, substance abuse, and other conditions. Employees must be able to perform the necessary functions of a job with "reasonable accommodations." Reasonable accommodations include modifications to the workplace or conditions of employment so that a worker with a disability can perform the job. Accommodations also include auxiliary aids for individuals who are deaf or hard of hearing or who are blind (EEOC n.d.d). See table 20.1 for examples of auxiliary aids.

Equal Pay

The **Equal Pay Act of 1963** amended the **Fair Labor Standards Act of 1938** (FLSA), which will be discussed in more detail later in the chapter. The Equal Pay Act (29 USC 206(d)) made it illegal to pay workers differently on the basis of sex. It regulates the concept of equal pay for men and women who perform similar work requiring similar skills, effort, and responsibility under similar working conditions. These four compensable factors are compared to ensure that pay is equal (EEOC n.d.e).

Genetics

Title II of the **Genetic Information Nondiscrimination Act of 2008** (GINA) prohibits health insurers and employers from discriminating against an individual or employee on the basis of genetic information in hiring, promotion, discharge, pay, fringe benefits, job training, classification, referral, and other aspects of employment. GINA restricts access and disclosure of genetic information, as discussed in chapter 15. Genetic information includes information about an individual's genetic tests, family members' genetic tests, and manifestation of diseases or disorders in family members (family medical history); requests for or receipt of genetic services; or participation in research that includes genetic services by an applicant, employee, or his or her family members (29 CFR 1635.3(c)(1)).

National Origin

Discrimination based on national origin refers to treating someone differently because he or she is from a certain part of the country or world. The EEOC states the following regarding national origin:

It is illegal to discriminate against an individual because of birthplace, ancestry, culture, or linguistic characteristics common to a specific ethnic group. A rule requiring that employees speak only English on the job may violate Title VII unless an employer shows that the requirement is necessary for conducting business. If the employer believes such a rule is necessary, employees must be informed when English is required and the consequences for violating the rule (EEOC n.d.f.).

The **Immigration Reform and Control Act of 1986** (8 USC 1101) requires employers to assure that employees hired are legally authorized to work in the United States. The act also contains anti-discrimination provisions outline four types of unlawful conduct which include citizenship or immigration status discrimination, national origin discrimination, unfair documentary practices during the Form I-9 process, and retaliation. However, an employer who requests employment verification only for individuals of a particular national origin, or individuals who appear to be or sound foreign, may violate both the Civil Rights Act and Immigration Reform and Control Act; verification must be obtained from all applicants and employees. Employers who impose citizenship requirements or give preferences to U.S. citizens in hiring or employment opportunities also may violate this act. A Form I-9 must be completed and maintained for each employee and should include original documents for identity verification. The Department of Homeland Security and the Social Security Administration operate an E-verify system which allows employers to electronically verify employment eligibility for workers.

Related to anti-discrimination and national origin, Title VI of the Civil Rights Act emphasizes that no person, because of race, color, or national origin, should be excluded from participation in or discriminated against by any program receiving federal financial assistance. While the focus of Title VI is on persons with **limited English proficiency** (LEP), aspects of the law are applicable to employees as well. LEP individuals are those who do not speak English as the primary language and have a limited ability to read, speak, write, or understand English. This is typically accessed during an oral interview with the patient during the history of present illness. Title VI applies to any healthcare organization or entity that receives federal funding. The Department of Health and Human Services (HHS) provides LEP guidance to healthcare organizations in determining how to comply with Title VI, including the obligation to translate vital materials such as informed consents for LEP persons. It suggests healthcare organizations take steps to ensure that interpreters are available upon request and that they understand issues of privacy, confidentiality, and security of patient information (HHS Office for Civil Rights 2004).

Sex and Sexual Harassment

It is unlawful to discriminate on the basis of sex (gender) in any aspect of employment. The term "sex" in the Civil Rights Act was expanded by the **Pregnancy Discrimination Act of 1973**, which prohibits discrimination against pregnancy, childbirth, or related medical conditions. These conditions must be handled like any other medical condition, and the individual must be afforded the same protections that would be granted a non-pregnant person in terms of accommodations, if necessary.

The EEOC defines sexual harassment as unwelcome sexual advances, requests for sexual favors, and other verbal or physical harassment of a sexual nature (EEOC n.d.g.). When unwanted sexual action by one individual to another interferes with work performance by creating an intimidating, hostile, or offensive work environment, a claim of sexual harassment may be made. Claims may also be made if an adverse employment decision is made which leads to demotion or termination. Comments made in general about women can be considered sexual harassment (EEOC n.d.). The harasser may be a man or a woman and can be a supervisor, co-worker, or nonemployee or other agent of the organization. If sexual harassment is reported, the employer must take action in order to avoid legal risk.

Check Your Understanding 20.1

Instructions: Indicate whether the following statements are true or false (T or F).

1. If an employee discovers he is carrying the gene that causes colon cancer, his insurance company can deny him insurance.

2. The DOL can waive the requirement for a Form I-9 for some workers.

3. A hospital has the right to deny employment to an applicant if that individual seeks reasonable accommodations to perform the job function.

4. Sexual harassment can only be claimed if both workers are the same gender.

5. Employers must handle the conditions of pregnancy and childbirth, or related medical conditions, in the same manner as they handle medical conditions afforded an individual who seeks employment.

Labor Laws

In addition to the employment laws related to an employee's civil rights and protection against discrimination, there are labor laws designed to protect employees' rights to a safe and healthful work environment. These laws address wages and overtime, compensation and benefits, and union activity. These laws are not enforced by the EEOC, but are workforce laws that prohibit discrimination or regulate workplace issues. Worker's Compensation and the Family and Medical Leave Act (FMLA) and OSHA are all examples of well-known laws not enforced by EEOC.

Wages and Overtime

The Fair Labor Standards Act (FLSA) (29 USC 201) has been amended a number of times since its original enactment in 1938. It addresses minimum wage and overtime pay as related to private and public employment. It establishes the federal minimum wage rate. It also sets standards that prescribe child labor requirements such as the age limitations on hiring children. For example, it restricts the number of hours a child under the age of 16 years can work and forbids children under the age of 18 years to work in jobs identified as too dangerous.

The act sets the minimum wage standard and defines which employees may be exempt from the standards. The FLSA is enforced by the Department of Labor (DOL) Wage and Hour Division. **Exempt employees** include individuals identified as professionals, administrators, or salespeople. Managers and supervisors are generally considered exempt employees as well. Exempt employees are typically paid a base salary regardless of the number of hours worked. **Nonexempt employees** must be paid at least the minimum wage up to 40 hours, and time and a half for any hours worked over 40. The FLSA has record-keeping requirements that establish minimum elements which must be maintained on each employee as well as retention of payroll and other employment-related wage records. Additionally there are guidelines for meal and sleep breaks based on the number of hours worked.

Accurate time records must be kept. Healthcare facilities have much flexibility because of the scheduling of healthcare workers such as nurses. The DOL has a fact sheet specific to hospitals and healthcare which outlines common industry problems, including failure to pay for hours worked.

Compensation and Benefits

Compensation is a complex issue and includes all direct and indirect pay. In addition to wages and mandatory benefits such as unemployment insurance and workers' compensation, the types of benefits offered to employees may vary but include

- Medical insurance
- Dental insurance
- Life insurance
- Accidental death insurance
- Short- and long-term disability
- Child care
- Elder care
- Retirement plans
- Paid-time off (vacation time)
- Paid sick time
- Longevity pay

These benefits are often included in a flexible benefits plan or cafeteria plan, which allows employees to choose from among the listed benefits.

Retirement plans are governed by federal law. The **Employee Retirement Income Security Act of 1974 (ERISA)** (29 USC 1001 et seq.) sets minimum standards for most voluntarily established pension and health plans in private industry to provide protection for individuals in these plans.

Insurance benefits are also governed by federal laws and regulations. The **Consolidated Omnibus Budget Reconciliation Act of 1986** (COBRA 1986) provides temporary continued health insurance for those who have lost coverage because of termination (except for gross misconduct), reduction in hours of employment, death of the covered employee divorce from the covered employee, covered employee becoming Medicare eligible and for a dependents status loss under the plan. An alternative to COBRA coverage is provided by the Health Insurance Portability and Accountability Act of 1996 (HIPAA). HIPAA provides rights and protections for participants and beneficiaries in group health plans. HIPAA includes protections for coverage under group health plans that limit exclusions for preexisting conditions; prohibit discrimination against employees and dependents based on their health status; and allow a special opportunity to enroll in a new plan to individuals in certain circumstances. HIPAA may also allow the purchase of individual coverage if no group health plan coverage is available, and have exhausted COBRA or other continuation coverage. The request for special enrollment must be made within 30 days of loss of job-based coverage (DOL 2015).

Unions

According to the US Department of Labor's Bureau of Labor Statistics report for 2015, 11.1 percent of employed wage and salary workers were union members, down from previous years. The total number of unionized workers in 2015 was 14.8 million, with 13 percent of those union members listed in the category of healthcare support occupations (Department of Labor Bureau of Labor Statistics 2016). Members include all types of healthcare workers, such as nurses, physicians, and those who work in departments such as health information management (HIM).

Unions that represent healthcare workers include the Service Employees International Union (SEIU); the American Federation of State, County and Municipal Employees (AFSCME), which represents healthcare workers in public healthcare facilities; the American Federation of Teachers (AFT) healthcare division; and the Teamsters Union healthcare division. Examples of issues for healthcare workers are minimum staffing, overtime pay, and recruitment as well as other contract issues common to all types of workers. With the increasing number of healthcare workers, the healthcare arena is a focus area for growth for unions, especially with the decline in blue-collar membership. Employees join and support unions because they feel a need to protect their jobs and want a formal method of communicating with management. Wages and benefits are commonly the primary issues for negotiation between management and unionized employees.

The **National Labor Relations Act of 1935** (NLRA; also known as the Wagner Act) (29 USC 151-169) regulates union and employer relations in the private sector. Section 7 of the act gives employees the right to self-organize and to form, join, or assist labor organizations. It allows employees to bargain collectively through whomever they choose as their representative and to engage in other activities for mutual aid protection. The law was expanded by the **Labor-Management Relations Act of 1947** (29 USC 141 et seq.), which amended the Wagner Act to prohibit unfair labor practices on the part of unions and to allow the President of the United States to stop strikes in cases that might impact national health and safety.

While the act established worker rights related to union activity and membership, it also identified behaviors considered to be unfair labor practices. For example, employers cannot keep employees from forming or joining a union, and employers must bargain with union representatives in good faith. See table 20.2 for a list of worker rights and unfair labor practices.

National Labor Relations Board

The **National Labor Relations Board** (NLRB) is an independent federal agency that safeguards employees' rights to engage in union activity. It oversees union elections and handles unfair labor practices committed by private sector employers and unions. For many years, healthcare organizations were not included under the NLRA, because of the concern that healthcare services could be disrupted. The NLRB assumed jurisdiction over hospitals in 1974. Sometimes the union represents more people in the organization than those who actually pay dues and are members of the union.

Labor unions exist in many healthcare facilities, and the administration and unions must work together in collaboration. The person most responsible for the operation of the union contract on a day-to-day basis is the supervisor, and training of supervisors and departmental management is important to ensure good relationships between employees and management while providing effective and efficient patient care. When union organizing begins in an organization, there are regulations about what can be done.

An election following NLRB regulations is conducted to determine whether a union will be authorized to bargain and negotiate a labor contract with the management, as well as which employees will be part of the bargaining unit that will be covered. The contract spells out details of the relationship between management and the employees. According to Dunn (2010), contracts deal with matters such as union recognition, management rights, union security, wages, conditions, hours of work, vacations, holidays, leaves of absence, seniority, promotions, and similar terms and conditions of employment. Pension issues and healthcare benefits are important in today's climate as employers attempt to lower their expenditures for employees and retirees.

Collective Bargaining

During **collective bargaining**, a contract is negotiated that sets forth the relationship between the employees and the healthcare organization. In a unionized facility, management must be very careful to

Table 20.2 Worker rights and unfair labor practices

Private Sector Workers Rights
• Organize a union to negotiate with your employer concerning your wages, hours, and other terms and conditions of employment.
• Form, join or assist a union.
• Bargain collectively through representatives of employees' own choosing for a contract with your employer setting your wages, benefits, hours, and other working conditions.
• Discuss your terms and conditions of employment or union organizing with your co-workers or a union.
• Take action with one or more co-workers to improve your working conditions by, among other means, raising work-related complaints directly with your employer or with a government agency, and seeking help from a union.
• Strike and picket, depending on the purpose or means of the strike or the picketing.
• Choose not to do any of these activities, including joining or remaining a member of a union.

Unfair Labor Practices—Employer	Unfair Labor Practices—Union
• Prohibit you from soliciting for a union during non-work time, such as before or after work or during break times; or from distributing union literature during non-work time, in non-work areas, such as parking lots or break rooms.	• Threaten you that you will lose your job unless you support the union.
• Question you about your union support or activities in a manner that discourages you from engaging in that activity.	• Refuse to process a grievance because you have criticized union officials or because you are not a member of the union.
• Fire, demote, or transfer you, or reduce your hours or change your shift, or otherwise take adverse action against you, or threaten to take any of these actions, because you join or support a union, or because you engage in concerted activity for mutual aid and protection, or because you choose not to engage in any such activity.	• Use or maintain discriminatory standards or procedures in making job referrals from a hiring hall.
• Threaten to close your workplace if workers choose a union to represent them.	• Cause or attempt to cause an employer to discriminate against you because of your union-related activity.
• Promise or grant promotions, pay raises, or other benefits to discourage or encourage union support.	• Take other adverse action against you based on whether you have joined or support the union.
• Prohibit you from wearing union hats, buttons, t-shirts, and pins in the workplace except under special circumstances.	
• Spy on or videotape peaceful union activities and gatherings or pretend to do so.	

Source: Department of Labor National Labor Relations Board 2011.

abide by the contract in matters of discipline when employees do not follow the organization's rules and in handling employee grievances or complaints. The human resources department is available to assist, but the manager is responsible for the daily activities of the department. The manager will work closely with the union steward to handle disciplinary issues.

Every healthcare organization will have some type of **grievance procedure** to handle situations such as violation of a work rule or other condition of employment. This procedure begins with the employee and the supervisor. In a unionized environment, a **union steward** represents the employee. It is important for supervisors and management to know the grievance procedure and to be trained in how to handle disciplinary issues. Issues may relate to insubordination or refusal to obey orders, absenteeism, failure to follow work rules, and so on. Good recordkeeping will provide the information needed to back up supervisory actions. The employee has the right to due process (as discussed in chapters 3, 8, and 19), which means that employers must be sure that procedural requirements spelled out in either the personnel procedure manual or the union contract are followed. Issues that are not settled may be submitted to **arbitration** (hearings by a third party).

Downsizing and Layoffs

Another issue that must be handled carefully is downsizing or layoffs. Seniority is protected by most union contracts and has become a problem in healthcare organizations with poorly written job descriptions. In a layoff issue, for example, a cafeteria worker with more seniority could bump a clerical employee in the HIM department. Job descriptions are important tools of management, but in a unionized system with seniority protections, qualifications including specific experience must be included in job descriptions.

State Laws

State labor laws may be fashioned after federal labor laws, or a state law may establish its own version of the law. Many states have enacted "right to work" laws that specify that a worker does not have to join a labor union to keep or land a job. Federal labor law is considered minimum law. A state may enact stricter labor laws or labor laws that go beyond the federal laws. If the state law is considered stricter than the federal law, the state law will preempt the federal law.

The Occupational Safety and Health Administration (OSHA)

In 1970 Congress passed the Occupational Safety and Health Act (29 CFR 1910) to help employers reduce injuries, illnesses, and deaths on the job. The act established the Occupational Safety and Health Administration (OSHA) under the auspices of the Department of Labor for the purpose of providing leadership in occupational safety and health. OSHA is responsible for setting and enforcing workplace safety standards, and providing information, training, and assistance to employers and workers, as summarized in figure 20.2 (DOL OSHA 2015a). OSHA regulations enable states to seek approval from OSHA to administer their own occupational safety and health programs at the state level. At least 25 states have approved plans. OSHA maintains a list of these states and effective dates of the plans and a link to the plans on the OSHA website.

OSHA works closely with the Centers for Disease Control and Prevention (CDC) in identifying best practices for the management of diseases and injuries that may affect employees in the workplace. OSHA standards and CDC guidelines for conditions or situations commonly found in healthcare settings that may affect healthcare workers include numerous hazardous chemicals, equipment, and waste products—for example, hazardous chemicals or equipment used in laboratories and radiology and waste products like body fluids and tissues related to patient treatment. The standards and guidelines spell out in detail how such products are to be handled as well as what employers must communicate to healthcare workers regarding the safety and disposal of the products.

Figure 20.2	**OSHA responsibilities**

- Encourages employers and employees to reduce workplace hazards and to implement new safety and health management systems or improve existing programs
- Develops mandatory job safety and health standards and enforces them through worksite inspections, and, sometimes, by imposing citations, penalties, or both
- Promotes safe and healthful work environments through cooperative programs including the Voluntary Protection Programs, OSHA Strategic Partnerships, and Alliances
- Establishes responsibilities and rights for employers and employees to achieve better safety and health conditions
- Supports the development of innovative ways of dealing with workplace hazards
- Establishes requirements for injury and illness recordkeeping by employers, and for employer monitoring of certain occupational illnesses
- Establishes training programs to increase the competence of occupational safety and health personnel
- Provides technical and compliance assistance, and training and education to help employers reduce worker accidents and injuries
- Works in partnership with states that operate their own occupational safety and health programs
- Supports the consultation programs offered by all 50 states, the District of Columbia, Puerto Rico, Guam, Northern Mariana Islands, and the Virgin Islands

Because of healthcare workers' increased exposure to viruses, microorganisms such as human immunodeficiency virus (HIV) and hepatitis B and C viruses, and other bloodborne pathogens, the Occupational Exposure to Bloodborne Pathogens standard (29 CFR 1910.1030) was enacted in 1991. Subsequently, in 2000 Congress passed the Needlestick Safety and Prevention Act (2000), which directed OSHA to revise the bloodborne pathogen standard to require employers to establish an exposure control plan that includes controls to eliminate or minimize employee risk as a result of a needlestick or other sharps-related injury (DOL OSHA 2011).

Employer Responsibility and Employee Rights

Employers have a duty under OSHA standards to provide employees with a safe working environment, especially in a healthcare setting. Noncompliance with the standards puts employers at risk for violations resulting in citations and fines. Employees also have a duty to comply with OSHA standards and report problems, follow safety rules, and wear protective equipment if required to do so. Employers and employees may appeal negative decisions under certain situations. Overall, employers must

- Follow all relevant OSHA safety and health standards
- Find and correct safety and health hazards
- Inform employees about chemical hazards through training, labels, alarms, color-coded systems, chemical information sheets, and other methods
- Notify OSHA within eight hours of a workplace fatality or when three or more workers are hospitalized
- Provide required personal protective equipment at no cost to workers
- Keep accurate records of work-related injuries and illnesses

- Post OSHA citations, injury and illness summary data, and the OSHA "Job Safety and Health—It's the Law" poster in the workplace where workers will see them
- Not discriminate or retaliate against any worker for using his or her rights under the law (DOL OSHA 2014a)

The OSHA recordkeeping regulation requires employers to keep detailed records on serious occupational injuries and illnesses (29 CFR 1904). Recordkeeping requirements are defined in the 2001 Occupational Injury and Illness Recording and Reporting Requirements ("the Recordkeeping rule") which was revised in 2014 and implemented January 1, 2015 (DOL OSHA 2015b).

Under OSHA, employees have the right to

- Working conditions that do not pose a risk of serious harm
- Receive information and training (in a language workers can understand) about chemical and other hazards, methods to prevent harm, and OSHA standards that apply to their workplace
- Review records of work-related injuries and illnesses
- Get copies of test results done to find and measure hazards in the workplace
- File a complaint asking OSHA to inspect their workplace if they believe there is a serious hazard or that their employer is not following OSHA rules. When requested, OSHA will keep all identities confidential
- Use their rights under the law without retaliation or discrimination. If an employee is fired, demoted, transferred, or discriminated against in any way for using their rights under the law, they can file a complaint with OSHA. This complaint must be filed within 30 days of the alleged discrimination (DOL OSHA 2014a)

OSHA Inspections

OSHA inspections are usually unannounced; however, under special circumstances, an employer may be given a 24-hour notice of a pending inspection. An employee's representative must also be informed of the advance notice by the employer or OSHA. Circumstances that warrant an advance notice include the following:

- Imminent danger situations that require correction as soon as possible
- Accident investigations where the employer has notified the agency of a fatality or catastrophe
- Inspections that must take place after regular business hours or that require special preparation
- Cases where notice is required to ensure that the employer and the employee representative or other personnel will be present
- Cases where an inspection must be delayed for more than five working days when there is good cause
- Situations in which the OSHA Area Director determines that advance notice would produce a more thorough or effective inspection (DOL OSHA 2015b)

OSHA is responsible for inspecting more than 111 million workplaces, and thus it has set inspection priorities based on the worst situations. These priorities are listed in figure 20.3.

In healthcare organizations, adherence to OSHA standards is absolutely required as a means to minimize legal risk from the standpoint of delivering quality patient care and protecting employees from harm. Healthcare organizations require employees to complete training on a variety of OSHA-related

Figure 20.3	OSHA inspection priorities

Imminent Danger

Imminent danger situations receive top priority. An imminent danger is any condition where there is reasonable certainty that a danger exists that can be expected to cause death or serious physical harm immediately or before the danger can be eliminated through normal enforcement procedures. If a compliance officer finds an imminent danger situation, he or she will ask the employer to voluntarily abate the hazard and remove endangered employees from exposure. Should the employer fail to do this, OSHA, through the regional solicitor, may apply to the Federal District Court for an injunction prohibiting further work as long as unsafe conditions exist.

Catastrophes and Fatal Accidents

Second priority goes to the investigation of fatalities and accidents resulting in a death or hospitalization of three or more employees. The employer must report such catastrophes to OSHA within 8 hours. OSHA investigates to determine the cause of these accidents and whether existing OSHA standards were violated.

Complaints and Referrals

Third priority goes to formal employee complaints of unsafe or unhealthful working conditions and to referrals from any source about a workplace hazard. The act gives each employee the right to request an OSHA inspection when the employee believes he or she is in imminent danger from a hazard or when he or she thinks that there is a violation of an OSHA standard that threatens physical harm. OSHA will maintain confidentiality if requested, inform the employee of any action it takes regarding complaints, and, if requested, hold an informal review of any decision not to inspect.

Programmed Inspections

Programmed inspections are aimed at specific high-hazard industries, workplaces, occupations, or health substances, or other industries identified in OSHA's current inspection procedures. OSHA selects industries for inspection on the basis of factors such as the injury incidence rates, previous citation history, employee exposure to toxic substances, or random selection.

Follow-up Inspections

A follow-up inspection determines if the employer has corrected previously cited violations. If an employer has failed to abate a violation, the compliance officer informs the employer that he or she is subject to "Failure to Abate" alleged violations. This involves proposed additional daily penalties until the employer corrects the violation.

Source: DOL OSHA 2015b.

subjects as well as discrimination in the workplace, sexual harassment, and HIPAA privacy and security issues. HIM and informatics professionals, while not involved with patient care, are still required to participate in training activities as deemed relevant to their position in the organization.

Check Your Understanding 20.2

Instructions: Indicate whether the following statements are true or false (T or F).

1. The Fair Labor Standards Act (FLSA) establishes the maximum wage for employees.

2. Healthcare organizations are not allowed to have union employees.

3. The Consolidated Omnibus Budget Reconciliation Act of 1986 (COBRA) requires employers to provide health insurance benefits to employees.

4. A supervisor does not need to be familiar with union practices in the healthcare facility.

5. Hospital employers must provide healthcare workers with information regarding what to do if the worker is accidentally stuck with a needle that has been used on a patient.

Scenario 20

The Acme Medical Group is a provider for wellness and occupational medicine. Acme has contracts to do pre-employment physicals, OSHA screening and reviews, and other drug and injury assessments for the local fire department. You have the current position of HIIM and HR director at Acme Medical Group and are custodian of records for all of the testing and OSHA compliance. You have a HIM student intern for the summer and ask him to review the records to see if he can create a database to help monitor the exposure levels of the fire department workers to various chemicals. He discovers that some of the old data are unavailable and that one of the workers at Acme has gone back and created dummy files of old testing data. The student presents his findings to you at his exit conference.

1. What should the HIIM director do?
2. What course of action should Acme Medical Group take?
3. What are the potential liabilities for the HIIM director?
4. What are the potential liabilities for Acme Medical Group?

References

Department of Health and Human Services Office for Civil Rights. 2004. Guidance to federal financial assistance recipients regarding Title VI prohibition against national origin discrimination affecting limited English proficient persons. http://www.hhs.gov/.

Department of Labor. n.d. Health plans and benefits: Portability of health coverage (HIPAA). http://www.dol.gov/.

Department of Labor Employee Benefits Security Administration. 2015. COBRA An employee's guide to health benefits. http://www.dol.gov/ebsa/pdf/cobraemployee.pdf.

Department of Labor Bureau of Labor Statistics. 2016. Union members—2015. http://www.bls.gov/.

Department of Labor National Labor Relations Board. 2011. Employee rights under the National Labor Relations Act. http://www.nlrb.gov.

Department of Labor Occupational Safety and Health Administration. 2011. OSHA's Bloodborne Pathogens Standard. https://www.osha.gov/OshDoc/data_BloodborneFacts/bbfact01.pdf.

Department of Labor Occupational Safety and Health Administration. 2014a. At a glance OSHA. https://www.osha.gov/Publications/3439at-a-glance.pdf.

Department of Labor Occupational Safety and Health Administration. 2014b. OSHA's Record Keeping Rule. https://www.osha.gov/recordkeeping2014/index.html.

Department of Labor Occupational Safety and Health Administration. 2015a. All about OSHA. https://www.osha.gov/Publications/all_about_OSHA.pdf.

Department of Labor Occupational Safety and Health Administration. 2015b. OSHA inspections. http://www.osha.gov/.

Dunn, R.T. 2010. *Healthcare Management*, 9th ed. Chicago: Health Administration Press.

Equal Employment Opportunity Commission. 2009. Federal Laws Prohibiting Job Discrimination Questions and Answers. https://www.eeoc.gov/facts/qanda.html.

Equal Employment Opportunity Commission. n.d.a. Overview. http://www.eeoc.gov/.

Equal Employment Opportunity Commission. n.d.b. Uniform guidelines on employee selection procedures. http://www.uniformguidelines.com/.

Equal Employment Opportunity Commission. n.d.c. Age discrimination. http://www.eeoc.gov/.

Equal Employment Opportunity Commission. n.d.d. Disability discrimination. http://www.eeoc.gov/.

Equal Employment Opportunity Commission. n.d.e. Equal pay/compensation discrimination. http://www.eeoc.gov/.

Equal Employment Opportunity Commission. n.d.f. National origin discrimination. http://www.eeoc.gov/.

Equal Employment Opportunity Commission. n.d.g. Sexual harassment. http://www.eeoc.gov/.

Joint Commission. n.d. Health Equity topics. https://www.jointcommission.org/topics/health_equity.aspx.

Society for Human Resources Management. 1978. Uniform Guidelines on Employee Selection Procedures of 1978. www.shrm.org/legalissues/federalresources.

Cases, Statutes, and Regulations Cited

29 CFR 1635.3(c)(1): Genetic Information Nondiscrimination Act of 2008.

29 CFR 1904: Occupational Safety and Health Administration regulations.

29 CFR 1910: Occupational Safety and Health Act of 1970.

29 CFR 1910.1030: Bloodborne pathogens. 1991.

8 USC 1101: The Immigration Reform and Control Act of 1986.

29 USC 141 et seq.: Labor-Management Relations Act of 1947.

29 USC 151-169: National Labor Relations Act of 1935.

29 USC 201: The Fair Labor Standards Act of 1938.

29 USC 206(d): Equal Pay Act of 1963.

29 USC 621-34: Age Discrimination in Employment Act of 1967.

29 USC 1001 et seq.: Employee Retirement Income Security Act of 1974.

42 USC 12101 et seq.: Americans with Disabilities Act of 1990 and Amendments Act of 2008.

Consolidated Omnibus Budget Reconciliation Act of 1986. Public Law 99–272.

Needlestick Safety and Prevention Act of 2000. Public Law 106–480.

Glossary

A

Abbreviation: Shortened form of a word or phrase; in healthcare, when there is more than one meaning for an approved abbreviation, either only one meaning should be used or the context in which the abbreviation is to be used should be identified

Abuse (healthcare): Provider, supplier, and practitioner practices that are inconsistent with accepted sound fiscal, business, or medical practices and that may directly or indirectly result in unnecessary costs to the program, improper payment, services that fail to meet professionally recognized standards of care or are medically unnecessary, or services that directly or indirectly result in adverse patient outcomes or delays in appropriate diagnosis or treatment

Acceptance: Agreeing to an offer, reflecting a meeting of minds on terms of a contract

Access: One of the rights protected by the Privacy Rule, the right of access allows an individual to inspect and obtain a copy of his or her own protected health information that is contained in a designated record set, such as a health record; also an information security term that refers to the ability to enter an electronic system and make use of the data within it

Access report: Proposed by the Department of Health and Human Services in the May 31, 2011, Notice of Proposed Rulemaking, it would allow individuals (upon request) to receive a listing from covered entities with EHRs of every person who viewed the individuals' designated record set during the previous three years

Accountable Care Organization: Groups of providers and suppliers meeting certain criteria that work together to manage and coordinate care for Medicare fee-for-service beneficiaries

Accounting of disclosures: A list of all disclosures made of a patient's health information; Section 164.528 of the Privacy Rule states that an individual has the right to receive an accounting of certain disclosures made by a covered entity within the six years prior to the date on which the accounting was requested

Accreditation Council for Graduate Medical Education (ACGME): Accrediting body for medical schools that sets practice standards for graduates of medical school

Accuracy: The extent to which information reflects the true, correct, and exact description of the care that was delivered with respect to both content and timing

Act of God: Natural disaster, such as an earthquake or a flood, that is not human related

Active record: A health record of an individual who is a currently hospitalized inpatient or an outpatient

Actual causation: Determined by the "but–for" test: but for the defendant's action, the result would not have happened

Addendum: *See* **Amendment**

Addition of entries: Changes to the health record in the form of late entries, amendments, or addenda

Addressable specification: The implementation specifications of the HIPAA Security Rule that are designated "addressable" rather than "required"; to be in compliance with the rule, the covered entity must implement the specification as written, implement an alternative, or document that the risk for which the addressable implementation specification was provided either does not exist in the organization or exists with a negligible probability of occurrence

Adhesion contract: An agreement that may be unenforceable because unequal bargaining power between the parties forces the weaker party to agree to unfavorable terms

Administrative agency: An executive branch agency; source of administrative law

Administrative agency tribunal: A form of alternative dispute resolution in which a tribunal is created by statute or the Constitution to hear a dispute arising from administrative law

Administrative data: Coded information contained in secondary records, such as billing records, describing patient identification, diagnoses, procedures, and insurance

Administrative information: Information used for administrative and healthcare operation purposes such as billing and quality oversight

Administrative law: Rules and regulations created by administrative agencies

Administrative safeguards: A set of nine standards defined by the HIPAA Security Rule: security management functions, assigned security responsibility, workforce security, information access management, security awareness and training, security incident reporting, contingency plan, evaluation, and business associate contracts and other arrangements

Administrative simplification: The original intent of HIPAA—the streamlining and standardization of the healthcare industry's nonuniform and seemingly inefficient business practices, such as billing and creating standards for the electronic transmission of data

Admissibility: Evidence that is allowed to be admitted in a court of law

Admission of facts: A discovery method in which a party elicits from the opposing party certain admissions that will diminish the amount of time and money that would otherwise be spent proving those facts

Adoption: A legal status in which the parental rights and responsibilities of one set of parents are legally terminated and a new parental relationship is established by law

Advance directive: A legal document that specifies an individual's healthcare wishes in the event that he or she has a temporary or permanent loss of competence

Adverse patient occurrence (APO): An occurrence such as admission for adverse results of outpatient management, readmission for complications, incomplete management of problems on previous hospitalization, or unplanned removal, injury, or repair of an organ or structure during surgery; covered entities must have a system for concurrent or retrospective identification through medical chart–based review according to objective screening criteria

Advisory opinion: Opinions about the application of the Office of the Inspector General's fraud and abuse authorities to the requesting party's existing or proposed business arrangement

Affidavit of merit: A measure to deter excessive or frivolous litigation. It is required by some jurisdictions especially in medical malpractice claims whereby an expert witness must attest in an affidavit that in the opinion of the expert witness a standard of care has been breached

Affiliated covered entities: Legally separate covered entities, affiliated by common ownership or control; for purposes of the Privacy Rule, these legally separate entities may refer to themselves as a single covered entity

Affirmative defenses: Those defenses for which the defendant bears the burden of proving he or she is entitled to rely on them

Against medical advice (AMA): When a patient discharges himself or herself before a physician has determined it to be medically appropriate

Age Discrimination in Employment Act of 1967: A law that protects individuals 40 years or older from employment discrimination

Agency: Where individuals appear to others to be agents or representatives of the hospital or entity in which the individuals are providing services

Agency for Healthcare Research and Quality (AHRQ): Government agency whose purpose was and still is to build private–public partnerships to conduct and support research

Age of majority: In most states, the age of 18; an individual generally must have reached the age of majority in order to be considered a competent adult

Agent: Person designated by an individual (principal) to make certain decisions or perform certain acts on the individual's behalf.

AHIC: *See* **American Health Information Community**

AHIMA: *See* **American Health Information Management Association**

Allied health professional: A credentialed healthcare worker who is not a physician, nurse, psychologist, or pharmacist (for example, a physical therapist, dietitian, social worker, or occupational therapist)

Altered authorization: Authorization is required, but one or more standard authorization elements may be omitted

Alternative dispute resolution: Ways of resolving a dispute or lawsuit other than through the court system, including arbitration, mediation, or resolution through an administrative agency

AMA: *See* **American Medical Association**

Amendment: Synonymous with addendum; a type of late entry in which information is added to support or clarify a previous entry and that often requires additional space for documentation

Amendment request: The right of individuals to ask that a covered entity amend their health records, as provided in Section 164.526 of the Privacy Rule

American Board of Medical Specialties: Not-for-profit organization that assists 24 approved medical specialty boards in the development and use of standards in the ongoing evaluation and certification of physicians

American Health Information Community (AHIC): A public-private federal advisory committee associated with the Office of the National Coordinator that makes recommendations to the secretary on how to accelerate adoption of interoperable electronic health information technology

American Health Information Management Association (AHIMA): The professional membership organization for managers of health information services and healthcare information systems as well as coding services; provides accreditation, advocacy, certification, and educational services

American Medical Association (AMA): A national professional membership organization for physicians that distributes scientific information, informs members of legislation related to health and medicine, and represents the medical profession's interests in national legislative matters

American Medical Informatics Association (AMIA): A professional organization of health informatics and information management personnel, biomedical informatics professionals, educators, and others

American National Standards Institute (ANSI): An organization that governs standards in many aspects of public and private business; developer of the Health Information Technology Standards Panel

American Recovery and Reinvestment Act of 2009 (ARRA): Federal legislation that included significant funding for health information technology and provided for significant changes to the HIPAA Privacy Rule

American Society for Testing and Materials (ASTM): A national organization whose purpose is to establish standards on materials, products, systems, and services

Americans with Disabilities Act of 1990: Law that ensures equal opportunity for, and elimination of discrimination against, persons with disabilities

AMIA: *See* **American Medical Informatics Association**

Analysis: Review of health record for proper documentation and adherence to regulatory and accreditation standards

ANSI: *See* **American National Standards Institute**

Answer: A defendant's response to a legal complaint, which may take the form of a denial, an admission, a plea of ignorance to the allegations, additional legal actions, or a request for dismissal

Antitrust: Referring to laws that protect the public against trusts and monopolies that are so large they have the power to control a market, and thereby restrict free trade and freedom of choice

APO: *See* **Adverse patient occurrence**

Apology statutes: State laws that, to varying degrees, deem apologies by healthcare providers to patients and their relatives following unanticipated medical outcomes to be inadmissible as evidence in court

Appeal: The next stage in the litigation process after a court has rendered a verdict; must be based on alleged errors or disputes of law rather than errors of fact

Appellant: The party appealing a case, also known as the petitioner

Appellate courts: Courts that hear appeals on final judgments of the state trial courts or federal trial courts

Appellee: The party against whom a case is appealed, also known as the respondent

Applied ethics: A practical application of moral standards or philosophical examination of moral situations or issues

Arbitration: A form of alternative dispute resolution in which a dispute is submitted to a third party or a panel of experts outside the judicial trial system

Assault: A form of intentional tort that involves conduct that causes *apprehension* of a harmful or offensive contact instead of actual contact

Assumption of risk: An affirmative defense that bars a plaintiff from recovering on his or her negligence claim if the defendant proves that the plaintiff: 1. had actual knowledge of a danger, 2. understood and appreciated the risks associated with the danger, and 3. voluntarily exposed himself or herself to those risks

ASTM: *See* **American Society for Testing and Materials**

Attestation: Applying a signature to documentation, thus showing authorship

Attorney in fact: Agent authorized by an individual to make certain decisions, such as healthcare determinations, according to a directive written by the individual

Audit trail: A record that shows who has accessed a computer system, when it was accessed, and what operations were performed

Authenticated evidence: Evidence that appears to be relevant and has been shown to have a baseline authenticity or trustworthiness

Authentication: Verification of a record's validity (that is, it is the record of the individual in question and it is what it purports to be) and, therefore, its reliability and truthfulness as evidence; also a security mechanism to validate the identity of a user in an electronic system

Authenticity: The genuineness of a record, that it is what it purports to be; information is authentic if proved to be immune from tampering and corruption

Authorization: A patient's permission to disclose protected health information (PHI); the form or detailed document that gives covered entities permission to use PHI for specified purposes, generally other than for treatment, payment, or health care operations, or to disclose PHI to a third party specified by the individual

Authorized agent: Individual or organization such as credential verification organization granted responsibility by a hospital to query or report to the National Practitioner Data Bank

Authorship: The origination or creation of recorded information attributed to a specific individual or entity acting at a particular time

Auto-attestation: *See* **Auto-authentication**

Auto-authentication: A process by which the failure of an author to review and affirmatively either approve or disapprove an entry within a specified time period results in authentication

Automatic log-off: A security procedure that causes a computer session to end after a predetermined period of inactivity, such as 10 minutes

Autonomy: A core ethical principle centered on the individual's right to self-determination that includes respect for the individual; in clinical applications, the patient's right to determine what does or does not happen to him or her in terms of healthcare

Autopsy: A postmortem examination to determine cause of death

B

Bailiff: The person responsible for maintaining order and decorum in the court, as well as managing the schedule of the judge; depending on state law, the bailiff may or may not be required to also be a peace officer

Batch signing: Attesting to multiple entries or orders at one time

Battery: Intentional and nonconsensual contact with a person

Behavioral health: A broad array of psychiatric services provided in acute, long-term, and ambulatory care settings; includes treatment of mental disorders, chemical dependency, mental retardation, and developmental disabilities as well as cognitive rehabilitation services

Behavioral healthcare information: Information related to treatment for conditions such as mental disorders, mental retardation, and other developmental disabilities

Belmont Report: A statement of ethical principles to prevent the unethical use of human subjects in research, sponsored by the Department of Health and Human Services

Bench trial: A trial without a jury

Beneficence: A legal term that means promoting good for others or providing services that benefit others, such as releasing health information that will help a patient receive care or will ensure payment for services received

Beneficiary and Family Centered-Quality Improvement Organizations (BFCC-QIOs): Perform the quality of care (medical case) reviews and medical necessity reviews

Benefits: Healthcare services for which the healthcare insurance company will pay

Best evidence rule: A rule under which in order to prove the contents of a writing, recording, or photograph, the original writing, recording, or photograph is required; protects against intentional perjury or faulty memory

Billing advocates: Individuals who advocate on behalf of patients to negotiate and lower their medical bills

Bioethics: A discipline that addresses matters of life and death in the use of biological and medical technology

Biometric identification system: A security system that analyzes biological data about the user, such as a voiceprint, fingerprint, handprint, retinal scan, faceprint, or full-body scan

Birth certificate: Paperwork that must be filed for every live birth, regardless of where it occurred

Birth defects registries: Database that includes information on newborns with birth defects, usually maintained by the state

Blanchard-Peale Ethics Check: A reputable decision-making guideline

Board of directors: The elected or appointed group of officials who bear ultimate responsibility for the successful operation of a healthcare organization

Board of trustees: *See* **Board of directors**

Boilerplate: Standard contract provisions

Breach: Defined by HITECH a as an "unauthorized acquisition, access, use or disclosure of PHI which compromises the security or privacy of such information" (American Recovery and Reinvestment Act of 2009, Title XIII—Health Information Technology, Subtitle D Sections 13400, 13402.)

Breach notification: An American Recovery and Reinvestment Act requirement that mandates the notification of individuals following the unauthorized use or disclosure of their protected health information, as the information's security or privacy may be compromised

Breach of confidentiality: A type of claim based on the special relationship—fiduciary in nature—between patients and healthcare providers

Breach of contract: Violation of one of more terms of a contract that can result in a lawsuit

Breach of duty: A failure to exercise reasonable care under the given circumstances, either by acting or failing to act

Brief: A legal document prepared by each party's attorney for a case heard before an appellate or supreme court

Burden of proof: The task of sufficiently proving or establishing the requisite degree of belief for each element of a case; usually belongs to the plaintiff

Business associate: A person or organization other than a member of a covered entity's workforce that performs functions or activities on behalf of or affecting a covered entity that involve the use or disclosure of individually identifiable health information

Business associate agreement: A written and signed contract that allows covered entities to lawfully disclose protected health information to business associates such as consultants, billing companies, accounting firms, or others that perform services for the provider, provided that the business associate agrees to abide by the provider's requirements to protect the information's security and confidentiality

Business record: A record that is made and kept in the usual course of business, at or near the time of the event recorded

Business records exception: A rule under which a record is determined not to be hearsay if it was made at or near the time by, or from information transmitted by, a person with knowledge; it was kept in the course of a regularly conducted business activity; and it was the regular practice of that business activity to make the record

Bylaws: Internal rules of an organization or company

C

CAMH: *See* **Comprehensive Accreditation Manual for Hospitals**

Cancer registry: Records maintained by many states for the purpose of tracking the incidence (new cases) of cancer

Capacity: Indicates that an individual is mentally competent and is in control of himself or herself.

Captain of the ship: Case law holding physicians solely responsible for all aspects of the patient's care, including care provided by hospital staff.

Case law: The body of law that is created when, as the result of a dispute, a court renders a decision

Case management: 1. The ongoing, concurrent review performed by clinical professionals to ensure the necessity and effectiveness of the clinical services being provided to a patient; 2. A process that integrates and coordinates patient care over time and across multiple sites and providers, especially in complex and high-cost cases; 3. The process of developing a specific care plan for a patient that serves as a communication tool to improve quality of care and reduce cost

Cause of action: Facts that give the plaintiff[s] the right to some type of legal remedy

CCHIT: *See* **Certification Commission for Health Information Technology**

Center for Democracy & Technology: A nonprofit public interest organization that promotes privacy in communications technologies; it houses the Health Privacy Project

Center for Quality Improvement and Patient Safety (CQuiPS): Established within AHRQ to oversee a number of quality and patient safety programs including the yearly publication of the National Healthcare Quality and Disparities Report Program. These reports share trends in patient safety, and data on quality and access to healthcare on a yearly basis

Centers for Medicare and Medicaid Services (CMS): Division of the Department of Health and Human Services responsible for developing healthcare policy and administering the Medicare program and federal portion of the Medicaid program

Certification Commission for Health Information Technology (CCHIT): An independent, nonprofit group formed and funded in 2004 to compare products submitted by vendors against current standards

CEs: *See* **Covered entities**

CFR: *See* **Code of Federal Regulations**

Charitable immunity: A doctrine that shields hospitals (as well as other institutions) from liability for negligence because of the belief that donors would not make contributions to hospitals if they thought their donation would be used to litigate claims, combined with concern that a few lawsuits could bankrupt a hospital

Chief of staff: The physician designated as leader of a healthcare organization's medical staff

CIA: *See* **Corporate Integrity Agreement**

Circuit courts: Federal appellate courts distributed throughout the United States, including the District of Columbia and US territories, so that each court represents a specific number of the district courts

Circumstantial evidence: Evidence that is not directly from an eyewitness or participant and requires some reasoning to prove a fact

Civil law: Noncriminal law

Civil Monetary Penalties Act (CMP): Section 1128A of the Social Security Act, passed in 1981 as one of several administrative remedies to combat increases in healthcare fraud and abuse, which authorizes the secretary and inspector general of the Department of Health and Human Services (HHS) to impose civil monetary penalties, assessment, and program exclusions on individuals and entities whose wrongdoing causes injury to HHS programs or their beneficiaries

Civil procedure: The rule and parameters that govern civil (noncriminal) cases

Claims management program: Can help prevent or reduce financial loss in the occurrence of an adverse event.

Class action: A type of lawsuit involving multiple plaintiffs, often a group of consumers filing suit against a large and generally powerful entity for alleged wrongdoing

Clayton Act: Federal antitrust statute that exempts union activities from antitrust laws and prohibits discriminatory pricing practices, tying arrangements, and mergers and acquisitions that reduce competition

Clerk of courts: A government official responsible for officially maintaining documents associated with legal actions filed in a court system

CLIA: *See* **Clinical Laboratory Improvement Amendments**

Clinical Laboratory Improvement Amendments (CLIA): A law that provides that clinical laboratories are to disclose test results or reports only to "authorized persons"—unless state law defines them otherwise, defined by the law as the person who orders the test

Cloning: Includes placing information on the wrong encounter or wrong patient, entering information that does not reflect the current situation and failing to customize it to the appropriate patient, omitting the identity of the original author of the information, and using information without the original author's knowledge or permission

Closing argument: The point in a trial after both sides have presented and rested their cases when each side presents an argument that seeks to compel the jury to find in favor of its client

CME: *See* **Continuing medical education**

CMP: *See* **Civil Monetary Penalties Act**

COBRA: *See* **Consolidated Omnibus Budget Reconciliation Act of 1986**

Code of ethics: A statement of ethical principles regarding business practices and professional behavior

Code of Federal Regulations (CFR): A publication of the regulations issued by administrative agencies, or administrative laws

Collateral source payment: Payment a plaintiff in a tort case receives from a source other than the defendant(s), can be from multiple sources

Collective bargaining: A process through which a contract is negotiated, which sets forth the relationship between the employees and the healthcare organization

Common law: The body of law (that is, judicial or case law) that is created when a court renders a decision as the result of a dispute

Common rule: A federal law that imposes specific requirements designed to protect participants (human subjects) in research, relates to Institutional Review Boards

Communicable disease: A disease that can be transmitted from an infected person, animal, or inanimate reservoir to a susceptible person or host by either direct or indirect contact

Community benefit standard: To achieve and maintain tax-exempt status with the Internal Revenue Service, a healthcare facility must provide a certain amount of uncompensated care and engage in activities that benefit its community

Comparative negligence: A defendant is able to demonstrate that the plaintiff's conduct contributed in part to the injury the plaintiff suffered

Compensation: All direct and indirect pay, including wages, mandatory benefits, and benefits such as medical insurance, life insurance, child care, elder care, retirement plans, and longevity pay

Compensatory damages: Damages in which the plaintiff is compensated for losses incurred; actual damages

Competent adult: An individual who has reached the age of majority and is mentally and physically competent to tend to his or her own affairs; may consent to treatment and may authorize the access or disclosure of his or her health information

Complaint: The document that is filed with a court in order to commence a lawsuit

Completeness: An element of a legally defensible health record; the health record is not complete until all its parts are assembled and the appropriate documents are authenticated according to medical staff bylaws

Compliance: 1. The process of establishing an organizational culture that promotes the prevention, detection, and resolution of instances of conduct that do not conform to federal, state, or private payer healthcare program requirements or the healthcare organization's ethical and business policies; 2. The act of adhering to official requirements

Compliance officer: An individual responsible for overseeing an organization's compliance program and ensuring that the program promotes ethical business practices and conformity to federal, state, and private payer program requirements

Compound authorization: An authorization that combines informed consent with an authorization for the use and/or disclosure of protected health information

Comprehensive Accreditation Manual for Hospitals (CAMH): Accreditation manual published by the Joint Commission

Comprehensive Alcohol Abuse and Alcoholism Prevention, Treatment, and Rehabilitation Act of 1970: Federal statute that provides specific and highly particularized safeguards for the protection of information relating to the diagnosis, treatment, or referral for treatment of conditions relating to drug abuse or other substance abuse

Computer key: A number unique to a specific individual for purposes of authentication

Computer virus: The most common and virulent forms of intentional computer tampering; types may include file infectors, system or boot-record infectors, and macro viruses

Conditioned authorization: Requires authorization in order to receive treatment or some other service or benefit

Conditions of Participation: The standards that govern providers receiving Medicare and Medicaid reimbursements

Confidential communications: As defined by HIPAA, a request that protected health information be routed to an alternative location or by an alternative method; must be honored by health plans under HIPAA

Confidentiality: A legal and ethical concept that establishes the healthcare provider's responsibility for protecting health records and other personal and private information from unauthorized use or disclosure

Confidentiality of Alcohol and Drug Abuse Patient Records Regulation: Regulation enacted for the purpose of encouraging individuals to seek substance abuse treatment without fear of their health information being disclosed

Conflict of interest: A conflict between private or personal interests and the official responsibilities of a person in a leadership position

Conflict of laws: An inconsistency between the laws of different states arising from a legal action that involves the territory of more than one jurisdiction

Consent: 1. A patient's acknowledgment that he or she understands a proposed intervention, including that intervention's risks, benefits, and alternatives; 2. A patient's agreement that protected health information can be disclosed; the document that provides a record of the patient's consent

Consideration: An element necessary for a valid contract; what each party will receive from the other party in return for performing the obligations described in the contract

Consolidated Omnibus Budget Reconciliation Act of 1986 (COBRA): The federal law requiring every hospital that participates in Medicare and has an emergency room to treat any patient in an emergency condition or active labor, whether or not the patient is covered by Medicare and regardless of the patient's ability to pay; COBRA also requires employers to provide continuation benefits to specified workers and families who have been terminated but previously had healthcare insurance benefits

Constitution: A document that defines and lays out the powers of a government; considered the supreme law of that government

Constitutional law: Body of law that deals with the amount and types of power and authority that governments are given

Consultation: The response by one healthcare professional to another healthcare professional's request to provide recommendations or opinions regarding the care of a particular patient or resident

Consumer Coalition for Health Privacy: Affiliated with the Health Privacy Project, this organization was created to educate and empower healthcare consumers on privacy issues at the various levels of government and consists of patients and consumer advocacy organizations

Consumer Health Information Bill of Rights: Created by the American Health Information Management Association (AHIMA); furthers the organization's commitment to support and protect people's rights regarding their health information

Context-based access control: The most stringent type of access control, which takes into account the person attempting to access the data, the type of data being accessed, and the *context* of the transaction in which the access attempt is made

Contingency fee: A lawyer's fee that is paid based on a percentage of the money awarded to the client; this fee is commonly one-third of the total recovery

Contingency planning: A plan for recovery in the event of a power failure, disaster, or other emergency that limits or eliminates access to facilities and electronic protected health information (ePHI); an important component of protecting ePHI

Continuing medical education (CME): Activities such as accredited sponsorship, nonaccredited sponsorship, medical teaching, publications that advance medical care, and other learning experiences, proof of which is required for a physician to maintain certification

Contract: 1. A legally enforceable agreement; 2. An agreement between a union and an employer that spells out details of the relationship of management and the employees

Contract law: The body of civil law relating to agreements between parties, most often in the context of business or commercial relationships

Contributory negligence: An individual's conduct contributed in part to the injury that the individual suffered

Coroner: Typically, an appointed or elected official, who may or may not be a physician, who is responsible for investigating suspicious deaths

Corporate code of conduct: A part of the compliance plan that expresses the organization's commitment to ethical behavior

Corporate compliance: Refers to adherence to the laws and regulations passed by official regulating bodies as well as general principles of ethical conduct

Corporate compliance programs: Programs that became common after the Federal Sentencing Guidelines reduced the fines and penalties to organizations found guilty of healthcare fraud if the organization has a fraud prevention and detection program in place; the programs also help organizations identify problems and improve performance

Corporate integrity agreement (CIA): A compliance program imposed by the government that involves substantial government oversight and outside expert involvement in the organization's compliance activities and is generally required as a condition of settling a fraud and abuse investigation

Corporate negligence: A doctrine under which hospitals may be held liable in their own right

Corporation: An organization created as an artificial and legally distinct being under the authority of state statute

Correct Coding Initiative (CCI): A national initiative designed to improve the accuracy of Part B claims processed by Medicare carriers

Counterclaim: A claim by a defendant against a plaintiff

Countersignature: Authentication by a second provider that signifies review and evaluation of the actions and documentation, including authentication, of a first provider

Court of Claims: A federal or state court in which legal actions against the government are brought

Court order: A document issued by a judge that compels certain actions, such as testimony or the production of documents such as health records

Court reporter: An individual who is present during the entire course of a trial and is responsible for providing a verbatim transcript of the trial

Covered entities (CEs): Persons or organizations that must comply with the HIPAA Privacy and Security Rules; include healthcare providers, health plans, and healthcare clearinghouses

Credentialing: The process of reviewing and validating the qualifications (degrees, licenses, and other credentials) of physicians and other licensed independent practitioners for the purpose of granting medical staff membership to provide patient care services

Credentials verification organization (CVO): An organization that verifies healthcare professionals' backgrounds, licensing, and schooling and tracks continuing education and other performance measures

Creditor: Anyone who regularly, and in the ordinary course of business, meets one of the following criteria: 1. obtains or uses consumer reports in connection with a credit transaction; 2. furnishes information to consumer reporting agencies in connection with a credit transaction; or 3. advances funds to, or on behalf of, someone (except for funds for expenses that are incidental to a service provided by the creditor to that person)

Criminal law: A type of law in which the government is a party prosecuting an accused who has been charged with violating a criminal statute or regulation

Criminal negligence: Reckless disregard for another individual's safety or, stated differently, willful indifference to a harm that could result from an act

Criminal procedure: Procedural law that guides criminal cases

Cross appeal: An appeal in which both the respondent and the petitioner file appeals

Cross-claim: A claim by one party against another party who is on the same side of the main litigation

Cryptography: The study of encryption and decryption techniques

Cultural competence: How an organization, through its policies and human behaviors and attitudes, functions effectively in cross-cultural situations

Custodian: *See* **Custodian of health records**

Custodian of health records: The person designated as responsible for the operational functions of the development and maintenance of the health record and who may certify through affidavit or testimony the normal business practices used to create and maintain the record

Cut, copy, paste: *See* Cloning

CVO: *See* **Credentials verification organization**

Cyber attack: A deliberate and often systematic attempt to gain unauthorized access to a device or network

D

Damages: Monetary compensation awarded by a court to an individual injured in a civil action through the wrongful act of another party

Darling case: Often credited as the landmark case for extending liability for negligence to hospitals (*Darling v. Charleston Community Memorial Hospital*)

Data encryption: A form of technical security used to ensure that data transferred from one location on a network to another are secure from anyone eavesdropping or seeking to intercept them

Data governance: The "enterprise authority that ensures control and accountability for enterprise data" (Johns 2015.)

Data security: The process of keeping data, both in transit and at rest, safe from unauthorized access, alteration, or destruction

Data stewardship: The responsibilities and accountabilities associated with managing, collecting, viewing, storing, sharing, disclosing, or otherwise making use of personal health information (AMIA 2007)

Data use agreement: An agreement between a covered entity and a researcher stipulating that the researcher will receive only a limited data set for research, public health, or healthcare operations

DDS: *See* **Disability determination services**

Death certificate: As directed by state law, paperwork that must be completed when someone dies; generally filled out by the funeral director or another person responsible for internment or cremation of remains and signed by the physician, who provides the cause of death

Deemed status: Enables a Joint Commission–accredited healthcare organization to use its accreditation status in lieu of a separate Medicare or Medicaid Conditions of Participation healthcare organization certification process

Defamation: False communication about a person to someone else that harms the person's reputation

Default judgment: An automatic judgment by the court against the defendant that is made when the defendant fails to respond to a complaint within the time frame specified by the court

Defendant: The individual or organization that is the object of the lawsuit, and against whom a lawsuit is brought; wrongdoer

Deficit Reduction Act of 2005 (DRA): A law enacted in 2006 that transformed the nature of compliance programs from voluntary to mandatory; failure to comply may result in the affected entity being ineligible to receive Medicaid payments

Deidentified information: Information from which personal characteristics have been stripped and that, as a result, neither identifies nor provides a reasonable basis to believe it could identify an individual

Deletion: Permanent elimination of information from a document

Deliberations: The secret conversation of a jury before it renders a decision or verdict

Demonstrative evidence: Actual objects, pictures, models, and other devices that are supposedly intended to clarify the facts for the judge and jury

Deontology: The obligation to perform your duty

Department of Health and Human Services (HHS): The federal agency that oversees Medicare, Medicaid, and other health and essential human services

Deponent: A person directed by subpoena to appear at an appointed time and place to testify under oath at a deposition

Deposition: A formal proceeding by which the oral testimonies of individuals are obtained as part of the discovery process

Designated health services: Services defined by the Federal Physician Self-Referral Statute (Stark Law), which prohibits physicians from ordering certain services for patients from entities with which the physician or an immediate family member has a financial relationship

Designated record set: A group of records maintained by or for a covered entity encompassing medical records and billing records about individuals and enrollment, payment, claims adjudication, and case or medical management record systems maintained by or for a health plan used, in whole or in part, by or for the covered entity to make decisions about individuals

Destruction of records: The act of breaking down the components of a health record into pieces that can no longer be recognized as parts of the original record; for example, paper records can be destroyed by shredding, and electronic records can be destroyed by magnetic degaussing

Deterministic algorithm: Compares values in various database fields (for example, date of birth, race, marital status) to detect exact or partial matches

Diabetes registries: Database that includes cases of patients with diabetes for the purpose of assisting in the management patient care and research

Digital signature: A type of e-signature that encrypts the document (represented by a series of numbers), identifies who performed the encryption (that is, the person who is authenticating), and validates and detects whether any subsequent changes have been made to the document

Digitized signature: An image of a handwritten signature created by signature pads, scanning, or digital photography

Direct evidence: "Real, tangible or clear evidence of a fact, happening or thing that requires no thinking or consideration to prove its existence" (ALM Media Properties 2012)

Directed verdict: A request made by an attorney for the judge to determine that a case is over and rule favorably to the requesting party, even without the opposition presenting its case

Disability determination services (DDS): State agencies responsible for providing to the Social Security Administration medical evidence to determine whether a resident of a state is or is not disabled under the Social Security disability law

Disaster recovery planning: A plan for securing electronic protected health information (ePHI) in the event of a disaster that limits or eliminates access to facilities and ePHI

Discharge analysis: A detailed review of the health record at or following discharge

Discharge summary: A recapitulation of an individual's stay at a healthcare facility that is used along with the postdischarge plan of care to provide continuity of care upon discharge from the facility

Disclosure: The act of making information known; the release of confidential health information about an identifiable person to another person or entity; release, transfer, provision of access to, or divulging in any other manner of information outside the entity holding the information (45 CFR 160.103) (*See also* **Release of information**)

Discoverability: Limitations on the ability of parties to discover pretrial information held by another party

Discovery: The next pretrial stage after the commencement of a lawsuit, which allows all parties (generally via their legal counsel) to use various strategies to discover or obtain information held by other parties and, subsequently, to assess the strengths and weaknesses inherent in each party's case

Disposition: The removal of records from a record storage system, whether through destruction, transfer, or loss

Dismissal: Termination of a legal proceeding

Distributive justice: The fair apportionment of resources to all patients, considering several factors including ability to pay, need, equity, and potential benefit of resources

District courts: The first and lowest level in the federal court system

Diversity: Differences including, but not limited to, age, ethnicity, gender, religious beliefs, sexual orientation, socioeconomic status, and physical abilities

Diversity jurisdiction: A form of court that enables parties from different states to engage in a lawsuit in federal court if the suit fulfills the following obligations: 1. *no* plaintiff can be from the same state as *any* of the defendants and 2. the amount in controversy must be at least $75,000

DNR: *See* **Do not resuscitate (DNR) order**

Do not resuscitate (DNR) order: A specific type of advance directive in which an individual states that healthcare providers should not perform CPR if the individual experiences cardiac arrest or cessation of breathing

Documentary evidence: Evidence in written form, not oral (original records, letters, e-mails, photographs), used to prove a fact included in the information imparted (such as medical record documentation that describes a patient fall)

Documentation templates: Functionalities in EHRs that already have some phrases in place, but allow for the standardized collection of specific data through features such as drop-down menus that providers can select from to describe a patient's condition, or to describe or order treatment

DPOA: *See* **Durable power of attorney**

DRA: *See* **Deficit Reduction Act of 2005**

Drug Abuse Prevention, Treatment, and Rehabilitation Act of 1972: Federal statutes that provide specific and highly particularized safeguards for the protection of information relating to the diagnosis, treatment, or referral for treatment of conditions relating to drug abuse or other substance abuse

Due diligence: A legally acceptable level of care required of members of corporate boards of directors

Due process: The right of individuals to fair treatment under the law

Due process of law: The guarantee provided under the Constitution and the Bill of Rights that laws will be reasonable and not arbitrary and allow for challenges to a law's content and substance

Duplicate billing: The practice of submitting more than one claim for the same item or service

Durable power of attorney (DPOA): A power of attorney that remains in effect even after the principal is incapacitated; can be drafted to take effect only when the principal becomes incapacitated

Durable power of attorney for healthcare decisions (DPOA-HCD): A legal instrument through which a principal appoints an agent to make healthcare decisions on the principal's behalf in the event the principal become incapacitated

Duty of loyalty: A requirement of members of corporate boards of directors; placing the interests of the corporation ahead of one's own personal interests

Duty of responsibility: A requirement of members of corporate boards of directors; acting with due care in exercising their duties

Duty to warn: The legal obligation of a health professional to disclose information to warn an intended victim when a patient threatens to harm an individually identifiable victim or victims, and the psychiatrist or other mental health provider believes that the patient is likely to actually harm the individual(s)

E

Economic credentialing: Granting medical staff privileges to a provider based on volume of services rather than quality of care

Economic damages: *See* **Special damages**

e-Discovery: Pretrial legal process used to describe the methods by which parties will obtain and view electronically stored information

EEOC: *See* **Equal Employment Opportunity Commission**

eHealth Initiative: A private organization that involves many groups working on the improvement of health information through information technology and health information exchange

EHR: *See* **Electronic health record**

Electronic health record (EHR): A computerized record of health information and associated processes; an electronic record of health-related information on an individual that conforms to nationally recognized standards and that can be created, managed, and consulted by authorized clinicians and staff across more than one healthcare organization

Electronic medical record (EMR): An electronic record of health-related information on an individual that can be created, gathered, managed, and consulted by authorized clinicians and staff within a single healthcare organization

Electronic protected health information (ePHI): Under HIPAA, all individually identifiable information that is created or received electronically by a healthcare provider or any other entity subject to HIPAA requirements

Electronic Records Express: A program implemented by the Social Security Agency and state Disability Determination Services that enables providers to submit records related to disability claims to a secure website

Electronic signature: Technological corollary to the handwritten signature in a paper record; any representation of a signature in digital form, including an image of a handwritten signature. Authentication of a computer entry can be completed via a digitized image of one's signature, a biometric identifier, a secret code or password, or a digital signature that is linked to the user's name, credentials, and access rights to verify the identity of the signer in the system and create an individual signature on the record.

Electronic Signatures in Global National Commerce Act (E-SIGN): An act passed in 2000 that gives e-signatures the same legality as handwritten signatures where interstate commerce is involved and that provides guidance on how records may be stored and retained electronically

Electronically stored information (ESI): Data or documents used in digital format that are created, stored, manipulated, and communicated electronically through the use of computer hardware and software

E/M codes: *See* **Evaluation and management (E/M) codes**

Emancipated minor: One who is under the age of majority and is self-supporting, and whose parents have surrendered their rights of custody, care, and support

Embryonic stem cell research: Embryonic stem cells harvested from unused donated fertilized embryos and used for research purposes

Emergency medical condition (EMC): a health condition that could result in serious harm or death if not treated immediately

Emergency Medical Treatment and Active Labor Act (EMTALA): A 1986 law enacted as part of the Consolidated Omnibus Reconciliation Act largely to combat "patient-dumping"—transferring, discharging, or refusing to treat indigent emergency department patients because of their inability to pay

Emotional distress: May include manifestations such as sleeplessness, anxiety, irritability, or the emotional inability to perform activities or go places that a plaintiff was capable of prior to the event for which a lawsuit has been filed

Employee health record: A record kept on an employee as part of employment that contains any and all information related to such items as medical tests, drug tests, examinations, physical abilities, immunizations, screenings required by law, biohazardous exposure, and physical limitations

Employee nondisclosure agreement: A contract between employer and employee in which the employee promises not to divulge specified information, subject to disciplinary action or termination

Employee Retirement Income Security Act of 1974 (ERISA): An act that sets minimum standards for most voluntarily established pension and health plans in private industry in order to provide protection for individuals in these plans

EMR: *See* **Electronic medical record**

EMTALA: *See* **Emergency Medical Treatment and Active Labor Act**

Encryption: A technique used to ensure that data transferred from one location on a network to another are secure from eavesdropping or interception

Enforcement rule: A rule that created standardized procedures and substantive requirements for investigating complaints and imposing civil monetary penalties (CMPs) for HIPAA violations, as well as a uniform compliance and enforcement mechanism that addresses *all* of the Administrative Simplification regulations, including privacy, security, and transactions and code sets

Enterprise master patient index (EMPI): Tracks patients in integrated healthcare systems that increasingly consist of multiple care sites and a variety of information systems

Enterprise risk management: a structured process that focuses on identifying and eliminating the financial impact and volatility of a portfolio of risks rather than on risk avoidance alone

Entity authentication: The corroboration that an entity is the one claimed (HHS n.d.); the computer reads a predetermined set of criteria to determine whether the user is who he or she claims to be

ePHI: *See* **Electronic Protected Health Information**

Equal Employment Opportunity Act of 1972: An act that, in combination with Title VII of the Civil Rights Act, prohibits discrimination based on age, race, color, sex, religion, or national origin

Equal Employment Opportunity Commission (EEOC): Enforces the Equal Employment Opportunity Act, Title VII of the Civil Rights Act, the Immigration Reform and Control Act, the Fair Labor Standards Act, and the Americans with Disabilities Act, among others; investigates job discrimination complaints and can bring federal lawsuits against employers

Equal Pay Act of 1963: An act that regulates the concept of equal pay for men and women who perform similar work requiring similar skills, effort, and responsibility under similar working conditions

Equity: A form of judgment in which the defendant is required to do or to refrain from doing something

ERISA: *See* **Employee Retirement Income Security Act of 1974**

ESI: *See* **Electronically stored information**

E-SIGN: *See* **Electronic Signatures in Global National Commerce Act**

Ethical decision-making model: A model of ethical decision making that provides specific steps that can be used to approach any ethical decision

Ethical principles: Set of four principles to assist healthcare professionals in addressing healthcare related dilemma (*See also* **Autonomy, Beneficence, Nonmaleficence, Justice**)

Ethics: A field of study that deals with moral principles, theories, and values; in healthcare, a formal decision-making process for dealing with the competing perspectives and obligations of the people who have an interest in a common problem

Evaluation and management (E/M) codes: *Current Procedural Terminology* codes that describe patient encounters with healthcare professionals for assessment counseling and other routine healthcare services

Evidence: The means by which the facts of a case are proved or disproved

Exculpatory contract: An agreement that may be unenforceable; seeks to excuse a party in advance from any potential liability

Executive branch: The branch of government charged with enforcing laws, including the issuance of regulations by administrative agencies, with ultimate executive-branch power vested in the chief executive (the president of the United States on the federal level and the governor of each state at the state level)

Exempt employee: An employee for whom minimum wage and overtime regulations do not apply

Expert witness: An individual with expertise in a certain subject who is called to testify in a case

Express consent: Consent that is communicated through words, regardless of whether those words are written or spoken

External security threat: A security threat caused by individuals or forces outside the organization

F

Facility: A building necessary in the provision of health services (for example, hospitals, nursing homes, and ambulatory care centers)

Facility directory: A directory of patients being treated in a healthcare facility

FACTA: *See* **Fair and Accurate Credit Transactions Act**

Failure Mode Effect and Criticality Assessment (FMECA): A methodology for determining the cause of sentinel events

Fair and Accurate Credit Transactions Act (FACTA): An act that requires advance employee (i.e., patient) authorization for a consumer reporting agency to share medical information with employers for employment or insurance purposes; it also requires financial institutions and creditors to develop and implement written identity theft programs that identify, detect, and respond to red flags that may signal the presence of identity theft

Fair Labor Standards Act of 1938 (FLSA): An act that provides regulations for wages and overtime

False Claims Act: The government's primary litigation tool for combating fraud, which provides that anyone who "knowingly" submits false claims to the government is liable for damages up to three times the amount of the erroneous payment plus mandatory penalties between $5,500 and $11,000 for each false claim submitted

False cost reports: A way of increasing Medicare payments inappropriately

False imprisonment: The intentional confinement of another person against that person's will

Federal Anti-Kickback Statute: A statute that establishes criminal penalties for individuals and entities that knowingly and willfully offer, pay, solicit, or receive remuneration in order to induce business for which payment may be made under any federal healthcare program

Federal Information Processing Standards (FIPS): Outlines approved security functions, approved protection profiles, approved random number generator, and approved key establishment techniques

Federal Physician Self-Referral Statute (Stark Law): A law that prohibits physicians from ordering designated health services for Medicare (and to some extent Medicaid) patients from entities with which the physician or an immediate family member has a financial relationship; also known as the Stark Law

Federal Policy for the Protection of Human Subjects (Common Rule): Regulations that govern research on human subjects

Federal Rules of Civil Procedure (FRCP): The rules governing civil cases at the trial level in federal courts

Federal Rules of Criminal Procedure (FRCrP): The rules governing criminal cases at the trial level in federal courts

Federal Rules of Evidence (FRE): Rules governing evidence used in cases presented in federal court because they involve federal laws

Federal Trade Commission (FTC) Act: Federal antitrust statute that gives the Federal Trade Commission broad powers to act against organizations engaging in unfair methods of competition, or unfair or deceptive acts that affect commerce

Felony: A crime such as murder, larceny, rape, or assault that is more serious in nature than a misdemeanor; under federal law and many state statutes, a felony is punishable by a minimum of imprisonment exceeding one year

Fetal death: The death of a fetus of a particular weight or gestation, frequently 500 grams or more or 22 or more completed weeks of gestation, though the weight and week gestation may vary from state to state

Fiduciary duty: Obligation to act in the best interest of another party based on a special relationship of trust, confidence, or responsibility in certain obligations

Firewall: Hardware or software devices that examine traffic entering and leaving a network and prevent some traffic from entering or leaving based on established rules; can be used to describe the software that protects computing resources or to describe the combination of the software, hardware, and policies that protect the resources

FLSA: *See* **Fair Labor Standards Act of 1938**

FMECA: *See* **Failure Mode Effect and Criticality Assessment**

Focused professional practice evaluation: A time-limited period during which an organization evaluates and determines a practitioner's professional performance of privileges; it occurs in all requests for new privileges and when there are concerns regarding the provision of safe, high-quality care by a current medical staff member

FOIA: *See* **Freedom of Information Act of 1967**

For-profit corporation: Tax status that allows a company to distribute its income to the shareholders, directors, officers, and other individuals for their private gain

For-profit organization: The tax status assigned to business entities that are owned by one or more individuals or organizations and that earn revenues in excess of expenditures that are subsequently paid out to the owners or stockholders

Foreseeability: An indication that the defendant's actions would result in the plaintiff's injury

Fraud: A false representation of fact or a failure to disclose a fact that is material (relevant) to a healthcare transaction that results in damage to another party that reasonably relies on the misrepresentation or failure to disclose Intentional deception or misrepresentation that the individual or entity makes knowing that the misrepresentation could result in some unauthorized benefit to the individual, the entity, or some other party (NHCAA)

Fraud Enforcement and Recovery Act of 2009 (FERA): Expands both the potential for liability under the False Claims Act (FCA) and the government's investigative powers, and it eliminates the requirement that a person has to present a false claim to a US government officer or employee, or a member of the US armed services, in order to be liable under the FCA

FRCP: *See* **Federal Rules of Civil Procedure**

FRE: *See* **Federal Rules of Evidence**

Freedom of Information Act of 1967 (FOIA): A law covering the right of disclosure to and access by the public regarding federal agency records

Fundraising: Money-generating activities that benefit a HIPAA-covered entity and are subject to the HIPAA Privacy Rule

G

Garnishment: A method of collecting a monetary award in which a certain percentage of the defendant's wages are routinely set aside and paid to the plaintiff toward full satisfaction of the judgment

General consent: A form that covers routine diagnostic procedures and medical treatment by hospital staff, as well as other activities such as release of information for treatment purposes and disposal of human tissue and body fluids

General damages: Damages that naturally and necessarily flow from a tort and directly result from the tort

General jurisdiction: Courts that hear more serious criminal cases (for example, felonies) or civil cases that involve large amounts of money; may hear all matters of state law except for those cases that must be heard in courts of special jurisdiction

Genetic Information Nondiscrimination Act of 2008 (GINA): Federal legislation that prohibits discrimination by health insurers and employers based on genetic information

Good Samaritan statute: State law or statute that protects healthcare providers from liability for not obtaining informed consent before rendering care to adults or minors at the scene of an emergency or accident

Governing Board: *See* **Board of directors**

Grievance: A formal written description of a complaint or disagreement

Grievance procedures: The steps employees may follow to seek resolution of disagreements with management on job-related issues

Gross negligence: Very great or excessive negligence that implies an extreme departure from the ordinary standard of care and shows a reckless disregard for the rights of others

H

Handwritten signature: The most common method for authenticating paper health records

HCQIA: *See* **Health Care Quality Improvement Act**

Health Care Decisions Act: Legislation, usually by states, that encourages the making and enforcement of advance healthcare directives and provides a means for making healthcare decisions for those who have failed to plan

Health Care Fraud Prevention and Enforcement Action Team: A joint HHS and DOJ initiative to combat Medicare and Medicaid fraud. This team is using real-time data analysis to investigate healthcare fraud cases, rather than a prolonged subpoena and account analyses, resulting in much shorter periods of time between fraud identification, arrest and prosecution

Health Care Quality Improvement Act (HCQIA): A 1986 act that requires facilities to report professional review actions on physicians, dentists, and other facility-based practitioners to the National Practitioner Data Bank (NPDB)

Healthcare Research and Quality Act of 1999: Created the federal Agency for Healthcare Research and Quality

Healthgrades: an independent organization online resource that provides profiles and ratings on numerous hospitals and physicians in the United States

Health informatics and information management (HIIM): Refers to the individuals responsible for managing healthcare data and information in paper or electronic form and controlling its collection, access, use, exchange, and protection through the application of health information technology

Health information: The data generated and collected as a result of delivering care to a patient

Health information exchange (HIE): Electronic movement of health-related information among organizations within a region or community that facilitates access to and retrieval of clinical data in support of safe, timely, efficient, and effective patient-centered care; an organization or entity that forms to create an electronic framework to connect physicians to pharmacies, hospitals, and other healthcare entities

Health information handler (HIH): Organization or entity that handles information on behalf of a provider

Health information management (HIM) department: Healthcare facility department responsible for the management and safeguarding of information in paper and electronic form

Health Information Management Systems Society (HIMSS): A national membership association that provides leadership in healthcare for the management of technology, information, and change

Health Information Organization (HIO): An organization that oversees and governs the exchange of health-related information among organizations according to nationally recognized standards

Health Information Security and Privacy Collaboration (HISPC): An organization for exchanging ideas and developing solutions to promote interoperability

Health information technology (HIT): The technical aspects of processing health data and records, including classification and coding, abstracting, registry development, storage, and so on

Health Information Technology for Economic and Clinical Health (HITECH) Act: Federal legislation that was passed as a portion of the American Recovery and Reinvestment Act; contains changes to the HIPAA Privacy Rule

Health Insurance Portability and Accountability Act of 1996 (HIPAA): A law enacted by Congress on August 21, 1996, governing various aspects of health information; federal legislation enacted to provide continuity of health coverage, control fraud and abuse in healthcare, reduce healthcare costs, and guarantee the security and privacy of health information

Health Level 7 (HL7): An international organization of healthcare professionals dedicated to creating standards for the exchange, management, and integration of electronic information

Health Privacy Project: A nonprofit organization whose mission is to raise public awareness of the importance of ensuring health privacy in order to improve healthcare access and quality

Health record: Individually identifiable data, in any medium, that are collected, processed, stored, displayed, and used by healthcare professionals; documents the care rendered to the patient and the patient's healthcare status

Healthcare Information Technology Standards Panel (HITSP): An organization developed under the auspices of the American National Standards Institute (ANSI) to deal with the many issues of privacy and security as the United States Nationwide Health Information Network develops

Healthcare Integrity and Protection Data Bank (HIPDB): A database maintained by the federal government to provide information on fraud-and-abuse findings against US healthcare providers

Health literacy: Degree of capacity that an individual has to not only read health information, but to "obtain, process, and understand basic health information and services needed to make appropriate health decisions"

Health Plan Report Card: A website that provides information on hundreds of health plans

Hearsay: A written or oral statement made outside of court that is offered in court as evidence

HHS: *See* **Department of Health and Human Services**

HIE: *See* **Health information exchange**

Highly sensitive health information: Certain types of patient information that require special handling in regard to access, requests, uses, and disclosures due to the nature of the information

HIH: *See* **Health information handler**

HIIM: *See* **Health informatics and information management**

Hill-Burton Act: A 1946 act that provided hospitals and certain other healthcare facilities money for construction and modernization as long as the facilities agreed to provide a reasonable volume of services to those unable to pay and to make their services available to all persons residing in the area of the facility

HIM: *See* **Health information management (HIM) department**

HIMSS: *See* **Health Information Management Systems Society**

HIO: *See* **Health Information Organization**

HIPAA: *See* **Health Insurance Portability and Accountability Act of 1996**

HIPAA Privacy Rule: Federal regulations created to implement the privacy requirements within the administrative simplification subtitle of the Health Insurance Portability and Accountability Act of 1996 and safeguard identifiable health information

HIPAA Security Rule: Federal regulations created to implement the security requirements within the administrative simplification subtitle of the Health Insurance Portability and Accountability Act of 1996

HISPC: *See* **Health Information Security and Privacy Collaboration**

Histocompatibility: Compatibility of donor and recipient tissues

History: Pertinent information about a patient, including chief complaint, past and present illnesses, family history, social history, and review of body systems

HITSP: *See* **Healthcare Information Technology Standards Panel**

HIV: *See* **Human immunodeficiency virus**

HL7: *See* **Health Level 7**

Hold harmless/indemnification clause: Contract clause that either transfers liability or establishes the assumption of liability by a particular party to the contract

Homeland Security Act: A 2002 act with the goal of preventing terrorist attacks in the United States while reducing the vulnerability of terrorism, minimizing its damages, and assisting in recovery from attacks in the United States; gives government authorities the right to access information needed to investigate and deter terrorism

Horizontal restraint of trade: Situation in which competitors agree to fix prices, divide the market, and attempt to exclude others from competing in the same market

Hospice care: Palliative care provided to terminally ill patients, often in their home or residential living facility

House staff: A physician in training who is continuing his or her medical education in a residency program and working with specialists to obtain higher-level skills and experience treating patients

Human Genome Project: A multiyear project that ended in 2003 in which all human DNA was identified and mapped

Human immunodeficiency virus (HIV): The virus that causes acquired immunodeficiency syndrome (AIDS)

Hung jury: A verdict where neither a conviction nor an acquittal is achieved

Hybrid entity: An entity that performs both covered and noncovered functions under the Privacy Rule; for example, a university that educates students and maintains student educational records is not covered by the Privacy Rule. However, the same university that operates a medical center is covered by the Privacy Rule, as it meets the definition of "healthcare provider."

Hybrid health record: A health record that uses a combination of paper and electronic formats

I

Identity and access management (IAM): The security discipline that enables the right individuals to access the right resources at the right times for the right reason

Identity theft: A crime in which an individual's personal information is stolen, often through the ease of obtaining data in electronic environments

I'm Sorry Laws: *See* **Apology Statutes**

Immigration Reform and Control Act of 1986: A law that requires employers to ensure that employees hired are legally authorized to work in the United States

Immunity: A defense to tort liability that is extended to a particular group of persons or entities

Immunization registry: Registries implemented in many states as a way to collect and maintain vaccination records on children—and in some cases, adults—in an effort to promote disease prevention and control

Implant registries: Database for tracking the performance of implants, including complications, deaths, and defects resulting from implants, as well as implant longevity

Implied consent: Consent for medical treatment that is communicated through a person's conduct or some other means besides words

Improper payment: has been defined by the federal government as any payment that should not have been made or that was made in an incorrect amount (including overpayments and underpayments) under statutory, contractual, administrative, or other legally applicable requirements

In camera inspection: A form of inspection in which the judge personally reviews disputed records in his or her chambers and decides whether the records are discoverable or admissible in the case

Inactive records: Records that are not used often, generally because patient encounters have ceased due to death or other factors, but must be retained either as a reference or because they have not reached the required retention period

Incidence: New cases of a particular disease or condition in a particular population

Incident report: The means through which occurrences that are inconsistent with a healthcare facility's routine patient care practices or operations are documented

Incident reporting: A process for identifying and responding to adverse events and other occurrences that are inconsistent with the standard of care

Incidental uses and disclosures: Occur as part of a permitted use or disclosure and are a component of doing business

Incidents: Patient safety events that reached the patient, whether or not there was harm involved

Incompetent adult: An individual who is at or above the age of majority and becomes incapacitated due to illness or injury, either permanently or temporarily; another person should be designated to make decisions for that individual, including decisions about the use and disclosure of the individual's protected health information

Indemnification clause: *See* **Hold harmless**

Individual: According to the HIPAA Privacy Rule, a person who is the subject of protected health information

Infliction of emotional distress: A common law tort for intentional conduct that results in extreme emotional distress, such as sleeplessness, anxiety, irritability, or the emotional inability to perform activities or go places that the plaintiff was capable of prior to the event

Information governance: Strategic management of enterprise electronic information, including the standards, policies, and procedures for access, use, and control of that information

Information system (IS): An automated system that uses computer hardware and software to record, manipulate, store, recover, and disseminate data (that is, a system that receives and processes input and provides output); often used interchangeably with "information technology"

Informative relationship: Characterized by the provider who dispenses information, but the patient who makes the decisions

Informed consent: A type of consent in which the patient should have a basic understanding of which medical procedures or tests may be performed as well as the risks, benefits, and alternatives for those tests or procedures

Initials: An authentication method for paper health records that may be permitted in lieu of a full signature as long as the initials are readily identifiable as the author's through a signature legend on the same document

Injunction: Court order where one party to a contract is ordered to do or stop doing something in order to prevent irreparable harm to the other party

Injury: Physical and/or mental suffering

Inpatient: A currently hospitalized patient

Institute for Healthcare Improvement (IHI): A quality and safety improvement group

Institute of Medicine (IOM): A branch of the National Academy of Sciences whose goal is to advance and distribute scientific knowledge with the mission of improving human health

Institutional review board (IRB): A committee of at least five members with varying backgrounds that determines the acceptability of proposed human subjects research in accordance with institutional policies, applicable law, and standards of professional practice and conduct

Integrated health record: A system of health record organization in which all paper forms are arranged in strict chronological order and forms created by different departments are intermixed

Integrity: The state of being whole or unimpaired

Intentional threats: Attacks from outside the network or internal malicious actions by workforce members

Intentional torts: Torts that involve a deliberate or intentional act

Internal security threat: A security threat caused by individuals or forces within an organization

Interoperability: The ability of different information systems and software applications to communicate and exchange data

Interpretive relationship: The provider supplies information to the patient, but only after knowing the patient's wishes, such as what is important to the patient and what his or her concerns are, resulting in shared decision making

Interrogatories: Discovery devices consisting of written questions given to a party, witness, or other person who has information needed in a legal case

Invasion of privacy: A form of tort based on the violation of a person's right to privacy

In vitro fertilization: The act of fertilization outside of the body

Involuntary civil commitment: Institutionalizing individuals against their wishes, such as when a provider admits a patient or prevents discharge if the patient is deemed a danger to self or others

IOM: *See* **Institute of Medicine**

IRB: *See* **Institutional review board**

IS: *See* **Information system**

J

Joinder: Action by a defendant to bring in ("join") an outsider as a codefendant

Joint and several liability: A principle that allows each defendant in a legal action to be held responsible for the entire amount of damages that a plaintiff is awarded, regardless of the defendant's degree of fault

The Joint Commission: An agency that develops standards for healthcare organizations and certifies healthcare organizations on the basis of adherence to those standards

Joint ventures: Partnerships created for a specific purpose and designed to have a limited lifespan

Judge: The person who presides over a trial and the courtroom and who makes critical decisions regarding the admissibility of evidence, which will guide the outcome of a case; in a trial without a jury, the judge also serves as the fact-finder

Judge-made law: *See* **Common law**

Judgment lien: A method of collecting judgment in which a defendant's property is encumbered and the debtor-defendant is prevented from taking any money from its sale until the judgment owed to the plaintiff has first been paid

Judicial branch: The branch of government responsible for interpreting the law and adjudicating disputes, thus creating common law

Judicial law: The body of law created as a result of court (judicial) decisions

Judicial search warrant: A judge's written order authorizing a law enforcement officer to conduct a search of a specified place and to seize evidence

Jurisdiction: The legal authority that a body possesses to make decisions

Jury: The fact-finding body that hears evidence given by the parties, if they testify, and other witnesses; observes evidence presented by both sides; hears the opening statements and closing arguments of each side; and decides facts based on the perceived credibility of the evidence, but does not decide law

Jury instructions: The legal instructions given to the jury by the judge

Justice: The impartial administration of policies or laws that takes into consideration the competing interests and limited resources of the individuals or groups involved

K

Knowing standard: A method of determining Federal Claims Act liability, requiring that the provider must have knowingly submitted the false claim

L

Labor-Management Relations Act of 1947: A law that amended the Wagner Act to prohibit unfair labor practices on the part of unions and allows the president to stop strikes in cases of national health and safety

Late entry: An addition to the health record in which a pertinent entry was missed or was not written in a timely manner

Law: Set of governing rules designed to protect citizens living in a civilized society, establish order, provide parameters for conduct, and define the rights and obligations of the government and its citizens

Lay witness: An individual's testifying based on his or her own observations of the situation(s) that prompted the case at hand

LCD: *See* **Local Coverage Decisions**

Leapfrog Group: A voluntary program founded in 2000 that is composed of a consortium of major companies and other entities that are responsible for purchasing health care coverage for employees; the program encourages the public to report outcomes and runs a Hospital Rewards program to reward providers for improving quality, safety, and affordability

Learned intermediary: A defense doctrine used most often by pharmaceutical companies and medical device manufacturers that says companies have a duty to warn physicians directly about potential adverse effects caused by their products; in doing so, the physician (or other user of the product) becomes a "learned intermediary" who interprets the information and advises patients appropriately

Legal guardian: Individual designated by the court system to assume legal responsibility for another individual

Legal health record (LHR): The form of a health record that is the legal business record of the organization and serves as evidence in lawsuits or other legal actions; what constitutes an organization's legal health record varies depending on how the organization defines it

Legal hold: A court order that suspends the processing or destruction of paper or electronic records; also known as a preservation order, preservation notice, or litigation hold

Legibility: An aspect of the quality of provider entries; if an entry cannot be read, it must be assumed that it cannot be used or was not used in the patient care process

Legislative branch: The branch of government charged with enacting laws in the form of statutes through the Senate and the House of Representatives

LEP: *See* **Limited English proficiency**

LHR: *See* **Legal health record**

Liability: 1. A legal obligation or responsibility that may have financial repercussions if not fulfilled; 2. An amount owed by an individual or organization to another individual or organization

Libel: Defamation in a written form

Licensed independent practitioner (LIP): Professionals such as physician assistants or nurse practitioners who are allowed by state laws and licensing regulations to practice without direction of a physician

Licensure: The legal authority or formal permission from authorities to carry on certain activities that by law or regulation require such permission (applicable to institutions as well as individuals)

Limited data set: Protected health information that excludes direct identifiers of the individual and the individual's relatives, employers, or household members but still does not deidentify the information

Limited English proficiency (LEP): Limited English speaking skills as identified in Title VI of the Civil Rights Act

Limited jurisdiction: Refers to courts that hear cases pertaining to a particular subject matter (for example, landlord-tenant or juvenile cases), that involve crimes of lesser severity (for example, misdemeanors), or involve civil matters of lesser dollar amounts

LIP: *See* **Licensed independent practitioner**

Litigation: The legal proceedings that accompany a lawsuit

Litigation trigger: Untoward event or events and organization identifies that they feel may lead to litigation

Living will: A document executed by a competent adult that expresses that individual's wishes to limit treatment measures when specific health-related diagnoses or conditions exist

Local Coverage Decisions (LCD): Medicare coverage restrictions at the state level

Local Coverage Determination (LCD): New format for LMRPs: Coverage rules, at a fiscal intermediary (FI) or carrier level, that provide information on what diagnoses justify the medical necessity of a test; LCDs vary from state to state

Locum tenens: When a healthcare practitioner or individual fills in for another for a given length of time

Long form consent: In the context of human subjects research, a consent form that includes all of the informed consent requirements included in the Common Rule

M

Malicious software: Software whose purpose is to harm or destroy legitimate software

Malfeasance: A wrong or improper act

Malpractice: The misconduct of professional persons, including healthcare providers, attorneys, accountants, and others

Marketing: Communication about a product or service that encourages the recipient to purchase or use that product or service

Master patient index (MPI): A patient-identifying directory that serves as a link to the patient record or information, facilitates patient identification, and assists in maintaining a longitudinal patient record from birth to death

Meaningful Use (MU): A requirement per the American Recovery and Reinvestment Act for healthcare providers to receive Medicare and Medicaid incentive payments; emphasizes collection of electronic data in the electronic health record (EHR) and subsequent use of EHR functionalities for tracking, reporting, and patient-care purposes

Mediation: A form of alternative dispute resolution in which a dispute is submitted to a third party and the outcome is decided by agreement of the parties

Medical device: Anything that is used in treatment or diagnosis that is not a drug such as an instrument, apparatus, or other article that is used to prevent, diagnose, mitigate, or treat a disease or to affect the structure or function of the body, with the exception of drugs

Medical device reporting: The Food and Drug Administration (FDA) requires that deaths and severe complications thought to be due to a device must be reported to the FDA and the manufacturer

Medical emergency: Severe injury or illness (including pain); definition depends on healthcare insurer

Medical ethics: A specific type of applied ethics that draws upon moral principles and applies those to relevant scenarios or situations in the delivery of healthcare

Medical examiner: Typically a physician with pathology training given the responsibility by a government, such as a county or state, for investigating suspicious deaths

Medical identity theft: A type of identity theft and financial fraud that involves the inappropriate or unauthorized misrepresentation of one's identity to obtain medical goods or services, or to obtain money by falsifying claims for medical services

Medical malpractice: A type of action in which the plaintiff must demonstrate that a physician–patient, nurse–patient, therapist–patient, or other healthcare provider–patient relationship existed at the time of the alleged wrongful act

Medical malpractice insurance: Insurance that protects a party from claims of medical negligence or other tortious injury arising out of care provided to patients

Medical necessity: As defined by Medicare, "services or supplies that are needed for the diagnosis or treatment of your medical condition, meet the standards of good medical practice in the local area, and aren't mainly for the convenience of you or your doctor" (Medicare.gov/Glossary)

Medical plagiarism: Using information without the original author's knowledge or permission

Medical screening exam (MSE): An evaluation of a patient's health condition

Medical staff: The staff members of a healthcare organization who are governed by medical staff bylaws; may or may not be employed by the healthcare organization

Medical staff bylaws: Standards governing the practice of medical staff members that are typically voted on by the organized medical staff and the medical staff executive committee and then approved by the facility's board; medical staff members must abide by these bylaws in order to continue practicing in the healthcare facility

Medical staff executive committee: A body composed of those elected representative members of the medical staff who are authorized to act on behalf of the medical staff

Medicare: A program that provides healthcare services to qualified individuals

Medicare Administrative Contractors: private health insurers that have been awarded a geographic jurisdiction to process Medicare Parts A and B medical claims and Durable Medical Equipment claims for Medicare Fee-for-Service beneficiaries

Medicare and Medicaid Patient and Program Protection Act: A 1987 act that expanded information contained in the NPDS

Medicaid Integrity Contractors: CMS contractors responsible for detecting and deterring fraud and abuse in the Medicaid program, including the review of Medicaid provider activities, auditing claims, identifying overpayments, and providing education on Medicaid program integrity issues

MedWatch: *See* **Safety Information and Adverse Event Reporting Program**

Mental examination: A discovery method in which an individual may request an independent mental examination, particularly if the mental condition of an individual is in question

Metadata: Data about data; generally refers to information about an electronic data element's content, including means of creation, purpose, time and date of creation, author, revisions, placement on a network, and standards used

Minimum necessary: A "need to know" filter that is applied to limit access to a patient's PHI and to limit the amount of PHI used, disclosed, and requested

Minor: An individual who is under the age of majority (usually 18 years of age) who has not been legally emancipated (declared an adult) by the court

Misdemeanor: A crime that is less serious than a felony and is generally punishable by a fine or imprisonment other than in a penitentiary

Misfeasance: Relating to negligence or improper performance during an otherwise correct act

Mitigation: Required by the Privacy Rule (45 CFR 164.530(f)), the lessening as much as possible of harmful effects that result from the wrongful use and disclosure of protected health information; possible courses of action may include an apology, disciplinary action against the responsible employee or employees (although such results will not be able to be shared with the wronged individual), repair of the process that resulted in the breach, payment of a bill or financial loss that resulted from the infraction, or gestures of goodwill and good public relations (such as a gift certificate) that may assuage the individual

Morals: An individual's code relating to what is right or wrong in human behavior

Moral values: Principles formed through the influence of family, culture, religion, and society

Motion to quash: A document filed with the court that asks the judge to nullify a subpoena

MPI: *See* **Master patient index**

N

National Alliance for Health Information Technology (NAHIT): A partnership of government and private sector leaders from various healthcare organizations that worked toward using technology to achieve improvements in patient safety, quality of care, and operating performance; founded in 2002; ceased operations in 2009

National Association of Medical Staff Services: Recommends 13 criteria for review that should be included in the medical staff bylaws, rules and regulations and other governance documents. The credentialing review should also detect professional incompetence, malevolence, behavioral problems, and other red flags

National Benefit Integrity Medicare Drug Integrity Contractor: CMS contractor responsible for detecting and preventing fraud, waste, and abuse in the Medicare Part C (Medicare Advantage) and Part D (Prescription Drug Coverage) program on a national level

National Cardiovascular Data Registry: A database supported by Medicare and maintained by the American College of Cardiologists that requires hospitals that are reimbursed by Medicare for implantable cardiac defibrillators to submit data on patients who receive implants to the registry

National Instant Criminal Background Check System (NICS): Federal Bureau of Investigation's national criminal database that is populated by information from state law enforcement agencies and certain covered entities that report limited information on individuals who have been involuntarily committed to a mental institution or otherwise have been determined by a lawful authority to be a danger to themselves or others

National Committee for Quality Assurance (NCQA): An organization with credentialing standards that requires verification from the primary source of information on the medical staff application; accredits managed care organizations

National Committee on Vital and Health Statistics (NCVHS): An advisory group to Congress and the Department of Health and Human Services regarding health policy

National Coverage Decisions: Medicare coverage restrictions at the national level

National Coverage Determination (NCD): An NCD sets forth the extent to which Medicare will cover specific services, procedures, or technologies on a national basis. Medicare contractors are required to follow NCDs

National Human Genome Research Institute: A division of the National Institutes of Health that discusses the issues and questions around the Human Genome Project and how the information and technology will affect standards of patient care

National Labor Relations Act of 1935 (Wagner Act): A law that established conditions for collective bargaining, listed unfair labor practices, and created the National Labor Relations Board (NLRB) to oversee union elections and handle situations of unfair labor practices; also known as the Wagner Act

National Labor Relations Board (NLRB): An organization that governs the activities between employers and unions and assumed jurisdiction over hospitals in 1974

National Patient Safety Goals: A set of goals published each year by the Joint Commission and designed to improve patient safety in specific healthcare areas identified as problematic by the Sentinel Event Advisory Group

National Practitioner Data Bank (NPDB): A data bank created by the 1986 Health Care Quality Improvement Act that collects malpractice, disciplinary, and credentialing information on physicians, dentists, and other facility-based practitioners

National Quality Strategy: A strategy that has three aims and six priorities that have guided HHS, CMS, and AHRQ program development related to improving the delivery of healthcare services, patient outcomes, and overall population health

National Regulatory Commission: A body that has oversight responsibility for the medical use of ionizing radiation and to which medical events must be reported

National Research Act of 1974: An act that required the Department of Health, Education, and Welfare (now the Department of Health and Human Services) to codify its policy for the protection of human subjects into federal regulations and created a commission that generated the Belmont Report

Nationwide Health Information Network (NHIN): A term that refers to the building blocks or foundation for interoperability; the physical and national network components that make electronic health records interoperable

NCQA: *See* **National Committee for Quality Assurance**

NCVHS: *See* **National Committee on Vital and Health Statistics**

Near misses (or close calls): Patient safety events that did not reach the patient

Negligence: A type of tort in which the defendant does not necessarily intend to cause harm but harm is a foreseeable consequence of his or her conduct

Next-of-kin: An individual who, by virtue of his or her relationship to the patient (such as a spouse, adult child, parent, or adult sibling), may make healthcare decisions on the patient's behalf

NHIN: *See* **Nationwide Health Information Network**

NLRB: *See* **National Labor Relations Board**

No-fault insurance: A term used to describe any type of insurance contract under which insured individuals are indemnified for losses by their own insurance company, regardless of fault in the incident generating losses

Nominal damages: Damages awarded simply to recognize wrongdoing by the defendant when there is no substantial injury suffered by the plaintiff that necessitates compensation or the plaintiff has failed to demonstrate a dollar amount

Noncompete agreement: A contract provision in which an employee or contractor agrees not to compete directly or work for a competitor for a certain period of time after leaving his or her employment or contracting position

Non compos mentis: Not of sound mind

Noncustodial parent: A parent who does not have custody of a child or children as designated by the court system in cases of divorce or legal separation

Nondisclosure agreement: An agreement relating to the confidentiality and privacy of patient information that employees may be required to sign as a condition of employment

Noneconomic damages: Damages that are not monetary in nature; an issue targeted by tort reforms

Nonexempt employee: An employee for whom overtime and minimum wage regulations do apply; nonexempt employees must be paid at least the minimum wage up to 40 hours and time and a half for any hours worked over 40

Nonfeasance: A type of negligence meaning failure to act

Nonmaleficence: A legal principle that means "first do no harm"

Nonrepudiation: The claim that guarantees that the source of the health record documentation cannot deny later that he or she was the author.

Not-for-profit corporation: A corporation that may not distribute its income for the private gain of individuals

Not-for-profit organization: An organization that is not owned by individuals whose profits are retained by the organization and reinvested back into the organization for the benefit of the community it serves

Notice of Privacy Practices (NPP): A statement (mandated by the HIPAA Privacy Rule) issued by a healthcare organization that informs individuals of the uses and disclosures of patient-identifiable health information that may be made by the organization, as well as the individual's rights and the organization's legal duties with respect to that information

Notifiable diseases: Communicable diseases that must be reported to the state for the purpose of tracking outbreaks and preventing spread of the disease

NPDB: *See* **National Practitioner Data Bank**

O

Occupational Safety and Health Administration (OSHA): Federal Occupational Safety and Health Administration (OSHA) regulations ensure that an employee (or designated representative) is given access to his or her own medical and exposure records within 15 days of a request

Occupational safety and health record: As part of employment, a record kept on an employee that contains any and all information related to such items as medical tests, drug tests, examinations, physical abilities, immunizations, screenings required by law, biohazardous exposure, and physical limitations

Occurrence screening: A method for identifying risk through health record review according to objective screening criteria

OCR: *See* **Office for Civil Rights**

Offer: A communicated promise by a party to a contract to either do or not do something if the other party agrees to do or not do something

Office for Civil Rights (OCR): An office within the Department of Health and Human Services (HHS) that is responsible for enforcing civil rights laws that prohibit discrimination on the basis of race, color, national origin, disability, age, sex, and religion by healthcare and human services entities over which the Office for Civil Rights (OCR) has jurisdiction, such as state and local social and health services agencies, hospitals, clinics, nursing homes, or other entities receiving federal financial assistance from HHS; this office also has the authority to investigate alleged violations of the HIPAA Privacy Rule

Office of Inspector General (OIG): Branch of the Department of Health and Human Services (HHS) with responsibility for audits, investigations, inspections, and other activities to protect the integrity of HHS programs and their beneficiaries

Office of the National Coordinator for Health Information Technology (ONC): An office created in 2004 by the federal government to "provide leadership for the development and nationwide implementation of an interoperable health information technology infrastructure to improve the quality and efficiency of health care and the ability of consumers to manage their care and safety" (Office of the Secretary for HHS 2005)

OHCA: *See* **Organized Healthcare Arrangement**

OIG: *See* **Office of Inspector General**

ONC: *See* **Office of the National Coordinator for Health Information Technology**

Ongoing professional practice review: Documenting data on credentialed staff on an ongoing basis rather than at the two-year reappointment process

Open records laws: Laws that define what information is subject to public disclosure and are used to deny Freedom of Information Act (FOIA) requests that include protected health information; also known as public records, sunshine law, or freedom of information laws

Opening statement: The beginning of a trial in which each side outlines the evidence that will be heard

Opinion: A court's written determination that outlines the facts of the case and the legal theories followed in reaching an outcome

Oral argument: The form of argument used, instead of a trial, in appellate courts, state supreme courts, US circuit courts, and the US Supreme Court

Ordinary negligence: Failure to exercise ordinary care under same or similar circumstances

Organ Procurement and Transplantation Network (OPTN): Facilitates patient and donor organ matching opportunities

Organ procurement organization: Nonprofit organizations who are responsible for the evaluation and procurement of donor organs for organ transplantation

Organized healthcare arrangement (OHCA): An agreement characterized by two or more covered entities that share protected health information to manage and benefit their common enterprise and are recognized by the public as a single entity (HHS 2003)

OSHA: *See* **Occupational Safety and Health Administration**

Outpatient: A patient currently being seen in an ambulatory care, clinic, or physician setting who is not admitted to a hospital as an inpatient

Overcoding: Billing for services at a level of complexity that is higher than the service actually provided or documented (also see Upcoding)

Owner: An individual who owns shares or stock in a corporation or company

Ownership: In healthcare, the person to whom the health record belongs (traditionally, the healthcare provider)

P

Partial/modified comparative negligence: Allows a plaintiff to recover only if the plaintiff's negligence is "not greater than" or "not as great as" the defendant's negligence

Parties: In a lawsuit, the plaintiff and the defendant, accompanied by their respective attorneys unless they are providing legal representation for themselves

Partnership: A legal business entity in which two or more parties agree to share the risk and rewards of the entity

Password: A sequence of characters used to verify that a computer user requesting access to a system is actually that particular user

Paternalism: A medical professional's opinion on how the patient should act that often threatens to supersede a patient's autonomy

Paternalistic relationship: Where the provider is the medical authority and the patient is the passive recipient

Patient Care Partnership (patient rights): A group developed by the American Hospital Association that helps patients understand their expectations, rights, and responsibilities when receiving hospital services

Patient-centered care: Care that is "respectful of and responsive to individual patient preferences, needs, and values and ensuring that patient values guide all clinical decisions" (Institute of Medicine. 2000.)

Patient matching: Accurately connecting a patient to his or her medical information

Patient portals: Provider-hosted "secure websites where patients can access their medical history and often certain information from their EHR"

Patient Protection and Affordable Care Act (PPACA): A federal statute that was signed into law on March 23, 2010. Along with the Health Care and Education Reconciliation Act of 2010 (signed into law on March 30, 2010), the act is the product of the healthcare reform agenda of the Democratic 111th Congress and the Obama administration

Patient rights: *See* **Patient Care Partnership**

Patient Safety: Refers to making patient care continually safer by reducing harm and preventable mortality

Patient Safety and Quality Improvement Act of 2005: A law intended to improve patient safety by encouraging clinicians and hospitals to voluntarily report their confidential quality and patient safety data on events that adversely affected patients

Patient Safety Organizations (PSOs): Public and private data organizations that collect, analyze, and aggregate patient safety data at the local, regional, national levels

Patient safety work product: Any data, reports, records or written or oral material developed by the provider or the PSO for patient safety purpose

Patient Self-Determination Act: A law that became effective in 1991 requiring healthcare institutions that bill Medicare or Medicaid for services to provide adult patients with information about the various types of advance directives

Patriot Act: A 2001 law enacted to deter and punish terrorist acts in the United States and around the world and to enhance law enforcement investigations; gives government authorities the right to access information needed to investigate and deter terrorism

Pay for performance: Programs that reward quality and safety in hospitals and by providers in an attempt to align quality and outcomes with payment

Peer review: A broad range of activities undertaken by a peer review committee to ensure that a facility provides quality care, which may include such activities as the review of quality and safety issues and determinations of medical staff credentials

Peer Review Organizations (PROs): Conduct utilization review of hospital services and review of medical necessity of care

Per se antitrust violation: Activities that are automatically considered to be antitrust violations

Peremptory challenge: A process through which attorneys may excuse jurors for unstated reasons

Personal health record (PHR): An electronic or paper health record maintained and updated by an individual for himself or herself

Personal identification number (PIN): A private electronic password or code

Personal representative: A person with legal authority to act on behalf of another individual and who is treated the same as the individual regarding the use and disclosure of the individual's protected health information

Person or entity authentication: Requires the implementation of procedures to verify that a person or entity seeking access to ePHI is the person or entity they claim to be

Persuasive authority: The principle by which courts that are not bound by precedent to follow one another may nonetheless look to one another's decisions for guidance

Petition for writ of certiorari: The process by which a party submits a request for the Supreme Court to hear a case

Petitioner: The party appealing a case, also known as the appellant

PGP: *See* **Pretty good privacy**

PHI: *See* **Protected health information**

Phishing: When someone impersonates a business or other known entity to attempt to have the user provide personal information

PHR: *See* **Personal health record**

Physical examination: A discovery method in which a party may request an independent physical examination, particularly if the physical or mental condition of a party is in question; for example, a defendant may request that a physical examination be performed on the plaintiff in a personal injury lawsuit if the nature and extent of the injuries being claimed are in question

Physical safeguards: A set of four standards defined by the HIPAA Security Rule: facility access controls, workstation use, workstation security, and device and media controls

Physician order(s): A type of documentation within the health record that provides mandatory instructions regarding medical interventions such as treatments, ancillary medical services, tests and procedures, medications, or seclusion and restraint

Physician–patient privilege: The legal protection from confidential communications between physicians and patients related to diagnosis and treatment being disclosed during civil and some misdemeanor litigation

Piercing the corporate veil: An exception to corporate immunity in which the owners of a corporation may be liable for particularly bad acts such as fraud or crime

PIN: *See* **Personal identification number**

PKI: *See* **Public key infrastructure**

PL: *See* **Public law**

Plaintiff: The individual who initiates a lawsuit to enforce either his or her rights or another's obligations

Pleadings: Limited documents that emanate from parties involved in a lawsuit, such as complaints and answers, and are central to the litigation process

Power of attorney: A legal instrument used by a principal (person) to grant legal authority to one or more agents to make certain legal and financial decisions on behalf of the principal

Precedent: A legal doctrine stating that local courts within a court system are bound to follow (apply) the decisions of higher courts in the same court system in order to determine the outcome of a case, as long as the fact pattern of the case in the higher court is similar to that of the current case; also known as *stare decisis*

Preemption: A legal doctrine that requires a covered entity to comply with federal law when federal and state law conflict (that is, federal law preempts contrary state law)

Pregnancy Discrimination Act of 1973: An expansion of Title VII of the Civil Rights Act that requires that pregnancy and related conditions be handled like any other medical condition

Preponderance of evidence: Evidence proving it is "more likely than not" that each element of the case was met and that the defendant committed the alleged wrongdoing

Prescription drug monitoring program: A program implemented by most states in an effort to identify inappropriate and illegal activities involving controlled prescription drugs

Pretrial conference: A meeting between the parties, their attorneys, and the court in which the upcoming trial and potential settlement negotiations are discussed

Pretty good privacy (PGP): A type of encryption software that uses public key cryptology and digital signatures for authentication

Primary data source (in healthcare): A record developed by healthcare professionals in the process of providing patient care

Primary source verification: Verification of healthcare practitioners' (physician) credentials as part of the credentialing process for medical staff privileges

Principal: Individual who signs a power of attorney giving an agent (person designated by the principal) to make certain decisions for the principal.

Privacy: The quality or state of being hidden from, or undisturbed by, the observation or activities of other people or freedom from unauthorized intrusion; in healthcare-related contexts, the right of a patient to control disclosure of personal information

Privacy Act of 1974: A law that requires federal agencies to safeguard personally identifiable records and provides individuals with certain privacy rights

Privacy and Security Solutions for Interoperable Health Information Exchange Project: A project sponsored by the Agency for Healthcare Research and Quality "to assess variations in organization-level business practices, policies, and state laws that affect electronic health information exchange and to identify and propose practical ways to reduce the variation to those 'good' practices that will permit interoperability while preserving the necessary privacy and security requirements set by the local community" (Dimitropoulos 2007, ES-7)

Privacy board: A group formed by a HIPAA-covered entity to review research studies in which authorization waivers are requested and to ensure the HIPAA privacy rights of research subjects

Privacy officer: A position mandated under the HIPAA Privacy Rule—covered entities must designate an individual to be responsible for developing and implementing privacy policies and procedures

Privacy Rule: *See* **Health Insurance Portability and Accountability Act of 1996**

Private law: The branch of law concerned with the rules and principles that define rights and duties among people and among private businesses

Privilege: A concept that certain specified communications are secret and cannot be forcibly revealed except under special circumstances, for example protects confidential communications between provider and patient related to diagnosis and treatment from disclosure during civil and some criminal misdemeanor litigation

Privileged communication: Communication shared between two parties—such as physician and patient, clergy and parishioner, husband and wife, and attorney and client—that is considered privileged; may be defined by state law

Privilege statutes: Laws that legally protect confidential communications between a provider (e.g., physician, psychologists, marital therapist) and a patient from disclosure during civil and some criminal misdemeanor litigation

Pro se: In a lawsuit, an individual who represents himself or herself in lieu of having an attorney

Procedural due process: Applies due process to the federal and state governments; provides that the government shall not take a person's life, liberty, or property without due process of law; procedural due process intends fair processes and procedures

Procedural law: The court's rules that guide a lawsuit from the time it begins through completion, whether it culminates in a trial or ends with a settlement or dismissal

Procreation: The beginning of life

Production of documents: A discovery method initiated by a subpoena duces tecum, which requests that an individual bring documents or other records to court

Professional ethics: Codes that are designed to provide guidance about the ethical conduct of a profession

Professionalism: The conduct or qualities that characterize or mark a profession or a professional person

Professional Standards Review Organizations (PSROs): Ensure that hospital services for Medicare and Medicaid patients were medically necessary and appropriate

Program Safeguard Contractors: CMS program integrity contractors responsible for detecting fraud and abuse in Medicare Parts A and B prior to establishment of Zone Program Integrity Contractors

Protected health information (PHI): A term defined in the HIPAA Privacy Rule as "individually identifiable health information that is transmitted by electronic media, maintained in electronic medium, or transmitted or maintained in any other form or medium" (45 CFR 160.103)

Provider Self-Disclosure Protocol: A mechanism for providers to voluntarily disclose self-discovered evidence of potential fraud to the OIG. This protocol gives providers the opportunity to avoid the costs and disruptions associated with a Federal investigation and civil or administrative litigation

Proximate causation: An event sufficiently related to a legally recognizable injury so as to be held as the cause of that injury; an act that results in injury through a natural, direct, uninterrupted consequence and without which the injury would not have occurred

Psychotherapy notes: Behavioral health notes recorded by a mental health professional that document or analyze the content and impressions of conversations that are part of private counseling sessions; they are not part of the health record and do not contain information such as diagnosis, prescriptions, treatment modalities, and test results

Public key infrastructure (PKI): A key system with two keys, a private key and a public key

Public law (PubL): The branch of law concerned with the federal, state, or local government and its relationship to individuals and business organizations; the most familiar form of public law is criminal law

Public record laws: Laws that provide public disclosure upon request of any information of any public body in a state, except as otherwise exempt by state regulations

Punitive damages: Damages that exceed compensatory damages and serve to punish the defendant(s)

Pure comparative negligence: Permits a plaintiff to recover for the percentage of the defendant's negligence

Q

QIO: *See* **Quality improvement organization**

Qualified clinical data registry: An entity that collects clinical data and submits it to CMS on behalf of health care providers such as physicians or physician group practices who are voluntarily participating in the federally sponsored Physician Quality Reporting System (PQRS)

Quality: "Doing the right thing, at the right time, in the right way, for the right person—and having the best possible results" (AHRQ)

QualityCheck.org: The Joint Commission publishes hospital core performance measurement data on this website

Quality improvement: The overall processes a facility has in place to make sure healthcare is safe, effective, patient centered, timely, efficient, and equitable

Quality improvement organization (QIO): Community-based organization selected by the Centers for Medicare and Medicaid Services to conduct quality-related activities

Quality Innovation Network-Quality Improvement Organizations (QIN-QIOs): These groups work with providers, stakeholders, and Medicare beneficiaries to improve patient safety, reduce harm, engage patients and families, and improve clinical care at the local and regional levels

Qui tam relator: The "whistleblower" provisions of the False Claims Act provide that private persons, known as relators, may enforce the act by filing a complaint, under seal, alleging fraud committed against the government

R

Ransomware: Distinct from malware in that it attempts to deny access to a user's data, by encrypting the data with a key known only to the hacker. When the ransom is paid the user is given a decryption key which allows access to the user's data

RBAC: *See* **Role-based access control**

Reasonably prudent person: A hypothetical person that a community believes exhibits ideal behavior in a particular situation and can differ from one situation to another

Recovery Audit Contractors (RACs): Private organizations utilized by the Department of Health and Human Services to identify underpayments and overpayments associated with services paid under the Medicare program; RACs are paid a contingency fee based on the amount of overpayments and underpayments identified

Red Flags Rules: A provision under the Fair and Accurate Credit Transaction Act (FACTA) that requires financial institutions and creditors—including many healthcare organizations—to develop and implement written programs that identify, detect, and respond to red flags that may signal the presence of identity theft

Red flags: Suspicious documents, information, or behaviors that indicate the possibility of identity theft

Redisclosure: Disclosure by a healthcare organization of information that was created by and received from another entity

Regional Health Information Organization (RHIO): A health information organization that brings together healthcare stakeholders within a defined geographic area and governs health information exchange among them for the purpose of improving health and care in that community

Registry: A database including information about a particular disease or condition; more information is obtained for registries than is required for communicable diseases

Relator: Private persons who may enforce the False Claims Act by filing a complaint, under seal, alleging fraud committed against the government

Release of information (ROI): The act of making information known; the release of confidential health information about an identifiable person to another person or entity; release, transfer, provision of access to, or divulging in any other manner of information outside the entity holding the information (45 CFR 160.103) (*see also* **Disclosure**); the process of disclosing protected health information from the health record to another party

Referral: For Medicare Part B services means "the request by a physician for the item or service", for all other Medicare and Medicaid services, "the request or establishment of a plan of care by a physician which includes the provision of the designated health service" (42 USC 1395(h)(5)(A))

Relevant evidence: Evidence having a tendency to make the existence of any fact more probable or less probable

Remuneration: The transfer of anything of value, directly or indirectly, overtly or covertly, in cash or in kind such as kickbacks, bribes, and rebates.

Report cards: Comparative data about healthcare providers reported on websites such as healthgrades.com or by organizations such as the National Committee for Quality Assurance and Centers for Medicare and Medicaid Services

Request for admissions: A discovery method that asks the opposing party in litigation to admit to certain facts so the facts do not have to be proven

Request restrictions: Under the Privacy Rule, the right of an individual to request that a covered entity limit the uses and disclosures of protected health information to carry out treatment, payment, or healthcare operations

Requests: Ways in which access, use, and disclosure of patient information are made, which may include mail, telephone, physical presence of the requester, fax, or e-mail

Required specification: The implementation specifications of the HIPAA Security Rule that are designated "required" rather than "addressable"; required standards must be present for the covered entity to be in compliance

Res ipsa loquitur: Latin for "the thing speaks for itself"; an exception to the plaintiff having the burden of proof in which the facts or circumstances accompanying an injury may raise a presumption, or at least permit an inference, of negligence on the part of the defendant or some other individual who is charged with negligence and the burden of proof is shifted to the defendant

Res judicata: Latin for "a matter already judged"; a legal doctrine that bars litigation between the same parties on matters already determined in a former lawsuit

Rescue doctrine: Principle that if a tortfeasor creates a circumstance that places a victim in danger, the tortfeasor is liable not only for the harm caused to the victim but also for the harm caused to any person injured in an effort to rescue that victim

Resolution agreements: Settlements compelling an entity to perform obligations per the agreements (often including payments) and to submit reports to HHS for three years

Respondeat superior: Latin for "let the master answer"; the doctrine under which a hospital holds itself responsible for the actions of its employees provided those individuals were acting within the scope of their employment or at the hospital's direction at the time of the activity in question

Respondent: The party against whom a petition is filed on appeal

Restraint: A device or drug that restricts a patient's freedom of movement and is not related to diagnosis or treatment, protecting a patient from falling out of bed, or permitting a patient to participate in activities without the risk of harm

Restraints and seclusion: Ways of managing behavior; the right of patients to be free from non–medically necessary restraints and seclusion is protected under the Medicare Conditions of Participation

Retaliation and waiver: Rights protected under the Privacy Rule. To ensure the integrity of individuals' right to complain about alleged Privacy Rule violations, covered entities are expressly prohibited from retaliating against anyone who exercises his or her rights under the Privacy Rule, assists in an investigation by the Department of Health and Human Services or other appropriate investigative authority, or opposes an act or practice that he or she believes is a violation of the Privacy Rule; individuals cannot be required to waive the rights that they hold under the Privacy Rule in order to obtain treatment, payment, or eligibility for enrollment or benefits

Retention: A mechanism for storing records, providing for timely retrieval, and establishing the length of time that various types of records will be retained by the healthcare organization

Retention schedule: A timeline for records retention based on factors such as federal and state laws, statutes of limitations, age of patient, competency of patient, accreditation standards, AHIMA recommendations, and operational needs

Retraction: Appropriate deletion of information in an electronic environment

Retrieval: Quick location of requested records and information needed for patient care or other uses

Revenue cycle: The supervision of all administrative and clinical functions that contribute to the capture, management, and collection of patient service revenues

Revisions: Corrections or alterations to the health record

RHIO: *See* **Regional Health Information Organization**

Right-based ethics: A code based on the idea that every individual has certain rights

Risk analysis: The process of identifying which risks should be proactively addressed and which risks are lower in priority

Risk and opportunity identification: Refers to a systematic means of identifying potential risks. The process should include a review of adverse events, committee reports, root cause analysis, patient satisfaction surveys and various other tools

Risk control techniques: Prevent or reduce the chances or effects of a loss occurrence

Risk evaluation: The final step in the risk management process, which involves evaluating each piece of the process to determine whether objectives are being met

Risk exposure or identification: A systematic means of identifying potential losses that requires an understanding of the facility's business, legal, organizational, and clinical components

Risk financing: Methods used to pay for the costs associated with claims and other expenses—most commonly, liability insurance

Risk management: The processes in place to identify, evaluate, and control risk; defined as the organization's risk of accidental financial liability

Risk treatment: The application of risk control and risk financing techniques to determine how a risk should be treated, often aimed at preventing or reducing the chances or effects of a loss occurrence

ROI: *See* **Release of information**

Role-based access control (RBAC): A control system in which access decisions are based on the roles of individual users as part of an organization

Root cause analysis: A structured method of identifying the physical, human and/or organizational causes of an event, how the causes contributed to the event, and developing a process to prevent reoccurrence of the event.

Rubber signature stamp: A type of authentication for paper records; stamp must be used only by the person identified by the stamp in accordance with laws, standards, and regulations

Rule of reason analysis: Court determination of whether an antitrust violation exists; includes analysis of affected geographic markets, product or service involved, nature of the industry, motivation of the alleged illegal activity, and impact of the activity on the industry

S

Safe harbor exception: Activities designated by the Office of Inspector General as not subject to prosecution and protect the organization from civil or criminal penalties

Safe Harbor method: The removal of 18 specified identifiers about an individual or the individual's relatives, employers or household members to de-identify protected health information

Safe Medical Devices Act (SMDA): A federal program that requires reporting to the Food and Drug Administration (FDA) and the product manufacturer of the medical device any occurrences that have or may have contributed to serious illness, serious injury, or death

Safety Information and Adverse Event Reporting Program (MedWatch): The FDA's electronic system for reporting of adverse consequences relate to medical devices

SAMHSA: *See* **Substance Abuse and Mental Health Services Administration**

Scalability: The concept that based on the size of the CE, the threshold of compliance varies

Scribe: A person who documents in the health record for the provider

Search and retrieval fees: Fees to cover the costs associated with reviewing requests, or searching for and retrieving PHI (such as locating and reviewing the PHI in the record, and segregating and preparing the requested PHI)

Seclusion: "The involuntary confinement of a patient alone in a room or area from which the patient is physically prevented from leaving." It can only be used in response to violent or self-destructive behavior (42 CFR 482.13 2012.)

Secondary data: When data from a record are used for purposes other than what was intended

Secondary liability: A healthcare organization is liable to patients for the torts of its employees (including nurses and employed physicians) under the doctrine of *respondeat superior* (Latin for "let the master answer")

Secure date: Data that cannot be intercepted, copied, modified, or deleted while in transit or at rest in a file system (for example, on a disk or tape)

Security: 1. The means to control access and protect information from accidental or intentional disclosure to unauthorized persons and from unauthorized alteration, destruction, or loss; 2. The physical protection of facilities and equipment from theft, damage, or unauthorized access; collectively, the policies, procedures, and safeguards designed to protect the confidentiality of information, maintain the integrity and availability of information systems, and control access to the content of these systems

Security incident: An event in which the security of a system was breached or threatened

Security officer or chief security officer: An individual responsible for overseeing privacy policies and procedures

Sentinel event: An unexpected occurrence involving death or serious physical or psychological injury, or the risk thereof (Joint Commission 2006)

Separation of powers: Among the three branches of federal and state governments, the authority of each is limited in order to inhibit the ability of any one branch of government to become autocratic

Service: The means by which a defendant is notified of a lawsuit

Settlement: Determining the outcome of a legal case between the parties without pursuing the matter through to trial

Shadow record: A duplicate record kept for the convenience of the provider or facility; it usually is an exact duplicate of the original health record and should not contain documentation that is not in the original record

Shareholder (stockholder): A person who holds a share or shares of stock in a corporation or company

Sherman Antitrust Act: First passed in 1890, one of several antitrust laws that collectively make it illegal to restrain trade through contracts or conspiracies and prohibit price fixing and mergers that lessen competition, enforced by the Federal Trade Commission (FTC) and the Department of Justice (DOJ)

Short form consent: In the context of human subjects research, a written document stating that the elements of informed consent required by the Common Rule have been orally presented to and understood by the subject or the subject's legally authorized representative

Slander: Defamation in an oral form

SMDA: *See* **Safe Medical Devices Act**

Social media: A collection of online technologies and practices that people use to share opinions, insights, experiences, and perspectives; often used by healthcare organizations as marketing tools and mechanisms to communicate with consumers or patients

Social Security Administration (SSA): A division of the federal government that administers rehabilitation and disability services for people suffering from physical or mental disabilities that affect their ability to work or return to work in a timely manner

Sole proprietorship: A legal business entity in which a single owner elects not to insulate his or her personal assets through the use of a corporation or other legal form

Special damages: Arrive out of the special character, condition, or circumstances of the event or person injured

Special jurisdiction: A type of court in which particular areas of the law have been carved out for resolution (for example, small claims, domestic relations, juvenile, or probate courts)

Specific performance: A court order that requires the party that breached a contract to honor its contractual obligations

Spoliation: Intentional destruction, mutilation, alteration, or concealment of information relevant to a legal proceeding

SSA: *See* **Social Security Administration**

Stand-alone authorization: An authorization for the use or disclosure of one's protected health information that is separate from an informed consent for treatment or participation in a research study

Standalone PHR: Information provided by the patient and which is present either on paper, on the patient's computer or thumb drive, or in an Internet repository of the patient's choosing

Standard of care: What an individual is expected to do or not do in a particular situation, established by statute or ordinance, judicial decision, professional associations, or by practice; in healthcare professions, it is the exercise of reasonable care by healthcare professionals with similar training and experience in the same or similar communities

Stare decisis: Latin for "let the decision stand"; a legal doctrine stating that local courts within a court system are bound to follow (apply) the decisions of higher courts in the same court system in order to determine the outcome of a case, as long as the fact pattern of the case in the higher court is similar to that of the current case

Stark Law: *See* **Federal Physician Self-Referral Statute**

State action: When a private entity such as a hospital takes on the characteristics of a public organization; the private organization is then held to government standards such as due process

Statistical/mathematical algorithm: Assigns weights to data that nearly match, determining the probability that two records are those of the same patient

Statute of limitations: A statutory enactment that places time limits on certain claims

Statute of repose: Statute enacted to add new provisions, subject to certain exceptions, that provide a maximum amount of time within which to discover and file a claim; maximum or absolute limitations

Statutory law: Law based on statutes, which are created by the legislative branch of the government (the House of Representatives and the Senate)

Sterilization: Procedures that prevent conception by permanently altering the reproductive organs of the patient, thereby rendering them sterile

Steward: The person responsible for ensuring the integrity and security of electronic information and records (*see also* **Custodian of health records**)

Stewardship: Refers to responsibility for ensuring the integrity (accuracy, completeness, timeliness) and security (protection of privacy as well as protection from tampering, loss, or destruction) within the context of electronic information and records management

Strict liability: A theory under which a person is responsible for the damage and loss caused by his or her acts and omissions regardless of fault

Structured settlement: An arrangement by which the claim is paid in installments rather than in one lump sum settlement

Subject matter jurisdiction: A form of jurisdiction based on the content or substantive area of the case being brought

Subpoena: Legal order that commands an individual to give testimony or commands the production, inspection, copying, testing, or sampling of books, documents, electronically stored information, or tangible items

Subpoena ad testificandum: A subpoena that primarily seeks an individual's testimony

Subpoena duces tecum: A subpoena instructing the recipient to bring documents and other records to a deposition or to court

Substance Abuse and Mental Health Services Administration (SAMHSA): A division of the Department of Health and Human Services that, in 2004, published a document explaining the relationship between HIPAA and the Alcohol and Drug Abuse Regulations regarding confidentiality and release of information

Substantive due process: Guarantees that laws are fair, reasonable, and not arbitrary; allows for challenges to a law's content and substance

Substantive law: Law that defines the rights and obligations that arise between two or more parties, such as torts and contracts

Sudden emergency doctrine: Relieves a person of liability if, without prior negligence on his or her part, that person is confronted with a sudden emergency and acts as an ordinarily prudent person would act under the circumstances

Summons: A document that gives the defendant notice of the lawsuit and explains the defendant's procedural obligations

Sunshine laws: *See* **Open records laws, Public records laws**

Supplemental Medical Review Contractor: CMS contractor responsible for performing and/or providing support for a variety of tasks aimed at lowering improper payment rates and increasing efficiencies of the medical review functions of the Medicare and Medicaid programs

Supremacy Clause: A clause of the US Constitution that states that federal law is supreme over any conflicting state law

Supreme courts: Courts of final decision making, which exist at both the federal and state levels; other courts must abide by decisions of the supreme courts

Syndromic surveillance: Refers to monitoring nonspecific clinical information that may indicate a bioterrorism-associated disease before a specific diagnosis is made

System security: Totality of safeguards including hardware, software, personnel policies, information practice policies, disaster preparedness, and oversight of these components; protects both the system and the information contained within from unauthorized access from without and from misuse from within; enables the entity or system to protect the confidential information it stores from unauthorized access, disclosure, or misuse, thereby protecting the privacy of the individuals who are the subjects of the stored information

T

Technical safeguards: Security measures that are based on technology rather than on administration or physical security, including access control, unique user identification, automatic logoff, and encryption and decryption

Technology neutral: Specific technologies are not prescribed in the rules, which allows the use of the latest and appropriate technology

Telehealth: The use of digital technologies to deliver medical care, health education, and public health services, by connecting multiple users in separate locations (for example, videoconferencing, transmission of still images, patient portals, remote monitoring of vital signs)

Telemedicine: Defined by the American Telemedicine Association as "the use of medical information exchanged from one site to another via electronic communications to improve patients' health status" (American Telemedicine Association. n.d.)

Telephone callback procedures: A form of entity authentication in which a modem dials into the system and a special callback application asks for the telephone number from which the call was placed

Term of art: Word or phrase with a specific meaning in a defined subject, such as PHI (protected health information) in HIPAA

Termination of access: An administrative safeguard that is used when an employee changes job position, takes on new job roles or duties, or terminates employment with the organization

Tethered PHR: Personal health record that is connected via a secure electronic portal to an organization's information system, such as a healthcare provider's EHR

Therapeutic privilege: A doctrine that has historically allowed physicians to withhold information from patients in limited circumstances

Timeliness: The completion of a health record within timelines established by legal and accreditation standards and by organizational policy and medical staff bylaws

Title VII of the Civil Rights Act of 1964: A law that, in combination with the Equal Employment Opportunity Act of 1972, prohibits discrimination based on age, race, color, sex, religion, or national origin

Tokens: Devices such as key cards that are inserted into doors or computers in order to gain entry

Tolled: Delay, suspend, or hold off effect of a statute

Tort: A civil wrong for which the law provides a remedy in the form of a lawsuit to recover damages

Tort law: Law that involves the right of an individual, corporation, or other legal entity to recover damages for a loss caused by the defendant (tortfeasor or wrongdoer)

Tort reform: The variety of measures intended by legislatures to overhaul the justice system; with regard to medical malpractice, such reforms are intended to diminish the number of lawsuits and large jury verdicts, stabilize the market, and ultimately reduce premiums for physicians

Tortfeasor: Wrongdoer, defendant

TPO: *See* **Treatment, payment, and healthcare operations**

Transfer of health records: The movement of a record from one medium to another (for example, from paper to microfilm or to an optical imaging system) or to another records custodian

Transplant registries: Database of patients who need organs as well as databases of potential donors

Trauma registry: A registry designed to identify the types of traumatic injuries incurred in the state, currently required by 37 states

Traumatic injury: A wound or injury included in a trauma registry

Treatment, payment, and healthcare operations (TPO): Collectively, these three actions are functions of a covered entity that are necessary for the covered entity to successfully conduct business; thus, many of the Privacy Rule's requirements are relaxed or removed where protected health information is needed for purposes of treatment, payment, or healthcare operations

Trial: The stage in a lawsuit after the pretrial phase if the parties do not negotiate a settlement and the case is not dismissed

Trial courts: The first and lowest level of the US federal court system or of a state court system

Trier of fact: Judge or jury responsible for deciding factual issues

Triggers: *See* **Litigation trigger**

Trojan horse: A destructive piece of programming code that hides in another piece of programming code that looks harmless, such as a macro or an e-mail message

Types of requests: The ways in which requests for access, use, and disclosure of patient information are made, which may include mail, telephone, physical presence of the requester, fax, or e-mail

U

UHCDA: *See* **Uniform Health-Care Decisions Act**

Ultra vires act: A decision by a corporation's governing body or executives that goes beyond the express or implied powers of the corporation; such an act is usually void and can result in personal liability if financial loss results, if it was taken with the knowledge that the action was beyond the scope of power, or if it was made in bad faith

Unavoidable accident: An occurrence that could not have been foreseen or anticipated in the exercise of ordinary care and that results without the fault or negligence of either the defendant or the plaintiff

Unbundling: A billing practice in which providers use multiple procedure codes for a group of procedures instead of the appropriate comprehensive code in order to inappropriately maximize reimbursement

Unconditioned authorization: Authorization is not required in order to receive treatment or some other service or benefit

Uniform Anatomical Gift Act: An act that provides suggested standards for all aspects of organ donation, including who may make anatomical gifts and how intent to make anatomical gifts should be expressed—designed to create uniformity in this area across all 50 states

Uniform Durable Power of Attorney Act: Federal statute that provides a mechanism for individuals to deal with their property in the event of incapacity

Uniform Electronic Transactions Act: Federal statute that makes electronic transactions as enforceable as paper transactions, removing barriers to electronic commerce and increasing trust associated with electronic business transactions

Uniform Guidelines on Employee Selection Procedures: A set of guidelines published by the Equal Employment Opportunity Commission to guide selection of employees; the overriding principle is that selection of employees must be made on qualifications related to job performance

Uniform Health-Care Decisions Act (UHCDA): A model law created in 1993 that provides that an individual may give an oral or written instruction to a healthcare provider that remains in force even after the individual loses capacity, and suggests decision-making priority for that individual's surrogates

Uniform Photographic Copies of Business and Public Records as Evidence Act (UPA): Federal statute, with state versions, that makes admissible as evidence the reproduction of any record that has been retained in the regular course of business and kept by a process that accurately reproduces the original in any medium; supports the transition from paper to electronic storage of information

Unintentional threats: Include employee errors that may result from lack of training in proper system use. When users share their password, respond to phishing, or download information from a non-secure Internet site, for example, they create the potential for a breach in security

Union steward: A representative of the employee in a unionized environment

Unique identifier: A combination of characters and numbers assigned and maintained by the security system and used to track individual user activity; user ID

United States Code (USC): The compilation of all federal statutes

United States Supreme Court: The court of final decision-making. It hears appeals most commonly from the federal appellate (circuit) courts and occasionally from state supreme courts in matters involving federal statutes or the US Constitution

Unsafe conditions: circumstances that increase the probability of a patient safety event occurring (AHRQ n.d.b.)

Unusual event: A type of event that often must be reported to the state; may include unexpected occurrences resulting in death or serious injury unrelated to the natural course of a patient's illness or underlying condition, an incident resulting in the abuse of a patient, medication errors, transfusion errors, transfusion reactions, falls resulting in fractures, wrong patient/wrong site surgical procedures, and operative complications

Upcoding: Billing for services at a level of complexity that is higher than the service actually provided or documented (*also see* **Overcoding**)

USC: *See* **United States Code**

US Constitution: Document that defines and lays out the powers of the three branches of the federal government

Use: HIPAA definition with respect to individually identifiable health information, the sharing, employment, application, utilization, examination, or analysis of such information within an entity that maintains such information (45 CFR 160.103)

User: An individual with rights to use a particular secured system or access a particular physical area

User-based access control (UBAC): A security mechanism used to grant users of a system access based on the identity of the user (HHS n.d.)

Uses, disclosures, and requests: The three types of situations in which protected health information is handled and the Privacy Rule governs

Utilitarianism: An ethical theory based on the idea that the best option in an ethical decision relates to which choice provides the greatest advantage or benefits the greatest number of people

Utilization review: The process of determining whether the medical care provided to a specific patient is necessary according to preestablished objective screening criteria at time frames specified in the organization's utilization management plan

V

Vendors: Outside companies such as consultants and those who sell equipment and supplies, perform release-of-information functions, provide laundry or food services, or repair equipment that have a presence in a healthcare facility and may or may not be business associates

Verdict: The decision rendered by the jury at the end of a trial; in criminal cases, in order to convict or acquit a defendant, a unanimous vote is required

Version management: The manner in which an organization handles the numerous versions that may exist of a document or collection of data

Vertical restraint of trade: Situation in which two or more entities at different levels in a distribution chain act together to restrain trade

Vicarious liability: *See* **Secondary liability**

Virtue-based ethics: A theory of ethics that focuses on the happiness found in our intrinsic characteristics and virtues

Viruses: Common types are classified as file infectors, which attach to program files so that when a program is loaded the virus is also loaded; system or boot-record infectors, which infect system areas of diskettes or hard disks; and macro viruses, which infect Microsoft applications, inserting unwanted words or phrases

Vital record: Records concerned with births, deaths, marriages, divorces, abortions, and late fetal deaths; each state requires that a certificate be completed that verifies the vital event

Voir dire: The process through which a jury is selected

Vulnerabilities: Weaknesses that impact security of systems and networks

W

Wagner Act: *See* **National Labor Relations Act of 1935**

Waived authorization: Individual HIPAA authorization is not required for the use and disclosure of information for research

Waiver of privilege: An exception to physician–patient privilege that occurs when a party claims damages for a mental or physical injury; the party thereby waives his or her right to confidentiality to the extent that it is necessary to determine whether the mental or physical injury is due to another cause

Warranties: Statements of fact in a contract that are made by one party to induce another party to enter into the contract

Waste: Over-utilization or inappropriate utilization of services and misuse of resources

Weight of the evidence: The amount of consideration the judge or jury gives a particular record or piece of evidence when deciding the factual issues of the case

WEP: *See* **Wired equivalent privacy**

Whistleblower: An individual who discloses wrongdoing by an organization to the authorities or to the public

Wired equivalent privacy (WEP): A form of encryption used to authenticate the sender and the receiver of messages over networks, particularly when the Internet is involved in the data transmission; should provide authentication (both sender and recipient are known to each other), data security (safe from interception), and data nonrepudiation (data sent have arrived unchanged)

Workers' compensation: Legislation that ensures that employees who are injured on the job or become ill as a result of a job are provided with some means of support while recovering from their illness or injuries

Workforce: Under the HIPAA Privacy Rule, employees, volunteers, trainees, and other persons, whether paid or not, who work for and are under the direct control of the covered entity

Workstation: A computer designed to accept data from multiple sources in order to assist in managing information for daily activities and to provide a convenient means of entering data as desired by the user at the point of care

Worm: A special type of computer virus that stores and then replicates itself

Writ: A formal written order issued by one with administrative or judicial jurisdiction over a case

Writ of execution: A method of collecting judgment that directs the appropriate law enforcement official to seize the defendant's real or personal property to satisfy the debt owed to the plaintiff

Wrongful death: A distinct claim with a separate statute of limitations that may be filed in addition to a tort claim in order to compensate the deceased individual's survivors

Z

Zone Program Integrity Contractors: CMS contractors that replaced Program Safeguard Contractors and are responsible for detecting, investigating, and deterring fraud, waste, and abuse in seven zones for Medicare Parts A and B, Durable Medical Equipment Prosthetics, Orthotics, and Supplies, Home Health and Hospice

Index

legal doctrine of preemption, 254–255
medical device reporting, 404
minimum necessary requirement, 232–233
mitigation, 256–257
noncustodial parents' rights of access, 344
on-site record reviews, 371
policies and procedures, 255–256
privacy and security rules complaint process, 259
privacy of patient information, 208–210
release of PHI without authorization, 360
request restrictions, 249
requests for payment purposes, 364
research uses and disclosures of PHI, 251–254
retaliation and waiver, 257
right to request information, 374
ROI reimbursement and fee structure, 373
scope and anatomy of, 206–207
terminology, 215–218
tracking and accounting of disclosures of PHI, 374
uses and disclosures of patient's authorization, 222–230
workforce, defined, 345
workforce training and management, 256
private law, 34
privilege, 83–85
between patients and other providers, 85
waiver of, 84–85
privileged communication, 7, 83–84
privilege statutes, 348
procedural due process, 35
procedural law, 50
professional ethics, 14
professionalism, 19
Program Safeguard Contractors (PSCs), 457
pro se, 52
protected health information (PHI), 3, 198, 211, 213–215, 339, 411. *See also* electronic protected health information (ePHI)
access, uses, and disclosures of, 221, 244–250, 305, 308, 332, 340–348, 341, 344–345, 345, 347, 348, 358, 359, 363, 364, 366, 368–371, 392, 395, 398, 407–408, 429
amendment request, 246–247
commercial uses and disclosures of, 231–232
disclosure of, 216, 225
HITECH breach notification requirement, 290
individual rights, 243–249
release without authorization, 360, 362, 384, 388, 403–404
request for, 216
requesting access to one's own, 245–246
requesting disclosure of HIV/AIDS, 352
requests for health information, 216
research uses and disclosures of, 251–254

safeguards necessary for protecting, 367
search and retrieval fees, 246
Security Rule regulation, 265, 267, 269
test for determining whether information, 213
tracking and accounting of disclosures of, 374
Provena Covenant Medical Center v. Department of Revenue, 124
Provider Self-Disclosure Protocol, 461
proximate causation, 102
psychotherapy notes, 222, 347
public and private collaborations, 1
public health reporting, 2, 248
public key cryptography, 303
public key infrastructure (PKI), 303
public law, 34
public records laws, 360
punitive damages, 103, 116
pure comparative negligence, 105

Q

Quackenbush case, 155–156
qualified clinical data registry (QCDR), 410
QualityCheck.org, 432
quality healthcare, 416
quality improvement in healthcare, 2, 416, 427–433. *See also* patient safety
government focus on patient safety, 429–431
organization and operation of quality and patient safety management, 433
Quality Improvement Organizations (QIOs), 429
Quality Innovation Network- Quality Improvement Organizations (QIN-QIOs), 430
qui tam relators, 442

R

ransomware, 287
reasonably prudent person, 101
Recovery Audit Contractors (RACs), 457–458
red flag, 291
Red Flags Rule, 291
redisclosures, 230
Reese v. Bd. of Directors of Memorial Hosp. of Laramie Co., 104
referral, 447
Regional Perinatal Intensive Care Centers (RPICC) data, 409
reimbursement
coding and, 29
fee-for-service reimbursement models, 1, 366, 441, 456–457
ROI, 373
third-party, 2
release of information (ROI), 340, 367–377
determining appropriateness of disclosure, 371–372